Cutaneous Metastases

Dimitra Koumaki
Marios Papadakis
Stamatios Gregoriou
Editors

Cutaneous Metastases

Decoding Dermatological Challenges in Cancer Care

Springer

Editors
Dimitra Koumaki
Department of Dermatology and Venereology
University Hospital of Heraklion
Heraklion, Greece

Stamatios Gregoriou
Department of Dermatology and Venereology, Andreas Sygros Hospital
National and Kapodistrian University of Athens, Medical School of Athens
Athens, Greece

Marios Papadakis
Associate Professor & Head of Department, Department of Plastic, Reconstructive & Aesthetic Surgery
Faculty of Medicine, University of Thessaly
Larissa, Greece

ISBN 978-3-032-26763-4 ISBN 978-3-032-26764-1 (eBook)
https://doi.org/10.1007/978-3-032-26764-1

This Springer imprint is published by the registered company Springer Nature Switzerland AG
The registered company address is: Gewerbestrasse 11, 6330 Cham, Switzerland

Preface

Cutaneous metastases occupy a very special, if not often overlooked, place in the spectrum of metastatic malignancies, finding itself at the intersection of the fields of dermatology, oncology, pathology, radiology, and surgery. While they are relatively rare when compared to other metastases, skin metastases have very significant diagnostic, prognostic, and therapeutic implications. In some instances, they may be the first presentation of an underlying malignancy, while in other instances, they may indicate disease progression with a very poor prognosis.

As the survival rate of patients with cancer continues to rise due to improvements in oncologic treatments and earlier diagnosis, there has been an increasing number of patients with cutaneous manifestations of metastases. Therefore, dermatologists and many other medical professionals continue to find themselves faced with the dilemma of identifying, diagnosing, and treating patients with cutaneous metastases, despite the scarcity of resources on this subject available today.

The current book, *Cutaneous Metastasis*, was developed as a response to all these identified gaps. The current book aims to serve as a comprehensive resource that addresses the whole gamut of cutaneous metastatic diseases. From the basic principles of definition, epidemiology, pathogenesis, and presentation of cutaneous metastatic diseases to the more sophisticated approaches of diagnosis, histopathology, imaging studies, management, and future studies, all the chapters that follow are carefully developed to focus on the relevance of the material.

Particular attention is given to the different primary tumors responsible for cutaneous metastases, and these include gynecologic, gastrointestinal, thoracic, breast, genitourinary, hematologic, neuroendocrine, pediatric, sarcomatous, and central nervous system cancers, besides metastases from an occult primary source. The special emphasis given in certain chapters, including those concerning dermoscopy, new modalities for diagnosing cancers, molecular pathology, and measures related to quality of life/prognosis, is indicative of the dynamic development in this area. Also adding significant clinical content is the provision for extensive case studies.

This book is designed for use by dermatologists, oncologists, pathologists, surgeons, radiologists, residents, fellows, and all other clinicians caring for cancer patients. Its intended purposes are not only the facilitation of proper diagnosis and patient management but also the stimulation of further research in the recently emerged field of study concerning skin metastasis.

We would like to thank all contributing authors for their extraordinary level of expertise, dedication, and commitment to excellence, as well as Springer for their support in completing this ambitious project. Our sincere hope is that our book volume will become a valuable resource and stimulant for further progress in the field of understanding and managing cutaneous metastatic disease.

Heraklion, Greece Dimitra Koumaki
Larissa, Greece Marios Papadakis
Athens, Greece Stamatios Gregoriou

Contents

Part I

Introduction

1 Definition of Cutaneous Metastases

Katerina Grafanaki

Abstract

Cutaneous metastases (CM) are defined as the spread of malignant cells from a primary internal cancer to the skin, resulting in secondary tumor deposits within the dermis or subcutaneous tissue. Despite their reported incidence of only 0.7–10% among cancer patients, CM carry significant clinical implications, as they may serve as the first indicator of an undiagnosed malignancy, herald tumor recurrence, or reflect advanced disseminated disease. The development of CM is a complex, multistep process involving hematogenous or lymphatic dissemination, direct tumor extension, and, rarely, iatrogenic implantation, facilitated by molecular mechanisms such as epithelial–mesenchymal transition, tumor–microenvironment interactions, and immune evasion.

The clinical spectrum of cutaneous metastases is broad, encompassing classic nodular lesions as well as inflammatory, sclerodermoid, vascular, and dermatomal patterns, including distinctive entities such as carcinoma erysipelatoides, carcinoma en cuirasse, carcinoma telangiectoides, alopecia neoplastica, and the characteristic umbilical metastasis known as Sister Mary Joseph's nodule. Because these lesions frequently mimic benign dermatologic conditions or primary cutaneous tumors, accurate diagnosis requires careful clinicopathologic correlation supported by histopathology, immunohistochemistry, and imaging studies. Early recognition is critical, as CM may provide a visible clue to internal malignancy and disease progression.

Keywords

Cutaneous metastases · Skin metastasis · Internal malignancy · Dermatologic oncology · Paraneoplastic dermatoses · Metastatic pathways · Hematogenous spread · Lymphatic dissemination · Carcinoma erysipelatoides · Carcinoma en cuirasse · Sister Mary Joseph's nodule · Alopecia neoplastica · Zosteriform metastases · Acral metastases · In-transit metastases · Skin cancer diagnosis

1.1 Introduction

The skin can serve as a diagnostic mirror, revealing underlying internal malignancies through a spectrum of manifestations. These cutaneous signs may represent either direct or indirect effects of cancer. Direct effects arise from local invasion or metastatic spread of tumor cells to the skin, compromising normal tissue architecture and function. Indirect effects, by contrast, result from remote interactions between the tumor and

K. Grafanaki (✉)
Department of Dermatology-Venereology, School of Medicine, University of Patras, Patras, Greece
e-mail: grafanaki@upatras.gr

D. Koumaki et al. (eds.), *Cutaneous Metastases*, https://doi.org/10.1007/978-3-032-26764-1_1

host systems, giving rise to paraneoplastic syndromes—nonmetastatic skin findings associated with internal neoplasia [1–3].

Although relatively uncommon (occurring in approximately 9–10% of cases), cutaneous manifestations carry substantial clinical significance [4–6]. They may represent the first sign of an otherwise occult cancer in an apparently healthy patient or may indicate tumor recurrence, underscoring the failure of eradication. Among these, cutaneous metastases (CM) are particularly important as they signal systemic dissemination and are often associated with poor prognosis. While the reported prevalence of skin involvement in cancer patients ranges from 0.7% to 10.4%, recognizing these manifestations is crucial for early diagnosis, appropriate staging, and timely intervention [7–10].

Accurate identification requires an understanding of the patterns, routes of spread, pathophysiology, and distinctive clinical variants of CM, as well as their differentiation from primary skin cancers, paraneoplastic dermatoses, and reactive conditions. Such knowledge is essential in dermatologic oncology, where skin findings may serve as critical diagnostic and prognostic tools.

1.2 Cutaneous Metastases

Definition Cutaneous metastasis is defined as the spread of malignant cells from a primary internal cancer to the skin, resulting in secondary tumor deposits within the dermis or subcutaneous tissue. These lesions represent hematogenous, lymphatic, or direct extension of the malignancy and indicate systemic dissemination of disease. However, rare cases deviate from these routes, manifesting in atypical or iatrogenic locations.

Cutaneous metastases are most frequently associated with cancers of the breast, lung, gastrointestinal (GI) tract, gynecologic organs, endocrine system, head and neck, and hematologic malignancies. While rare compared with visceral metastases, their recognition is clinically significant because they may be the first sign of an internal cancer, the earliest indicator of recurrence, or a marker of advanced systemic disease [11]. Additionally, CM involving dual primary malignancies with concurrent cutaneous metastatic involvement have been reported [12].

1.2.1 Mechanisms of Spread

Metastasis is a complex, multistep biological process involving detachment from the primary tumor, invasion, intravasation, circulation, extravasation, and proliferation at distant sites [7, 8]. Tumor cells may disseminate through blood and lymphatic systems, often simultaneously due to their anatomical interconnections [9, 10].

Most metastases to the skin occur near the primary tumor, governed by anatomical proximity, lymphatic drainage, or tissue-specific affinity. However, distant CM can occur and may manifest in unexpected locations [13, 14].

1.2.1.1 Hematogenous Spread

The most frequent route of cutaneous metastasis is hematogenous dissemination, particularly in carcinomas such as lung, kidney, and colon adenocarcinomas [10, 13, 15, 16] (Fig. 1.1). Tumor cells intravasate into the bloodstream and are carried to the skin, especially to regions with rich vascularization such as the scalp, face, and trunk. This mechanism often results in the formation of nodular metastases, which are typically firm, painless, and rapidly enlarging [15, 16].

On a molecular level, hematogenous spread involves epithelial–mesenchymal transition (EMT), degradation of the extracellular matrix, and intravasation mediated by matrix metalloproteinases and integrins [17]. Once in the circulation, tumor cells can evade immune surveillance via interactions with platelets and endothelial adhesion molecules [17, 18].

1.2.1.2 Lymphatic Spread

Lymphatic dissemination is another significant pathway, especially in tumors of the breast, stomach, and cervix, where cancer cells migrate through lymphatic vessels to reach dermal lymphatics [13, 15, 16]. This route frequently results

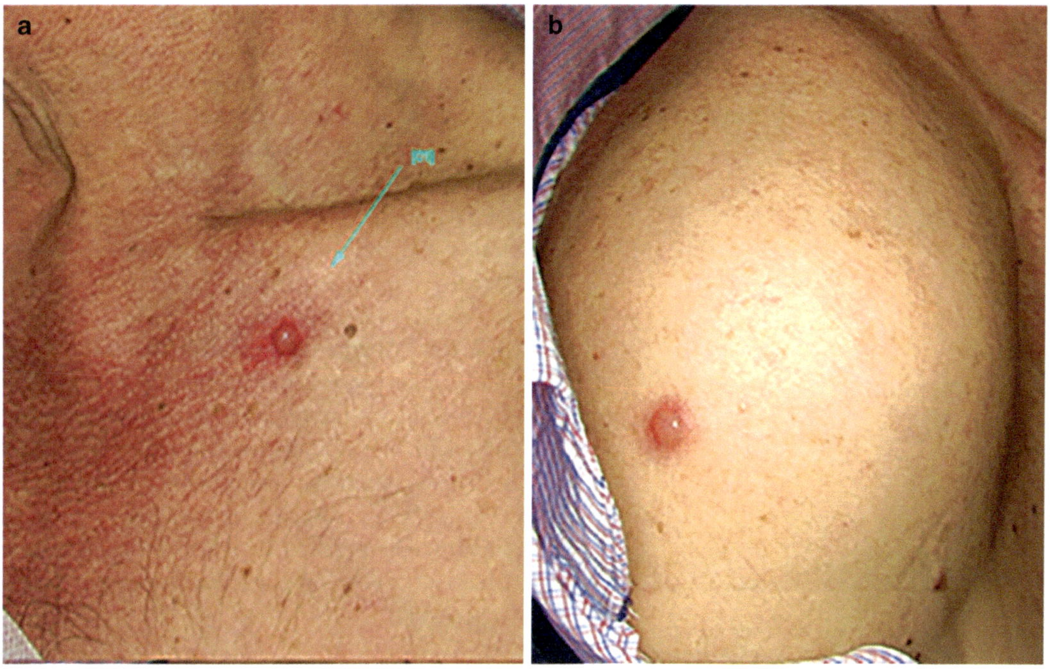

Fig. 1.1 Colorectal adenocarcinoma and cutaneous metastases presenting as painful, rapidly enlarging pink, shiny papules and nodules on the sternum (**a**) and upper extremities (**b**). (All figures: Courtesy of the archive of Dr. Katerina Grafanaki)

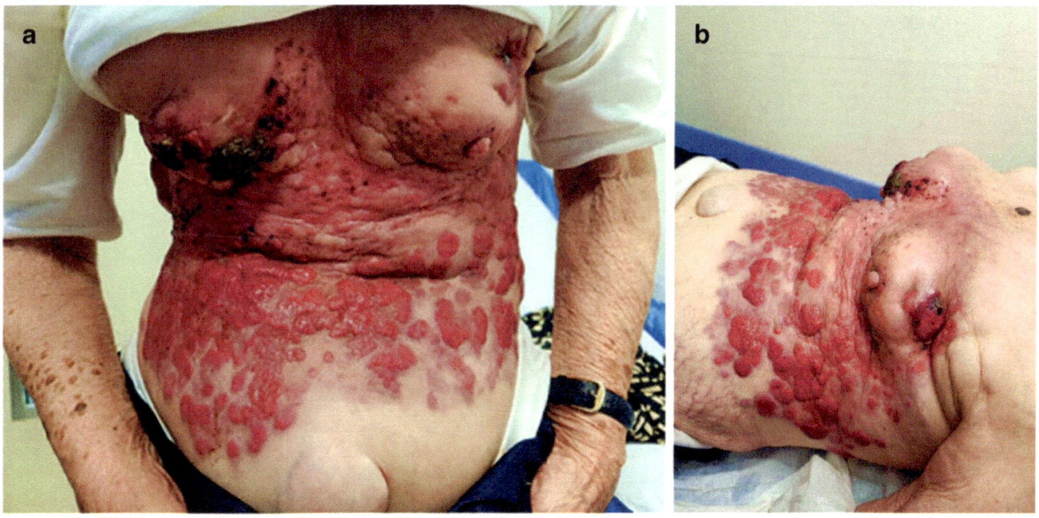

Fig. 1.2 Cutaneous metastases from breast cancer presenting as multiple firm, red-to-flesh–colored exophytic papules and nodules on the chest, extending to the abdomen (**a**) and laterally across the trunk (**b**)

in inflammatory-type cutaneous metastases, characterized by erythematous plaques or diffuse induration, sometimes mimicking cellulitis or lymphangitis carcinomatosa [10, 15].

In breast cancer, for example, tumor emboli in lymphatic vessels lead to clinical manifestations like carcinoma en s or carcinoma telangiectoides [15, 19] (Figs. 1.2 and 1.3). Lymphatic spread is also implicated in Sister Mary Joseph's nodule—a periumbilical metastasis commonly from gastrointestinal or gynecologic cancers, thought to involve both lymphatic and hematogenous mechanisms [20, 21].

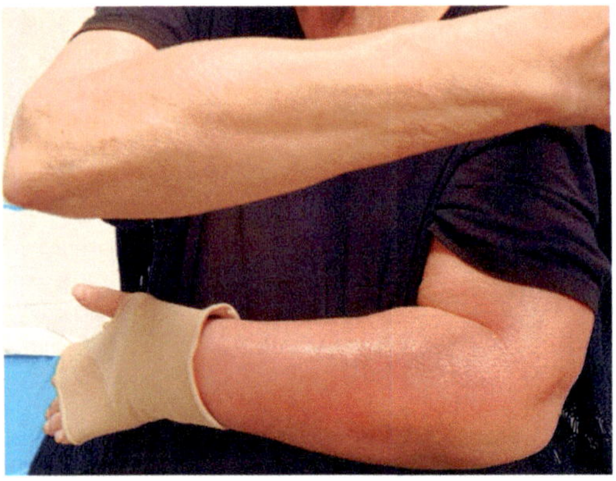

Fig. 1.3 Erysipelatoides cutaneous metastasis

1.2.1.3 Direct Extension

Direct contiguous invasion from underlying malignancies to the skin is relatively uncommon but can occur in tumors located close to the dermis, such as head and neck, breast, or parotid gland carcinomas [15, 16, 22]. These metastases often present in areas adjacent to the primary tumor and are associated with a worse prognosis due to extensive local invasion [16].

1.2.1.4 Iatrogenic Implantation

Surgical or procedural implantation is a rare but documented route of spread, especially in cases of needle biopsy, catheter placement, or surgical incisions involving tumor-bearing tissues [16] (Fig. 1.4). For instance, port site metastases in laparoscopic procedures or scar metastases after breast or colorectal cancer surgeries have been reported [10].

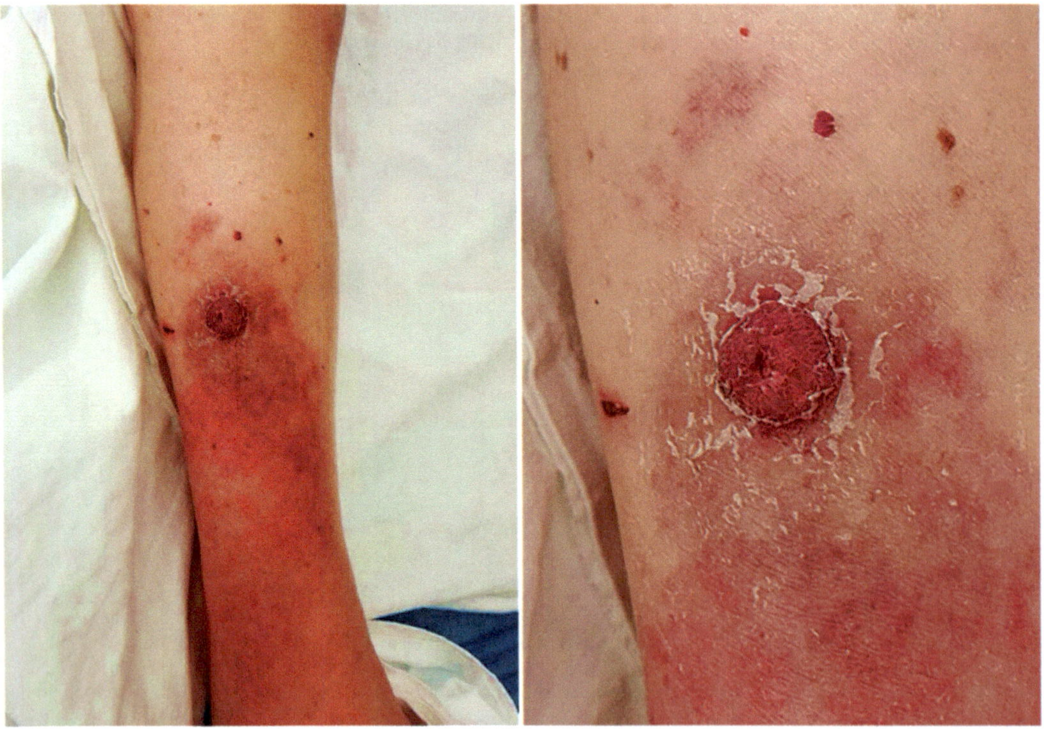

Fig. 1.4 Rare, cutaneous in-transit metastases from Merkel cell carcinoma on the lower legs' skin, upon iatrogenic dissemination

1.2.1.5 Embryonic Remnants and Anatomical Weak Points

Certain cutaneous metastases exploit embryonic remnants or natural anatomical weak points. The umbilicus, for example, is a well-known site for metastatic spread due to its embryological connections with the peritoneal cavity via the umbilical vein and ligament remnants [10, 20]. This explains the occurrence of Sister Mary Joseph's nodule, which frequently originates from gastric, ovarian, or pancreatic carcinomas [21, 23].

1.2.1.6 Molecular Mechanisms Facilitating Metastasis

The metastatic process is orchestrated by intricate molecular signaling cascades. Key players include EMT regulators, chemokines (e.g., CXCL12/CXCR4), adhesion molecules (e.g., E-cadherin, integrins), and angiogenic factors like VEGF [17, 18]]. Breast cancer metastasis, in particular, demonstrates subtype-specific tropism and mechanisms, such as triple-negative tumors displaying higher rates of cutaneous involvement due to loss of adhesion and aggressive migratory behavior [18].

Moreover, recent reviews underscore the importance of the tumor microenvironment, immune evasion, and exosome-mediated premetastatic niche formation in determining cutaneous metastatic patterns [16, 24, 25].

1.2.2 Clinical Presentations and Epidemiology

Large retrospective studies report skin metastases in about 5–10% of patients with internal malignancies [6, 8, 26]. Cutaneous metastases may be the first sign of malignancy in 1–7% of cases, particularly in breast, lung, or renal carcinomas [6, 8, 26, 27]. Brownstein and Helwig analyzed 724 cases and emphasized gender-specific primary sites: lung and kidney in men and breast in women [13].

Clinically, metastatic lesions often appear as firm nodules, sometimes grouped or ulcerated, and may present on old surgical scars or sites of trauma. Coloration varies, ranging from flesh colored to black [14, 27]. In men, lesions typically localize to the head, neck, and trunk, while in women, they are concentrated on the anterior chest and abdomen [13, 28].

1.2.3 Distinctive Clinical Presentations of Cutaneous Metastases (CM)—Clinical Spectrum

Cutaneous metastases represent a heterogeneous group of skin manifestations secondary to internal malignancies, most often indicating advanced systemic disease. Their morphology and distribution vary according to the primary tumor type, anatomical site, and route of dissemination. Several characteristic clinical patterns have been described. Recognizing these variants is crucial, as CM may represent the first sign of an undiagnosed malignancy or signal disease progression. Because of their polymorphic nature and potential for misdiagnosis, histopathological confirmation is essential for any suspicious lesion, particularly in patients with a history of internal cancer.

1.2.3.1 Nodular Metastases

The nodular variant is the most common CM presentation. Lesions typically appear as firm, flesh-colored to erythematous papules or violaceous papules or nodules, which may be solitary or multiple [29]. They are usually painless but may ulcerate in advanced stages [10, 15, 16]. Distribution correlates with the site of primary tumor [5, 30]. Breast carcinoma commonly metastasizes to the chest wall, while gastrointestinal malignancies often involve the abdominal skin [13, 15, 31]. Lung, renal, and gastrointestinal tumors frequently manifest nodular CM via hematogenous spread [10, 15] (Figs. 1.1 and 1.5).

1.2.3.2 Carcinoma Erysipelatoides

The inflammatory or carcinoma erysipelatoides variant presents as erythematous, indurated, warm plaques with well-demarcated borders, closely mimicking cellulitis or erysipelas. It is most often associated with inflammatory breast

Fig. 1.5 Newly diagnosed lung cancer with a painful, erythematous, inflamed, encapsulated cutaneous metastatic nodule extending to the dorsal surface of the ribs

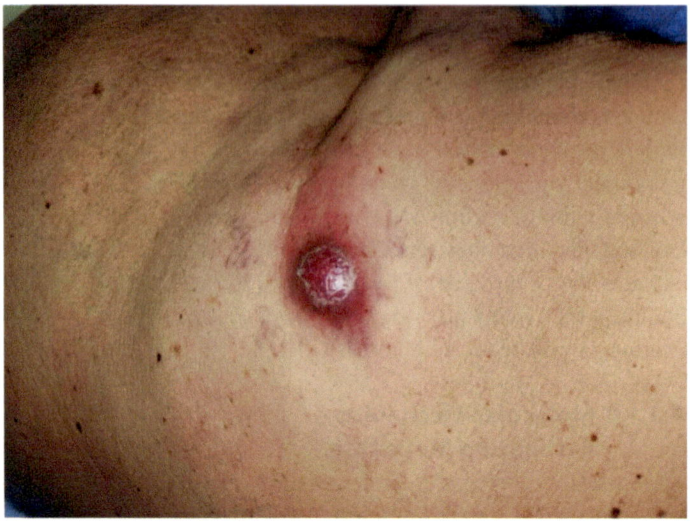

carcinoma but has also been described in gastric, uterine, and rectal cancers [2, 14, 27]. Misdiagnosis as infection is common, often leading to delayed treatment, and resistance to antibiotic therapy in such patients should raise suspicion [2]. Carcinoma erysipelatoides arises due to lymphatic invasion by tumor cells, therefore needs biopsy diagnosis confirmation [10, 15, 16] (Fig. 1.3).

1.2.3.3 Carcinoma En Cuirasse

Named for its resemblance to a breastplate, carcinoma en cuirasse presents as a woody induration or sclerodermoid plaque, most often on the anterior chest wall [32]. It is commonly associated with breast cancer and reflects extensive dermal fibrosis and lymphatic obstruction [2, 10, 13, 15, 33, 34]. Histologically, tumor cells may be seen in a linear "Indian-file" pattern within dermal collagen [33]. The skin may become bound to underlying structures, reflecting advanced disease (Fig. 1.6).

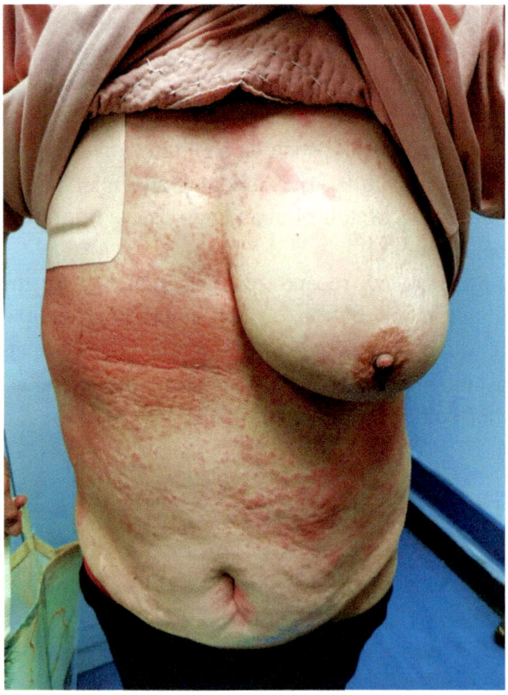

Fig. 1.6 Carcinoma en cuirasse

1.2.3.4 Carcinoma Telangiectoides

The telangiectatic form manifests as violaceous macules, papules, or plaques with prominent telangiectasias or a pseudovascular appearance. Most cases are associated with breast carcinoma and result from dermal vascular or lymphatic invasion by tumor emboli [15, 16]. Biopsy is crucial to distinguish it from benign vascular proliferations.

1.2.3.5 Zosteriform and Inflammatory Patterns

A rare presentation of CM involves a zosteriform distribution, where metastatic lesions follow a dermatomal pattern and mimic the vesicular eruption of herpes zoster [10, 15]. This atypical manifestation may represent the first sign of an underlying malignancy and is generally associated with a poor prognosis. This is reported most frequently in cancers of the breast, lung, lymphoma, squamous cell carcinoma, urinary, and gastrointestinal tract [35]. Proposed mechanisms include perineural or lymphatic dissemination and, less commonly, Koebner's phenomenon in skin previously affected by herpes zoster [36]. Because of its resemblance to varicella-zoster infection, misdiagnosis is common and may delay appropriate oncologic evaluation [15, 16, 37].

1.2.3.6 Alopecia Neoplastica

When metastases affect the scalp, they may present as areas of nonscarring alopecia with underlying indurated plaques or nodules, termed alopecia neoplastica. Most often seen with breast, lung, and gastrointestinal primaries, these lesions can mimic inflammatory conditions, such as alopecia areata or cicatricial alopecias [10, 15, 16, 27, 38, 39].

1.2.3.7 Umbilical Metastasis (Sister Mary Joseph's Nodule)

Umbilical metastasis, classically referred to as Sister Mary Joseph's nodule, represents a rare but highly suggestive manifestation of periumbilical cutaneous metastasis. It is most frequently associated with primary malignancies from gastric, ovarian, pancreatic, and colorectal cancers [20, 21, 40–42]. It is considered a clinical hallmark of advanced intra-abdominal malignancies which appear as a firm, often ulcerated periumbilical nodule or mass in the periumbilical region. The metastatic spread occurs through lymphatic and hematogenous dissemination, or along embryonic ligamentous remnants such as the falciform ligament and the urachus [20, 21]. These nodules are typically firm, vascular, and histologically adenocarcinomas [43, 44].

1.2.3.8 Genital and Perianal CM

Though rare, CM to the scrotum, penis, vulva, or perianal region have been documented, especially from colorectal, bladder, and cervical carcinomas These may present as ulcerated plaques, nodules, or verrucous lesions, often mistaken for primary dermatoses or infections. Their presence can be a sign of aggressive disease [45–48] (Fig. 1.7).

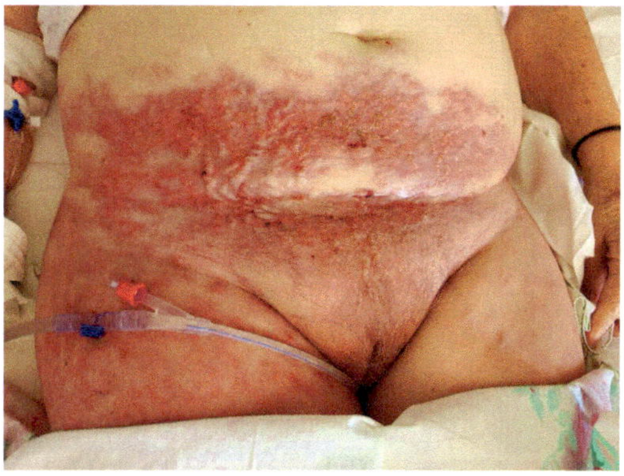

Fig. 1.7 Cutaneous metastases from unknown primary site. Biopsy showed malignant epithelial neoplasm of the pelvic region of the iliac and inguinal lymph nodes

1.2.3.9 Facial Involvement (Including Nasal Tip)

Metastases to the face are rare (<0.5% of CM) but reported, including cases from melanoma, small cell lung cancer (SCLC), colon adenocarcinoma, and tonsillar squamous cell carcinoma [6, 22, 48, 49]. Diagnosis may be delayed as lesions may go unnoticed or misdiagnosed as benign infectious or mucocutaneous conditions and require a high index of suspicion [50]. Histologic evaluation is mandatory due to disseminated disease and poor prognosis [51].

Nasal tip CM are sometimes referred to as "clown nose" sign [52–55]. They appear as red, violaceous or nodular lesions on the nasal tip and can mimic benign conditions such as nonmelanoma skin cancers (NMSCs) or rosacea (rhinophyma). Common primary cancers that spread to the nasal tip include lung, kidney, thyroid, cervical, liver, and esophageal carcinomas [55–57].

1.2.3.10 Unusual Morphologies and Mimics

A particularly rare variant, known as carcinoma hemorrhagiectoides, manifests as diffuse, violaceous, hemorrhagic plaques and has been described in cases of salivary duct carcinoma, with a characteristic "shield sign" [58].

CM may occasionally simulate benign lesions such as keratoacanthoma (Fig. 1.8), pyogenic granuloma, or inflammatory dermatoses like psoriasis or eczema [59, 60]. CM lesions arising in previously irradiated or scarred skin may further complicate diagnosis [15, 60] (Fig. 1.9).

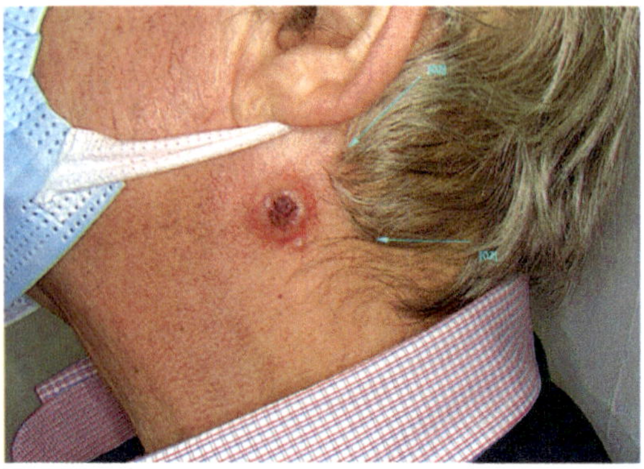

Fig. 1.8 Keratoacanthoma-like lesion in a patient with poorly differentiated colorectal adenocarcinoma, as CM

1.2.3.11 Acral Cutaneous Metastases: A Rare Clinical Entity

Acral CM are rare (< 0.1% of CM) metastases to the extremities, particularly the hands, feet, sole, fingers, toes, and nail beds [61–64]. Most often arising from lung, gastrointestinal, or breast cancers [29, 65, 66]. Acral metastases usually occur via hematogenous spread, as acral sites are vascular end zones, and their presence usually indicates a high tumor burden or disseminated disease [67]. Clinically, lesions present as tender, erythematous to violaceous nodules and are often misdiagnosed as infections or inflammatory dermatoses, delaying

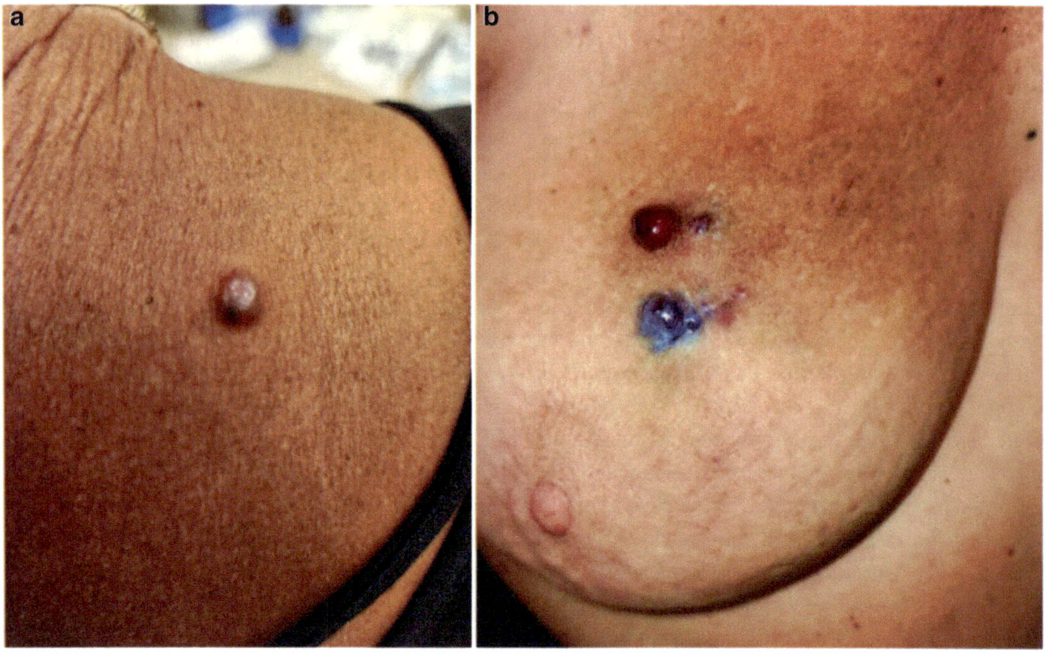

Fig. 1.9 Cutaneous angiosarcoma metastases on the back in a patient with prior breast irradiation; the primary angiosarcoma arose at the irradiated breast site

care [65, 68]. Dominant extremities may be more frequently involved due to higher perfusion, and their presence often indicates a poor prognosis.

1.2.3.12 In-Transit and Satellitosis Metastases

In-transit metastases are tumor deposits within dermal or subdermal lymphatics between the primary tumor and regional lymph nodes (Fig. 1.4). Although first described in melanoma, they also occur in cutaneous squamous cell carcinoma (cSCC), porocarcinoma [69], and breast cancer. Satellitosis refers to discrete tumor nodules within 2 cm of the primary lesion, whereas in-transit metastases arise beyond 2 cm but within the same anatomical region (Fig. 1.10).

Both patterns signal advanced disease and poorer outcomes [68–71]. Clinically, they present as multiple firm papules or nodules, sometimes coalescing into plaques, along the lymphatic drainage pathway; rare patterns such as diffuse vascular, intravascular, or folliculotropic involvement have been reported [72, 73]. Risk factors include tumor size, depth, lymphovascular invasion, and regional nodal disease [74–76]. In cSCC, the presence of satellitosis or in-transit metastases portends a worse prognosis and higher disease-specific mortality [71, 74, 77]. In melanoma, they may occur months to years after initial excision and are associated with increased recurrence risk [75, 78]. Because they signal advanced locoregional disease, their recognition is essential for accurate staging and may guide the use of sentinel node biopsy, regional therapies, or adjuvant systemic therapy [70, 75] (Table 1.1).

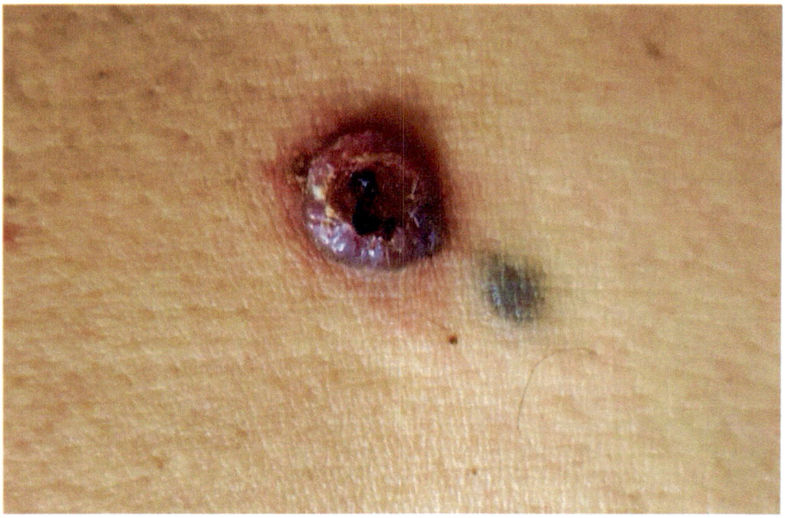

Fig. 1.10 Melanoma satellite metastasis

Table 1.1 Distinctive clinical presentations of cutaneous metastases (CM)

Clinical variant	Key clinical features	Common primary tumors	Pathogenesis
Nodular metastases	Firm, flesh-colored to erythematous or violaceous papules/nodules; solitary or multiple; may ulcerate in advanced stages	Breast (chest wall), GI (abdomen), lung, and renal	Most common CM; hematogenous spread; painless; correlates with primary tumor site
Carcinoma erysipelatoides	Erythematous, indurated warm plaques with sharp borders; mimics cellulitis/erysipelas; resistant to antibiotics	Breast (esp. inflammatory), gastric, uterine, and rectal	Lymphatic tumor spread; often misdiagnosed as infection; biopsy required
Carcinoma en cuirasse	Woody induration; sclerodermoid "breastplate" plaques; skin bound to deeper structures	Breast (chest wall)	Reflects dermal fibrosis and lymphatic obstruction; Indian-file pattern histology
Carcinoma telangiectoides	Violaceous macules, papules, plaques with telangiectasias; pseudovascular appearance	Breast	Dermal vascular/lymphatic invasion by tumor emboli; mimic benign vascular lesions
Zosteriform/ inflammatory CM	Lesions follow dermatomal distribution; mimic herpes zoster (vesicular/erythematous); painful	Breast, lung, GI, urinary tract, lymphoma, and SCC	Perineural or lymphatic dissemination; Koebner phenomenon; poor prognosis
Alopecia neoplastica	Nonscarring alopecia with underlying indurated scalp nodules/ plaques	Breast, lung, and GI	Mimics alopecia areata or cicatricial alopecia; biopsy essential
Umbilical metastasis (Sister Mary Joseph's nodule)	Firm, vascular, often ulcerated nodule/mass in periumbilical region	Gastric, ovarian, pancreatic, and colorectal	Advanced intra-abdominal malignancy; spread via lymphatics, hematogenous, or embryonic ligamentous remnants; usually adenocarcinoma histology
Genital/perianal CM	Ulcerated plaques, verrucous nodules; may mimic infections or primary dermatoses	Colorectal, bladder, and cervical	Rare; indicates aggressive disease; often misdiagnosed
Facial CM (incl. nasal tip)	Nodules or plaques; delayed diagnosis due to mimicry of benign conditions; nasal tip lesions red/ violaceous, "clown nose" sign	Melanoma, SCLC, colon, tonsillar SCC; nasal tip: Lung, kidney, thyroid, cervical, liver, and esophageal	Histology mandatory; facial CM indicates disseminated disease and poor prognosis; nasal tip lesions mimic NMSC or rhinophyma
Unusual morphologies and mimics	Rare forms: carcinoma hemorrhagiectoides (violaceous hemorrhagic plaques, "shield sign" in salivary duct carcinoma); CM mimicking keratoacanthoma, pyogenic granuloma, and psoriasis	Salivary duct carcinoma; others	CM in irradiated or scarred skin; wide morphological spectrum complicates diagnosis
Acral CM	Tender erythematous/violaceous nodules on hands, feet, nail beds; often misdiagnosed as infection	Lung, GI, and breast	Hematogenous spread to vascular end zones; dominant extremities more often involved; indicates disseminated disease and poor prognosis
In-transit/ satellitosis metastases	Firm papules/nodules along lymphatics between primary tumor and nodes; may form plaques	Melanoma, cutaneous squamous cell carcinoma, breast carcinoma, and porocarcinoma	Lymphatic tumor emboli; indicates advanced locoregional spread and poor prognosis

1.3 Diagnostic Work-Up and Imaging Correlation

The diagnosis of cutaneous metastases requires a multimodal approach integrating clinical, histopathologic, and imaging findings. Clinical examination, aided by dermoscopy, can provide early diagnostic clues. Dermoscopic features such as polymorphous vascular patterns and shiny white structures, while not pathognomonic, may raise suspicion for metastasis and warrant tissue confirmation [79–83].

The histological diagnosis of cutaneous metastasis is based on identifying a dermal infiltrate of malignant cells lacking connection to the epidermis, with immunohistochemistry guiding determination of the primary origin and differentiation from primary skin cancers. Marker panels help identify specific sources, such as breast (CK7, GCDFP-15), lung (TTF-1, CK7), or colorectal (CK20, CDX2) carcinomas [59, 84–87]. Clinical correlation with the patient's cancer history is essential, as in many cases—particularly breast and lung—cutaneous metastases may represent the first sign of disseminated disease. Cytology and biopsy remain the diagnostic gold standards: fine-needle aspiration cytology provides a minimally invasive and rapid method, while excisional or incisional biopsy yields adequate tissue for detailed immunohistochemical analysis [84, 85, 88, 89].

Imaging studies are essential for staging and systemic evaluation. The detection of cutaneous metastases should prompt comprehensive imaging with CT, PET/CT, or MRI to assess visceral spread and guide oncologic management [90–95]. Correlation across dermatology, pathology, and radiology optimizes diagnostic accuracy and treatment planning.

1.4 Prognostic Implications and Survival

Skin metastases usually indicate advanced systemic disease. Nonetheless, the latency between primary tumor diagnosis and skin involvement can be long—up to decades in rare cases like ocular melanoma [96–98]. Prognosis is generally poor, with skin metastasis signifying subclinical dissemination. However, early identification may lead to timely intervention, especially if metastasis is the presenting sign [16].

Prognostic impact depends on tumor type, burden, and timing of appearance. Metastases occurring synchronously with or before the primary tumor typically correlate with reduced survival [28]. More recent studies confirm that early cutaneous involvement often portends an aggressive disease course [99].

Beyond survival, skin metastases frequently mirror systemic disease progression, paralleling visceral tumor burden, and can therefore serve as a clinically valuable marker for disease monitoring [98, 100–102]. Recognizing these associations helps clinicians counsel patients, anticipate systemic progression, and adapt therapeutic strategies.

1.5 Management Considerations

The primary malignancy dictates the therapeutic approach. Excision of isolated skin metastases may be considered for diagnostic confirmation or palliation. Unlike paraneoplastic syndromes, resolution of cutaneous metastases is not typically achieved with systemic cancer therapy alone [7, 103]. Biopsy of any unexplained skin nodule, persistent ulcer, or indurated lesion remains a cornerstone in identifying occult internal malignancy [3].

1.6 Conclusion

Cutaneous metastases exhibit a wide spectrum of clinical manifestations ranging from nodules to plaques and inflammatory or vascular mimics. Recognizing these distinctive clinical presentations is critical, as they may provide the first clue to an undiagnosed malignancy or signal disease progression. Given the potential for misdiagnosis due to their polymorphic nature, histopathological evaluation remains essential in all suspicious cutaneous lesions, particularly in patients with a history of internal malignancy.

References

1. Griffiths C, Barker J, Bleiker T, Chalmers R, Creamer D. Rook's textbook of dermatology. 9th ed. Chichester: Wiley; 2016.
2. Cancer: principles & practice of oncology – NLM Catalog – NCBI. 2025. https://www.ncbi.nlm.nih.gov/nlmcatalog/101227521. Accessed Aug 6.
3. Brenner S, Tamir E, Maharshak N, Shapira J. Cutaneous manifestations of internal malignancies. Clin Dermatol. 2001;19:290–7. https://doi.org/10.1016/s0738-081x(01)00174-2.
4. Leonard N. Cutaneous metastases: where do they come from and what can they mimic? Curr Diagn Pathol. 2007;13:320–30. https://doi.org/10.1016/j.cdip.2007.05.011.
5. Spencer PS, Helm TN. Skin metastases in cancer patients. Cutis. 1987;39:119–21.
6. Lookingbill DP, Spangler N, Helm KF. Cutaneous metastases in patients with metastatic carcinoma: a retrospective study of 4020 patients. J Am Acad Dermatol. 1993;29:228–36. https://doi.org/10.1016/0190-9622(93)70173-q.
7. Kleyn CE, Lai-Cheong JE, Bell HK. Cutaneous manifestations of internal malignancy: diagnosis and management. Am J Clin Dermatol. 2006;7:71–84. https://doi.org/10.2165/00128071-200607020-00001.
8. Lookingbill DP, Spangler N, Sexton FM. Skin involvement as the presenting sign of internal carcinoma. A retrospective study of 7316 cancer patients. J Am Acad Dermatol. 1990;22:19–26. https://doi.org/10.1016/0190-9622(90)70002-y.
9. del Regato JA. Pathways of metastatic spread of malignant tumors. Semin Oncol. 1977;4:33–8.
10. Nashan D, Meiss F, Braun-Falco M, Reichenberger S. Cutaneous metastases from internal malignancies. Dermatol Ther. 2010;23:567–80. https://doi.org/10.1111/j.1529-8019.2010.01364.x.
11. Fernández-Antón Martínez MC, Parra-Blanco V, Avilés Izquierdo JA, Suárez Fernández RM. Cutaneous metastases of internal tumors. Actas Dermosifiliogr (Engl Ed). 2013;104:841–53. https://doi.org/10.1016/j.adengl.2012.06.031.
12. Junak M, Jecius H, Erdrich J. Cutaneous metastasis in the setting of both colon and Breast primary malignancies. Case Rep Gastrointest Med. 2020;2020:8852459. https://doi.org/10.1155/2020/8852459.
13. Brownstein MH, Helwig EB. Patterns of cutaneous metastasis. Arch Dermatol. 1972;105:862–8.
14. Poole S, Fenske NA. Cutaneous markers of internal malignancy. I. Malignant involvement of the skin and the genodermatoses. J Am Acad Dermatol. 1993;28:1–13. https://doi.org/10.1016/0190-9622(93)70001-a.
15. Alcaraz I, Cerroni L, Rütten A, Kutzner H, Requena L. Cutaneous metastases from internal malignancies: a clinicopathologic and immunohistochemical review. Am J Dermatopathol. 2012;34:347–93. https://doi.org/10.1097/DAD.0b013e31823069cf.
16. Strickley JD, Jenson AB, Jung JY. Cutaneous Metastasis. Hematol Oncol Clin North Am. 2019;33:173–97. https://doi.org/10.1016/j.hoc.2018.08.008.
17. Khan SU, Fatima K, Malik F, Kalkavan H, Wani A. Cancer metastasis: molecular mechanisms and clinical perspectives. Pharmacol Ther. 2023;250:108522. https://doi.org/10.1016/j.pharmthera.2023.108522.
18. Park M, Kim D, Ko S, Kim A, Mo K, Yoon H. Breast cancer metastasis: mechanisms and therapeutic implications. International journal of molecular sciences. 2022;23. Multidisciplinary digital publishing institute:6806. https://doi.org/10.3390/ijms23126806.
19. André F, Zielinski CC. Optimal strategies for the treatment of metastatic triple-negative breast cancer with currently approved agents. Ann Oncol. 2012;23(Suppl 6):vi46–51. https://doi.org/10.1093/annonc/mds195.
20. Tso S, Brockley J, Recica H, Ilchyshyn A. Sister Mary Joseph's nodule: an unusual but important physical finding characteristic of widespread internal malignancy. Br J Gen Pract. 2013;63:551–2. https://doi.org/10.3399/bjgp13X673900.
21. Girijala RL, Riahi RR, Cohen PR. Sister Mary Joseph nodule as a cutaneous manifestation of metastatic Appendiceal adenocarcinoma: case report and literature review. Cureus. 2018;10:e2244. https://doi.org/10.7759/cureus.2244.
22. Bari O, Cohen PR. Cutaneous metastasis from tonsillar squamous cell carcinoma: report and review of the literature. Cureus. 2017;9:e1122. https://doi.org/10.7759/cureus.1122.
23. Kurt S, Camuzcuoglu H, Camuzcuoglu A, Dicle N, Tinar S. Umbilical metastasis of serous component as a first sign of mixed type epithelial ovarian cancer. Eur J Gynaecol Oncol. 2009;30:455–7.
24. Zhou S, Ou H, Wu Y, Qi D, Pei X, Yu X, Hu X, Wu E. Targeting tumor endothelial cells with methyltransferase inhibitors: mechanisms of action and the potential of combination therapy. Pharmacol Ther. 2023;247:108434. https://doi.org/10.1016/j.pharmthera.2023.108434.
25. Brent MB. Pharmaceutical treatment of bone loss: from animal models and drug development to future treatment strategies. Pharmacol Ther. 2023;244:108383. https://doi.org/10.1016/j.pharmthera.2023.108383.
26. Brownstein MH, Helwig EB. Metastatic tumors of the skin. Cancer. 1972;29:1298–307.
27. Braverman IM. Skin manifestations of internal malignancy. Clin Geriatr Med. 2002;18:1–19. https://doi.org/10.1016/s0749-0690(03)00031-4.
28. Brodland DG, Zitelli JA. Mechanisms of metastasis. J Am Acad Dermatol. 1992;27:1–8. https://doi.org/10.1016/0190-9622(92)70146-7.
29. Schwartz RA. Cutaneous metastatic disease. J Am Acad Dermatol. 1995;33:161–82; quiz 183–186. https://doi.org/10.1016/0190-9622(95)90231-7.

30. Krathen RA, Orengo IF, Rosen T. Cutaneous metastasis: a meta-analysis of data. South Med J. 2003;96:164–7. https://doi.org/10.1097/01.SMJ.0000053676.73249.E5.
31. Souza B, de Castro E, Miyashiro D, Pincelli MS, Sanches JA. Cutaneous metastases from solid neoplasms – literature review. An Bras Dermatol. 2023;98:571–9. https://doi.org/10.1016/j.abd.2022.10.009.
32. Siddiqui MA, Zaman MN. Primary carcinoma en cuirasse. J Am Geriatr Soc. 1996;44:221–2. https://doi.org/10.1111/j.1532-5415.1996.tb02455.x.
33. Mehregan AH. Metastatic carcinoma to the skin. Dermatologica. 1961;123:311–25. https://doi.org/10.1159/000255148.
34. Mullinax K, Cohen JB. Carcinoma en cuirasse presenting as keloids of the chest. Dermatol Surg. 2004;30:226–8. https://doi.org/10.1111/j.1524-4725.2004.30071.x.
35. Savoia P, Fava P, Deboli T, Quaglino P, Bernengo MG. Zosteriform cutaneous metastases: a literature meta-analysis and a clinical report of three melanoma cases. Dermatol Surg. 2009;35:1355–63. https://doi.org/10.1111/j.1524-4725.2009.01241.x.
36. Xu L, Wang Y, Mu Y, Huang Q, Shuai W, Yang H. A case report of zosteriform cutaneous metastases from breast carcinoma. Clin Cosmet Investig Dermatol. 2024;17:205–9. https://doi.org/10.2147/CCID.S444101.
37. Williams LR, Levine LJ, Kauh YC. Cutaneous malignancies mimicking herpes zoster. Int J Dermatol. 1991;30:432–4. https://doi.org/10.1111/j.1365-4362.1991.tb03900.x.
38. Cohen I, Levy E. SCHREIBER H: Alopecia neoplastica due to breast carcinoma. Arch Dermatol. 1961;84:490–2. https://doi.org/10.1001/archderm.1961.01580150136023.
39. Baum EM, Omura EF, Payne RR, Little WP. Alopecia neoplastica–a rare form of cutaneous metastasis. J Am Acad Dermatol. 1981;4:688–94. https://doi.org/10.1016/s0190-9622(81)80201-0.
40. Bai X-L, Zhang Q, Masood W, Masood N, Tang Y, Cao C-H, Fu Q-H, Zhang Y, Gao S-L, Liang T-B. Sister Mary Joseph's nodule as a first sign of pancreatic cancer. World J Gastroenterol. 2012;18:6686–9. https://doi.org/10.3748/wjg.v18.i45.6686.
41. Premkumar M, Rangegowda D, Vyas T, Grover S, Joshi YK, Sharma C, Sahney A. Cholangicarcinoma presenting as a sister Mary Joseph nodule. ACG Case Rep J. 2016;3:209–11. https://doi.org/10.14309/crj.2016.52.
42. Fernández Fernández C, Manrique Municio A, Justo Alonso I, García Moreno V, Marcacuzco Quinto AA. Sister Mary Joseph nodule: analysis of a case series of umbilical metastases of diverse origin in a single Centre. Clin Surg. 2021;6:3086: 4.
43. Powell FC, Cooper AJ, Massa MC, Goellner JR, Su WP. Sister Mary Joseph's nodule: a clinical and histologic study. J Am Acad Dermatol. 1984;10:610–5. https://doi.org/10.1016/s0190-9622(84)80265-0.
44. Khan AJ, Cook B. Metastatic carcinoma of umbilicus: "Sister Mary Joseph's nodule.". Cutis. 1997;60:297–8.
45. Udkoff J, Cohen PR. Adenocarcinoma of the colon presenting with scrotal metastasis: case report and review of the literature. Dermatol Online J. 2016;22:13030/qt1jg0t4kw.
46. Boyd AS. Cutaneous metastasis from a vaginal squamouscellcarcinoma. JAADCaseRep. 2020;6:1135–7. https://doi.org/10.1016/j.jdcr.2020.08.038.
47. Hakami R, Alali MN, Alshammari T, AlShammari S, Alyahya Z, Ayesh M, AlSaad K, Abduljabbar A. A cutaneous metastasis of unresectable rectal adenocarcinoma: a case report and literature review. Int J Surg Case Rep. 2020;71:95–101. https://doi.org/10.1016/j.ijscr.2020.04.102.
48. Fyrmpas G, Barbetakis N, Efstathiou A, Konstantinidis I, Tsilikas C. Cutaneous metastasis to the face from colon adenocarcinoma. Case report. Int Semin Surg Oncol. 2006;3(2) https://doi.org/10.1186/1477-7800-3-2.
49. Barbetakis N, Samanidis G, Paliouras D, Samanidou E, Tzimorota Z, Asteriou C, Xirou P, Tsilikas C. Facial skin metastasis due to small-cell lung cancer: a case report. J Med Case Rep. 2009;3:32. https://doi.org/10.1186/1752-1947-3-32.
50. Singh D, Kapoor A, Singhal MK, Singh P, Kumar V, Kumar HS. Cutaneous metastasis involving face in breast cancer: a series of three patients. Clin Cancer Investig J. 2014;3:545–7.
51. Hashimi Y, Dholakia S. Facial cutaneous metastasis of colorectal adenocarcinoma. BMJ Case Rep. 2013;2013:bcr2013009875. https://doi.org/10.1136/bcr-2013-009875.
52. Zhao B, Chen L, Liao J, Xie Z, Lei X, Shen Z. Update of clown nose-like lesion, a Underrecognized manifestation of metastatic malignancies and genetic cancer predisposition syndromes. Front Medi. 2021;8 https://doi.org/10.3389/fmed.2021.673336.
53. Ledderose GJ, Englhard AS. Isolated nasal tip metastasis from esophageal squamous cell carcinoma: case report and literature review. Case Rep Otolaryngol. 2015;2015:246094. https://doi.org/10.1155/2015/246094.
54. Gault DT, Subbuswamy SG. Metastatic tumours of the nasal tip. Br J Plast Surg. 1985;38:570–4. https://doi.org/10.1016/0007-1226(85)90023-2.
55. Chau C-h, Siu W-t, Li M K-w. Nasal tip metastasis from esophageal carcinoma. Can J Surg/Journal Canadien De Chirurgie. 2002;45:224–5.
56. Dong A, Zuo C, Wang Y, Zhai Z, Wen W. Isolated nasal tip metastasis from esophageal squamous cell carcinoma. Clin Nucl Med. 2015;40:65–7. https://doi.org/10.1097/RLU.0000000000000387.
57. Al-Ani SA, Hernon C, Sillitoe AT, Burgess PA, Stanley PRW. An unusual skin metastasis: esophageal squamous cell carcinoma metastasizing to the nose following nasogastric tube suture. Plast Reconstr Surg. 2005;116:683–5. https://doi.org/10.1097/01.prs.0000175962.71043.9e.

58. Cohen PR, Prieto VG, Piha-Paul SA, Kurzrock R. The "shield sign" in two men with metastatic salivary duct carcinoma to the skin: cutaneous metastases presenting as carcinoma hemorrhagiectoides. J Clin Aesthet Dermatol. 2012;5:27–36.
59. Tinca AC, Lazar BA, Cozac-Szőke AR, Radu GN, Simion SP, Chiorean DM, Kosovski IB, et al. Cutaneous metastases-histological particularities of multifaceted entities. Dermatopathology (Basel, Switzerland). 2025;12:14. https://doi.org/10.3390/dermatopathology12020014.
60. Riahi RR, Cohen PR. Clinical manifestations of cutaneous metastases: a review with special emphasis on cutaneous metastases mimicking keratoacanthoma. Am J Clin Dermatol. 2012;13:103–12. https://doi.org/10.2165/11590640-000000000-00000.
61. Amadio PC, Lombardi RM. Metastatic tumors of the hand. J Hand Surg Am. 1987;12:311–6. https://doi.org/10.1016/s0363-5023(87)80299-x.
62. Baños-Arévalo AJ, López-Navarro N, Gallego-Domínguez E, Herrera E. Acral metastasis of the fingers: report of 2 cases. Actas Dermosifiliogr (Engl Ed). 2018;109:e1–4. https://doi.org/10.1016/j.adengl.2018.10.002.
63. Karamouzis MV, Ardavanis A, Alexopoulos A, Papadopoulou A, Apostolikas N, Rigatos G. Multiple cutaneous acral metastases in a woman with breast adenocarcinoma treated with pegylated liposomal doxorubicin: incidental or aetiological association? Eur J Cancer Care. 2005;14:267–71. https://doi.org/10.1111/j.1365-2354.2005.00573.x.
64. Wu CY, Gao HW, Huang WH, Chao CM. Infection-like acral cutaneous metastasis as the presenting sign of an occult breast cancer. Clin Exp Dermatol. 2009;34:e409–10. https://doi.org/10.1111/j.1365-2230.2009.03391.x.
65. Umana GE, Scalia G, Palmisciano P, Passanisi M, Da Ros V, Pompili G, Barone F, et al. Acrometastases to the hand: a systematic review. Medicina. 2021;57:950. https://doi.org/10.3390/medicina57090950.
66. Afshar A, Farhadnia P, Khalkhali H. Metastases to the hand and wrist: an analysis of 221 cases. J Hand Surg Am. 2014;39:923–932.e17. https://doi.org/10.1016/j.jhsa.2014.01.016.
67. Vijaya B, Sunila SV, Manjunath GV. Erythematous nodules of the hand: a rare site of metastatic breast carcinoma. Indian J Dermatol Venereol Leprol. 2011;77:695–8. https://doi.org/10.4103/0378-6323.86484.
68. Çiftdemir M, Ustabaşıoğlu FE, Çölbe SA, Üstün F, Usta U, Çiçin İ. Clinicopathological and prognostic characteristics of acral metastases in patients with malignant disease: a retrospective study. Acta Orthop Traumatol Turc. 2021;55:67–72. https://doi.org/10.5152/j.aott.2020.20052.
69. Barone H, O'Connor DM, Nathan NR, Sowerby L. Porocarcinoma of the ear found to have cutaneous in-transit and regional nodal metastasis: implications for management and importance of clinical examination. Dermatol Surg. 2024;50:107–8. https://doi.org/10.1097/DSS.0000000000003949.
70. Kumar AB, Jakub JW, Lester SC, Markovic SN, Baum CL. In-transit melanoma metastases: evaluation and management for the dermatologist. J Am Acad Dermatol. 2025;93:188–95. https://doi.org/10.1016/j.jaad.2025.03.005.
71. Marti-Marti I, Podlipnik S, Cañueto J, Ferrándiz-Pulido C, Deza G, Sanmartín O, Jaka A, et al. Prognostic factors for satellitosis or in-transit metastasis in cutaneous squamous cell carcinoma: a multicentric cohort study. J Am Acad Dermatol. 2023;89:119–27. https://doi.org/10.1016/j.jaad.2023.02.048.
72. Su S, Liu J, Jiang Y. Rare presentation of melanoma recurrences with diffuse subcutaneous intravascular lesions: a novel in-transit metastases pattern. Am J Dermatopathol. 2024;46:620–2. https://doi.org/10.1097/DAD.0000000000002735.
73. Paolino G, Panetta C, Didona D, Donati M, Donati P. Folliculotropic cutaneous metastases and Lymphangitis Carcinomatosa: when cutaneous metastases of breast carcinoma are mistaken for cutaneous infections. Acta Dermatovenerol Croatica: ADC. 2016;24:154–7.
74. Pahalyants, Vartan, Neil K. Jairath, Derek E. Maas, Shayan Cheraghlou, Soutrik Mandal, Steven Friedman, Maressa C. Criscito, et al. 2025. Satellitosis/in-transit metastasis in cutaneous squamous cell carcinoma: risk factors and the prognostic significance. J Am Acad Dermatol: https://doi.org/10.1016/j.jaad.2025.07.029.
75. Huibers A, Leong SP, Kashani-Sabet M, White RL, Vetto J, Schneebaum S, O'Donoghue C, et al. Identification of predictive factors for the development of in-transit metastasis in patients with melanoma. Ann Surg Oncol. 2025;32:3203–11. https://doi.org/10.1245/s10434-025-17084-4.
76. Hirotsu KE, Aasi SZ, Samson KK, Zheng C, Nazaroff JR, Voller LM, Ruiz ES, et al. Lymphovascular invasion is an independent predictor of metastasis and disease-specific death in cutaneous squamous cell carcinoma: a multicenter retrospective study. J Am Acad Dermatol. 2025;93:368–77. https://doi.org/10.1016/j.jaad.2025.04.029.
77. Klein JC, McKesey J, Srivastava D, Nijhawan RI. In transit metastases of cutaneous squamous cell carcinoma: a single institution case series. J Am Acad Dermatol. 2023;88:943–5. https://doi.org/10.1016/j.jaad.2022.11.020.
78. Peirano D, Donoso F, Vargas S, Hidalgo L, Agüero R, Uribe P, Mondaca S, Navarrete-Dechent C. Patterns of recurrence of cutaneous melanoma: a literature review. Dermatol Pract Concept. 2023;13:e2023304. https://doi.org/10.5826/dpc.1304a304.
79. Bono R, Giampetruzzi AR, Concolino F, Puddu P, Scoppola A, Sera F, Marchetti P. Dermoscopic patterns of cutaneous melanoma metastases. Melanoma Res. 2004;14:367–73. https://doi.org/10.1097/00008390-200410000-00006.
80. Chernoff KA, Marghoob AA, Lacouture ME, Deng L, Busam KJ, Myskowski PL. Dermoscopic findings in cutaneous metas-

tases. JAMA Dermatol. 2014;150:429–33. https://doi.org/10.1001/jamadermatol.2013.8502.
81. Kamińska-Winciorek G, Pilśniak A, Piskorski W, Wydmański J. Skin metastases in the clinical and dermoscopic aspects. Semin Oncol. 2022;49:160–9. https://doi.org/10.1053/j.seminoncol.2022.04.005.
82. Jaimes N, Halpern JA, Puig S, Malvehy J, Myskowski PL, Braun RP, Marghoob AA. Dermoscopy: an aid to the detection of amelanotic cutaneous melanoma metastases. Dermatol Surg. 2012;38:1437–44. https://doi.org/10.1111/j.1524-4725.2012.02438.x.
83. Simionescu O, Petrică M, Avram AM, Costache M, Scurtu LG, Tudorache SI, Iorga PG, Grigore M. Dermoscopy of skin metastases in advanced cancer—systemic (visceral, hematologic) and cutaneous. Front Med. 2024;11:1445811. https://doi.org/10.3389/fmed.2024.1445811.
84. Dumlao JK, Gatmaitan EL, Cubillan A, David JP, Villena S. Clinical and histopathologic profile of patients with cutaneous metastasis in a tertiary Hospital in The Philippines. Dermatopathology (Basel, Switzerland). 2022;9:392–407. https://doi.org/10.3390/dermatopathology9040046.
85. Wong CYB, Helm MA, Kalb RE, Helm TN, Zeitouni NC. The presentation, pathology, and current management strategies of cutaneous metastasis. N Am J Med Sci. 2013;5:499–504. https://doi.org/10.4103/1947-2714.118918.
86. Gschnell M, Volberg C, Hauser C, Krönig L. Cutaneous metastases: from epidemiology to therapy. JDDG: J Dtsch Dermatol Ges. 2024;22:974–93. https://doi.org/10.1111/ddg.15342.
87. Habermehl G, Ko J. Cutaneous metastases: a review and diagnostic approach to tumors of unknown origin. Arch Pathol Lab Med. 2018;143:943–57. https://doi.org/10.5858/arpa.2018-0051-RA.
88. Handa U, Kundu R, Dimri K. Cutaneous metastasis: a study of 138 cases diagnosed by fine-needle aspiration cytology. Acta Cytol. 2017;61:47–54. https://doi.org/10.1159/000453252.
89. Sharma P, Gupta R, Bhardwaj S. Fine needle aspiration cytology of cutaneous metastatic nodules: an institution based study. JK Sci J Med Educ Res. 2022;24:156–61.
90. Dolek A, Betul DS, Ciliz NO, Ozet G, Duran S. Comparative analysis of whole-body diffusion-weighted imaging and PET/CT in metastasis detection: a prospective study. Cureus. 2024;16:e74756. https://doi.org/10.7759/cureus.74756.
91. Lother D, Robert M, Elwood E, Smith S, Tunariu N, Johnston SRD, Parton M, et al. Imaging in metastatic breast cancer, CT, PET/CT, MRI, WB-DWI, CCA: review and new perspectives. Cancer Imaging. 2023;23:53. https://doi.org/10.1186/s40644-023-00557-8.
92. Ebner R, Sheikh GT, Brendel M, Ricke J, Cyran CC. ESR essentials: staging and restaging with FDG-PET/CT in oncology—practice recommendations by the European Society for Hybrid, molecular and translational imaging. Eur Radiol. 2025;35:1894–902. https://doi.org/10.1007/s00330-024-11094-8.
93. Wright CL, Miller ED, Contreras C, Knopp MV. Precision nuclear medicine: the evolving role of PET in melanoma. Radiol Clin North Am. 2021;59:755–72. https://doi.org/10.1016/j.rcl.2021.05.007.
94. Olthof EP, Bergink-Voorthuis BJ, Wenzel HHB, Mongula J, van der Velden J, Spijkerboer AM, Adam JA, et al. Diagnostic accuracy of MRI, CT, and [18F] FDG-PET-CT in detecting lymph node metastases in clinically early-stage cervical cancer – a nationwide Dutch cohort study. Insights Imaging. 2024;15:36. https://doi.org/10.1186/s13244-023-01589-1.
95. Cao J, Yirui X, Yang Y, Weifeng Z, Ang X. Comparative study of total-body PET and PET/MR in the diagnosis of liver metastases. Front Oncol. 2025;15 https://doi.org/10.3389/fonc.2025.1519107.
96. Lorigan JG, Wallace S, Mavligit GM. The prevalence and location of metastases from ocular melanoma: imaging study in 110 patients. AJR Am J Roentgenol. 1991;157:1279–81. https://doi.org/10.2214/ajr.157.6.1950883.
97. Ossowski L, Aguirre-Ghiso JA. Dormancy of metastatic melanoma. Pigment Cell Melanoma Res. 2010;23:41. https://doi.org/10.1111/j.1755-148X.2009.00647.x.
98. Komurcugil I, Arslan Z, Bal ZI, Aydogan M, Ciman Y. Cutaneous metastases different clinical presentations: case series and review of the literature. Dermatol Rep. 2022;15:9553. https://doi.org/10.4081/dr.2022.9553.
99. Queirós CS, Filipe PL, Soares de Almeida L. Cutaneous metastases from solid neoplasms in the 21st century: a retrospective study from a Portuguese tertiary care center. J Eur Acad Dermatol Venereol: JEADV. 2020;34:1218–24. https://doi.org/10.1111/jdv.16120.
100. Christ SM, Pohl K, Willmann J, Heesen P, Heusel A, Ahmadsei M, Kühnis A, et al. Patterns of metastatic spread and tumor burden in unselected cancer patients using PET imaging: implications for the oligometastatic spectrum theory. Clin Transl Radiat Oncol. 2024;45:100724. https://doi.org/10.1016/j.ctro.2024.100724.
101. Gor D, Ghimire B, Abbas O, Diab M, Gor D, Ghimire B, Abbas O, Diab M. Cutaneous metastases without a known primary: a clinical conundrum. Cureus. 2025;17 https://doi.org/10.7759/cureus.83591.
102. Cassalia F, Bolzon A, Ponzano M, Ventura L, Danese A, Del Fiore P, Belloni Fortina A, et al. The importance of reading the skin: cutaneous metastases of pancreatic cancer, a systematic review. J Clin Med. 2024;13:104. https://doi.org/10.3390/jcm13010104.
103. Gmitter TL, Dhawan SS, Phillips MG, Wiszniak J. Cutaneous metastases of colonic adenocarcinoma. Cutis. 1990;46:66–8.

Epidemiology of Cutaneous Metastasis

2

Antonios G. A. Kolios

Abstract

Cutaneous metastases are a relatively rare but clinically significant manifestation of internal malignancies. They typically indicate advanced disease and are associated with poor prognosis. This chapter provides a comprehensive overview of the epidemiology of cutaneous metastases, including incidence rates, timing of presentation, gender-based differences, ethnic and geographic variations, tumor-specific patterns, and histological subtypes. While breast cancer remains the most common source in women, melanoma, lung, and gastrointestinal cancers are leading contributors in men. Notably, in some cases, cutaneous metastasis may precede the diagnosis of the primary malignancy. Epidemiological data are limited by the rarity of the condition, diagnostic variability, and the retrospective nature of most studies.

Keywords

Cutaneous metastasis · Skin metastases · Internal malignancy · Epidemiology

A. G. A. Kolios (✉)
Department of Dermatology, University of Zurich, Zürich, Switzerland

Department of Dermatology, Inselspital, Bern University Hospital, University of Bern, Bern, Switzerland

Key Features

- Cutaneous metastases are relatively uncommon and may serve as an initial indicator of an underlying internal malignancy.
- Lesions frequently appear in anatomical proximity to the primary tumor, particularly when spread occurs via lymphatic routes.
- The propensity for cutaneous dissemination varies by tumor type, being highest in breast cancer and lowest in prostate cancer.
- In women, breast cancer and melanoma are the leading causes of skin metastases; in men, common sources include melanoma, head and neck cancers, lung, and colorectal carcinomas.
- The most typical clinical presentation is a firm, erythematous, non-tender nodule.

2.1 Introduction

Cutaneous metastases are an uncommon but clinically significant manifestation of internal malignancies. Their presence often indicates advanced stage cancer and is associated with a poor prognosis. While relatively rare overall, the incidence, distribution, and clinical implications of cutaneous metastasis vary by sex, tumor type, and ethnic population.

The skin is not necessarily a common site for metastatic spread but has prognostic implications and requires dermatological attention, as it can

D. Koumaki et al. (eds.), *Cutaneous Metastases*, https://doi.org/10.1007/978-3-032-26764-1_2

mimic more common skin diseases such as cysts, lipomas, or cellulitis, which could delay its diagnosis.

This chapter provides a comprehensive overview of the epidemiology of cutaneous metastases.

2.2 Clinical Relevance

Cutaneous metastases refer to the infiltration of malignant cells into the skin from a noncontiguous internal neoplasm. They are considered a marker of advanced disease and typically indicate a poor prognosis. Though relatively uncommon in the general oncologic population, their timely recognition is essential. Cutaneous metastasis may be the initial presentation of internal malignancy and is associated with a broad spectrum of morphologic features:

- It may alert the clinician to an undiagnosed internal malignancy.
- It often signals disease progression or recurrence.
- It may require urgent management due to bleeding, pain, or disfigurement.

2.3 General Incidence and Definition

Cutaneous metastases occur in approximately 1–10% of patients with internal malignancies, depending on the tumor type and population studied [1, 2], and overall account for around 2% of all skin tumors [3–5]. In large series, breast, lung, colon, and melanoma are consistently the most common primaries that metastasize to the skin (see Table 2.1). For example, in metastatic melanoma up to 45% of patients can develop skin metastasis.

The rarity and variable clinical presentation of cutaneous metastases can lead to delayed diagnosis. Most patients with cutaneous metastasis have advanced disease with Stage III–IV. On average cutaneous metastases develop 36 months after the diagnosis of a primary malignancy [6]. In less than 1% of cases, the cutaneous metastasis is the presenting sign of an internal malignancy.

Table 2.1 Cutaneous metastasis in patients with metastatic cancer

Primary malignancy	%
Melanoma	45
Breast	30
SCC (head and neck)	13
Endocrine glands	12.5
Esophagus	8.5
Urinary bladder	8
Gallbladder/bile ducts	5.5
Liver	5
Kidney	4.5
Colon/rectum	4.5
Ovary	4
Lung	2.5
Endometrium	2
Stomach	2
Pancreas	2
Uterine cervix	1
Prostate	<1
Testes	<1
Unknown	7.5

Adapted from Lookingbill et al. [1]

Additionally, it is important to account for the age of patients; for example, in children, the majority of cutaneous malignancies are due to leukemia, rhabdomyosarcoma, or neuroblastoma [7].

2.4 Timing of Occurrence

In most cases, skin metastases appear late in the disease course, often together with visceral spread. However, in a substantial subset of patients—up to 10%—cutaneous lesions may be the initial sign of malignancy, preceding the diagnosis of the primary tumor. This proportion is notably higher in men (up to 37%) than in women (around 6%) [3].

2.5 Gender-Based Distribution

The distribution of primary tumors leading to cutaneous metastases differs significantly between sexes, largely reflecting the prevalence of certain cancers (see Tables 2.2 and 2.3).

In woman breast carcinoma (70%) and malignant melanoma (12%) are the most common, whereas in men malignant melanoma (32%), head and neck (16%), lung (12%), and colon (11%) are the most common cancers causing cutaneous metastasis [3, 4].

The predominance of breast cancer in women as a cause of cutaneous metastasis may be due not only to its incidence but also to the superficial location of breast tumors and their proximity to skin [3, 4].

2.6 Ethnic and Geographic Variations

Significant differences in the rates and patterns of cutaneous metastases are observed across ethnic populations:

- A Taiwanese cohort identified an overall cutaneous metastasis rate of 1.02% among 12,146 patients with internal malignancies—markedly lower than rates in Caucasian populations. Breast cancer was still the leading cause, followed by lung and oral cancers, but the incidence of breast cancer was lower than in Caucasian cohorts [4].
- A Thai study reported a remarkably low incidence of 0.3% among 11,418 solid tumor patients, with breast cancer (36%) being the leading primary site, followed by head and neck and pancreatic cancers [5].

These findings underscore that genetic, environmental, and diagnostic factors may influence metastatic patterns and detection rates.

Table 2.2 Origin of cutaneous metastases stratified by gender (women)

Primary malignancy	%
Breast	70.7
Melanoma	12
Ovary	3.3
Oral cavity	2.3
Lung	2
Colon and rectum	1.3
Endometrium	1.3
Urinary bladder	1.3
Unknown	3

Adapted from Lookingbill et al. [1]

Table 2.3 Origin of cutaneous metastases stratified by gender (men)

Primary malignancy	%
Melanoma	32.3
Lung	11.8
Colon and rectum	11
Oral cavity	8.7
Larynx	5.5
Kidney	4.7
Upper gastro intestinal tract	3.9
Unknown	8.7

Adapted from Lookingbill et al. [1]

2.7 Tumor-Specific Patterns

Certain tumors such as melanoma, lung, renal, and colorectal cancers have a higher metastatic preference for the skin, whereas gastric, liver, or pancreatic cancers do not [8, 9].

- Melanoma has the highest rate of skin metastases among solid tumors (up to 45% in some series) [1, 10, 11].
- Lung cancer has the second highest rate of cutaneous metastases in men, ranging from 1.8% to 7.6%, often involving the head, neck, or chest [8].
- Breast cancer: in women the most common cancer metastasizing to the skin, with the chest wall and abdominal skin commonly affected.
- Colorectal carcinoma: several patients have metastases located at the site of incision after

colectomy. Metastases are most commonly found at the trunk, extremities, and perineum [1]. Sister Mary Joseph's nodules have an incidence of 1–3% in patients with intra-abdominal or pelvic malignancies. Most commonly seen in gastrointestinal (52%) and gynecologic (28%) cancers, and within gastrointestinal cancers, most commonly seen in stomach (45%), colorectal (29%), and pancreatic (17%) cancers [12, 13].
- Pancreatic cancer: skin metastases are rare (1–3%), but when present, skin metastases often involve the umbilicus (Sister Mary Joseph nodule) or head and neck, chest, abdomen, buttocks, scrotum, and labia [14–17]. In 58% of pancreatic cancer cases, cutaneous metastases preceded the primary diagnosis [18].
- Renal cancer is found at an advanced stage on initial presentation in 33% of cases, with metastasis in up to 18.4% of cases at the time of presentation due to its indolent course [19]. 4–8% of all cases of cutaneous metastases are due to kidney cancer, and skin involvement is seen in about 1.4% of cases of metastatic renal cell cancer. Clear cell renal cell cancer is the most common histologic subtype [1, 20, 21].
- Head and Neck Cancer: in patients with squamous cell carcinoma, distant skin metastases occur in up to 13% [10, 22].
- Hematologic malignancies can have extramedullary involvement of the skin as leukemia cutis. This accounts for acute myeloid leukemia (AML) and chronic lymphocytic leukemia (CLL) in 2–4% of patients as well as adult T-cell leukemia/lymphoma [23, 24].

2.8 Histologic Subtypes

Adenocarcinomas are the most likely histologic subtype resulting in cutaneous metastases across tumor types, e.g., ranging from 77% to 82% in breast cancer [1, 25]. Squamous cell carcinomas and poorly differentiated tumors also contribute, but less frequently [3, 4].

2.9 Site Distribution of Cutaneous Lesions

Lesions most frequently occur:

- In regions near the primary tumor (especially with lymphatic spread).
- On the anterior chest and abdomen in women.
- On the head, neck, and back in men.
- Umbilical region for gastrointestinal malignancies.
- Rarely, lesions appear in the scalp, eyelid, or genital areas, often raising initial diagnostic uncertainty [3].

2.10 Summary

Although several large retrospective series have provided valuable insights, obtaining robust epidemiologic data on cutaneous metastasis remains challenging. This rarity, coupled with their diverse clinical presentations and the need for histopathologic confirmation, contributes to underreporting and variability across studies. Furthermore, data are often derived from tertiary centers or dermatopathology services, which may not reflect broader population-based trends.

Cutaneous metastases, though uncommon, represent a clinically valuable marker of internal malignancy and are frequently underdiagnosed. The incidence, primary tumor distribution, and anatomical localization vary according to sex, ethnicity, and geographic region. Studies from East Asia suggest lower overall incidence rates, possibly reflecting differences in tumor biology, skin examination frequency, or reporting practices. Breast cancer remains the most common primary internal malignancy leading to cutaneous metastasis, but lung, GI, and head and neck cancers are also significant contributors. Larger, international, multi-center studies or registries are needed to better understand the epidemiology of cutaneous metastases.

References

1. Lookingbill DP, Spangler N, Helm KF. Cutaneous metastases in patients with metastatic carcinoma: a retrospective study of 4020 patients. J Am Acad Dermatol. 1993;29(2 Pt 1):228–36.
2. Rolz-Cruz G, Kim CC. Tumor invasion of the skin. Dermatol Clin. 2008;26(1):89–102. viii
3. Alcaraz I, Cerroni L, Rutten A, Kutzner H, Requena L. Cutaneous metastases from internal malignancies: a clinicopathologic and immunohistochemical review. Am J Dermatopathol. 2012;34(4):347–93.
4. Hu SC, Chen GS, Wu CS, Chai CY, Chen WT, Lan CC. Rates of cutaneous metastases from different internal malignancies: experience from a Taiwanese medical center. J Am Acad Dermatol. 2009;60(3):379–87.
5. Teyateeti P, Ungtrakul T. Retrospective review of cutaneous metastasis among 11, 418 patients with solid malignancy: a tertiary cancer center experience. Medicine (Baltimore). 2021;100(29):e26737.
6. Nashan D, Muller ML, Braun-Falco M, Reichenberger S, Szeimies RM, Bruckner-Tuderman L. Cutaneous metastases of visceral tumours: a review. J Cancer Res Clin Oncol. 2009;135(1):1–14.
7. Hussein MR. Skin metastasis: a pathologist's perspective. J Cutan Pathol. 2010;37(9):e1–20.
8. Kovacs KA, Hegedus B, Kenessey I, Timar J. Tumor type-specific and skin region-selective metastasis of human cancers: another example of the "seed and soil" hypothesis. Cancer Metastasis Rev. 2013;32(3–4):493–9.
9. Mueller TJ, Wu H, Greenberg RE, Hudes G, Topham N, Lessin SR, et al. Cutaneous metastases from genitourinary malignancies. Urology. 2004;63(6):1021–6.
10. Strickley JD, Jenson AB, Jung JY. Cutaneous metastasis. Hematol Oncol Clin North Am. 2019;33(1):173–97.
11. Wong CY, Helm MA, Helm TN, Zeitouni N. Patterns of skin metastases: a review of 25 years' experience at a single cancer center. Int J Dermatol. 2014;53(1):56–60.
12. Galvan VG. Sister Mary Joseph's nodule. Ann Intern Med. 1998;128(5):410.
13. Piura B, Meirovitz M, Bayme M, Shaco-Levy R. Sister Mary Joseph's nodule originating from endometrial carcinoma incidentally detected during surgery for an umbilical hernia: a case report. Arch Gynecol Obstet. 2006;274(6):385–8.
14. Kotsantis I, Economopoulou P, Dritsakos K, Oikonomopoulos N, Bakogeorgos M, Rapti C, et al. Extensive cutaneous metastases of pancreatic adenocarcinoma: a case report and review of the literature. Clin Case Reports. 2017;5(1):51–6.
15. Miulescu R, Balaban DV, Sandru F, Jinga M. Cutaneous manifestations in pancreatic diseases-a review. J Clin Med. 2020;9(8)
16. Ramachandran P, Boyapati L, Joseph G. Scalp metastasis as the first presentation of an underlying aggressive pancreatic cancer. J Investig Med High Impact Case Rep. 2020;8:2324709620931667.
17. Shi Y, Li SS, Liu DY, Yu Y. Cutaneous metastases of pancreatic carcinoma to the labia majora: a case report and review of literature. World J Gastrointest Oncol. 2020;12(11):1372–80.
18. Cassalia F, Bolzon A, Ponzano M, Ventura L, Danese A, Del Fiore P, et al. The importance of Reading the skin: cutaneous metastases of pancreatic cancer, a systematic review. J Clin Med. 2023;13(1)
19. Graves A, Hessamodini H, Wong G, Lim WH. Metastatic renal cell carcinoma: update on epidemiology, genetics, and therapeutic modalities. Immunotargets Ther. 2013;2:73–90.
20. Kovacs KA, Kenessey I, Timar J. Skin metastasis of internal cancers: a single institution experience. Pathol Oncol Res. 2013;19(3):515–20.
21. Hsieh JJ, Purdue MP, Signoretti S, Swanton C, Albiges L, Schmidinger M, et al. Renal cell carcinoma. Nat Rev Dis Primers. 2017;3:17009.
22. Pitman KT, Johnson JT. Skin metastases from head and neck squamous cell carcinoma: incidence and impact. Head Neck. 1999;21(6):560–5.
23. Agis H, Weltermann A, Fonatsch C, Haas O, Mitterbauer G, Mullauer L, et al. A comparative study on demographic, hematological, and cytogenetic findings and prognosis in acute myeloid leukemia with and without leukemia cutis. Ann Hematol. 2002;81(2):90–5.
24. Wagner G, Fenchel K, Back W, Schulz A, Sachse MM. Leukemia cutis – epidemiology, clinical presentation, and differential diagnoses. J Dtsch Dermatol Ges. 2012;10(1):27–36.
25. Gan EY, Chio MT, Tan WP. A retrospective review of cutaneous metastases at the National Skin Centre Singapore. Australas J Dermatol. 2015;56(1):1–6.

3 Pathogenesis of Cutaneous Metastases

Dimitra Koumaki, Georgios Evangelou,
Giannis Evangelou, and Stamatios Gregoriou

Abstract

Cutaneous metastasis of internal malignancies is an uncommon but clinically significant phenomenon in 0.6–10.4% of patients with cancer and is typically a marker of advanced disease. Skin metastasis's pathophysiology occurs through four primary mechanisms: hematogenous dissemination, lymphatic spread, direct implantation, and contiguous extension. Hematogenous dissemination correlates with intravasation of tumor cells, survival in the bloodstream, and extravasation within the dermal microvasculature, facilitated through angiogenic factors and immune evasion. Lymphatic spread is defined by lymphangiogenesis, stimulated by the tumor; matrix remodeling; and travel along lymphatic tracts, the result of which is regional nodal spread and possible extranodal spread to the skin. Direct implantation occurs as a consequence of surgical procedures or trauma, capitalizing on local immune suppression and inflammation secondary to wound healing. Contiguous extension is a local extension of the skin directly from underlying structures, usually for tumors close to the dermis. The umor microenvironment, including macrophages, fibroblasts, and adipocytes, is conducive to metastatic colonization, promoting angiogenesis, immune suppression, and tissue remodeling. Clinically, cutaneous metastases are variably morphologic—nodules, plaques, or ulcers—and may be the first manifestation of an occult cancer. Histopathologically, patterns of resemblance to the primary tumor are encountered. Cutaneous metastases in general portend a poor prognosis, with a survival of months. Early detection and histopathologic confirmation are essential to diagnosis and management.

Keywords

Cutaneous metastasis · Hematogenous spread · Lymphatic spread · Direct implantation · Contiguous extension · Tumor microenvironment · Angiogenesis · Immune suppression · Clinicopathology · Prognosis

D. Koumaki (✉) · G. Evangelou
Dermatology Department, University Hospital of Heraklion, Heraklion, Greece
e-mail: dkoumaki@yahoo.g

G. Evangelou
Computer Science Department, University of Crete, Heraklion, Greece

S. Gregoriou
Department of Dermatology and Venereology, Andreas Sygros Hospital, National and Kapodistrian University of Athens, Medical School of Athens, Athens, Greece

D. Koumaki et al. (eds.), *Cutaneous Metastases*, https://doi.org/10.1007/978-3-032-26764-1_3

3.1 Introduction

Cutaneous metastases are a significant clinical manifestation of metastatic cancer, resulting when malignant cells from internal primary cancers seed and populate the skin [1]. The pathogenesis is multifactorial and involves hematogenous spread, lymphatic spread, direct implantation after surgical or traumatic compromise, and contiguous growth from underlying tissues [2]. Tumor cell migration and survival are facilitated by dynamic interactions with the skin microenvironment, including angiogenesis—predominantly through vascular endothelial growth factor (VEGF)—immune evasion, and inflammation, which is commonly further aggravated by wound healing and local tissue trauma [3, 4]. Macrophages and subcutaneous tissue and dermal adipocytes also support tumor growth and survival, and immunosuppression related to age increases the risk for metastatic colonization, particularly in elderly patients (Fig. 3.1).

Cutaneous metastasis is a coordinated, organ-directed process, and the pattern of distribution will reflect that of the original tumor site and the preferred routes of metastasis. For example, breast carcinoma frequently metastasizes to the chest wall, and gastrointestinal cancers may manifest as an umbilical nodule (Sister Joseph nodule) by lymphatic or contiguous spread [1–4]. Histopathologically, cutaneous metastases are frequently dermal in origin and may demonstrate nodular, infiltrative, diffuse, or intravascular patterns of growth that are often very similar to the original malignancy [5–7]. Hematogenous spread is a dominant pathway, with tumor cells disseminating to local blood vessels, surviving in circulation through platelet shielding and immune checkpoint expression, and extravasating into the skin, where colonization is fostered by angiogenic and immunosuppressive factors. Clinical presentation is highly variable, and cutaneous metastases can be the presenting manifestation of an otherwise unsuspected internal malignancy; therefore, clinical suspicion must be high and histopathologic diagnosis rapid [8, 9].

Hematogenous dissemination is a major avenue by which primary tumors metastasize to the skin. It is a multifactorial multistep process involving invasion of cancer cells, intravasation,

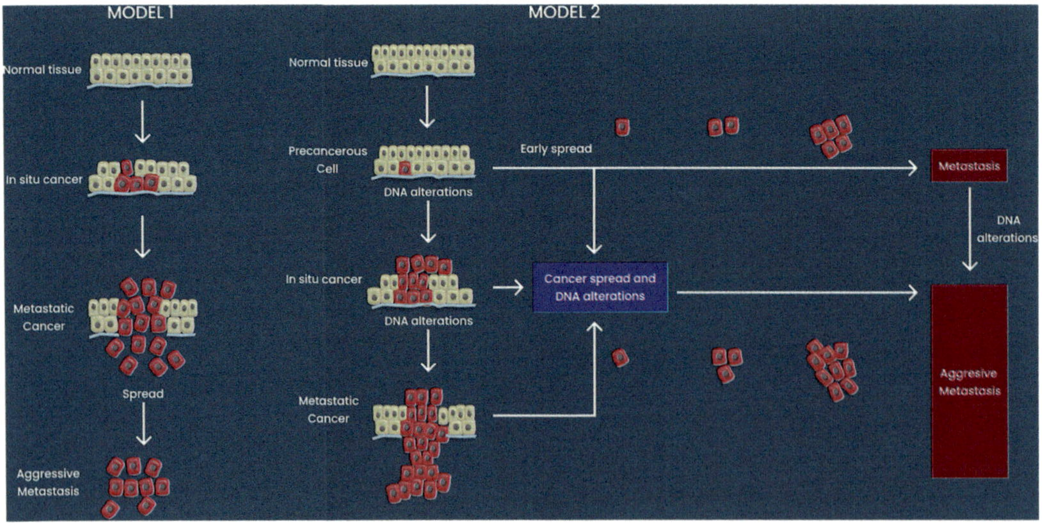

Fig. 3.1 This figure shows the two models proposed for cancer development and progression. In the classical human cancer model, metastasis is the final stage of the tumorigenic process (Model 1). By contrast, more recent evidence suggests an alternative model (Model 2), which posits that the activation of proteins for the epithelial-to-mesenchymal transition not only permits malignant transformation but also metastatic dissemination. Primary tumor cells, from this viewpoint, can disseminate at any point during cancer progression. (Source Sánchez-García [1] and Fernández-Antón et al. [2])

circulation, survival, immune evasion, extravasation, and ultimately colonization of the cutaneous microenvironment. Invasion by tumor cells begins with the local breakdown of the basement membrane and extracellular matrix by proteolytic enzymes such as matrix metalloproteinases. Macrophages present on tumors and inflammatory mediators facilitate the process of invasion by inducing angiogenesis (most significantly by VEGF) and creating a permissive environment for motility and invasion of tumor cells. Intravasation refers to the invasion of cancer cells into the blood vessels. Intravasation is regulated by complex interactions among cancer cells, endothelial cells, and perivascular macrophages. The metastatic tumor microenvironment of metastasis (TMEM) is an organized complex in which an overexpressing Mena cancer cell, a Tie2/VEGF-expressing macrophage, and an endothelial cell interact well, which makes highly efficient transendothelial migration possible [3, 8, 9]. Mesenchymal and amoeboid modes of migration are implicated, and paracrine signaling (e.g., CSF1/EGF axis) also promotes intravasation. Survival in circulation is a critical restrictive phase for metastatic cells. Circulating tumor cells (CTCs) encounter shear stress, matrix detachment, and immune recognition. Cloaking by platelets, display of immune checkpoint molecules, and secretion of immunosuppressive cytokines all help the CTCs evade destruction. Some of the CTCs survive to migrate to distant sites [10]. Immune evasion is mandatory for the progression of the metastatic cascade. The tumor cells exploit local and systemic immunosuppression, including VEGF-mediated inhibition of dendritic cell maturation and T-cell activity, and immunosuppressive myeloid cell recruitment. Immunosenescence and wound-healing type inflammation also increase metastatic seeding, particularly in older or post-operative individuals. Extravasation involves the arrest, adhesion, and transmigration of cancer cells into the endothelium at a distance [11–13]. Extravasation is governed by microvascular geometry, hydrodynamic forces, and cell surface expression of adhesion molecules (e.g., selectins and integrins) on tumor and endothelial cells. Adhesion sites for tumor cells and sites for diapedesis are the endothelial glycocalyx and intercellular clefts. Chemomechanical signaling in the guise of bidirectional biochemical interaction between tumor and endothelial cells controls cytoskeletal dynamics to attain transendothelial migration. Organ site colonization of the skin is controlled by the "seed and soil" model, whereby molecular compatibility between the cutaneous microenvironment and cancer cells determines metastatic success. Preemption of the skin by metastasis is generated by premetastatic niche formation that comprises recruitment of bone marrow-derived cells, deposition of extracellular matrix proteins, and local immunomodulation. Preemption of the skin by tumor-exosomes and soluble factor action also promotes metastatic colonization. Clinically, skin metastases may be the presenting feature of an occult cancer and are invariably a bad prognostic indicator. The process is highly selective and non-random, both reflecting tumor-intrinsic characteristics and the unique biology of skin as a metastatic organ. Understanding these processes is necessary for the development of targeted therapy that blocks the metastatic cascade at various levels.

Lymphatic spread is a significant pathway of cutaneous metastases for solid tumors, which involves a series of coordinated processes: 1. Invasion of local lymphatic vasculature by tumor cells: Cancer cells invade lymphatic capillaries by exploiting physiological mechanisms involved in leukocyte migration [14–16]. This is facilitated by tumor-induced lymphangiogenesis and VEGF-C and VEGF-D-mediated signaling through VEGFR-3, which expands and reorganizes lymphatic networks in the tumor's periphery and draining lymph nodes. Matrix metalloproteinases (MMPs) and ADAMs degrade the extracellular matrix and remodel intercellular junctions to create portals of entry for the tumor cells into lymphatic vessels. Adhesion molecules such as integrins and the hyaluronan-LYVE-1/CD44 axis permit firm adhesion and transmigration of the tumor cells across the lymphatic endothelium [17]. 2. Directional migration and transport to regional lymph nodes: Inside lymphatic vessels, tumor cells are guided by chemotactic, haptotactic, and durotactic signals—chemokine gradients (e.g., CCL21/CCR7) direct migration to lymphatic endothelium and draining lymph nodes. Integrins and the hyaluronan-LYVE-1/CD44 pathway also facilitate directional migration and retention in lymphatic channels. Tumor cells are then transported to regional lymph nodes, where they can proliferate to establish metastatic foci. 3. Cutaneous colonization and extranodal extension: Metastatic cells within lymph nodes can penetrate through the nodal capsule to invade nearby subcutaneous tissues and skin, a process known as extranodal extension. Extranodal extension due to tumor microenvironment composed of tumor-associated macrophages, fibroblasts, immune cells, and inflammatory mediators supports lymphatic invasion and metastatic colonization by promoting angiogenesis, immune evasion, and local immunosuppression. Wound healing and chronic inflammation also enhance the permissiveness of the skin for metastatic colonization [18, 19]. All of these mechanisms enable solid tumors to employ the lymphatic system for dissemination and cutaneous metastasis, with the tumor microenvironment playing a central role in controlling each step.

Direct implantation caused by trauma or surgery is an independent mechanism by which cutaneous metastasis of solid cancers occurs. By virtue of surgical procedures or traumatic injury, viable tumor cells can be physically transplanted into the skin or subcutaneous tissue [20]. This can be achieved via contaminated surgical instruments, gloves, or direct contact with tumor tissue itself, especially in compromised skin barrier cases. Wound healing creates an environment of inflammatory mediators, growth factors (especially VEGF), and activated macrophages, which collectively increase the survival of tumor cells, angiogenesis, and immune evasion [21–24]. Local immunosuppression and increased vascular permeability also increase the growth and development of metastatic cells in the implantation site. This is a clinical relevance process in cases of cutaneous metastases along areas of surgical scars, areas of drainage, or areas of previous trauma. The pathway is supplemented by the induction of immunosuppressive cells (such as myeloid-derived suppressor cells and regulatory T cells) and suppression of natural killer cell activity, suppressing anti-tumor immunity and promoting metastatic growth. Inflammatory cytokines and tissue remodeling of wound healing are commandeered by tumor cells, distinguishing direct implantation from hematogenous and lymphatic spread, which are vascular or lymphatic dissemination-dependent.

Continuous extension is one of the modes of cutaneous metastasis wherein malignant cells from an underlying solid tumor invade the skin directly from contiguous underlying tissues such as subcutaneous tissue, fascia, muscle, or serosal surfaces. This is most frequently seen in cancers adjacent to the skin, such as breast carcinoma, chest wall tumors, and abdominal cancer presenting as umbilical metastasis (Sister Joseph nodule). The pathophysiology involves the following sequence: tumor cells invade through the basement membrane and move along tissue planes by being assisted by proteolytic enzymes (mainly matrix metalloproteinases), which degrade extracellular matrix molecules. The local inflammation response, especially following surgery, injury, or chronic inflammation, may further promote tumor cell migration by reorganizing the tissue structure as well as immune surveillance. Tumor-associated macrophages and angiogenic factors such as VEGF contribute to a tumor-favorable microenvironment that includes tumor growth, neovascularization, and immunosuppression. Subcutaneous adipocytes also have the ability to activate tumor growth in lymph node-involvement conditions. Histologically, contiguous extension cutaneous metastases are typically observed as nodular, infiltrative, or diffuse dermal patterns, which often replicate the primary neoplasm morphology. This is in contrast to hematogenous or lymphatic spread, which would result in more diffuse or multifocal cutaneous involvement. Clinically, such metastases can manifest as rapidly enlarging, firm, painless nodules or plaques, and their presentation may be imitated by benign dermatologic disorders. Detection of contiguous extension is significant as it usually indicates far-advanced local disease and may influence prognosis and treatment [25–28].

The goal of this textbook on cutaneous metastasis is to present the clinical variability of their cutaneous appearance across metastatic tumors originating from different tissues, to raise clinicians' awareness of including cutaneous metastasis in the differential diagnosis, and to provide an overview of current treatment options and palliative care for affected patients.

References

1. Sánchez-García I. The crossroads of oncogenesis and metastasis. N Engl J Med. 2009;360(3):297–9. https://doi.org/10.1056/NEJMcibr0808031. PMID: 19144947
2. Fernández-Antón Martínez MC, Parra-Blanco V, Avilés Izquierdo JA, Suárez Fernández RM. Cutaneous metastases of internal tumors. Actas Dermosifiliogr. 2013;104(10):841–53. https://doi.org/10.1016/j.ad.2012.06.005. Epub 2012 Jul 30. PMID: 22853962.
3. Brodland DG, Zitelli JA. Mechanisms of metastasis. J Am Acad Dermatol. 1992;27(1):1–8. https://doi.org/10.1016/0190-9622(92)70146-7. PMID: 1619054
4. Otsuka I. Cutaneous metastasis after surgery, injury, lymphadenopathy, and peritonitis: possible mechanisms. Int J Mol Sci. 2019;20(13):3286. https://doi.org/10.3390/ijms20133286. PMID: 31277406
5. Hussein MR. Skin metastasis: a pathologist's perspective. J Cutan Pathol. 2010;37(9):e1–20. https://doi.org/10.1111/j.1600-0560.2009.01469.x. Epub 2009 Nov 17. PMID: 19922483.
6. Strickley JD, Jenson AB, Jung JY. Cutaneous Metastasis. Hematol Oncol Clin North Am. 2019;33(1):173–97. https://doi.org/10.1016/j.hoc.2018.08.008. PMID: 30497674
7. BCE S, Miyashiro D, Pincelli MS, Sanches JA. Cutaneous metastases from solid neoplasms – literature review. An Bras Dermatol. 2023;98(5):571–9. https://doi.org/10.1016/j.abd.2022.10.009. PMID: 19922483.
8. Alcaraz I, Cerroni L, Rütten A, Kutzner H, Requena L. Cutaneous metastases from internal malignancies: a clinicopathologic and immunohistochemical review. Am J Dermatopathol. 2012;34(4):347–93. https://doi.org/10.1097/DAD.0b013e31823069cf. PMID: 22617133
9. Dieterich LC, Tacconi C, Ducoli L, Detmar M. Lymphatic vessels in cancer. Physiol Rev. 2022;102(4):1837–79. https://doi.org/10.1152/physrev.00039.2021. Epub 2022 Jun 30. PMID: 35771983.
10. Jackson DG. Lymphatic trafficking of immune cells and insights for cancer metastasis. Clin Exp Metastasis. 2024;41(4):381–6. https://doi.org/10.1007/s10585-023-10229-3. Epub 2023 Aug 22. PMID: 37606814.
11. Leong SP, Pissas A, Scarato M, Gallon F, Pissas MH, Amore M, Wu M, Faries MB, Lund AW. The lymphatic system and sentinel lymph nodes: conduit for cancer metastasis. Clin Exp Metastasis. 2022;39(1):139–57. https://doi.org/10.1007/s10585-021-10123-w. Epub 2021 Oct 15. PMID: 34651243.
12. Wang Z, Li Z, Sun X, Men W, Xu Y. Cellular components of tumor microenvironment: understanding their role in lymphatic metastasis of tumors. Front Pharmacol. 2024;15:1463538. https://doi.org/10.3389/fphar.2024.1463538. eCollection 2024. PMID: 39726782.
13. Alitalo A, Detmar M. Interaction of tumor cells and lymphatic vessels in cancer progression. Oncogene. 2012;31(42):4499–508. https://doi.org/10.1038/onc.2011.602. Epub 2011 Dec 19. PMID: 22179834.
14. Nathanson SD. Insights into the mechanisms of lymph node metastasis. Cancer. 2003;98(2):413–23. https://doi.org/10.1002/cncr.11464. PMID: 12872364
15. Sleeman JP, Thiele W. Tumor metastasis and the lymphatic vasculature. Int J Cancer. 2009;125(12):2747–56. https://doi.org/10.1002/ijc.24702. PMID: 19569051
16. Rezzola S, Sigmund EC, Halin C, Ronca R. The lymphatic vasculature: an active and dynamic player in cancer progression. Med Res Rev. 2022;42(1):576–614. https://doi.org/10.1002/med.21855. Epub 2021 Sep 5. PMID: 34486138.
17. Viúdez-Pareja C, Kreft E, García-Caballero M. Immunomodulatory properties of the lymphatic endothelium in the tumor microenvironment. Front Immunol. 2023;14:1235812. https://doi.org/10.3389/fimmu.2023.1235812. eCollection 2023. PMID: 37744339.
18. Zhou H, Lei PJ, Padera TP. Progression of metastasis through lymphatic system. Cells. 2021;10(3):627. https://doi.org/10.3390/cells10030627. PMID: 3380895
19. Farnsworth RH, Achen MG, Stacker SA. The evolving role of lymphatics in cancer metastasis. Curr Opin Immunol. 2018;53:64–73. https://doi.org/10.1016/j.coi.2018.04.008. Epub 2018 Apr 23. PMID: 29698919.
20. Cheng X, Zhang H, Hamad A, Huang H, Tsung A. Surgery-mediated tumor-promoting effects on the immune microenvironment. Semin Cancer Biol. 2022;86(Pt 3):408–19. https://doi.org/10.1016/j.semcancer.2022.01.006. Epub 2022 Jan 20. PMID: 35066156.
21. Rolz-Cruz G, Kim CC. Tumor invasion of the skin. Dermatol Clin. 2008;26(1):89–102, viii. https://doi.org/10.1016/j.det.2007.08.004. PMID: 180237734.
22. Jaros J, Hunt S, Mose E, Lai O, Tsoukas M. Cutaneous metastases: a great imitator. Clin Dermatol. 2020;38(2):216–22. https://doi.org/10.

1016/j.clindermatol.2019.10.004. Epub 2019 Oct 25. PMID: 32513401.
23. Guanziroli E, Coggi A, Venegoni L, Fanoni D, Ercoli G, Boggio F, Veraldi S, Berti E, Gianotti R, Ferrero S, Del Gobbo A. Cutaneous metastases of internal malignancies: an experience from a single institution. Eur J Dermatol. 2017;27(6):609–14. https://doi.org/10.1684/ejd.2017.3142. PMID: 29160213
24. Mueller TJ, Wu H, Greenberg RE, Hudes G, Topham N, Lessin SR, Uzzo RG. Cutaneous metastases from genitourinary malignancies. Urology. 2004;63(6):1021–6. https://doi.org/10.1016/j.urology.2004.01.014. PMID: 15183939
25. Queirós CS, Filipe PL, Soares de Almeida L. cutaneous metastases from solid neoplasms in the 21st century: a retrospective study from a Portuguese tertiary care center. J Eur Acad Dermatol Venereol. 2020;34(6):1218–24. https://doi.org/10.1111/jdv.16120. Epub 2020 Jan 30. PMID: 31788857.
26. Vernemmen AIP, Li X, Roemen GMJM, Speel EM, Kubat B, Hausen AZ, Winnepenninckx VJL, Samarska IV. Cutaneous metastases of internal malignancies: a single-institution experience. Histopathology. 2022;81(3):329–41. https://doi.org/10.1111/his.14705. Epub 2022 Jul 20. PMID: 35758186.
27. Kamińska-Winciorek G, Pilśniak A, Piskorski W, Wydmański J. Skin metastases in the clinical and dermoscopic aspects. Semin Oncol. 2022;49(2):160–9. https://doi.org/10.1053/j.seminoncol.2022.04.005. Epub 2022 May 3. PMID: 35589424.
28. El-Kenawi A, Hänggi K, Ruffell B. The immune microenvironment and cancer metastasis. Cold Spring Harb Perspect Med. 2020;10(4):a037424. https://doi.org/10.1101/cshperspect.a037424. PMID: 31501262

Clinical Presentation of Cutaneous Metastases

4

Ana-Maria Forsea

Abstract

Cutaneous metastases (CM) are uncommon yet clinically significant indicators of internal malignancy, frequently signifying advanced disease and poor prognosis. In a subset of patients, they may be the initial manifestation of an undiagnosed cancer or mark recurrence. CM can arise from a wide spectrum of primary tumors and display varied clinical morphologies. Their appearance is shaped by the biology and site of the primary tumor, as well as patient-specific factors. Anatomic distribution follows vascular and lymphatic drainage patterns, with common sites including the chest wall, abdomen, and scalp. Morphologically, CM may present as nodules, plaques, tumor masses, or mimic inflammatory, infectious, or vascular conditions, such as cellulitis, herpes zoster, or vasculitis. Rare forms include carcinoma erysipelatodes, carcinoma en cuirasse, telangiectatic metastases, and alopecia neoplastica. Recognizing these diverse patterns is essential for prompt diagnosis and management. Early identification directly impacts treatment decisions, alleviates patient distress, and may influence survival outcomes.

Keywords

Cutaneous metastases · Clinical morphology · Metastatic cancer · Clinical diagnosis · Skin presentation

4.1 Introduction

Cutaneous metastases (CM) are uncommon but carry major clinical and prognostic significance. Their presence typically signals advanced-stage disease, often with poor survival outcomes. In up to 30% of cases, they may be the presenting sign of internal neoplasia [1, 2], or they may signal the recurrence of a previously treated cancer. While the incidence of CM in oncologic patients is estimated to range from 0.7% to 10% [3–5], their prevalence may increase in the future, as cancer survival rates improve due to new innovative oncological therapies. Their presence and progression severely impact the patients' quality of life, as psycho-sociological suffering from stigma and disfigurement adds to the pain and discomfort. For all these reasons, prompt recognition of CM is of critical importance for improving the patients' prognosis, management, and quality of life. The clinicians should be well aware of the various clinical presentations of CM.

A.-M. Forsea (✉)
Department of Oncologic Dermatology, Elias University Hospital Bucharest, Carol Davila University of Medicine and Pharmacy, Bucharest, Romania

Dermatology Department, Health and Medical University Potsdam, Potsdam, Romania

D. Koumaki et al. (eds.), *Cutaneous Metastases*, https://doi.org/10.1007/978-3-032-26764-1_4

4.2 Clinical Presentation of CM

The clinical aspect of CM depends on the type, biology, and site of the primary tumor, as well as of the patients' particularities, including age, sex, and previous medical history. CM can arise from primary skin tumors, such as melanoma, squamous cell carcinoma, but also Merkel cell carcinoma, angiosarcoma, or the rare skin adnexal malignant neoplasms; from internal organ solid malignancies or from hematologic malignancies like lymphomas and leukemias. Metastatic skin involvement is most frequently associated with breast, lung cancer and melanoma, and less commonly with other primaries such as colon, ovary, and head-and-neck cancers [3, 6–8]. In women, breast cancer predominates; in men, lung cancer and melanoma are leading sources of CM.

4.3 Location

The anatomical distribution of CM is influenced by the location of the primary tumor, patterns of vascular and lymphatic drainage, and surgical or radiation history. Metastases reach the skin via hematogenous, lymphatic routes, through direct extension along anatomic structures such as fascia or nerve sheaths, or through iatrogenic dissemination following invasive procedures [7, 9]. Commonly involved sites include the anterior chest wall—particularly in breast carcinoma and also in lung cancer; the abdomen—especially in gastrointestinal tract and genitourinary system cancers; scalp; and neck—which are frequent locations for metastases from visceral malignancies such as the lung or gastrointestinal tract [8–10]. The *scalp* is a notable predilection site for metastases from lung, kidney, and breast cancers, likely due to its rich vascular supply [11–13]. *Umbilical metastases*, known as Sister Mary Joseph nodules, typically originate from intra-abdominal or pelvic malignancies [6, 14]. Postoperative scars, radiation fields, and sites of prior trauma may also serve as loci for tumor implantation [3, 5, 8, 15]. While the *trunk* is most frequently affected overall, *extremity involvement* is relatively rare and often indicates advanced systemic disease [16, 17]. Metastases can appear solitary or multiple and may follow dermatomal or linear patterns when associated with lymphatic spread [8, 18].

Understanding these distribution patterns can aid in timely recognition and diagnosis, either of an unknown primary visceral tumor, or of the progression of a previously treated cancer, in all cases bringing a crucial contribution to prompt management and to improving prognosis.

4.4 Morphologic Patterns

CM manifest in a remarkably broad morphological spectrum and consequently may be misdiagnosed for a wide range of dermatoses [6]. Moreover, more than one pattern may present in the same patient. Awareness of the clinical appearances—both common and rare—is essential for proper early diagnosis.

4.5 The Most Frequently Encountered Patterns

Nodular Lesions Firm, often painless nodules or papules arising in the dermis or subcutis are the most frequent presentation of CM [19]. They may be skin-colored, erythematous, violaceous, bluish, or pigmented, occasionally ulcerating or bleeding. Black, blue, or gray hues suggest the presence of melanin pigment and are often found in melanoma metastases. Metastatic nodules may be solitary or multiple, varying in size from less than one to several centimeters [6, 10]; the lesions may coalesce into plaques or even larger subcutaneous masses (Figs. 4.1 and 4.2). The overlying epidermis is usually intact and stretched in early lesions, while secondary erosion, ulceration, or necrosis may develop later in larger progressive lesions. Pain and bleeding are later symptoms. The nodular metastases appear more often in skin areas in the proximity of the primary tumor, but widespread dissemination, linear disposition along dermatomeres or lymphatic vascular structures, or even isolated emergence at distant locations (e.g., fingertip metastases from lung cancers) are possible [2, 6, 8, 9, 17].

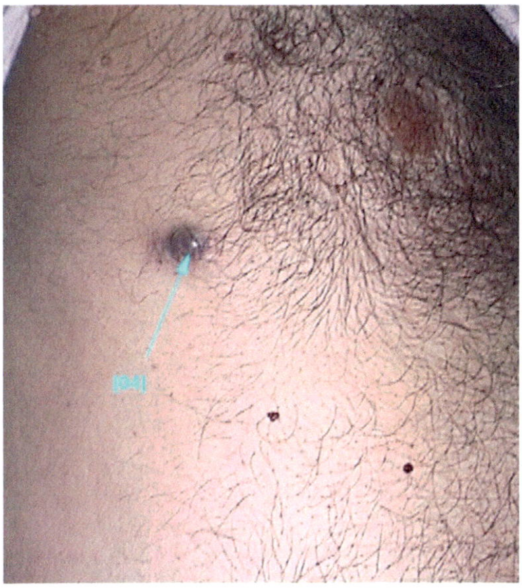

Fig. 4.1 Nodular metastases of melanoma on trunk

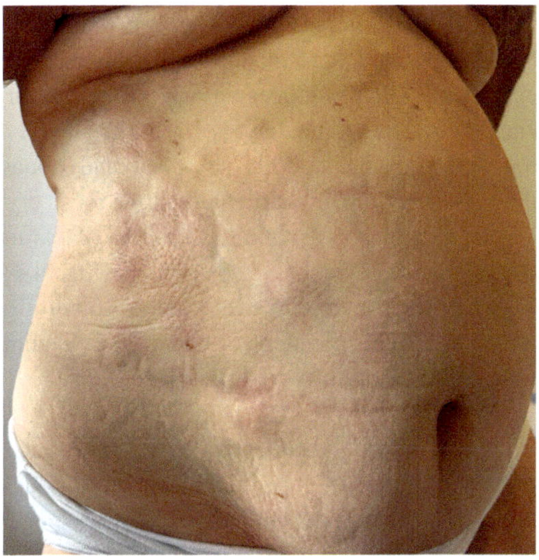

Fig. 4.2 Deep subcutaneous nodules and infiltrative masses on the abdominal wall - metastases of biliary carcinoma

Smaller, early nodules may mimic benign entities, such as cysts, lipomas, dermatofibromas, or hemangiomas. Ulcerated nodules should be differentiated from primary skin neoplasms. Multiple nodules should be differentiated from inflammatory processes such as various forms of nodular panniculitis [6].

Tumoral Masses with Ulceration and Erosions CM may present as tumoral masses that grow rapidly and, in advanced stages, develop necrosis and ulcerate, with bleeding, exudate, crusting, and malodor. They may be asymptomatic initially, but pain and discomfort appear later, often as they become superinfected [9, 10, 20].

Plaques and Flat Lesions CM may present as elevated, variably infiltrated plaques, skin-colored or erythematous, or erythemato-violaceous, sometimes resulting from the coalescence of multiple papules. They may have an infiltrative aspect and can be single or multiple, extending over variably large surfaces. They can mimic eczematous rashes, drug-induced exanthema, psoriasis, or extensive tinea corporis [9, 21, 22].

Carcinoma erysipelatodes Also known as *inflammatory metastatic carcinoma, carcinoma erysipeloides,* or *carcinomatous lymphangitis*, carcinoma erysipelatodes is a distinct clinical manifestation of CM, caused by malignant cells spread through dermal lymphatic vessels and characterized by erythematous, indurated plaques that resemble infectious processes such as erysipelas or cellulitis [6, 19, 23, 24]. The affected skin typically appears erythematous to violaceous and is firm on palpation, with well-demarcated borders; it may become thickened or exhibit a *peau d'orange* appearance due to tumor-induced lymphatic obstruction (Fig. 4.3). Lesions may be mildly warm to the touch and are often asymptomatic, though occasionally sensations of tightness, tenderness, or burning may occur. This pattern of CM most commonly occurs on the anterior chest wall, most frequently in patients with a history of breast carcinoma, but may also stem from cancers of the lung, intra-abdominal or pelvic organs; it frequently arises in or near previously irradiated areas or surgical scars.

The pathogeny of this type of CM consists of the metastatic obstruction of the dermal lymphatic vessel networks [24]. Correspondingly, malig-

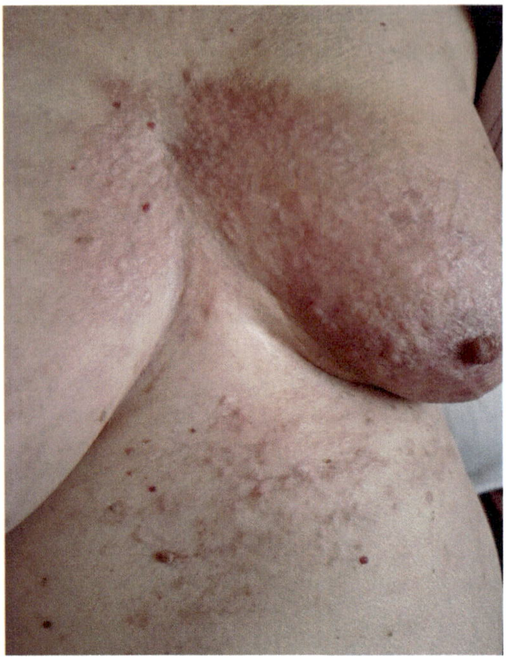

Fig. 4.3 Carcinoma erysipelatodes—wide erythematous infiltrative plaque of the left breast, with *peau d'orange* aspect, mimicking cellulitis; satellite micro-nodules over a widespread area on the upper abdominal wall. Recurrence of mammary carcinoma of the left breast, following incomplete resection

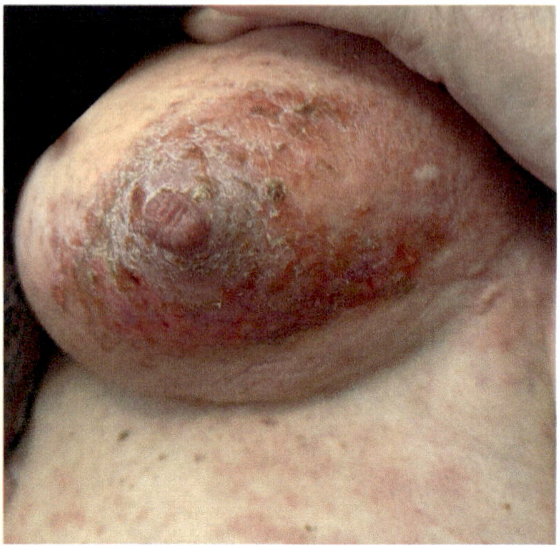

Fig. 4.4 Carcinoma "*en cuirasse*" - hard, sclerodermoid infiltration of the right breast, with fibrous retraction of the central, periareolar area. Recurrence of right mammary carcinoma

nant cell emboli within dermal lymphatic vessels, without significant inflammatory infiltrate, are visible on the histology of skin biopsies [19].

Carcinoma erysipelatodes can develop synchronously with the primary malignancy, but most commonly emerges months to years later and may be the first clinical indication of locoregional recurrence or distant metastasis. The progressive course, poor response to antibiotic therapy, subdued symptoms and lack of fever or leukocytosis help distinguishing it from acute infectious processes like cellulitis or erysipelas and should prompt further investigation. Prompt recognition is critical, as misdiagnosis can lead to delays in appropriate oncological treatment.

Carcinoma "en cuirasse" This is a rare form of CM marked by diffuse, sclerodermoid infiltration of the skin and subcutaneous tissue, most commonly seen in advanced breast carcinoma, but also in lung, stomach, and other visceral neoplasms [1, 6, 25, 26]. Clinically, it presents as a broad, indurated, hard plaque—typically over the chest wall—that produces an armor-like appearance, hence the name "*en cuirasse*". The overlying skin appears smooth, stretched and bound down, often with hyperpigmentation, focal erythema, telangiectasias, or a *peau d'orange* texture due to dermal lymphatic obstruction (Fig. 4.4). The affected area spreads widely, sometimes across the neck, shoulders, or upper arms, leading to restricted mobility and discomfort.

The condition frequently arises in or near prior mastectomy scars or radiation fields, though it can also occur independently. Histologically, it is characterized by dense dermal fibrosis with scattered malignant cells and frequent lymphovascular invasion [19]. Carcinoma *en cuirasse* is often misdiagnosed as morphea, scleroderma, or radiation-induced changes, particularly in its early stages. Its development indicates extensive metastatic disease and is associated with poor prognosis [2, 19, 26]. Skin biopsy, ideally including deep dermal tissue, is essential for diagnosis and should be performed promptly in any patient with an oncological history presenting with new, progressive sclerodermoid plaques.

Telangiectatic metastases Also known as *carcinoma telangiectaticum,* these are a rare but distinctive form of CM, characterized by prominent, dilated telangiectatic vessels on the background of erythematous to violaceous patches or plaques [1, 6, 9, 19]. These lesions may mimic angiomas or trauma-induced ecchymoses (Fig. 4.5). Most commonly seen in breast carcinoma, they typically develop on the anterior chest wall, but may occur elsewhere. The skin may be slightly indurated or atrophic, and lesions can remain asymptomatic or be associated with mild tenderness. Biopsy reveals dermal or subdermal metastatic tumor cells disrupting local vasculature and inducing vascular dilation but also angiogenesis, which accounts for their marked telangiectatic appearance [2, 19, 27].

Alopecia Neoplastica This variant of scalp CM presents as circumscribed areas of alopecia, often indurated, with a violaceous or erythematous hue. They may resemble alopecia areata or tinea capitis in early stages, but also lupus erythematosus or, in more advanced stages, scleroderma or other scarring alopecias [9, 11–13, 19]. Scalp metastases often originate from internal malignancies such as breast, lung, or gastrointestinal carcinomas [28]. Clinically, the affected area appears as a smooth or variably infiltrated plaque, with hair thinning or complete hair loss. Infiltration and epidermal changes may be absent or subtle at the beginning, making early recognition challenging. As disease progresses, the lesion may become indurated—possibly to sclerodermoid aspect, erythematous, or tender, sometimes with telangiectasias or ulceration, and follicular invasion makes alopecia irreversible (Fig. 4.6). Biopsy reveals tumor cell infiltration of the dermis and follicular structures, often with follicular destruction, confirming the metastatic nature of the lesion. Awareness of this rare presentation is crucial in patients with a history of malignancy, but not only, as this type of CM has been reported as a presenting sign of an occult neoplasia [28].

Zosteriform (Dermatomal) Pattern CM may cluster along a dermatome, mimicking herpes zoster [1, 5, 6, 29]. Individual lesions may take various appearances, such as papules, nodules, vesicles, or even bullae. They can be skin-colored, erythematous, violaceous, or purpuric, but also pigmented like in melanoma. Melanoma seems the most frequent source of this particular pattern of metastatic distribution [30], but other cancers such as breast, lung, or gastrointestinal tract have also been reported. Zosteriform metastases may sometimes be painful like herpes infections and are not uncommonly misdiagnosed initially as herpes zoster; most often, however, they are asymptomatic, and together with the prolonged and persistent course and papular or nodular appearance, this is a helpful clue towards the correct clinical interpretation (Fig. 4.7).

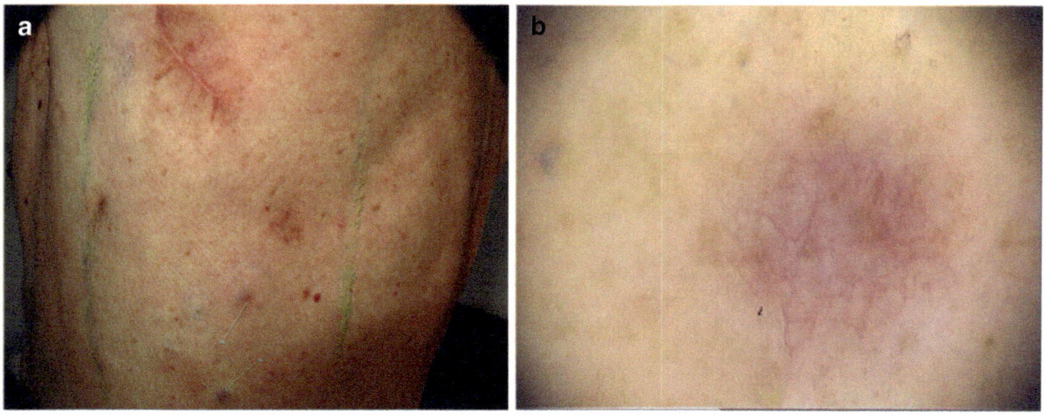

Fig. 4.5 Telangiectatic metastases (metastases of lung adenocarcinoma). (**a**) Violaceous plaques and flat dermal nodules, resembling hematomas, on the left thoracic wall in a male patient; (**b**) Dermoscopic aspect of one of the lesions, revealing telangiectasias on the background of a slightly livid hue. Metastases of lung adenocarcinoma

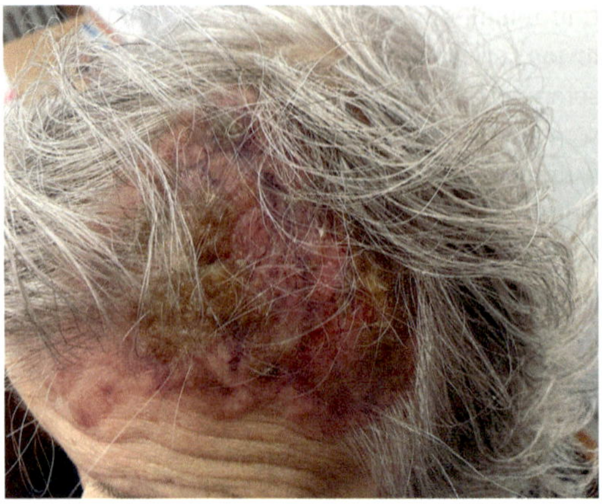

Fig. 4.6 Alopecia neoplastica - a sharp demarcated, infiltrated and indurated alopecic plaque on the frontotemporal area of a female patient. Metastases from ipsilateral mammary carcinoma

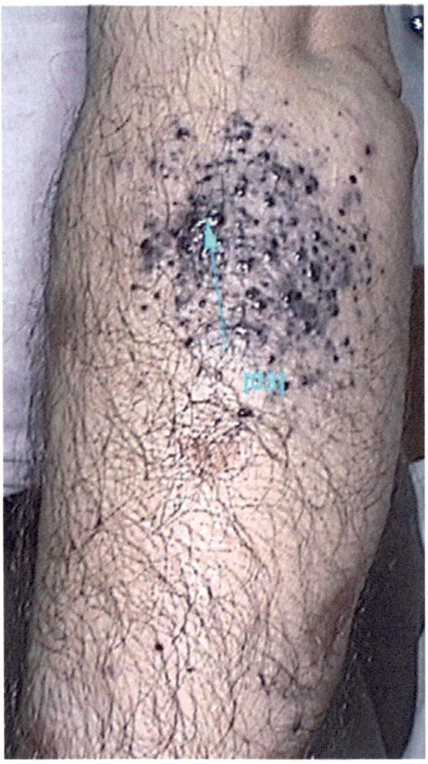

Fig. 4.7 Zosteriform metastases on the forearm, from subungual melanoma

4.6 Rare Presentations

Keratoacanthoma-Like Nodules This is a rare presentation of CM, as skin-colored or erythematous nodules with *central keratin-filled craters*, resembling keratoacanthoma. They may be the presenting sign of an occult neoplasia and have been reported in lung, esophageal, and breast cancers, among others [6, 31, 32].

Umbilical Metastasis (Sister Mary Joseph Nodule) This presents as a firm, often painless, periumbilical nodule, and it represents CM most commonly from intra-abdominal or pelvic malignancies such as gastric, pancreatic, colorectal, or ovarian carcinoma [2, 3, 6, 19, 33]. Clinically, it appears as a solitary, indurated nodule that may be skin-colored, violaceous, or erythematous and can range from a few millimeters to several centimeters in diameter. The surface may be smooth, occasionally mimicking benign lesions like epidermal inclusion cysts or umbilical hernias, or it can be friable, exudative, with crusting and ulceration. The lesion often signals widespread metastatic disease, associated with poor prognosis. Diagnosis is confirmed by biopsy, revealing adenocarcinoma cells consistent with the primary tumor.

Subungual Metastases These occur rarely, under nails or in the adjacent nail folds, presenting as painful, erythematous-violaceous nodules, edema, or deformity of the distal phalanx, mimicking infections or glomus tumors [17, 22, 34, 35].

Vascular (Angioma-Like) Lesions These present as rapidly growing, firm, reddish nodules with high vascularity that may resemble pyogenic granulomas or hemangiomas and may bleed easily. They are reported mostly as CM from poorly differentiated visceral neoplasms [6, 36].

Diffuse or Infiltrative Patterns Rarely, CM present as diffuse erythema, edema, or widespread infiltration, even with sclerodermoid induration, of a broad region—without discrete nodules or tumoral masses [1, 2, 8, 9, 19].

Ulcerative, Bullous, Purpuric, or Vasculitis-Like Lesions CM may occasionally present as bullous, purpuric, vesicular, or vasculitis-like lesions, often mimicking inflammatory dermatoses, and challenging early recognition [19, 37]. *Bullous metastases* manifest as tense or flaccid blisters overlying erythematous or indurated skin and arise due to tumor invasion at the dermo-epidermal junction or tumor-induced lymphatic obstruction. *Purpuric or hemorrhagic metastases* present as violaceous macules, petechiae, or ecchymotic patches and are typically the result of intravascular tumor emboli or tumor-induced coagulopathy, making them easily misinterpreted as vascular or hematologic disorders [36]. Metastases mimicking *leukocytoclastic vasculitis* may present as palpable purpura, hemorrhagic bullae, or ulcerated papules; biopsy in such cases typically reveals dermal tumor infiltration rather than true vessel wall inflammation—a key distinction from true vasculitis [34, 38].

4.7 Conclusion

CM exhibit a wide range of clinical appearances, often mimicking benign or inflammatory skin conditions. Early recognition is essential, as CM may be the first sign of an internal malignancy or disease progression. Clinicians should maintain a high level of suspicion, particularly in patients with known cancer, to ensure timely diagnosis and appropriate management. Prompt biopsy and awareness of atypical presentations can significantly impact prognosis and patient quality of life.

References

1. Kamińska-Winciorek G, et al. Skin metastases in the clinical and dermoscopic aspects. Semin Oncol. 2022;49(2):160–9.
2. Murina A, Allen A. Paraneoplastic Dermatoses and Cutaneous Metastases. Clin Geriatr Med. 2024;40(1):177–95.
3. Queirós CS, Filipe PL, de Almeida LS. Cutaneous metastases from solid neoplasms in the 21st century: a retrospective study from a Portuguese tertiary care center. J Eur Acad Dermatol Venereol. 2020;34:1218–24.
4. Sakhri S, et al. Cutaneous metastasis as a first presentation of lung carcinoma: a case series. J Med Case Rep. 2023; https://doi.org/10.1186/s13256-023-04029-2.
5. Strickley JD, Jenson AB, Jung JY. Cutaneous metastasis. Hematol Oncol Clin North Am. 2019;33(1):173–97.
6. Jaros J, et al. Clinical presentation, CM: a great imitator. Clin Dermatol. 2020;38(2):216–22.
7. Kovács KA, et al. Tumor type-specific and skin region-selective metastasis of human cancers: Another example of the "seed and soil" hypothesis. Cancer Metastasis Rev. 2013;32:493–9.
8. Lookingbill DP, Spangler N, Sexton FM. Skin involvement as the presenting sign of internal carcinoma: a retrospective study of 7316 cancer patients. J Am Acad Dermatol. 1990;22:19–26.
9. Betlloch-Mas I, et al. Cutaneous metastases of solid tumors: demographic, clinical, and survival characteristics. Cureus. 2021;13(11):e19970.
10. Choate EA, Nobori A, Worswick S. Cutaneous metastasis of internal tumors. Dermatol Clin. 2019;37(4):545–54.
11. Chiu CS, et al. Malignant cutaneous tumors of the scalp: a study of demographic characteristics and histologic distributions of 398 Taiwanese patients. J Am Acad Dermatol. 2007;56(3):448–52.
12. Lambertini M, et al. Scalp clinical presentation, CM: a warning bell. Curr Prob Cancer. 2021; https://doi.org/10.1016/j.currproblcancer.2021.100714.
13. Salemis NS, et al. Scalp metastasis as the first sign of small-cell lung cancer: management and literature review. Int Surgery. 2014;99:325.
14. Tollan CJ, Moyes C, Malyon A. Rare cutaneous metastasis from sarcomatoid carcinoma of lung. BMJ Case Rep. 2021;14(3):e240731.
15. Giudice G, et al. Cutaneous metastases of melanoma affecting exclusively skin graft donor and receiving sites: a novel clinical presentation. Dermatol Surg. 2018;44(3):464–6.

16. Alkhayat H, Hong CH. Cutaneous metastases from non-small cell lung cancer. J Cutan Med Surg. 2006;10:304–7.
17. Cohen PR. Metastatic tumors to the nail unit: subungual metastases. Dermatol Surg. 2001;27(3):280–93.
18. Viegas PS, et al. Clinical presentation, CM: a review of 74 cases 1. J Am Acad Dermatol. 2004;50(3):P68.
19. Chairatchaneeboon M, Kim EJ. Cutaneous paraneoplastic syndromes. In: Kang S, et al., editors. Fitzpatrick's dermatology, 9e. New York: McGraw-Hill Education; 2019.
20. Mollet TW, Garcia CA, Koester G. Skin metastases from lung cancer. Dermatol Online J. 2009;15:1.
21. Iliescu CA, et al. Atypical presentation of rapidly progressive cutaneous metastases of clear cell renal carcinoma: a case report. Medicina (Kaunas). 2024;60(11):1797.
22. Souza BDCE, et al. Cutaneous metastases from solid neoplasms—literature review. Anais Brasileiros de Dermatologia. 2023;98(5):571–9.
23. Mekheal E, et al. Carcinoma erysipeloides: an underdiagnosed phenomenon of cutaneous metastases of breast cancer. Am J Case Rep. 2023;24:e937843.
24. Prat L, et al. Cutaneous lymphangitis carcinomatosa in a patient with lung adenocarcinoma: case report and literature review. Lung Cancer. 2013;79:91–3.
25. Lin Y, Zhou S, He W. Clinicopathological diagnosis of morphea-like carcinoma en cuirasse in the neck: a rare presentation of lung cancer. Diagn Pathol. 2025;20(1):16.
26. Salemis NS, Christofyllakis C, Spiliopoulos K. Primary breast carcinoma en cuirasse. A rare presentation of an aggressive malignancy and review of the literature. Breast Dis. 2020;39(3–4):155–9.
27. Dobson CM, et al. Telangiectatic metastatic breast carcinoma in face and scalp mimicking cutaneous angiosarcoma. J Am Acad Dermatol. 2003;48(4):635–6.
28. Paolino G, et al. Alopecia neoplastica as a sign of visceral malignancies: a systematic review. J Eur Acad Dermatol Venereol. 2019;33(6):1020–8.
29. Tsai PY, Lo Y. Rare cutaneous manifestation of zosteriform cutaneous metastases of lung cancer: Two cases and literature review. Kaohsiung J Med Sci. 2024;40:768–9.
30. Savoia P, et al. Zosteriform Clinical presentation, CM: a literature meta-analysis and a clinical report of three melanoma cases. Dermatol Surg. 2009;35(9):1355–63.
31. Reich A, et al. Keratoacanthoma-like cutaneous metastasis of lung cancer: a learning point. Acta Derm Venereol. 2006;86:459–60.
32. Sławińska M, et al. Keratoacanthoma-like cutaneous metastases as the frst presentation of lung cancer. Polish Arch Intern Med. 2017;127:66–7.
33. Karaja S, et al. Cutaneous metastases of invasive lobular breast cancer as the first clinical manifestation: a case report. J Int Med Res. 2025;53(2):3000605251314804.
34. Babacan NA, et al. A case of multifocal skin metastases from lung cancer presenting with vasculitic-type cutaneous nodule. Indian J Dermatol. 2015;60:213.
35. Sweldens K, et al. Lung cancer with skin metastases. Dermatology. 1992;185:305–6.
36. Dereure O, Guilhou JJ, Guillot B. An unusual clinical pattern of cutaneous metastasis: target-like lesions. Br J Dermatol. 2003;148(2):361.
37. Alcaraz I, et al. Cutaneous metastases from internal malignancies: a clinicopathologic and immunohistochemical review. Am J Dermatopathol. 2012;34(4):347.
38. Demircioğlu D, et al. Livedoid cutaneous metastasis of signet-ring cell gastric carcinoma. J Cutan Pathol. 2021;48(6):785–8.

5 Dermoscopic Appearance of Skin Metastases

Danica Tiodorovic and Aimilios Lallas

Abstract

Cutaneous metastases (CM), which originate from a broad spectrum of primary tumors, represent a significant diagnostic challenge. They account for roughly 0.7–9% of all metastatic occurrences. Although they are typically associated with the advanced stage of malignancy, they can occasionally serve as the initial visible sign of an otherwise silent internal cancer. As their clinical features can differ significantly, distinguishing CMs from other skin conditions is often challenging, leading to diagnostic difficulties for both dermatologists and oncologists. When examined dermoscopically, melanoma-related CMs are most often pigmented and tend to display a structureless blue or brown pattern. On the other hand, cutaneous metastases from internal organs are usually non-pigmented. The great majority of CM from visceral organs, as well as non-pigmented melanoma CM, show on dermoscopy linear serpentine vessels and a white, structureless pattern. Since the presence of CMs can have profound implications for both prognosis and treatment choice, accurate and timely recognition is essential for effective patient management.

Keywords

Cutaneous metastases · Dermoscopy · Melanoma · Internal malignancy

5.1 Background

Diagnosing CM arising from various primary cancers remains a complex and often challenging task. Reports from autopsy analyses of cancer patients show that the occurrence of CMs can range significantly, with rates spanning from 0.2% up to 9% [1–3]. These secondary skin lesions may present simultaneously with the primary tumor or develop at different stages following the initial diagnosis. In some cases, CMs can be among the earliest indicators of cancer, while in others, they emerge during the later phases of disease progression. Remarkably, they can sometimes serve as the first observable sign of a previously undetected malignancy [1, 2, 4]. Early identification of these lesions plays a crucial role in guiding treatment decisions and can significantly impact patient prognosis.

D. Tiodorovic (✉)
Clinic of Dermatology, University Clinical Centre of Nis, Nis, Serbia

Medical Faculty of Nis, University of Nis, Nis, Serbia

A. Lallas
Medical School, Aristotle University, Thessaloniki, Greece

D. Koumaki et al. (eds.), *Cutaneous Metastases*, https://doi.org/10.1007/978-3-032-26764-1_5

5.2 Clinical Presentations

Cutaneous metastases often begin with subtle signs that can easily be missed without a high degree of clinical suspicion. They most frequently present as nodules, followed by plaques and ulcers, typically appearing either as solitary or multiple lesions [5, 6]. Early lesions are often painless, erythematous papules that are freely mobile, which may gradually evolve into inflammatory nodules. These lesions are frequently misdiagnosed as benign conditions, such as cysts, lipomas, fibromas, or adnexal neoplasms, or in other cases as malignant lesions including basal cell carcinoma or primary melanomas [6, 7].

Identifying the origin of the primary cancer based on the clinical appearance of CMs is rarely feasible. However, the anatomical site of the skin metastasis may offer a clue, as these lesions often arise near the location of the primary tumor. CMs are typically firm on palpation due to involvement of the dermis or lymphatic system [8]. When pigmentation is present, it most often suggests a metastatic melanoma [3, 9]. Besides melanoma, the most frequently observed primary cancers responsible for CMs vary by gender. In men, melanoma is the leading cause, followed by cancers of the lung, colon, oral cavity, and kidney. In women, breast cancer predominates as the primary source of skin metastases, with colorectal, lung, kidney, ovarian cancers, and melanoma also commonly implicated. When focusing on pediatric patients, rhabdomyosarcoma and neuroblastoma represent the most common primary tumors associated with skin metastases [5].

5.3 Dermoscopic Features

Although dermoscopy is widely used to assess numerous skin conditions, whether pigmented or not, there is a scarcity of research focused on its effectiveness in diagnosing cutaneous metastases. Moreover, detailed dermoscopic criteria for distinguishing CMs from different primary sources remain largely undefined. Regarding dermoscopic evaluation, recent research has placed growing emphasis on these features to enhance accurate identification, since both oncologists and dermatologists have frequently misdiagnosed them. This challenge stems partly from their uncommon presentation and/or lack of recognition, as well as the broad spectrum of conditions included in the differential diagnosis [3–5].

Cutaneous metastases from melanoma (CMM) are among the most frequently observed types of skin metastases. Depending on the source, they are reported to occur in approximately 2–20% of melanoma cases [9, 10]. In 2–8% of patients, CMM may even represent the initial clinical sign of metastatic spread [11]. These lesions are characterized by considerable variability in both their clinical presentation and dermoscopic appearance. CMM often appears as small, pigmented, or flesh-colored nodules or papules and can easily mimic benign skin conditions. Their broad clinical and dermoscopic variability makes early recognition particularly challenging. Accurate diagnosis is further complicated by the need to distinguish them from primary melanomas, benign melanocytic proliferations, and various non-melanoma skin tumors [9, 11].

Regarding dermoscopic features of CMM, the literature remains limited, consisting primarily of isolated case reports and small case series [9–11]. However, a recent multi-center study conducted by the International Dermoscopy Society (IDS) represents the most extensive investigation to date, involving a large cohort of patients. The study included participating centers from numerous countries, such as Austria, Italy, Serbia, Spain, Greece, France, Germany, Australia, Japan, the United States, Argentina, Belgium, Poland, Sweden, Croatia, Israel, North Macedonia, Brazil, Romania, and Turkey, all specifically focused on cutaneous metastases [3].

Regarding the first publication on CMM, Bono et al. analyzed 130 CMM in 32 patients, comparing them with various benign and malignant skin lesions [12]. They evaluated nine dermoscopic features and identified saccular and vascular patterns, marked by polymorphic and winding vessels, along with pigmentary halos and peripheral gray spots, as the most indicative of CMM. The saccular pattern reflects junctional nests of atypical melanocytes and appears as sharply bordered, brownish-red to blue-gray globules. The homogeneous pattern shows diffuse gray-blue to black pigmentation without distinct structures. Amelanotic metastases are often subtle and difficult to detect due to their dermal location, presenting as vascular structures, such as dotted, corkscrew, serpentine, arborizing, or hairpin vessels, as well as milky-red areas [12]. Avilés-Izquierdo et al. focused on color-based classifications (blue, pink, brown, and mixed), finding that 75% of 150 cases exhibited a monochromatic pattern, with key features including peripheral light brown halos, gray spots, and atypical polymorphic vessels [9].

The first dermoscopic evaluation of CMM associated with clinicopathological melanoma characteristics was implemented by Kostaki et al. [13]. They studied 42 melanoma patients and identified five dermoscopic patterns in CMM: saccular, amelanotic, homogenous, vascular, and polymorphic. The most frequent patterns were homogenous (30.95%) and amelanotic (28.57%). Homogeneous features predominated in satellite metastases and were more common in superficial spreading melanomas, while amelanotic patterns appeared mostly in in-transit metastases. Saccular patterns were associated with thinner melanomas (<2 mm), whereas vascular structures were observed only in metastases from tumors with a Breslow index of 2–4 mm. Homogeneous and amelanotic patterns were exclusive to lesions thicker than 4 mm. Vascular structures were more frequent in deeper tumors, while nevus-like features were associated with thinner primaries [13].

A recently published multi-center study by the IDS represents the largest series to date on dermoscopic features of CM, including 632 histologically confirmed lesions in 583 patients [3]. Among them, 474 were melanoma metastases, with 260 classified as locoregional and 56 as distant; location data were missing in 128 cases. Overall, 52.2% of CMs were locoregional, and 26.7% were distant, challenging the prevailing view that CMs are mostly locoregional, even in melanoma. In this study, most CMM were pigmented, predominantly showing structureless areas of blue (63.6%), brown (57.2%), and white (68.6%). The primary diagnostic challenge is distinguishing pigmented CMM from blue nevi, especially in the head and neck regions, where both conditions commonly occur. In practice, vascular structures, recent onset, and patient history support differentiation. Non-pigmented CMM revealed a structureless white pattern and linear serpentine vessels [3] (Fig. 5.1).

Cutaneous metastases from solid tumors are relatively rare, occurring in approximately 0.7–9% of cases of metastatic disease. Typically, patients already have a known malignancy when skin metastases appear, but in up to one-third of cases, the skin lesion is the first indication of cancer [14, 15]. Kovács et al. reported an even higher rate—43% of patients presented with skin metastases as the initial or concurrent sign of malignancy, surpassing previous estimates of 22–23% [8]. The interval between primary tumor diagnosis and skin metastasis ranges from weeks to over a decade, with some cases documented as late as 13 years. Often, skin metastases signify cancer recurrence, and 79% of patients have simultaneous visceral metastases. Clinically, CM manifestations are diverse and may mimic inflammatory conditions, benign tumors, or other malignant skin lesions [6–8].

The most frequently reported dermoscopic feature of CM from visceral cancers is a vascular pattern characterized by irregular, polymorphic vessels [3, 12]. Structureless pink or white areas have also been described. About half of non-melanoma skin cancer metastases exhibit a combination of red and white (52.63%) or red, white, and irregular vessels (52.63%) [14, 15]. In breast cancer, pigmented patterns resembling melanoma have been observed. Metastases from ovarian cancer and chronic leukemia are almost exclusively structureless (100% and 98.95%, respectively). The structureless white pattern is a strong indicator of cutaneous metastasis, present in 81.26% of cases ($p < 0.001$) [14, 15].

Chernoff et al. studied 20 outpatients with biopsy-confirmed cutaneous metastases from various primary cancers, including breast (6 cases), colorectal [3], thyroid [2], ovarian [2], and others, such as endometrial, gastric, lung, bladder, peritoneal, melanoma, and leiomyosar-

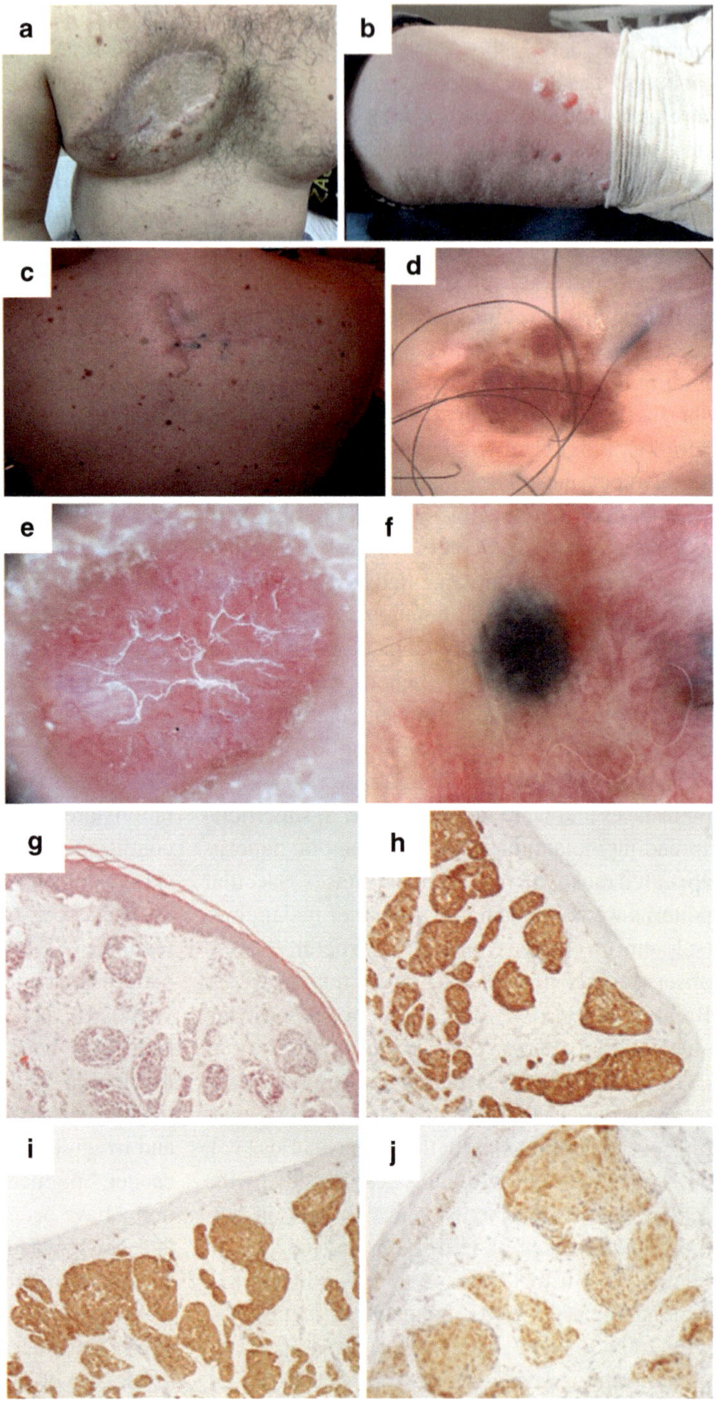

Fig. 5.1 Clinical, dermoscopical, and pathohistological presentations of melanoma CM. (**a**, **b**) Multiple non-pigmented locoregional CMs; (**c**) Multiple pigmented locoregional CMs; (**d**) CM dermoscopically revealing saccular pattern; (**e**) Non-pigmented CM showing structureless white pattern with linear serpentine vessels; (**f**) Pigmented CM revealing structureless blue pattern; (**g**) Well-circumscribed neoplastic nests within the dermis (H&E, x10); (**h**) Immunohistochemical staining revealing *HMB45* positivity (IHH, ×10); (**i**) Neoplastic cells positive for *Melan-A* (IHH, ×10; (**j**) Neoplastic cells positive for *S-100* (IHH, ×20)

coma [15]. Most patients (12/20) presented with new nodules near the primary tumor site, while the remaining 8 showed papules or plaques. The predominant dermoscopic feature was a vascular pattern, observed in all 17 non-pigmented lesions. Specifically, 88% displayed discrete vessels, mainly serpentine or linear, and 12% showed pink, homogeneous, structureless areas. Among the three pigmented lesions (all breast cancer metastases), various melanocytic patterns were noted [15].

A Sister Mary Joseph nodule (SMJN) is a rare umbilical metastasis typically diagnosed clinically in patients with known malignancies whose origin is histologically confirmed [16]. SMJN indicates a poor prognosis and most often arises from intra-abdominal or pelvic cancers. Ge et al. reported a rare case associated with esophageal squamous cell carcinoma, dermoscopically revealing a polymorphous vascular pattern of serpentine, dotted, and comma-shaped vessels beneath a white veil [17]. In men, SMJN most commonly originates from gastrointestinal cancers, while in women, ovarian and gastrointestinal tumors are the primary sources [17].

The previously mentioned IDS study analyzed 632 cutaneous metastases (CMs) from various non-melanoma cancers: breast cancer (59 patients), gastrointestinal tract (GIT, 25), lung (21), renal, Merkel cell carcinoma [6], ovarian [4], thyroid [2], squamous cell carcinoma (20), and basal cell carcinoma [2] [3]. Of these, 51.1% were pigmented, while 48.9% were non-pigmented, indicating a high proportion of amelanotic CMs. Most non-melanoma CMs were non-pigmented with prominent vascular features. Linear serpentine vessels were the most common vessel type, found in 56.3% of all CMs and nearly all metastases of lung (Fig. 5.2) and breast cancer (Fig. 5.3). The structureless white pattern dominated overall (84.2%). Ulceration was noted in 11.1% of CMs, most frequently in squamous cell carcinoma (31.2%), GIT (24%), and lung (23.8%) metastases. The recurring combination of structureless white areas with linear serpentine vessels may serve as a valuable diagnostic clue to differentiate CMs from other skin lesions (Figs. 5.4 and 5.5). This study also revealed a high frequency of distant CMs on the trunk, head, and neck. Melanoma metastases mainly appeared on the head and neck, while distant CMs from breast, lung, GIT, and renal cancers commonly involved the trunk and head/neck regions. For GIT and lung cancers—especially in men—the head and scalp were the predominant sites, contrasting with breast cancer in women, where the anterior chest wall was most common. This highlights the importance of considering primary tumor type and patient gender when assessing CM locations [3].

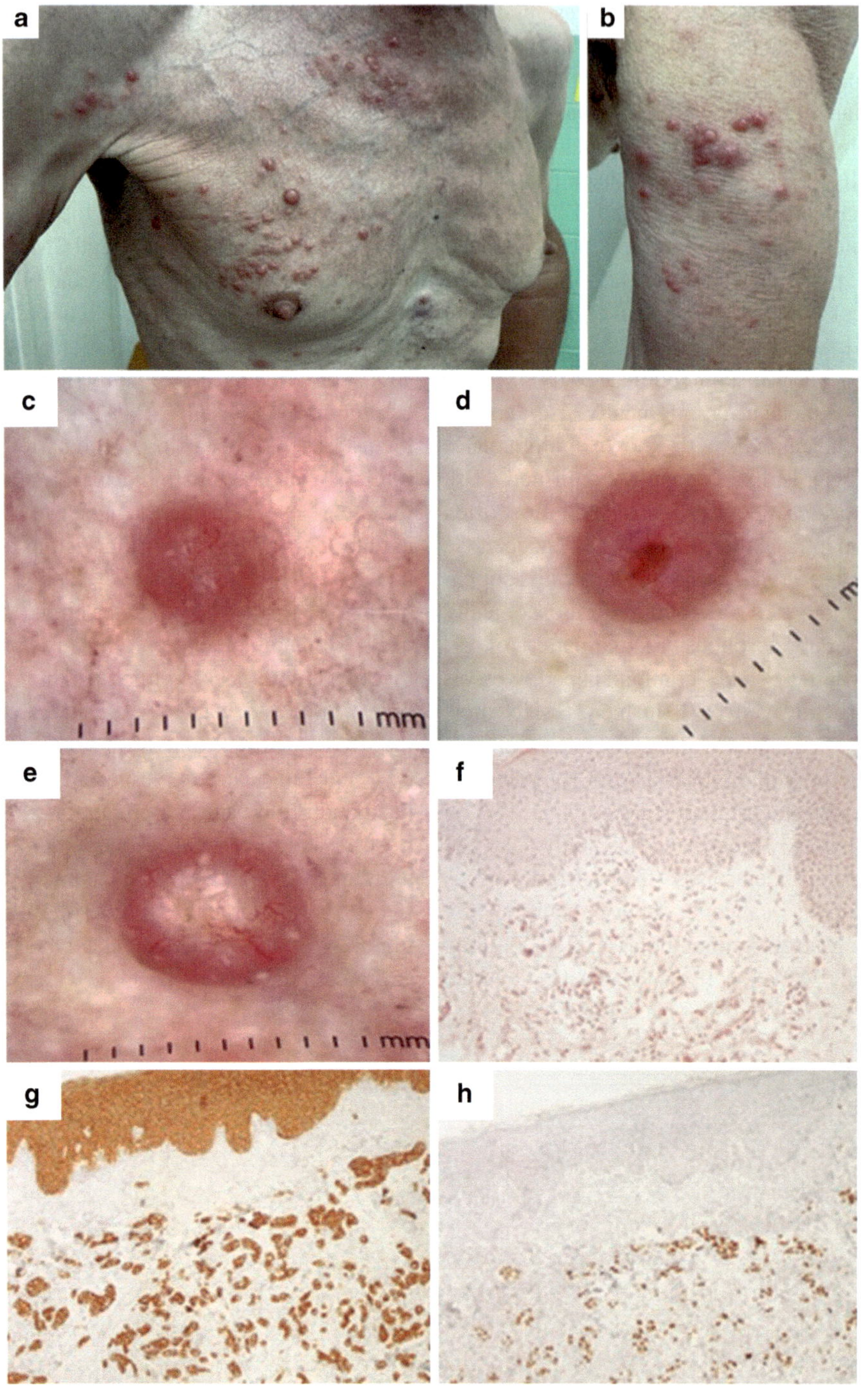

Fig. 5.2 Clinical, dermoscopical, and pathohistological presentations of lung CM. (**a**, **b**) Multiple non-pigmented papules and nodules on thorax and left arm; (**c–e**) Structureless red pattern with linear serpentine vessels associated with erosion in lesion (**d**) and whitish lines in lesions (**c**, **d**); (**f**) Low-differentiated adenocarcinoma cells within the dermis (H&E, ×10); (**g**, **h**) Immunohistochemical staining revealing both *CK AE1/AE3* and *TTF* positivity, confirming pulmonary origin (IHH, ×10)

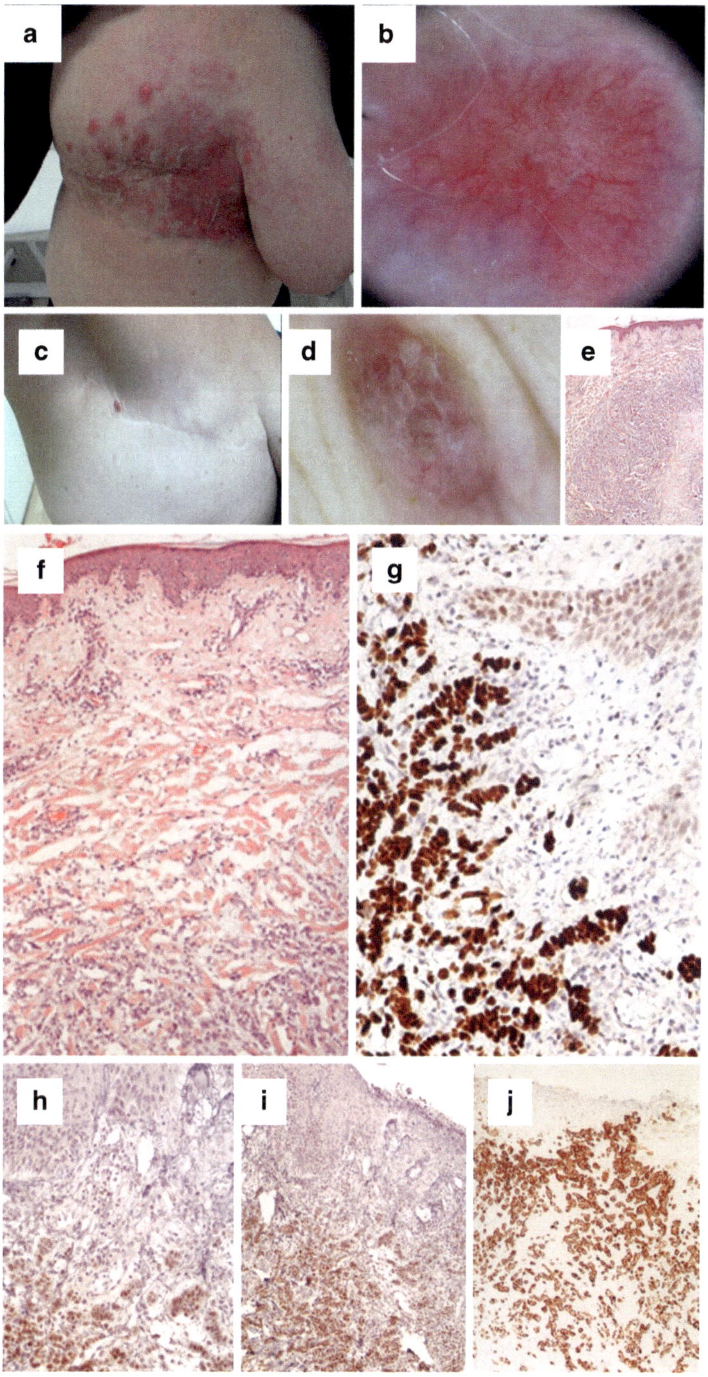

Fig. 5.3 Clinical, dermoscopical, and pathohistological presentations of breast CM. (**a**) Multiple non-pigmented locoregional CMs; (**b**) Non-pigmented CM revealing structureless white pattern with linear serpentine vessels; (**c**) Solitary non-pigmented CM; (**d**) Non-pigmented CM showing structureless white pattern with linear serpentine vessels; (**e**) Neoplastic cells of breast CM (H&E, ×10); (**f**) Infiltrating ductal breast carcinoma metastasis (H&E, ×10); (**g**) Immunohistochemical staining revealing *GATA3* positivity (IHH, ×20); (**h**) Neoplastic cells positive for *estrogen* (IHH, ×20); (**i**) Neoplastic cells positive for *estrogen* (IHH, ×10); (**j**) *CK7* positivity of neoplastic cells (IHH, ×10)

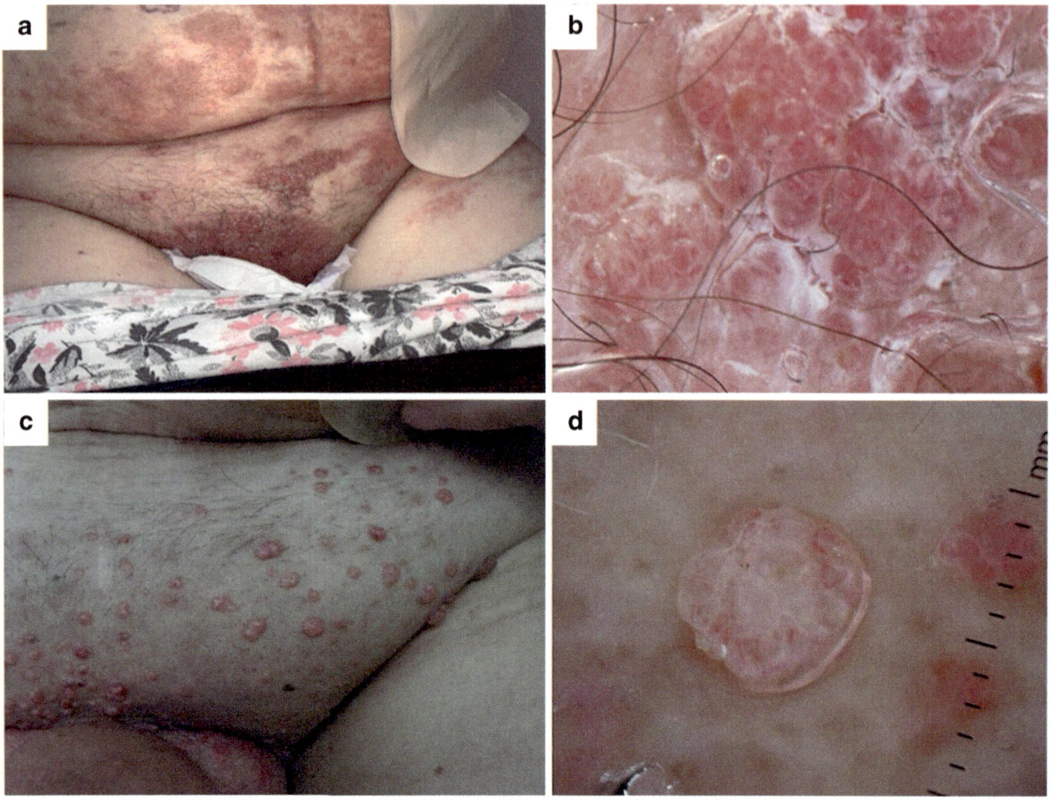

Fig. 5.4 Clinical and dermoscopical presentations of two patients with colon cancer CM. (**a**) Multiple non-pigmented papules on abdomen; (**b**) Non-pigmented CM showing structureless red pattern with linear serpentine vessels; (**c**) Multiple non-pigmented papules on abdomen; (**d**) Non-pigmented CM showing structureless white pattern with linear serpentine vessels

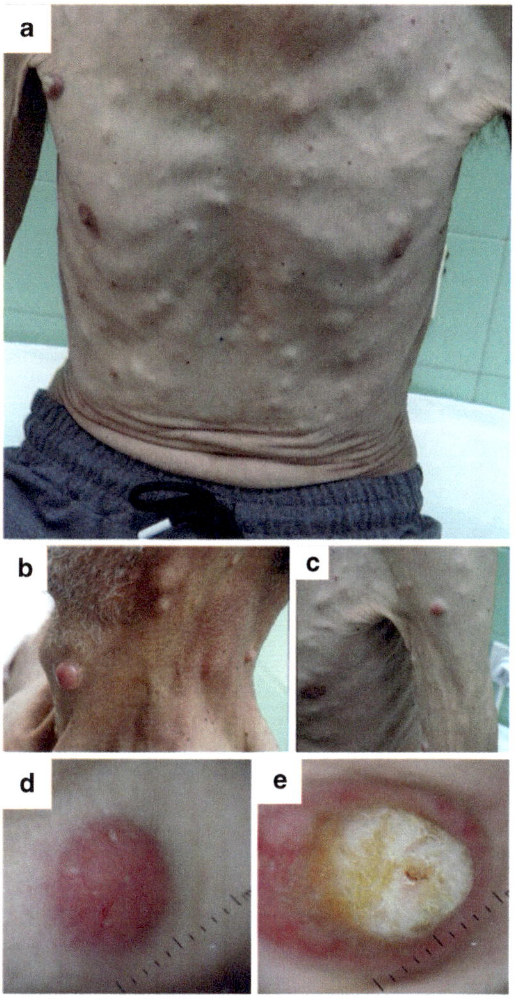

Fig. 5.5 Clinical, dermoscopical presentation of lung CM. (**a**–**c**) Multiple nodular and subcutaneous CM on trunk, arms, and neck; (**d**) Dermoscopic evaluation shows a structureless red pattern with linear serpentine vessels; (**e**) Dermoscopy reveals a structureless white and red pattern with linear serpentine vessels

5.4 Conclusion

Cutaneous melanoma metastases remain a significant diagnostic challenge, yet accurate and timely identification is critical for appropriate staging and treatment, particularly as the American Joint Committee on Cancer has integrated CMM into the latest TNM classification for melanoma. Dermoscopically, melanoma-related CMs are most often pigmented and tend to display a structureless blue or brown pattern, while CMs from internal organs are usually non-pigmented. Both CMs from internal organs and non-pigmented melanoma CMs typically show linear serpentine vessels and a white structureless pattern on dermoscopy. Key clinical information, such as a patient's oncological history, recent onset of lesions, changes in lesion size, and lesion location, plays a vital role in distinguishing these metastases from other skin conditions. Dermoscopy is an invaluable tool in identifying solitary cutaneous metastases. Our findings highlight the importance of routine, focused dermoscopic examinations of lesions, with special attention to sites prone to distant metastases, including the head and neck region for renal, breast, lung, and gastrointestinal cancers, as well as the frontal thoracic area in breast cancer patients.

References

1. Lookingbill DP, Spangler N, Sexton FM. Skin involvement as the presenting sign of internal carcinoma. A retrospective study of 7316 cancer patients. J Am Acad Dermatol. 1990;22(1):19–26.
2. Lookingbill DP, Spangler N, Helm KF. Cutaneous metastases in patients with metastatic carcinoma: a retrospective study of 4020 patients. J Am Acad Dermatol. 1993;29(2 Pt 1):228–36.
3. Tiodorovic D, Stojkovic-Filipovic J, Marghoob A, et al. Dermatoscopic patterns of cutaneous metastases: a multicentre cross-sectional study of the International Dermoscopy Society. J Eur Acad Dermatol Venereol. 2024;38(7):1432–8.
4. Krathen RA, Orengo IF, Rosen T. Cutaneous metastasis: a meta-analysis of data. South Med J. 2003;96(2):164–7.
5. Souza BCE, Miyashiro D, Pincelli MS, Sanches JA. Cutaneous metastases from solid neoplasms – literature review. An Bras Dermatol. 2023;98(5):571–9.
6. Gschnell M, Volberg C, Hauser C, Krönig L. Cutaneous metastases: From epidemiology to therapy. J Dtsch Dermatol Ges. 2024;22(7):974–93.
7. Nashan D, Müller ML, Falco MB, et al. Cutaneous metastases of visceral tumours: a review. J Cancer Res Clin Oncol. 2009;135:1–14.
8. Kovács KA, Kenessey I, Tímár J. Skin metastasis of internal cancers: a single institution experience. Pathol Oncol Res. 2013;19(3):515–20.
9. Avilés-Izquierdo JA, Ciudad-Blanco C, Sánchez-Herrero A, et al. Dermoscopy of cutaneous melanoma

metastases: a color-based pattern classification. J Dermatol. 2019;46(7):564–9.
10. Savoia P, Fava P, Nardò T, et al. Skin metastases of malignant melanoma: a clinical and prognostic survey. Melanoma Res. 2009;19(5):321–6.
11. Braun RP, Rabinovitz HS, Oliviero M, et al. Dermoscopy of pigmented skin lesions. J Am Acad Dermatol. 2005;52(1):109–21.
12. Bono R, Giampetruzzi AR, Concolino F, et al. Dermoscopic patterns of cutaneous melanoma metastases. Melanoma Res. 2004;14(5):367–73.
13. Kostaki M, Plaka M, Moustaki M, et al. Cutaneous melanoma metastases: Clinical and dermoscopic findings. J Eur Acad Dermatol Venereol. 2023;37(5):941–4.
14. Simionescu O, Petrică M, Avram AM, et al. Dermoscopy of skin metastases in advanced cancer-systemic (visceral, hematologic) and cutaneous. Front Med (Lausanne). 2024;11:1445811.
15. Chernoff KA, Marghoob AA, Lacouture ME, et al. Dermoscopic findings in cutaneous metastases. JAMA Dermatol. 2014;150(4):429–33.
16. Abu-Hilal M, Newman JS. Sister Mary Joseph and her nodule: historical and clinical perspective. Am J Med Sci. 2009;337(4):271–3.
17. Ge JS, Yang JH, Chen CP, et al. Dermoscopic characterization and image study of a Sister Mary Joseph nodule in patient with esophageal cancer. Dermatol Sin. 2016;34(4):192–5.

6 Other Noninvasive Techniques for Diagnosing Skin Metastasis

Stamatina Verykiou

Abstract

Cutaneous metastases occur in approximately 5–10% of cancer patients and may indicate disease progression or, in some cases, could present as the first sign of malignancy. Although traditional non-invasive imaging techniques such as MRI, CT, PET-CT, and ultrasound remain widely used, their role is largely complementary to histological evaluation of the lesion. More recently, advanced non-invasive techniques have emerged to improve diagnostic accuracy. Techniques like high-frequency ultrasound, reflectance confocal microscopy, optical coherence tomography (OCT), and line-field confocal OCT can provide useful information in the assessment of suspicious lesions. Novel techniques such as Raman spectroscopy, multispectral and hyperspectral imaging, and electrical impedance spectroscopy are emerging diagnostic tools but so far remain largely experimental. Overall, these non-invasive modalities improve lesion detection, characterization, and monitoring but remain complementary tools. Histopathological examination continues to be the gold standard for definitive diagnosis.

Keywords

Cutaneous metastasis · Cancer · Diagnosis · Non-invasive · Reflectance confocal microscopy · Optical coherence tomography · Line-field confocal OCT · High-frequency ultrasound

Cutaneous metastases are a reasonably common manifestation of cancer and affect approximately 5–10% of all cancer patients [1]. Cutaneous metastases can be the first presentation of cancer or can present at a different stage during cancer care, from diagnosis to treatment and can signify disease progression and failure of response to treatment modalities [2]. Several non-invasive modalities have been used over the years to approach the diagnosis of cutaneous metastases, including more traditional methods such as magnetic resonance imaging (MRI), computed tomography (CT), positron emission tomography-computed tomography (PET-CT), and ultrasound. However, more recently and with the increase in novel techniques for the diagnosis of cutaneous metastatic disease.

The most utilized non-invasive methods to diagnose metastatic lesions, apart from dermoscopy are, undoubtedly, the traditional imaging modalities, such as computer tomography, ultrasound sonography, and MRI. These have been used for many years to assist the clinicians in

S. Verykiou (✉)
Consultant Dermatologist and Mohs Micrographic Surgeon, Limassol, Cyprus

D. Koumaki et al. (eds.), *Cutaneous Metastases*, https://doi.org/10.1007/978-3-032-26764-1_6

deciphering the characteristics of tumor. More recently, a number of emerging techniques have been established to aid the clinician in diagnosing cutaneous metastases. This chapter will evaluate and summarize the known and emerging techniques to diagnose cutaneous metastases.

6.1 Known Techniques in the Assessment of Cutaneous Metastases

Computed tomography (CT) and magnetic resonance imaging (MRI can be used to detect cutaneous metastases; however, their sensitivity and specificity depend on the clinical context and the characteristics of the lesions.

MRI, and more particularly with high-resolution surface coils, is particularly valuable for assessing the extent, depth, and anatomic connection of cutaneous metastases, where precise mapping of locoregional disease can guide surgical planning and treatment strategy. High-resolution MRI can delineate tumor margins and depth, which is useful for preoperative planning and for evaluating complex anatomic sites [3].

In cutaneous squamous cell carcinoma, MRI can detect perineural spread, which can influence management decisions [4].

MRI can also help differentiate between tumor types based on signal characteristics, although this alone is not enough to reach a confident diagnosis without histological examination [5]. In summary, the role of MRI in the diagnosis of cutaneous metastasis is rather adjunctive, with a focus to assess the distribution, depth, and local invasion of known or suspected lesions, rather than as a primary diagnostic tool.

CT is another modality used to assess suspicious lesions. CT imaging can be useful for identifying subcutaneous or cutaneous metastatic lesions, especially when they are not readily apparent on physical examination, and for assessing the extent of disease, particularly in patients with advanced malignancy [6].

CT is most commonly employed in the staging and surveillance of patients with high-risk skin cancers (such as melanoma, cutaneous squamous cell carcinoma, and Merkel cell carcinoma) to detect nodal and visceral metastases, and it may incidentally reveal cutaneous or subcutaneous metastases [7]. In summary, these two well-described modalities are more complementary to classical histologic evaluation rather than diagnostic of metastatic disease alone.

6.2 Newer Techniques for the Diagnosis of Skin Metastases

6.2.1 High-Frequency Ultrasound (FHUS)

High-frequency ultrasound refers to ultrasound imaging that utilizes sound waves with frequencies usually above 10 MHz and more commonly in the range of 20–100 MHz to achieve high spatial resolution for the visualization of superficial biological structures such as skin, eye, and small vessels. The increased frequency results in shorter wavelengths, which enhances axial and lateral resolution but reduces tissue penetration depth, making this modality particularly suited for detailed imaging of superficially located lesions [8].

High-frequency ultrasound (HFUS) plays an important adjunctive role in detecting skin metastases by providing high-resolution, real-time imaging of the skin and subcutaneous tissues. HFUS can differentiate metastatic lesions from benign skin nodules based on sonographic features such as hypoechogenicity, irregular shape, and, when combined with color Doppler, the presence of hypervascularity with multiple peripheral and internal vessels [9].

HFUS is particularly valuable for identifying non-palpable or subclinical metastatic deposits, including in-transit and satellite lesions, and for assessing the extent and depth of cutaneous involvement, which is critical for surgical planning and staging [10].

Compared to physical examination alone, HFUS demonstrates superior sensitivity for detecting small or deeply located metastases, especially in areas [11].

While HFUS improves diagnostic accuracy and can guide biopsy or management decisions, its specificity for distinguishing metastases from other malignant or benign lesions is enhanced when combined with Doppler assessment of vascularity [9].

However, HFUS should be assessed in combination with clinical and histopathological characteristics, as there is variability in diagnostic capability and need for further standardization of the outcomes [12].

6.2.2 Reflective Confocal Microscopy (RCM)

RCM is a novel way of assessing skin lesions in vivo using a laser to acquire a horizontal analysis of the skin at a cellular level. It has been used for the evaluation of pigmented and non-pigmented skin lesions but also pigmentary disorders and inflammatory skin diseases. The additional use of RCM for clinical examination and dermoscopy has shown to reduce the number of unnecessary biopsies by 50–70% [13] and hence the cost of skin lesion diagnosis [2] making RCM a useful addition to the diagnostic tool for a clinician in day-to-day practice.

RCM uses a laser source to emit an infrared monochromatic light (830 nm), which penetrates the tissue, allowing for the detection of the reflected signal back to a focal point. The sensitivity and specificity of RCM have been evaluated in several studies with sensitivity and specificity of 93.6% (92%–95%) and 82.7% (81–84%), respectively, across several skin cancers [14]. More recently, the combined use of dermoscopy and RCM has been proven to further increase the specificity and sensitivity in the diagnosis of skin cancers [15].

RCM has been used primarily in the connect of skin cancer diagnosis and has been proven to be a useful tool not only in the initial diagnosis but also to monitor the disease progression and recurrence. More recently, emerging evidence is to support the use of RCM in the diagnosis of cutaneous metastases. Alexandris et al. in a recent publication have summarized the use of RCM in the diagnosis of cutaneous metastatic disease [15]. A small number of mainly case reports have shown the benefit of using RCM as a diagnostic tool in cutaneous metastases. Richtig et al., in 2009, published a case report of using RCM for the quick and non-invasive diagnosis of cutaneous metastasis in a patient with a history of breast cancer [16]. However, the use of RCM poses a number of challenges in the diagnosis of metastatic disease. Initially, the penetration capability of RCM is restricted to 250 microns in depth, and as a result, more invasive tumors cannot be assessed using this technique. Additionally, the thickness of the overlying epidermis also restricts the use of RCM. Lesions located on hyperkeratotic parts of the body, such as the acral skin, are not easily assessed, as the penetration of RCM is insufficient for accurately assessing these lesions. Finally, the interpretation of the RCM-derived images requires the acquisition of dermatopathology skills and specific RCM-related clinician skills, limiting the use to a small number of dermatologists.

6.2.3 Optical Coherence Tomography

Optical Coherence Tomography (OCT) is a non-invasive imaging technique that uses low-coherence light to capture cross-sectional images of the tissue [17]. It works similarly to ultrasound, but instead of sound waves, it uses light waves.

In dermatology, OCT is used to visualize the skin structures in real time, non-invasively, with micrometer-scale resolution. OCT allows for the assessment of the morphological details of the epidermis, dermis, and adnexal structures down to about 1–2 mm in depth, depending on the system, without the need for a biopsy [18]. OCT uses a near-infrared wavelength that penetrates approximately 1–2 mm into the skin in depth. The backscatter of the emitted light is then collected and analyzed to allow for a detailed reconstruction of the images [19]. The most widespread use of OCT in dermatology has been the non-invasive diagnosis of skin cancer [20] but also in margin delineation prior to surgical procedures and monitoring for recurrences and response to different destructive treatment modalities, such as lasers, topical therapies, and PDT.

Optical Coherence Tomography (OCT) has emerged as a valuable non-invasive imaging tool in the diagnosis of cutaneous metastases. By providing high-resolution, cross-sectional images of skin architecture in real time, OCT allows for the visualization of structural changes associated with metastatic infiltration, such as disruption of normal dermal–epidermal junctions, increased dermal reflectivity, and the presence of atypical cellular aggregates. Although not a substitute for histopathological confirmation, OCT can assist clinicians in identifying suspicious lesions, guiding biopsy sites, and monitoring disease progression or response to treatment. Its ability to offer immediate insights without tissue excision makes it especially useful in patients with multiple lesions or those unsuitable for invasive procedures.

OCT has been studied more extensively in detecting choroidal metastases [21] and to monitor response after treatment. More recently, Hobelsberger et al. presented a case series of 61 lesions assessed with [22] OCT, LC-OCT, and dermoscopy that has demonstrated similar characteristics of the cutaneous metastases, such as epidermal ulceration, disruption of the dermoepidermal junction, hyporeflective areas and coiled, serpiginous, and branched vessel patterns [22]. Although OCT poses as a valuable adjunctive tool for the diagnosis of skin metastases, the role of this technique has not been fully established as of today.

6.2.4 LC-OCT

Line-field confocal optical coherence tomography (LC-OCT) is an advanced imaging modality that combines the benefits of traditional OCT with confocal microscopy, offering high-resolution, three-dimensional imaging of the skin at cellular-level detail. LC-OCT allows for better resolution compared to traditional OCT and also allows for the switching from horizontal to cross-sectional sections in real time. One of the advantages compared to the methodologies mentioned previously is that LC-OCT functions using both a lateral and axial resolution (around 1 μm) and penetrates up to 500 μm, enough for the sufficient visualization of the epidermis and superficial dermis. The principle and advantage of LC-OCT lie within the fact that it is a real-time technique with high resolution approaching histological evaluation.

Although the majority of the evidence for LC-OCT as an adjunctive tool to clinical examination is mainly in primary skin malignancies, such as basal cell carcinoma, squamous cell carcinoma, and malignant melanoma, there is emerging evidence suggesting the usefulness of the technique in diagnosing skin metastases. Bang et al. in a recent paper presented a case series using a multimodal device combining reflectance confocal microscopy (RCM) and OCT (which includes the principles of LC-OCT) that was able to non-invasively detect and characterize cutaneous metastases from breast cancer, identifying tumor foci and measuring tumor depth with good correlation to histopathology [23].

LC-OCT has also been shown to adequately visualize tumor nests, detect cellular atypia, and architectural disruption in a variety of malignant skin lesions, supporting its potential use in the diagnosis of cutaneous metastatic disease [24]. Although the use of LC-OCT in the diagnosis of cutaneous metastases is promising, the current literature is still sparse and limited to small case series and descriptive studies. There is, therefore, a need for larger, systematic investigation to establish the sensitivity, specificity, and diagnostic criteria of LC-OCT for skin metastases.

6.3 Experimental

Newer techniques have been developed to target and diagnose other tumor-related characteristics. For example, Raman spectroscopy, a technique developed to analyze how light interacts with chemical molecules, detects the vibration of molecules, allowing for the evaluation of the biochemical composition of a lesion. More specifically in dermatology, Raman spectroscopy detects DNA/RNA changes, protein structures, lipid profiles, and collagen signals, and the difference between these characteristics between normal and malignant cells allows for the detection of malignant lesions [25].

Another recently used technique is multispectral (MSI) and hyperspectral imaging (HIS). In simple terms, this technique works by detailing tissue absorption and reflection of light across different wavelengths allowing for assessment of the chemical and structural characteristics of the tissue which has been studied. Since cancerous or metastatic skin lesions often have changes in vascularization, distribution of melanin, and collagen array, this technique can differentiate between benign and malignant cells [26].

Electrical impedance spectroscopy (EIS) is a non-invasive technique that measures the electrical impedance of a material or biological tissue across a range of frequencies. In EIS, a small alternating current is applied to the tissue or sample, and the resulting voltage response is measured. The frequency-dependent impedance data provide information about the resistive and capacitive properties of the tissue, which reflect its composition, structure, and physiological state [27]. In clinical applications, EIS is used to characterize and differentiate tissues based on their dielectric properties. EIS can distinguish between malignant and benign tissues in breast and skin cancer diagnostics, as neoplastic tissues often exhibit distinct impedance capabilities compared to normal tissues [28].

Finally, artificial intelligence (AI) is rapidly developing, and AI programs are integrating into our day to day practice.

Artificial intelligence (especially deep learning) can analyze dermoscopic, confocal, OCT, or ultrasound images to detect patterns, measure features and therefore predict a malignant risk for lesions therefore supporting clinical decisions for diagnostic biopsy, excisions, or to delineate surgical margins [29].

Although these methods are using cutting-edge technology, to date their use is limited mainly by the fact that the interpretation requires a high level of expertise, which is not applicable to the average dermatologist, the high cost of the equipment, and the fact the technology is still evolving. However, these techniques and especially the integration of AI in the use of day-to-day equipment used to detect cutaneous metastases are a space rapidly evolving and soon to be integrated into daily use.

6.4 Summary

Non-invasive techniques used in the diagnosis of cutaneous metastases include dermoscopy, reflectance confocal microscopy (RCM), optical coherence tomography (OCT), high-frequency ultrasound (HFUS), and, advanced multimodal imaging devices that combine RCM and OCT (LC-OCT).

Reflectance confocal microscopy (RCM) provides cellular-level resolution of the epidermis and superficial dermis, allowing visualization of tumor cell aggregates and architectural disruption. Optical coherence tomography (OCT) offers deeper tissue imaging, useful for assessing tumor depth and extent. The combination of RCM and OCT (LC-OCT) in a single device has shown promise for in vivo characterization of cutaneous metastases, enabling identification of tumor foci and differentiation from benign lesions.

High-frequency ultrasound (HFUS) can be used to assess lesion depth and involvement of subcutaneous structures, though its specificity for metastases is limited compared to the other modalities such as RCM and OCT.

These modalities offer a new field in the diagnosis of cutaneous metastases, their use has been limited by the expertise required by the operator to accurately assess the images provided by the equipment but also the equipment cost. Some of the limitations of the use of the techniques mentioned above are summarized in Table 6.1.

While these non-invasive modalities can guide clinical suspicion and help decision-making in day-to-day clinical practice, histopathological confirmation remains the gold standard for diagnosis. Non-invasive imaging is particularly valuable for lesion triage, monitoring, and guiding

Table 6.1 Summary of non-invasive techniques for the diagnosis of cutaneous metastases

Modality	Principle	Resolution	Penetration	Advantages	Limitations
RCM	Reflectance confocal microscopy	~1 μm (cellular)	200–300 μm	High cellular detail, "virtual histology"	Limited depth, small field of view
OCT	Optical coherence tomography	~5–10 μm (tissue)	1–2 mm	Cross-sectional imaging, depth evaluation	Lower resolution than RCM, less cellular detail
LC-OCT	Line-field confocal optical coherence tomography	~1–3 μm	500 μm	Combines cross-sectional + en face images; high detail	Limited to superficial dermis, expensive equipment
HFUS	High-frequency ultrasound	~30–100 μm	Up to 10 mm	Measures thickness, deep nodules, margins	Operator-dependent, lacks cellular detail

biopsy site selection but cannot replace tissue diagnosis to date.

References

1. Strickley D. Cutaneous metastasis. Hematol Oncol Clin North Am. 2019;33:173–97.
2. Guitera P. In vivo reflectance confocal microscopy enhances secondary evaluation of melanocytic lesions. J Invest Dermatol. 2009;129:133–8.
3. Seyed Morteza Seyed Jafari D. Noncontrast-enhanced 3-Tesla MRI using surface coil as a complementary test for assessment of distribution and depth of locoregional cutaneous metastases of malignant melanoma. Melanoma Res. 2022;32(4):211–7.
4. Libson K. Use of imaging in cutaneous squamous cell carcinoma to detect high-risk tumor features, nodal metastasis, and distant metastasis: a systematic review. Dermatologic Surg. 2024;50(8):705–9.
5. Kawaguchi M. MR imaging findings for differentiating cutaneous malignant melanoma from squamous cell carcinoma. Eur J Radiol. 2020;132:132.
6. Dunnick R. Detection of subcutaneous metastases by computed tomography. J Comput Assist Tomogr. 1978;2(3):275–9.
7. Libson K. Use of imaging in cutaneous squamous cell carcinoma to detect high-risk tumor features, nodal metastasis, and distant metastasis: a systematic review. Dermatol Surg. 2024;50(8):705–9.
8. Belfiore MP. Usefulness of high-frequency ultrasonography in the diagnosis of melanoma: mini review. Front Oncol. 2021;11(11):673026.
9. Giovagnorio F. High-resolution and color doppler sonography in the evaluation of skin metastases. J Ultrasound Med. 2003;22(10):1017–22.
10. Bard L. High-frequency ultrasound examination in the diagnosis of skin cancer. Dermatol Clin. 2017;35(4):505–11.
11. Ulrich J. Ultrasound in dermatology. Part II. Ultrasound of regional lymph node basins and subcutaneous tumours. Eur J Dermatol. 2001;11(1):73–9.
12. Hobayan CGP. Diagnostic accuracy of high-frequency ultrasound for cutaneous neoplasms: a narrative review of the literature. Arch Dermatol Res. 2024;316(7):419.
13. Shahriari N. Reflectance confocal microscopy: principles, basic terminology, clinical indications, limitations, and practical considerations. J Am Dermatol. 2021;84:1–14.
14. Levine A. Introduction to reflectance confocal microscopy and its use in clinical practice. JAAD Case Rep. 2018;10(4):1014–23.
15. Alexandris D. Dermoscopy and novel non invasive imaging of cutaneous metastases. Adv Cancer Biol Metastasis. 2022;6(1):100078.
16. Richtig E. Reflectance confocal microscopy in early diagnosis of cutaneous metastases of breast cancer. Gynecol Oncol. 2009;115:510–1.
17. Huang D. Optical coherence tomography. Science. 1991;254:1178–81.
18. Boone MA. High-definition optical coherence tomography: a new tool for the diagnosis of skin tumors. Dermatology. 2016;21:298–305.
19. Welzel J. Optical coherence tomography in dermatology: a review. Skin Res Technol. 2001;7(1):1–9.
20. Mogensen M. Optical coherence tomography for imaging of skin and skin diseases. Semin Cutan Med Surg. 2009;28(3):196–202.
21. Arevalo E. Optical coherence tomography characteristics of choroidal metastasis. Ophthalmology. 2005;112(9):1612–9.
22. Hobelsberger S. Immediate diagnosis of cutaneous metastases with optical coherence tomography, line-field confocal optical coherence tomography and dermoscopy: a case series. JEADV. 2023;3:622–8.
23. Bang AS. Non-invasive, in vivo, characterization of cutaneous metastases using a novel multimodal RCM-OCT imaging device: a case-series. J Eur Acad Dermatol Venereol. 2022;36(11):2051–4.
24. Dubois A. Line-field confocal optical coherence tomography for high-resolution noninvasive imaging of skin tumors. J Biomed Opt. 2018;23(10):1–9.
25. Kendall C. Vibrational spectroscopy: a clinical tool for cancer diagnostics. Analyst. 2009;134(6):1029–45.

26. Lu G. Medical hyperspectral imaging: a review. J Biomed Opt. 2014;19(1):10901.
27. McGivney D. Quantitative imaging with electrical impedance spectroscopy. Phys Med Biol. 2012;57(22):302.
28. Braun RP. Electrical impedance spectroscopy in skin cancer diagnosis. Dermatol Clin. 2017;35(4):489–93.
29. Esteva A, Kuprel B, Novoa RA, Ko J, Swetter SM, Blau HM, Thrun S, Esteva A. Dermatologist-level classification of skin cancer with deep neural networks. Nature. 2017;542:115–8.
30. Witkowski AM. Improving diagnostic sensitivity of combined dermoscopy and reflectance confocal microscopy imaging through double reader concordance evaluation in telemedicine settings: a retrospective study of 1000 equivocal cases. PLoS One. 2017;12:e0187748.

Part II

Cutaneous Metastasis from Gynecological Cancers

Cutaneous Metastasis from Gynecological Cancers

7

Dominika Kwiatkowska and Adam Reich

Abstract

Gynecologic cancers (ovary, endometrium, and cervix) are relatively uncommon sources of cutaneous metastasis. Among internal malignancies with cutaneous metastases, ovarian cancer constitutes approximately 4% of cases, whereas uterine (endometrial) carcinoma contributes only 1%, while cervical carcinoma, despite its high incidence, very rarely metastasizes to the skin. The classic presentation of cutaneous metastases demonstrates as firm, dermal, or subcutaneous nodules. Lesions could be solitary or multiple, ranging from a few millimeters to centimeters in size, skin-colored, pink, or violaceous nodules. Cutaneous metastases from ovarian, endometrial, and cervical carcinomas typically signify widespread disease and are connected with a poor prognosis; however, recent advances in therapy are improving outcomes for these metastatic malignancies.

Keywords

Cervical cancer · Endometrial cancer · Metastases · Ovarian cancer · Skin

7.1 Introduction

Cutaneous metastases refer to the spread of internal malignancies to the skin. They occur in approximately 3–10% of all cancer patients and usually manifest late in the course of advanced disease [1]. In women, breast carcinoma is the most common source of skin metastases (accounting for 70% of cases), followed by colorectal and ovarian carcinomas [2, 3]. Gynecologic cancers (ovary, endometrium, and cervix) are relatively uncommon sources of cutaneous metastasis, but their recognition is clinically crucial. Among internal malignancies causing skin spread, ovarian cancer constitutes approximately 4% of cases, whereas uterine (endometrial) carcinoma contributes only 1% [4, 5]. Cervical carcinoma, despite its high incidence, very rarely metastasizes to the skin (reported in only 0.1–2% of cases) [6, 7].

Cutaneous metastases from ovarian, endometrial, and cervical carcinomas typically signify widespread disease (FIGO stage III–IV) and portend a poor prognosis [8, 9]. Early dermatologic recognition and biopsy of suspicious skin lesions can lead to prompt diagnosis and multidisciplinary management. This chapter reviews the cutaneous metastases from ovarian, endometrial, and cervical cancers, emphasizing a dermatologic perspective.

D. Kwiatkowska · A. Reich (✉)
Department of Dermatology, Faculty of Medicine, University of Rzeszów, Rzeszów, Poland

D. Koumaki et al. (eds.), *Cutaneous Metastases*, https://doi.org/10.1007/978-3-032-26764-1_7

7.2 Ovarian Cancer

7.2.1 Epidemiology and Pathogenesis

Ovarian carcinoma is the most lethal gynecologic malignancy and frequently disseminates intra-abdominally. Cutaneous metastases from ovarian cancer are uncommon, occurring in roughly 0.9–5.8% of ovarian cancer patients [10–12]. Improved survival of advanced ovarian cancer patients (due to modern therapies) may be contributing to a slight increase in the observed incidence of skin metastases in recent years [4]. Ovarian cancer primarily spreads by direct entry of tumor cells into the peritoneal cavity, as well as via lymphatic vessels to pelvic, para-aortic, inguinal, or supraclavicular lymph nodes and hematogenous spread to distant sites [4]. Accordingly, two major patterns of cutaneous metastasis are seen. Umbilical metastasis—Sister Mary Joseph's nodule (SMJNs)—resulting from transperitoneal spread to the umbilicus, often associated with diffuse peritoneal carcinomatosis and a surgical scar or lymphatic route metastases—implants that develop in abdominal incision scars or at laparoscopic port sites and metastases in skin overlying regions of lymphatic drainage (e.g., the inguinal region) [13–17]. Umbilical metastases and non-umbilical skin metastases have roughly equal frequency in ovarian cancer [18]. Notably, the risk of tumor seeding at surgical sites is about 1–2% in patients undergoing laparoscopy for malignancy, and ovarian cancer can occasionally metastasize to these trocar sites even when the disease is thought to be confined [19].

7.2.2 Clinical Presentation

Cutaneous metastases from ovarian carcinoma often present as firm, dermal or subcutaneous nodules. Lesions could be solitary or multiple, ranging from a few millimeters to centimeters in size, skin-colored, pink, or violaceous nodules [20]. The classic SMJN nodule appears as an umbilical tumor nodule, sometimes with a red or bluish hue, and can be associated with surrounding erythema from lymphatic spread (carcinomatous lymphangitis) [21]. Aside from the umbilicus, ovarian cancer commonly yields skin metastases at surgical scars. The scar metastases can present as nodular swelling or persistent non-healing granuloma-like lesions at the scar site months or years after surgery [19]. Ovarian metastases can occasionally present as diffuse papulonodular eruptions on the abdomen or even distant sites; rare patterns like carcinoma erysipeloides (an erythematous, cellulitis-like patch due to dermal lymphatic invasion) have been described, though more commonly with breast or gastric primaries [22]. Likewise, multiple grouped papules mimicking herpes zoster (so-called "herpetiform" or zosteriform metastases) have been reported in ovarian cancer skin spread [23]. These atypical presentations are infrequent but important for dermatologists to recognize in the appropriate clinical context.

7.2.3 Differential Diagnosis

The dermatologist should maintain a high index of suspicion for metastasis when evaluating new skin lesions in patients with known ovarian carcinoma or an abdominal malignancy. The differential diagnosis of an umbilical nodule is broad. Benign entities such as umbilical endometriosis (Villar's nodule) can closely mimic an umbilical metastasis, especially if the patient is a woman of reproductive age [24]. Umbilical endometriosis typically presents as a tender brown or purple papule that may bleed or swell with menses, whereas a Sister Mary Joseph's nodule tends to be firmer and not cycle-dependent. A metastasis in an abdominal surgical scar must be distinguished from post-surgical changes or suture granulomas [25]. In any doubtful lesion, a skin biopsy is essential for definitive diagnosis.

7.2.4 Management

When ovarian cancer skin metastases occur early in the disease course (e.g., an umbilical metastasis at initial diagnosis), they may respond well to chemotherapy and do not uniformly portend a dismal prognosis [4]. In contrast, late-stage cutaneous recurrences (developing after multiple prior treatments) often present as widespread nodules and indicate chemoresistant disease with a poorer outlook.

Surgical excision of the cutaneous lesion can be performed for diagnosis and local control, followed by systemic chemotherapy [26]. Long-term remissions have been documented in rare instances where the skin lesion was the only detectable metastasis and was completely resected. However, in the more common scenario of multiple or late-appearing cutaneous metastases (e.g., diffuse abdominal wall nodules arising after chemotherapy), cure is unlikely, and treatment is palliative [27]. External beam radiotherapy can provide local symptom relief for bleeding or painful skin lesions [28].

From a dermatologic standpoint, local adjunctive treatments for cutaneous metastases can also be considered in selected cases. Topical imiquimod, a toll-like receptor 7 agonist, has shown efficacy in treating superficial skin metastases of other cancers (such as breast cancer) and is being studied for metastases of ovarian cancer as well [29, 30]. Likewise, electrochemotherapy (intralesional or systemic administration of chemotherapy with local electric pulse application to enhance drug uptake) has been successfully used for palliative management of multiple cutaneous metastases in various cancers [31]. These modalities may be employed for unresectable cutaneous lesions to achieve local tumor control or symptom relief.

7.3 Endometrial Cancer

7.3.1 Epidemiology and Pathogenesis

Endometrial carcinoma (carcinoma of the uterine corpus) is the most common gynecologic malignancy in women, yet cutaneous metastasis from endometrial cancer is exceedingly rare [5]. The reported frequency is on the order of 0.8–1% of endometrial cancer cases [32]. In large retrospective studies, skin involvement from endometrial adenocarcinoma was found in only 1 out of 86 patients (~1.1%) [8]. Such metastases typically occur in patients with advanced disease (FIGO stage III–IV). The routes of spread for endometrial carcinoma include direct extension (into myometrium and surrounding pelvic tissues), lymphatic dissemination (to pelvic/para-aortic lymph nodes), and hematogenous spread (to distant organs such as lung, liver, and bone). Transtubal spread of tumor cells through the fallopian tubes into the peritoneal cavity can also occur, leading to intraperitoneal metastases analogous to ovarian cancer [33].

However, the anterior abdominal wall (skin and subcutis) remains an uncommon site for endometrial cancer metastasis. When cutaneous metastases do arise, they usually signify widespread hematogenous and lymphatic spread of an aggressive tumor. In a review done by Nienhaus et al., skin metastases of endometrial carcinoma never occurred in isolation—all reported cases had concurrent metastases to lungs, lymph nodes, or other intra-abdominal sites [32]. Thus, from a pathogenesis standpoint, cutaneous spread in endometrial cancer often represents part of a generalized metastatic cascade in a terminal disease phase.

7.3.2 Clinical Presentation

Cutaneous metastases from endometrial cancer often present as rapidly growing subcutaneous nodules on the trunk [34]. These lesions tend to be firm, reddish, or skin-colored nodules that can be asymptomatic or tender. The trunk is a common location, reflecting hematogenous or lymphatic seeding of tumor cells that have bypassed the usual pelvic confines. For example, the umbilical area may be involved: although Sister Mary Joseph's nodule is classically associated with ovarian or gastrointestinal cancer, rare cases of endometrial adenocarcinoma presenting with an umbilical metastasis have been documented [35]. More often, endometrial cancer skin metastases present as multiple nodules on the abdominal wall or distant cutaneous sites. In one reported case, a patient developed multiple subcutaneous nodules on the trunk, extremities, and scalp only 6 months after initial treatment of stage I endometrial carcinoma, heralding widespread recurrence [36]. These nodules can sometimes coalesce or ulcerate. Less commonly, cutaneous metastasis of endometrial carcinoma can appear on surgical scars. Implantation of a tumor at the site of hysterectomy incision (or drain sites) is rare but has been reported even years after the initial surgery [37]. For instance, an abdominal wall metastasis arising in a cesarean or hysterectomy scar may present as a firm mass in the scar line. A 14-year delayed recurrence of endometrioid carcinoma in an abdominal incisional hernia repair scar has been described, illustrating that dormant tumor cells can seed a scar and remain quiescent for years before growing [38]. Because of the rarity of cutaneous spread, endometrial carcinoma metastases have also been reported in unusual locations. Case reports document metastases to the scalp and distal extremities, although these are exceptional [39]. Any new rapidly enlarging tumor on the skin of a patient with a history of endometrial cancer should raise concern for metastasis.

7.3.3 Differential Diagnosis

In a woman with known endometrial cancer, a new skin nodule must be distinguished from benign dermatologic lesions. The differential diagnosis includes benign lipomas, epidermal inclusion cysts, dermatofibromas, or granulomas, which are far more common than metastases. If the lesions are multiple and rapid in onset, metastases should be strongly considered. If an abdominal wall lesion arises in a scar years after a hysterectomy, one should differentiate between a recurrence and benign scar tissue or desmoid tumor. In one case, a suspected desmoid (fibromatosis) at a hernia repair site was found on biopsy to harbor metastatic endometrial carcinoma cells [32]. Thus, performing a biopsy of any suspicious scar lesion is mandatory.

7.3.4 Management

The appearance of cutaneous metastases in endometrial cancer generally signifies FIGO stage IVB disease. Management, therefore, is typically palliative systemic therapy [40]. Radiation therapy can be utilized for localized control, especially if a skin lesion is bleeding or ulcerated. For instance, an ulcerating chest wall metastasis from endometrial cancer may be palliated with external beam radiotherapy to reduce tumor burden and improve wound care [41].

More recently, immunotherapy has become an important part of the management of advanced endometrial cancers. Dermatologic follow-up in these patients should include monitoring for new skin lesions and managing cutaneous adverse effects of systemic treatments. Immune checkpoint inhibitors frequently cause cutaneous immune-related adverse events, such as maculopapular rash (in 16–25% of patients) and lichenoid dermatitis (in 20%) [42]. Dermatologists should distinguish these drug eruptions from new metastases and treat them appropriately to allow the patient to continue life-prolonging therapy. In summary, cutaneous metastases from endometrial carcinoma, though rare, are a grave sign and require coordinated oncologic and dermatologic care to optimize patient outcomes and quality of life.

7.4 Cervical Cancer

7.4.1 Epidemiology and Pathogenesis

Carcinoma of the uterine cervix is a common malignancy worldwide, but cutaneous metastasis from cervical cancer is very rare. The incidence is estimated to be between 0.1% and 2% of cervical cancer patients [43]. In a large clinical series of 1190 cervical cancer cases, only 15 patients (1.3%) developed skin metastases [44]. The likelihood of skin involvement increases with advanced stage: for example, in that series, skin metastases occurred in 0.8% of stage I, 1.2% of stages II-III, and 4.8% of stage IV cases [44]. Histologic subtype influences the risk—adenocarcinoma and undifferentiated carcinoma of the cervix have a higher propensity to metastasize to skin than the more common squamous cell carcinoma (SCC). One analysis found cutaneous metastases in 5–6% of cervical adenocarcinoma cases versus <1% of squamous cases [6]. This may relate to the more aggressive systemic spread pattern of cervical adenocarcinomas. Cervical cancer typically spreads by local extension and lymphatic metastasis to pelvic and para-aortic lymph nodes. Distant hematogenous metastases (to lung, bone, and liver) can occur in advanced disease. Cutaneous metastases usually arise via lymphatic or hematogenous routes, often in the setting of widespread tumor burden.

7.4.2 Clinical Presentation

When cervical carcinoma metastasizes to the skin, the abdominal wall, vulvar region, and upper thighs are among the most commonly involved sites [45]. More than half of reported cases present with lesions on the lower abdomen, presumably due to metastasis from pelvic lymphatics or surgical tract seeding. The anterior abdominal wall (often near the suprapubic area or within old surgical scars from procedures like cesarean section or lymph node dissections) is frequently noted. The vulva or perineum may be involved either by direct contiguous spread from a locally advanced cervical tumor or via lymphatic spread to the external genital skin. Clinically, cutaneous metastases from cervical cancer typically present as nodules or tumor masses in or under the skin. In the Imachi et al. series, 86.7% of patients had nodular skin lesions (often dermal or subcutaneous nodules) [44]. These nodules are usually firm and round, and may be skin-colored or reddish-blue. Sometimes, there is a linear arrangement of nodules along lymphatic channels.

A striking but rare presentation of cervical cancer skin metastasis is the zosteriform pattern. There are reports of cervical cancer, particularly adenocarcinoma, metastasizing to the skin in a dermatomal distribution that mimics herpes zoster. In one such case, a 54-year-old woman with cervical adenocarcinoma developed grouped papules on the abdomen following a single sensory dermatome, initially misdiagnosed as shingles until a biopsy confirmed metastatic carcinoma [46]. This zosteriform presentation is extremely uncommon—only a handful of cases have been documented—but it underscores that metastases can occasionally take on pseudo-infectious appearances.

7.4.3 Differential Diagnosis

The differential diagnosis for suspected cutaneous metastases of cervical cancer includes benign dermatologic lesions and other malignancies. An enlarging red nodule in an old surgical scar could be a keloid or hypertrophic scar, although those usually stabilize rather than rapidly enlarge. If the lesion is ulcerated, squamous cell carcinoma arising in chronic scars (Marjolin ulcer) could be considered, but in a patient with a cervical SCC history, metastasis is more likely. Differentiating a metastatic squamous cell carcinoma in the skin from a new primary cutaneous squamous cell carcinoma can be challenging. Clues favoring metastasis include deep localization (dermal/subcutaneous nodules without epidermal origin), multiple lesions, and a known cervical cancer history [47]. Immunohistochemistry can aid this distinction. Ultimately, a biopsy is required for any new suspicious skin lesion in a patient with current or past cervical cancer, as it is the only way to confirm metastasis and exclude mimickers.

7.4.4 Management

Cutaneous metastasis from cervical carcinoma indicates systemic disease (stage IVB) and warrants systemic therapy. Historically, prognosis has been very poor—earlier studies labeled skin metastasis from cervix as a "preterminal event," with survival often only 1–6 months in many cases [48]. In Imachi et al., 12 of 15 patients died within 1 year, and the median survival was around 6 months despite treatment [44]. Recent advances in therapy are improving outcomes for metastatic cervical cancer.

Topical or intralesional therapies are less established in cervical cancer, but anecdotal use of imiquimod on superficial perineal metastases has been considered in palliative scenarios (by analogy to its use in other skin metastases). Most importantly, dermatologists should help manage the side effects of systemic treatments or radiation dermatitis in irradiated fields.

7.5 Dermoscopy

Dermoscopy is a non-invasive diagnostic tool that can aid in the evaluation of cutaneous metastases. Although there are no pathognomonic dermoscopic patterns unique to gynecologic metastases, certain features should raise suspicion of metastatic carcinoma in a patient with known cancer. Vascular structures are the hallmark dermoscopic finding in non-pigmented metastases [49]. In a study of 20 patients with cutaneous metastases, 88% of non-pigmented lesions showed discrete vascular patterns on dermoscopy [49]. The most common were serpentine (linear irregular) vessels, often arranged in an asymmetrical distribution. Other vessel types such as dotted vessels (tiny pinpoint dots) or arborizing telangiectasia can also be present, reflecting the rich neovasculature of metastases [50]. The background color of metastatic lesions on dermoscopy is usually pink, red, or whitish. Structureless areas of white or pink are often observed and correspond to dense tumor tissue and fibrosis in the dermis. Notably, a recent study found that white structureless area was present in over 80% of cutaneous metastases, which likely represents the fibrosis or scarring induced by the tumor.

In metastases from ovarian cancer, a combination of white and tan structureless zones was found in 100% of lesions, often accompanied by dotted vessels in about 43% [50]. For cervical or endometrial metastases (usually non-pigmented), similar patterns would be expected—predominantly vascular features with no pigment network. Pigmented metastases are very rare in gynecologic cancers (since these primaries are not melanocytic). In general, if a cutaneous metastasis is pigmented (brown or blue-black), one must consider either hemorrhage in the lesion or melanoma metastasis.

While dermoscopy is an adjunct, it is not definitive for diagnosing cutaneous metastases. Its greatest utility is in prompting recognition and biopsy.

7.6 Histopathology and Immunohistochemistry

Histopathologic examination remains the gold standard for diagnosing cutaneous metastases and determining their origin. A skin biopsy of a suspicious lesion typically reveals tumor cells in the dermis and/or subcutis, often without epidermal involvement (the epidermis is usually intact unless secondarily ulcerated).

The histopathology of cutaneous metastases mirrors the primary gynecologic tumor (glandular for ovarian/endometrial, squamous for cervical), and immunohistochemistry can confirm the tissue of origin (Tables 7.1 and 7.2). Markers like PAX8 are crucial for identifying Müllerian tumors, while p16 helps pinpoint an HPV-associated cervical cancer [51–53]. This is especially important when a patient presents with skin metastasis of unknown primary—the correct identification of a gynecologic origin can direct the search for an occult pelvic tumor and appropriate management.

Table 7.1 Histopathologic features of cutaneous metastases from gynecologic cancers

Primary cancer type	Histopathologic features
Ovarian Carcinoma (High-grade serous adenocarcinoma)	Dermal infiltrates of adenocarcinoma are arranged in nests, glandular formations, or solid sheets; cells exhibit pleomorphic, hyperchromatic nuclei; the presence of psammoma bodies is characteristic of serous subtypes. Typically no epidermal involvement unless ulceration occurs
Endometrial Carcinoma (Endometrioid adenocarcinoma)	Malignant glandular structures are irregularly distributed within the dermis/subcutis; cribriform architecture or solid areas with central necrosis may occur. Tumor cells appear columnar or polygonal, displaying moderate nuclear pleomorphism
Cervical Carcinoma (Squamous cell carcinoma)	Nests and cords of atypical squamous epithelial cells infiltrating dermis; keratin pearls and intercellular bridges are evident in well-differentiated lesions; poorly differentiated tumors may present as solid, cohesive sheets. Stromal desmoplasia is frequently observed; epidermal ulceration can occur with superficial extension

Table 7.2 Diagnostic immunohistochemical profiles in gynecologic cancer skin metastases

Primary cancer type	Key immunohistochemical markers
Ovarian Carcinoma (High-grade serous adenocarcinoma)	*Positive*: CK7, PAX8 (confirming Müllerian origin), WT1 (serous subtype), CA-125. ER/PR is frequently positive in endometrioid and low-grade serous subtypes; p53 shows an abnormal pattern *Negative*: CK20, TTF-1, GATA3 (excluding gastrointestinal, pulmonary, or breast origin)
Endometrial Carcinoma (Endometrioid adenocarcinoma)	*Positive*: CK7, PAX8, ER/PR (strongly expressed in most cases), Vimentin; focal CEA positivity possible. Mismatch repair proteins are lost in microsatellite instability-high (MSI-H) cases *Negative*: CK20, TTF-1, other non-gynecologic organ markers
Cervical Carcinoma (Squamous cell carcinoma)	*Positive*: p63, CK5/6 (indicating squamous differentiation), diffuse nuclear/cytoplasmic p16 expression (high-risk HPV association), and HPV-specific in-situ hybridization positive in relevant cases. Adenocarcinoma subtype shows overlapping CK7 and PAX8 positivity with ovarian/endometrial carcinomas but uniquely demonstrates p16 positivity. *Negative*: Markers specific to non-gynecologic squamous carcinomas (e.g., lung SCC markers)

7.7 Conclusion

Cutaneous metastases from ovarian, endometrial, and cervical cancers are rare clinical findings that signal advanced disease and carry significant prognostic implications. Table 7.3 summarizes the incidence and clinical patterns of cutaneous metastasis in gynecologic cancers. For the dermatologist, recognizing a suspicious skin lesion as a potential metastasis can lead to early diagnosis of an internal malignancy or prompt detection of disease progression in a cancer patient.

Table 7.3 Incidence and clinical patterns of cutaneous metastasis in gynecologic cancers

Primary tumor	Incidence of skin metastasis	Sites and patterns
Ovarian carcinoma (usually high-grade serous)	~0.9–5%; frequency increases with advanced stages	Umbilicus (Sister Mary Joseph's nodule); surgical scar implants; rarely carcinoma erysipeloides or diffuse papular presentations
Endometrial carcinoma (endometrioid adenocarcinoma)	<1% (rare occurrence)	Abdominal wall (particularly near hysterectomy scars); distant sites (scalp); typically firm nodules; rare zosteriform dermatomal pattern
Cervical carcinoma (squamous cell carcinoma)	~0.8–2% (rare)	Lower abdomen, groin, perineum, vulva, and upper thighs; multiple red-to-violaceous nodules or papules, occasionally forming confluent plaques; surgical scar implants

References

1. Lookingbill DP, Spangler N, Helm KF. Cutaneous metastases in patients with metastatic carcinoma. J Am Acad Dermatol. 1993;29:228–36.
2. Naser AMB, Zaki MS, Brunner M, et al. Cutaneous metastasis in internal malignancy. Egyptian Dermatol Online J. 2007;3:1.
3. Rolz-Cruz G, Kim CC. Tumor invasion of the skin. Dermatol Clin. 2008;26:89–102.
4. Otsuka I. Cutaneous metastases in ovarian cancer. Cancers (Basel). 2019;11(9):1292.
5. Damewood MD, Rosenshein NB, Grumbine FC, Parmley TH. Cutaneous metastasis of endometrial carcinoma. Cancer. 1980;46(6):1471–5.
6. Alrefaie SI, Alshamrani HM, Abduljabbar MH, Hariri JO. Skin metastasis from squamous cell carcinoma of the cervix to the lower extremities: case report and review of the literature. J Family Med Prim Care. 2019;8(10):3443–6.
7. O'Brian CJ, Crissman JD, Sowers JR. Carcinoma erysipeloides: review of the literature and report of a gastric primary. Cancer. 1979;44:641–8.
8. Krathen RA, Orengo IF, Rosen T. Cutaneous metastasis: a meta-analysis of data. South Med J. 2003;96:164–7.
9. McWhirter E, Bingham J, Staples M, et al. Scalp metastases from endometrial carcinoma: a rare presentation. Dermatol Rep. 2022;15:9553.
10. Kobayashi A, Shigemitsu S, Kamura T. Cutaneous metastases from ovarian carcinoma: analysis of clinicopathologic features. Gynecol Oncol Rep. 2015;14:44–7.
11. Dauplat J, Hacker NF, Nieberg RK, et al. Distant metastases in epithelial ovarian carcinoma. Cancer. 1987;1:1561–6.
12. Cormio G, Capotorto M, Di Vagno G, et al. Skin metastases in ovarian carcinoma: a report of nine cases and a review of the literature. Gynecol Oncol. 2003;90:682–5.
13. Nikolaou M, Zyli P, Stamenkovic S, Koniari K, Psachoulia C, Kalofonos HP. Sister Mary Joseph's nodule in advanced ovarian cancer. J Obstet Gynaecol. 2013;33:214–5.
14. Husein-El Ahmed H, Aneiros-Fernandez J, Arias-Santiago S, Naranjo-Sintes R. Sister Mary Joseph's nodule as a metastasis of ovarian adenocarcinoma. Int J Dermatol. 2010;49:1045–6.
15. Mimura T, Yagi Y, Asami Y, Miyamoto S, Iitsuka C, Onuki M, Ishikawa T, Kushima M, Matsumoto K, Sekizawa A. Sister Mary Joseph nodule in ovarian cancer: a case report and literature review. Kanto J Obstet Gynaecol. 2018;55:479–84.
16. Ohta S, Yamakawa Y, Hasegawa T, Tateno M, Matsui K. Advanced ovarian cancer with Sister Mary Joseph's nodule: a case report. Gan To Kagaku Ryoho. 2007;34:117–9.
17. Haneda T, Kimura T, Sarukawa M, Horiguchi D, Kohda H, Takigawa M. Ovarian carcinoma with Sister Mary Joseph's nodule. Hifu Rinsho. 2001;42:342–3.
18. Brustman L, Seltzer V. Sister Joseph's nodule: seven cases of umbilical metastases from gynecologic malignancies. Gynecol Oncol. 1984;19:155–62.
19. Ramirez PT, Wolf JK, Levenback C. Laparoscopic port-site metastases: etiology and prevention. Gynecol Oncol. 2003;91:179–89.
20. Craig CD, Iglesias DA, Watkins J, Coleman RL, Kilgore L, Ramirez PT. Extensive cutaneous metastases of ovarian cancer after prolonged response to liposomal doxorubicin. Gynecol Oncol Case Rep. 2013;5:64–6.
21. Tso S, Brockley J, Recica H, Ilchyshyn A. Sister Mary Joseph's nodule: an unusual but important physical finding characteristic of widespread internal malignancy. Br J Gen Pract. 2013;63:551–2.
22. Lee HC, Chu CY, Hsiao CH. Carcinoma erysipeloides from ovarian clear-cell carcinoma. J Clin Oncol. 2007;25(36):5828–30.
23. Rasi A, Tajziehchi L, Shaianfar N. Metastatic carcinoma of the ovary presenting as zosteriform lesions. Arch Iran Med. 2007;10(2):250–2.

24. Ashindoitiang JA, Canice Nwagbara VI, Ugbem TI, Ukam JS, Asuquo ME. Umbilical nodule, a rare presentation of primary cutaneous endometriosis: case report and literature review. Rare Tumors. 2024;12(16):20363613241285148.
25. Imperiale L, Marchetti C, Salerno L, Iadarola R, Bracchi C, Vertechy L, di Francesco L, Musella A, Bevilacqua E, Pennesi P, Palaia I, Panici PB. Nonabsorbable suture granuloma mimicking ovarian cancer recurrence at combined positron emission tomography/computed tomography evaluation: a case report. J Med Case Rep. 2014;8:202.
26. Trope CG, Elstrand MB, Sandstad B, Davidson B, Oksefjell H. Neoadjuvant chemotherapy, interval debulking surgery or primary surgery in ovarian carcinoma FIGO stage IV? Eur J Cancer. 2012;48:2146–54.
27. Nakai N, Okuzawa Y, Katoh N. Clinical usefulness of Mohs' chemosurgery for palliative purposes in patients with cutaneous squamous cell carcinoma with risk factors or without indication for surgery: three case reports. J Dermatol. 2015;42:405–7.
28. Demirci S, Yavas F, Ozsaran Z, Ozsaran A, Dikmen Y, Zekioglu O, Karabulut B, Aras AB. Palliative radiotherapy for the skin metastasis of ovarian cancer: a case report and review of the literature. Med Oncol. 2010;27:628–31.
29. Adams S, Kozhaya L, Martiniuk F, Meng TC, Chiriboga L, Liebes L, Hochman T, Shuman N, Axelrod D, Speyer J, Novik Y, Tiersten A, Goldberg JD, Formenti SC, Bhardwaj N, Unutmaz D, Demaria S. Topical TLR7 agonist imiquimod can induce immune-mediated rejection of skin metastases in patients with breast cancer. Clin Cancer Res. 2012;18(24):6748–57.
30. Stanley MA. Imiquimod and the imidazoquinolones: mechanism of action and therapeutic potential. Clin Exp Dermatol. 2002;27(7):571–7.
31. Craig CD, Iglesias DA, Watkins J, Coleman RL, Kilgore L, Ramirez PT. Extensive cutaneous metastases of ovarian cancer after prolonged response to liposomal doxorubicin. Gynecol Oncol Case Rep. 2013;19:64–6.
32. Nienhaus A, Rajakulendran R, Bernad E. Cutaneous metastasis of endometrial cancer and long-term survival: a scoping review and our experience. Diagnostics (Basel). 2023;13(15):2603.
33. Lookingbill DP, Spangler N, Sexton FM. Skin involvement as the presenting sign of internal carcinoma. A retrospective study of 7316 cancer patients. J Am Acad Dermatol. 1990;22(1):19–26.
34. Barbetakis N, Paliouras D, Asteriou C, Samanidis G, Kleontas A, Anestakis D, Kaplanis K, Tsilikas C. Cutaneous skull metastasis from uterine leiomyosarcoma: a case report. World J Surg Oncol. 2009;7:45.
35. Li Y, Guo P, Wang B, Jia YT. Sister Mary Joseph's nodule in endometrial carcinoma: a case report. World J Clin Cases. 2019;7(20):3358–63.
36. Fan Y, Deng H, Tian L, Wang J. Cutaneous metastases of endometrial carcinoma: report of an unusual case and literature review. Arch Gynecol Obstet. 2021;304(5):1127–33.
37. Meshikhes AN, Al-Badr SH, Sulais EA, Al-Qudaihi HM. Late metastatic endometrial carcinoma at the repair site of an abdominal wall incisional hernia. Saudi Med J. 2017;38(5):546–8.
38. Lorenz U, Gassel AM, Thiede A, Gassel HJ. Endometrial carcinoma recurrence in an abdominal scar 14 years after total hysterectomy. Gynecol Oncol. 2004;95(2):393–5.
39. M'rabet FZZE, Hottinger A, George AC, Tille JC, Mesbahi OE, Castiglione-Gertsch M, Bodmer A. Cutaneous metastasis of endometrial carcinoma: a case report and literature review. J Clin Gynecol Obstet. 2012;1:19–23.
40. Abu-Rustum N, Yashar C, Arend R, Barber E, Bradley K, Brooks R, Campos SM, Chino J, Chon HS, Chu C, et al. Uterine neoplasms, version 1.2023, NCCN clinical practice guidelines in oncology. J Natl Compr Cancer Netw. 2023;21:181–209.
41. Atallah D, el Kassis N, Lutfallah F, Safi J, Salameh C, Nadiri S, Bejjani L. Cutaneous metastasis in endometrial cancer: once in a blue moon—case report. World J Surg Oncol. 2014;12:86.
42. Wang E, Kraehenbuehl L, Ketosugbo K, Kern JA, Lacouture ME, Leung DYM. Immune-related cutaneous adverse events due to checkpoint inhibitors. Ann Allergy Asthma Immunol. 2021;126(6):613–22.
43. Brady LW, O'Neil EA, Farber SH. Unusual sites of metastases. Semin Oncol. 1977;4:59–64.
44. Imachi M, Tsukamoto N, Kinoshita S, Nakano H. Skin metastasis from carcinoma of the uterine cervix. Gynecol Oncol. 1993;48(3):349–54.
45. Basu B, Mukherjee S. Cutaneous metastasis in cancer of the uterine cervix: a case report and review of the literature. J Turk Ger Gynecol Assoc. 2013;14(3):174–7.
46. Sandeep A, Rajeshwari D, Eeshaan R, Aradhana R. Cutaneous metastases in a case of adenocarcinoma cervix with atypical presentation. Indian J Dermatopathol Diagn Dermatol. 2021;8(1):17–9.
47. Popovic A, Bojic MD, Bojic M, Vukmirovic F, Juskovic A. Cutaneous metastases of cervical cancer: a rare entity and possible mechanisms of dissemination. Postepy Dermatol Alergol. 2024;41(1):136–8.
48. Shen Y, Jin X, Zhu Y, He C. Clinical analysis of patients with skin metastasis of cervical squamous cell carcinoma. Chin Clin Oncol. 2024;13(3):35.
49. Chernoff KA, Marghoob AA, Lacouture ME, Deng L, Busam KJ, Myskowski PL. Dermoscopic findings in cutaneous metastases. JAMA Dermatol. 2014;150(4):429–33.
50. Simionescu O, Petrică M, Avram AM, Costache M, Scurtu LG, Tudorache SI, Iorga PG, Grigore M. Dermoscopy of skin metastases in advanced cancer-systemic (visceral, hematologic) and cutaneous. Front Med (Lausanne). 2024;11:1445811.
51. Zhao L, Guo M, Sneige N, Gong Y. Value of PAX8 and WT1 immunostaining in confirming the ovar-

ian origin of metastatic carcinoma in serous effusion specimens. Am J Clin Pathol. 2012;137(2):304–9.
52. Fujiwara M, Taube J, Sharma M, McCalmont TH, Kim J. PAX8 discriminates ovarian metastases from adnexal tumors and other cutaneous metastases. J Cutan Pathol. 2010;37(9):938–43.
53. da Mata S, Ferreira J, Nicolás I, Esteves S, Esteves G, Lérias S, Silva F, Saco A, Cochicho D, Cunha M, Del Pino M, Ordi J, Félix A. P16 and HPV genotype significance in HPV-associated cervical cancer-a large cohort of two tertiary referral centers. Int J Mol Sci. 2021;22(5):2294.

Part III

Cutaneous Metastases from Gastrointestinal Cancers

8 Cutaneous Metastases from gastrointestinal cancers: Liver cancer

Eirini Kavvalou

Abstract

Cutaneous metastases of hepatocellular carcinoma (HCC) are rare, accounting for only 0.2%–2.7% of all skin metastases, and occur in approximately 3% of patients with HCC. They most commonly appear on the face, scalp, chest, and shoulders, typically presenting as single or multiple firm, painless nodules. However, they may also appear as erythematous lesions, hemangioma-like, basal-cell carcinoma-like, cauliflower-like growths, pyogenic granuloma-like lesions, subcutaneous abscesses, warts, subcutaneous masses, or gingival masses. Needle tract implantations usually present as single or multiple round or oval nodules along the needle path, extending from the intraperitoneal space through the abdominal or intercostal muscles to the skin or subcutaneous tissue. The overall incidence of tumor seeding across all techniques ranges from 0.5% to 1%, with most studies reporting rates below 2%. Cutaneous metastases of cholangiocarcinoma (CC) are extremely rare, reported in only 0.4%–5.3% of cases. The incidence of catheter tract implantation and metastasis is approximately 3%. These metastases usually present as firm, painless to slightly tender subcutaneous nodules but may also appear as indurated papules or plaques, morphea-like lesions, ulcers or ulcerated nodules, erythematous macules, or abscesses.

Keywords

Hepatocellular carcinoma · Cholangiocarcinoma · Skin metastases · Cutaneous metastases · Liver metastases

8.1 Hepatocellular Carcinoma

8.1.1 Introduction and Epidemiology

Hepatocellular carcinoma (HCC) accounts for approximately 90% of primary liver cancers [1]. The most common site of HCC metastasis is the lung, followed by the abdominal lymph nodes, bones, and adrenal glands [1]. Cutaneous metastases of HCC are rare, representing only 0.2%–2.7% of all skin metastases [2]. There is a male predominance [3]. They develop in approximately 3% of patients with HCC [4]. Their occurrence as the initial manifestation of the disease is particularly uncommon, reported in only 1%–5% of cases, and is associated with a poor prognosis due to a high likelihood of widespread metastasis [2]. In one study, cutaneous metastases were found in 2.7% of patients with cirrhotic HCC, while none were observed in those with non-cirrhotic HCC [5]. The presence of skin metasta-

E. Kavvalou (✉)
University General Hospital of Heraklion, Heraklion, Greece

D. Koumaki et al. (eds.), *Cutaneous Metastases*, https://doi.org/10.1007/978-3-032-26764-1_8

ses is linked to a median survival time of less than 5 months [2]. HCC should be included in the differential diagnosis of carcinomas metastatic to the skin, even when there are no liver-related symptoms or when imaging (e.g., ultrasound or CT) does not reveal a primary hepatic lesion [5]. The head is the most frequently involved site for cutaneous and subcutaneous metastases [6].

8.1.2 Clinical Presentation

Cutaneous metastases of HCC) most commonly occur on the face, scalp, chest, and shoulders, presenting as single or multiple, firm, painless lesions, which may or may not exhibit ulceration [2, 7], crusting [7], or rapid growth [8]. In some cases, lesions appear as erythema without ulceration [9]. A study of 24 cases of non-iatrogenic subcutaneous metastases identified the scalp as the most frequent site of involvement [10]. These lesions often manifest as erythematous nodules ranging from 1 to 5 cm in diameter [2]. Occasionally, they present as necrotic or purulent lesions or with a hemangiomatous morphology, which may bleed profusely if incised or otherwise injured [2]. On the nose, HCC cutaneous metastasis may appear as a pearly violet nodule with overlying telangiectasias, mimicking basal-cell carcinoma [11], or as a multilobulated mass with central necrosis [12] (Fig. 8.1). In rare instances, these lesions exhibit rapid growth and develop a cauliflower-like appearance [13].

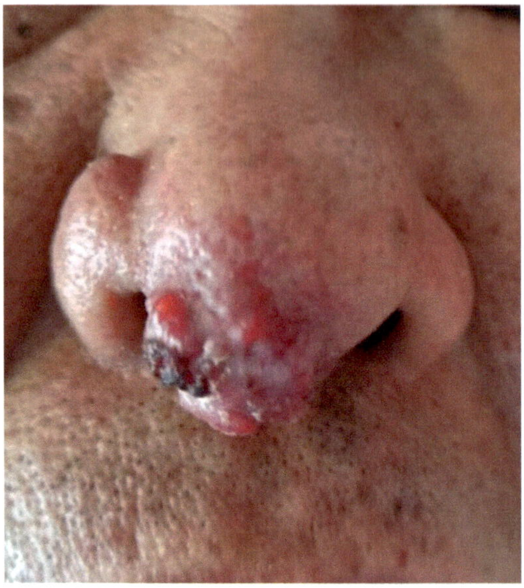

Fig. 8.1 Clinical presentation of cutaneous metastasis of HCC. Red infiltrative plaques with ulceration and scab on the nasal tip. (Taken from Li et al. [7]. © 2023)

HCC cutaneous metastases may also resemble pyogenic granulomas, particularly when appearing on the fingers as tender, erythematous nodules [14] (Fig. 8.2) or on the face as elastic, hard, dome-shaped nodules with a reddish, smooth surface [15]. Similar pyogenic granuloma-like lesions have also been reported on the abdomen, specifically in regions corresponding to previous therapeutic percutaneous ethanol injection (PEI) sites for HCC treatment [16] (Fig. 8.3). The red-

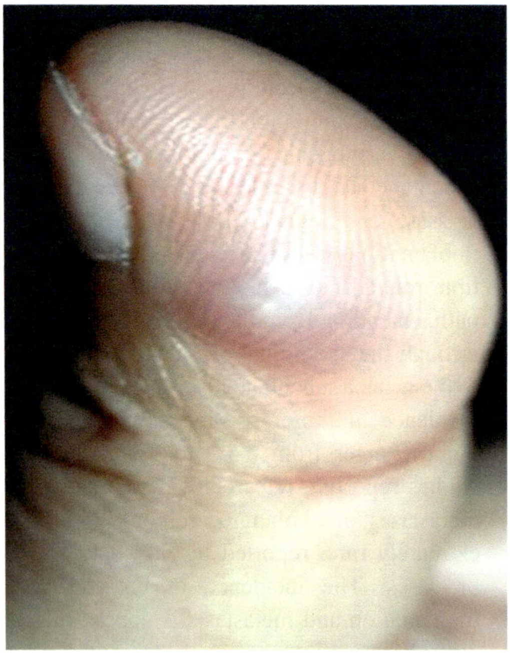

Fig. 8.2 Finger skin metastasis from HCC. (From Kim et al. [14], Copyright @ 2012 World Scientific)

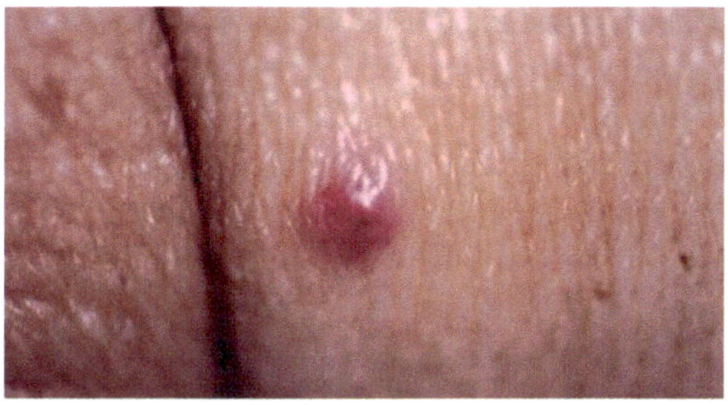

Fig. 8.3 A papule on the right waist. Cutaneous Seeding Following Percutaneous Ethanol Injection Therapy for HCC. (From Nagaoka et al. [29])

dish coloration of these lesions is likely due to the hypervascular nature of the tumor tissue [15]. In some instances, bone involvement has been observed [14]. Metastases to the hand are associated with poor prognosis, as they typically occur in the advanced stages of malignancy [14]. Patients with hand metastases generally have a median survival time of 5–6 months [14].

Another example of a cutaneous lesion serving as the initial manifestation of HCC is a subcutaneous abscess characterized by a hard, lobulated structure filled with hematic and purulent material [2].

Cutaneous metastasis of HCC may also present as a wart-like lesion near the nasal ala, which progressively enlarges into a large, nontender, pedunculated mass—measuring up to 5 cm—that may invade adjacent structures such as the gums [8]. The surface of such lesions is typically friable and prone to bleeding [8].

HCC metastasis has also been reported as presenting as an ulcerated plaque on the lower lip [17].

Another form of HCC metastasis is a subcutaneous mass (Fig. 8.4). Although subcutaneous metastasis of HCC is uncommon, it may present as the sole and initial manifestation of the disease. A case has been reported involving a subcutaneous mass in the occipital region of the scalp, invading the bone with both extra- and intracranial components [5]. Occasionally, the soft tissue mass may present as a fixed, nontender lesion on the forehead, mimicking a forehead hematoma [18]. Calvarial metastases have been reported in 0.4%–1.6% of patients with HCC [19]. This rare

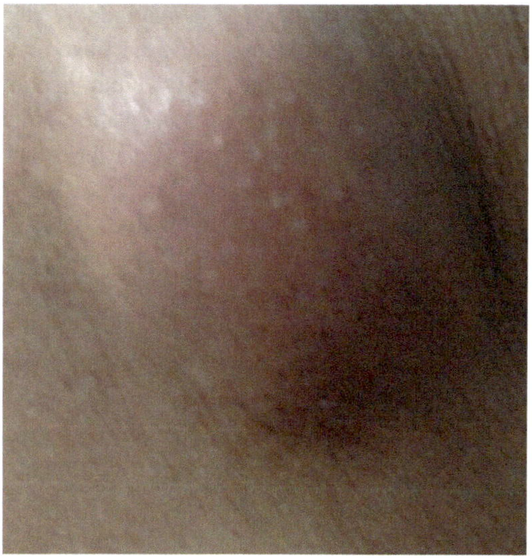

Fig. 8.4 Clinical appearance of nodular metastasis of HCC. (From Cazzato et al. [28])

manifestation often presents as cranial swelling [19]. Three growth patterns have been described in calvarial involvement: intracranial, extracranial, and a combination of both [19]. The extracranial growth pattern, in particular, may be mistaken for common scalp lesions such as trichilemmal cysts [19]. Therefore, preoperative imaging is essential in evaluating solitary head lesions [19].

Metastasis of primary HCC to the oral cavity is extremely rare, accounting for less than 1% of malignant oral neoplasms [20]. It may present as a progressively enlarging gingival mass, often accompanied by bleeding and detachment of necrotic tissue [20, 21].

8.1.3 Mechanisms of Cutaneous and Oral Metastasis

Skin metastases can occur through several mechanisms: hematogenous or lymphatic dissemination of neoplastic cells [2], direct infiltration, and implantation [7]. The face and scalp are frequently involved sites, likely due to the presence of arteriovenous shunts that allow tumor cells to spread via the inferior vena cava to the head and neck regions [8]. Oral metastasis from liver cancer primarily occurs through hematogenous dissemination [20]. Two major pathways have been proposed. The first is the portal hematogenous pathway, wherein liver tumors invade major hepatic vessels—such as the hepatic arteries and portal veins—with metastases often appearing in the lungs. The second pathway involves Batson's plexus, a network of valveless paravertebral veins. This system allows tumor cells to bypass the caval, portal, and pulmonary circulations, facilitating direct spread to the oral cavity [20].

The majority of subcutaneous metastases of HCC) originate from needle tracks or surgical wound contamination [5] (Fig. 8.5). Additionally, procedures such as radiofrequency ablation, ethanol ablation, transcatheter arterial chemoembolization, and postoperative liver transplantation have been associated with the development of cutaneous metastases [7]. Needle tract implantations typically present as single or multiple round or oval nodules along the needle path, extending from the intraperitoneal space through the abdominal or intercostal muscles to the skin or subcutaneous tissue [22]. The overall incidence of tumor seeding—across all techniques—ranges from 0.5% to 1%, with most studies reporting rates under 2% [22]. Several mechanisms have been proposed to explain tumor cell dissemination along the needle tract: viable tumor cells adhering to the needle and breaking off upon withdrawal, tumor cells being carried to the surface by reflux of blood or other fluids along the tract, and a sudden increase in intratumoral pressure, particularly during procedures such as radiofrequency ablation, forcing tumor cells into the needle tract [22].

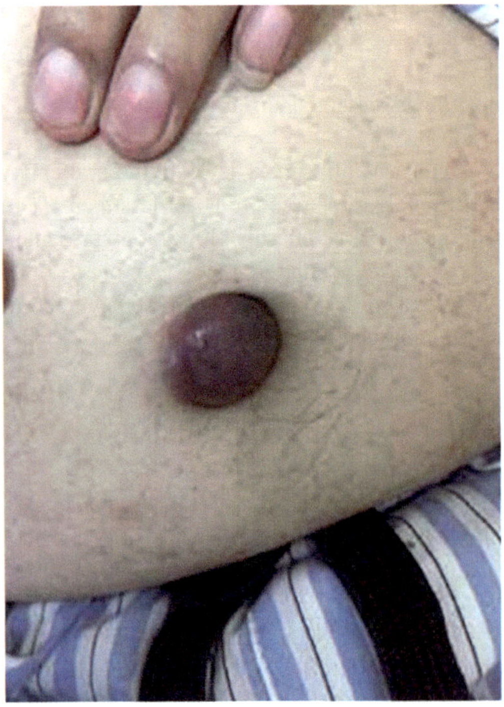

Fig. 8.5 Periumbilical cutaneous HCC metastasis in a 64-year-old man associated with abdominal surgical intervention. (From Hsu et al. [1], Copyright Elsevier (2024))

Port-site metastasis (PSM) is characterized by the direct implantation of malignant cells at a trocar insertion site following laparoscopic resection of an intra-abdominal tumor [1]. The pathogenesis of PSM is thought to involve two primary factors: pneumoperitoneum and direct tumor contamination [15]. During laparoscopic abdominal surgery with carbon dioxide (CO_2) insufflation, iatrogenic pneumoperitoneum may detach malignant cells from the tumor surface, allowing them to spread into the peritoneal cavity through aerosolization [15]. Several strategies have been proposed to prevent PSM, including stricter modifications of surgical techniques and intraperitoneal irrigation with chemotherapeutic agents [15]. Other promising methods, such as hyperthermic CO_2 insufflation and humidified CO_2 insufflation, have demonstrated efficacy in reducing peritoneal tumor spread in animal studies [15].

8.1.4 Histopathological and Immunohistochemical Findings

Histopathological examination of HCC skin metastases typically reveals malignant dermal cells. Hepatoid features—such as nests or cords of cells arranged in a trabecular or pseudoglandular pattern, sinusoidal formation, or the presence of bile—are observed in less than 50% of cases [3]. The identification of sinusoidal vessels can serve as an important diagnostic clue [17]. Tumor cells often appear polygonal, with abundant granular eosinophilic cytoplasm, an increased nuclear-to-cytoplasmic ratio, large round nuclei, and prominent nucleoli [17]. Atypical tumor cells separated by fibrous septae may also be seen [4]. Cytologically, the tumor cells may exhibit severe atypia and numerous mitotic figures, supporting their malignant nature [4]. Two distinct tumor cell types can be recognized: those with acidophilic cytoplasm and those with clear granular cytoplasm [4]. Mallory body-like cytoplasmic inclusions may also be present [4]. Additionally, histopathology may show epidermal necrosis with ulceration [7], although in some cases, the overlying epidermis appears slightly atrophic, with mild hyperkeratosis [11].

In the diagnosis of HCC), a range of immunohistochemical stains can be useful, including hepatocyte paraffin-1 (HepPar1), arginase-1 (Arg-1), glypican-3, polyclonal carcinoembryonic antigen (CEA), alpha-fetoprotein (AFP), cytokeratins (CK) 8 and 18, [17] Ki-67, villin [7], and mannan-3 [7]. HepPar1 has historically been regarded as the most sensitive marker for hepatocytes [17]. It is a monoclonal antibody that detects a formalin-resistant antigen specific to hepatocellular mitochondria, found in both normal and neoplastic hepatocytes [4]. HepPar1 demonstrates high specificity for HCC—greater than 90%—although it may also stain some extrahepatic malignancies [4]. Reported sensitivity for HCC ranges from 79% to 99.7% [4], with decreased sensitivity observed in poorly differentiated tumors [11]. Most hepatocytes and HCCs show a strong, coarse, granular cytoplasmic pattern for HepPar1 [11]. However, as HepPar1 can also be positive in certain adenocarcinomas and neuroendocrine tumors, additional immunostains such as CK7, CK20, chromogranin, synaptophysin, or INSM1 are recommended to support diagnostic accuracy [17]. While rarely a poorly differentiated adenocarcinoma may be CK7-/CK20—due to loss of specific marker expression, dual-negative staining is more consistent with HCC [17]. Polyclonal CEA (pCEA) and immunohistochemical stain, which cross-reacts with a CEA-like substance known as biliary glycoprotein present in the biliary canaliculi and ductal epithelium, are also useful in diagnosing metastatic HCC [11]. In HCC, pCEA typically stains in a canalicular pattern, characterized by short linear or branching linear staining between cells and dotlike positivity between adjacent cells [11]. The sensitivity of pCEA staining in HCC ranges shows between 70% and 100% [11]. Tumors that are less well differentiated have lower rates of positivity for pCEA: well-differentiated HCC shows pCEA positivity in 58%–100% of cases, moderately differentiated tumors show positivity in 25%–80% of cases, and poorly differentiated lesions show positivity in 0%–73% of cases [11]. Poorly differentiated HCC may exhibit diffuse cytoplasmic positivity rather than the characteristic canalicular pattern [11]. However, the specificity of the canalicular pattern of pCEA staining for HCC is exceptionally high, ranging from 97% to 100% [11]. In the context of a carcinoma, a canalicular pattern of pCEA positivity is considered specific for HCC [11]. Additionally, in cytologic specimens, pCEA staining has demonstrated a sensitivity of 82% and a specificity of 100% [11]. Tumor cells may also show positivity with periodic acid-Schiff (PAS) staining [11]. Immunohistochemical staining can reveal positivity for high molecular weight keratin (K903) [11]. Another useful immunohistochemical marker is CD10 (common acute lymphoblastic leukemia antigen, CALLA), a cell membrane metallopeptidase found in hematopoietic malignancies and various visceral carcinomas [11]. Similar to pCEA, it shows a canalicular staining pattern in both benign and malignant hepatocytes [11]. Although CD10 is less sensitive than pCEA, with reported positivity rates ranging from 40% to 68% in HCC, the canalicular pattern remains highly specific, approaching 100% [11]. Interestingly, there is a report of tumor cells from both a metastatic site and the liver staining positive for HMB-45 [23].

Immunostaining combined with albumin in situ hybridization (ISH) enhances the detection of metastatic HCC [3]. Albumin ISH, which detects albumin mRNA, is a reliable method for confirming hepatocellular differentiation, as albumin is synthesized exclusively by hepatocytes [24]. This technique demonstrates high sensitivity (93%–96%) and specificity (approaching 100%), although rare positivity has been reported in ovarian clear cell carcinoma and extrahepatic germ cell tumors with hepatoid features [24]. The combination of HepPar1 and albumin ISH offers high sensitivity and specificity for diagnosing HCC metastasis to the skin and is valuable in the differential diagnosis of poorly differentiated, cytokeratin-positive neoplasms [24].

It is important to illustrate the complementary molecular role of PET imaging alongside pathology, particularly when dual-tracer or multi-tracer PET is used in conjunction with pathology methods for cross-referencing and diagnostic confirmation [25].

8.1.5 Differential Diagnosis

Metastatic HCC) to the skin must be distinguished from other tumors, such as poorly differentiated squamous cell carcinoma, and metastatic tumors such as melanoma, adrenocortical carcinoma, renal cell carcinoma, cholangiocarcinoma, pancreatic islet cell tumor, carcinoid tumor, and poorly differentiated adenocarcinoma of the pancreas, colon, lung, stomach, esophagus, and urinary bladder [17].

HCC skin metastases can easily be mistaken for reactive cutaneous capillary endothelial proliferation (RCCEP), a common adverse event associated with camrelizumab treatment for advanced HCC [26]. During immunotherapy, the development of a large RCCEP-like lesion that fails to regress despite intensive treatment should raise the suspicion of possible skin metastasis [26].

8.1.6 Management

Surgery remains the first-line treatment for metastatic HCC to the skin, particularly for superficial lesions. Radiotherapy is a reasonable alternative in patients with advanced disease, poor performance status, or clinical scenarios where surgery is not feasible [5]. Partial response rates of 83.3% have been observed with radiation doses ranging from 8 to 64 Gy [5]. Following radiotherapy, the overall 6-month survival rate is 43.4%, and the 1-year survival rate is 22.8% [5]. Persistent cutaneous metastases can also be managed with transarterial embolization (TAE), which reduces lesion size and can be used in conjunction with systemic therapy for metastatic HCC [8]. For large primary tumors (>5 cm), systematic treatment is recommended both to prevent the development of cutaneous metastases and to improve prognosis following hepatectomy [9].

The hemorrhagic nature of metastatic HCC) has been widely reported. Patients with HCC and underlying cirrhosis often experience declining liver function, which disrupts the regulation of hemostasis at multiple levels. Decreased production of both coagulation factors and anticoagulant proteins contributes to an imbalance in hemostasis, resulting in a predisposition to both hypercoagulable and coagulopathic states. Additionally, thrombocytopenia due to increased splenic sequestration from splenomegaly has been described, further compounding bleeding risks. These factors can lead to excessive bleeding during surgical procedures [27].

8.2 Cholangiocarcinoma

8.2.1 Introduction and Epidemiology

Distant metastases of cholangiocarcinoma (CC) are common in patients with advanced disease and are associated with a poor prognosis [28]. Most cases of metastatic CC to the skin become clinically apparent within 3–30 months after the initial diagnosis [28]. The presentation of cutaneous metastases varies widely in anatomical location and clinical features, with a significant proportion involving either the scalp or the site of a previous percutaneous catheter [28]. Cutaneous metastases of CC are extremely rare, occurring in only 0.4–5.3% of cases [29]. In a few instances, cutaneous metastatic disease is the initial manifestation [28] and precedes the diagnosis of ductal CC [30]. Skin metastasis as the first sign of CC has been reported in approximately 27% of cases [31].

The incidence of catheter tract implantation metastasis has been reported to be approximately 3% [32]. The interval between drain placement and the diagnosis of cutaneous metastasis ranges from 3 to 30 months [32]. During this period, patients should be closely monitored for the development of subcutaneous metastasis along the catheter tract [32]. Some studies have suggested that catheter tract subcutaneous metastasis occurs more frequently in cases of well-differentiated CC [32].

8.2.2 Clinical Presentation

Cutaneous metastases of CC typically present as firm, painless to slightly tender subcutaneous nodules [28] (Fig. 8.6). Multiple nodules are observed in 46.4% of patients, while single nodules occur in 37.7% [29]. Most nodular lesions are covered by normal-appearing epithelium, which can lead to misdiagnosis as benign lesions [29]. Unique presentations have been reported, including multiple indurated plaques (Fig. 8.7) and papules on the chest, morphea-like lesions at the site of a percutaneous biliary drain exit, and a painless, indurated scalp ulcer with hemorrhagic crust [28]. Another unusual case involved a severely painful scalp metastasis that initially appeared as subcutaneous nodules and later recurred with spreading erythematous macules after irradiation [28]. Additional reported skin lesions include abscesses, ulcers [29], and ulcerated nodules [33].

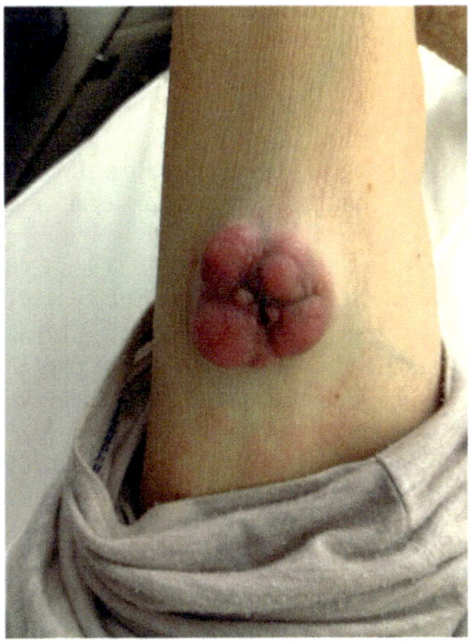

Fig. 8.6 Skin metastasis from cholangiocarcinoma. (Personal collection of Dr. D. Samonakis, University General Hospital of Heraklion, Greece)

8.2.3 Differential Diagnosis

The clinical differential diagnosis for CC metastases is broad and includes fibrous proliferation, panniculitis, granuloma, deposition diseases, infection, and abscess [28].

Biopsy pathology typically reveals a non-specific adenocarcinomatous appearance, and the immunohistochemical profile of CC is similarly non-specific, making clinical correlation essential for accurate diagnosis [28].

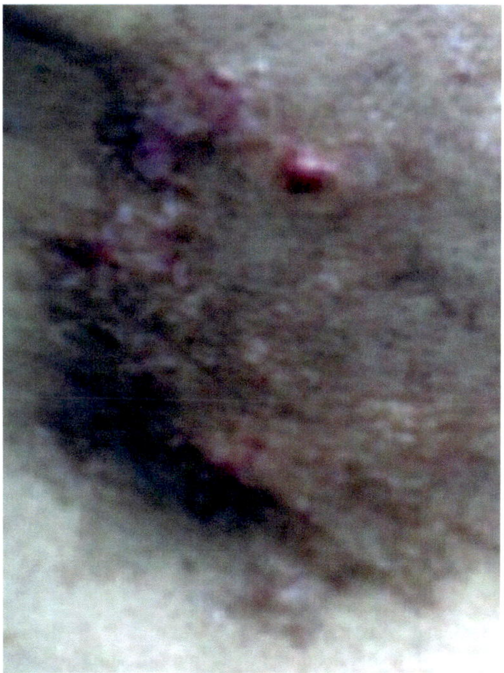

Fig. 8.7 A plaque in the periumbilical region of brownish color, with small tokens originating from the intrahepatic biliary tract. The 73-year-old male patient had been diagnosed five years earlier with intrahepatic cholangiocarcinoma. (From Cazzato et al. [28])

8.2.4 Immunohistochemical Findings

Primary cutaneous adenocarcinoma arising from adnexal structures is relatively rare, and distinguishing it from metastatic adenocarcinoma can be challenging [28]. In general, primary cutaneous carcinomas are more likely to express estrogen and progesterone receptors (ER/PR), GCDFP-15, CK15, p63, podoplanin (D2-40), and CK5/6 [28]. Combined positivity for p63, CK15, and podoplanin has been suggested as a strong indicator of primary cutaneous neoplasia, with p63 being the most sensitive marker and CK15 the most specific [28]. Notably, metastatic CC is negative for podoplanin and typically does not express p63 and CK5/6, although primary CC may occasionally express p63 [28]. While no immunohistochemical panel is pathognomonic for CC, tumors of biliary epithelial origin generally express CK7 and variably express CK20, while lacking CDX2 expression [28]. Immunohistochemical staining of a left temporal scalp skin nodule has shown positivity for CEA and CK 19 [29]. Additional staining demonstrates cytoplasmic positivity for cytokeratins 7–19, markers specific to biliary tract epithelium [34].

References

1. Hsu SW, Kao WY, Huang YM. Cutaneous metastasis from hepatocellular carcinoma: a rare cause of periumbilical bulging tumor. Asian J Surg. 2024;47(3):1472–4. https://doi.org/10.1016/j.asjsur.2023.11.136. Epub 2023 Dec 13. PMID: 38092597.
2. Amador A, Monforte NG, Bejarano N, Martí J, Artigau E, Navarro S, et al. Cutaneous metastasis from hepatocellular carcinoma as the first clinical sign. J Hepato-Biliary-Pancreat Surg. 2007;14(3):328–30. https://doi.org/10.1007/s00534-006-1141-1. Epub 2007 May 29. PMID: 17520212.
3. Gauger AJ, Li A, Fritz M, Katona TM, Alomari AK. Use of albumin in situ hybridization to diagnose cutaneous metastatic hepatocellular carcinoma with poorly differentiated features: a case report and review of the literature. Am J Dermatopathol. 2025;47(3):211–6. https://doi.org/10.1097/DAD.0000000000002854. Epub 2024 Oct 31. PMID: 39481028.
4. Terada T, Sugiura M. Metastatic hepatocellular carcinoma of skin diagnosed with hepatocyte paraffin 1 and a-fetoprotein immunostainings. Int J Surg Pathol. 2010;18(5):433–6. https://doi.org/10.1177/1066896908318743. Epub 2008 May 21. PMID: 18499685.
5. Tezcan Y, Koc M. Hepatocellular carcinoma with subcutaneous metastasis of the scalp. Radiol Oncol. 2011;45(4):292–5. https://doi.org/10.2478/v10019-011-0022-7. Epub 2011 Jul 20. PMID: 22933968; PMCID: PMC3423753.
6. de Agustín P, Conde E, Alberti N, Pérez-Barrios A, López-Ríos F. Cutaneous metastasis of occult hepatocellular carcinoma: a case report. Acta Cytol. 2007;51(2):214–6. https://doi.org/10.1159/000325720. PMID: 17425207.
7. Li S, Cai X, Yu K, Pan W. Nasal tip cutaneous metastasis of hepatocellular carcinoma: a case report. Clin Cosmet Investig Dermatol. 2023;(16):2893–7. https://doi.org/10.2147/CCID.S429480. PMID: 37869532; PMCID: PMC10590066.
8. Morishita A, Tani J, Oura K, Tadokoro T, Fujita K, Masaki T. Giant cutaneous metastasis from hepatocellular carcinoma. JGH Open. 2022;6(5):361–2. https://doi.org/10.1002/jgh3.12743. PMID: 35601124; PMCID: PMC9120903.
9. Jia J, Luo J, Zou B, Feng M, Liu L, Yu S, et al. Non-iatrogenic implantation of cutaneous metastasis from hepatocellular carcinoma. J Cancer Res Clin Oncol. 2023;149(4):1513–9. https://doi.org/10.1007/s00432-022-04030-0. Epub 2022 May 10. PMID: 35536361.
10. Huang YJ, Tung WC, Hsu HC, Wang CY, Huang EY, Fang FM. Radiation therapy to non-iatrogenic subcutaneous metastasis in hepatocellular carcinoma: results of a case series. Br J Radiol. 2008;81(962):143–50. https://doi.org/10.1259/bjr/81811976. PMID: 18238922
11. Royer MC, Rush WL, Lupton GP. Hepatocellular carcinoma presenting as a precocious cutaneous metastasis. Am J Dermatopathol. 2008;30(1):77–80. https://doi.org/10.1097/DAD.0b013e31815ea24f. PMID: 18212552
12. Isa NM, Bong JJ, Ghani FA, Rose IM, Husain S, Azrif M. Cutaneous metastasis of hepatocellular carcinoma diagnosed by fine needle aspiration cytology and Hep Par 1 immunopositivity. Diagn Cytopathol. 2012;40(11):1010–4. https://doi.org/10.1002/dc.21706. Epub 2011 May 11. PMID: 21563319.
13. Fang YR, Huang YS, Wu JC, Chao Y, Tsay SH, Chan CY, et al. An unusual cutaneous metastasis from hepatocellular carcinoma. Zhonghua Yi Xue Za Zhi (Taipei). 2001;64(4):253–7. PMID: 11458765
14. Kim JI, Song CH, Gong HS. Finger skin metastasis from hepatocellular carcinoma: a case report. Hand Surg. 2012;17(1):131–4. https://doi.org/10.1142/S0218810412720148. PMID: 22351551
15. Yamanishi K, Kishimoto S, Hosokawa Y, Yamada K, Yasuno H. Cutaneous metastasis from hepatocellular carcinoma resembling granuloma teleangiectaticum. J Dermatol. 1989;16(6):500–4. https://doi.org/10.1111/j.1346-8138.1989.tb01593.x. PMID: 2560782

16. Lee MC, Huang YL, Yang CH, Kuo TT, Hong HS. Cutaneous seeding of hepatocellular carcinoma due to percutaneous ethanol injection and masquerading as a pyogenic granuloma. Dermatologic Surg. 2004;30(3):438–40. https://doi.org/10.1111/j.1524-4725.2004.30120.x. PMID: 15008879
17. Queen D, Fisher J, Husain S, Linos K, Niedt GW, Samie FH. Cutaneous metastasis of hepatocellular carcinoma following liver transplantation. J Cutan Pathol. 2020;47(1):47–51. https://doi.org/10.1111/cup.13555. Epub 2019 Aug 22. PMID: 31381162.
18. Sanders K, Thomas A, Isache C, Siddiqi A. A rare case of metastatic hepatocellular carcinoma masquerading as a forehead hematoma. Case Rep Gastrointest Med. 2020;2020:8842936. https://doi.org/10.1155/2020/8842936. PMID: 33062352; PMCID: PMC7545472.
19. Polat G, Sade R. Calvarial mass confused with Trichilemmal cyst: hepatocellular cancer metastasis. J Craniofac Surg. 2017;28(2):e124–5. https://doi.org/10.1097/SCS.0000000000003298. PMID: 28005654
20. Kwon MJ, Ryu SH, Jo SY, Kwak CH, Yoon WJ, Moon JS, et al. A case of hepatocellular carcinoma presenting as a gingival mass. Korean J Gastroenterol. 2016;68(6):321–5. https://doi.org/10.4166/kjg.2016.68.6.321. PMID: 28025476
21. Pires FR, Sagarra R, Corrêa ME, Pereira CM, Vargas PA, Lopes MA. Oral metastasis of a hepatocellular carcinoma. Oral Surg Oral Med Oral Pathol Oral Radiol Endod. 2004;97(3):359–68. https://doi.org/10.1016/S1079210403006127. PMID: 15024361
22. de León FJ, Blanes MM, Albares MP, Berbegal L. Cutaneous metastasis from hepatocellular carcinoma after a percutaneous interventional procedure. Actas Dermosifiliogr. 2015;106(5):440–1. English, Spanish. https://doi.org/10.1016/j.ad.2014.10.014. Epub 2015 Jan 5. PMID: 25572905.
23. Gross JA, Perniciaro C, Gross DJ, Barksdale SK. Metastatic hepatocellular carcinoma to the skin staining positive with HMB-45. Am J Dermatopathol. 2012;34(1):110–2. https://doi.org/10.1097/DAD.0b013e3182104182. PMID: 22262362
24. Wood AJ, Lappinga PJ, Ahmed I. Hepatocellular carcinoma metastatic to skin: diagnostic utility of antihuman hepatocyte antibody in combination with albumin in situ hybridization. J Cutan Pathol. 2009;36(2):262–6. https://doi.org/10.1111/j.1600-0560.2008.01029.x. Epub 2008 Aug 24. PMID: 18727662.
25. Ho I, Chen S, Yip Y, Ho CL. The complementary role of PET to pathology in differentiating the primary origin of a malignant skin nodule from liver or lung. Nucl Med Mol Imaging. 2023;57(1):38–43. https://doi.org/10.1007/s13139-022-00777-z. Epub 2022 Oct 10. PMID: 36643947; PMCID: PMC9832204.
26. Liu J, Cao G, Zhang G, Liu S, Shi D. Nasal alar metastasis of advanced hepatocellular carcinoma misdiagnosed as reactive cutaneous capillary endothelial proliferation in a patient treated with camrelizumab and apatinib: a case report. J Gastrointest Oncol. 2023;14(3):1643–9. https://doi.org/10.21037/jgo-23-336. Epub 2023 Jun 25. PMID: 37435210; PMCID: PMC10331753
27. Ferraz VR, Vitorino-Araújo JL, Sementilli L, Neto JF, Veiga JC. Lesion in scalp and skull as the first manifestation of hepatocellular carcinoma. Case Rep Neurol Med. 2016;2016:2897048. https://doi.org/10.1155/2016/2897048. Epub 2016 Jun 14. PMID: 27403358; PMCID: PMC4923563.
28. Cazzato G, Colagrande A, Cimmino A, De Marco A, Romita P, Foti C, et al. Cutaneous metastases from primary liver cancers: the need for knowledge and differential diagnosis. Life (Basel). 2021;11(6):559. https://doi.org/10.3390/life11060559. PMID: 34198568; PMCID: PMC8231899.
29. Nagaoka Y, Nakayama R, Iwata M. Cutaneous seeding following percutaneous ethanol injection therapy for hepatocellular carcinoma. Intern Med. 2004;43(3):268–9. https://doi.org/10.2169/internalmedicine.43.268. PMID: 15098615
30. West KL, Selim MA, Puri PK. Cutaneous metastatic cholangiocarcinoma: a report of three cases and review of the literature. J Cutan Pathol. 2010;37(12):1230–6. https://doi.org/10.1111/j.1600-0560.2010.01619.x. Epub 2010 Sep 30. PMID: 20883451.
31. Hyun SY, Lee JH, Shin HS, Lee SW, Park YN, Park JY. Cutaneous metastasis from cholangiocarcinoma as the first clinical sign: a report of two cases. Gut Liver. 2011;5(1):100–4. https://doi.org/10.5009/gnl.2011.5.1.100. Epub 2011 Mar 16. PMID: 21461082; PMCID: PMC3065084.
32. Stergiopoulos C, Kountouras J, Kapetanakis N, Katsinelos P, Kokkali S, Tsapournas G, et al. Distant cutaneous metastasis preceding the diagnosis of ductal cholangiocarcinoma. J Eur Acad Dermatol Venereol. 2009;23(2):242–3. https://doi.org/10.1111/j.1468-3083.2008.02845.x. Epub 2008 Jun 11. PMID: 18554225.
33. Varma K, Singh A, Misra V. Cutaneous metastasis from cholangiocarcinoma presenting as thigh mass. J Clin Diagn Res. 2016;10(9):ED23–5. https://doi.org/10.7860/JCDR/2016/21524.8584. Epub 2016 Sep 1. PMID: 27790452; PMCID: PMC5071952
34. Geramizadeh B, Giti R, Malekhosseini SA. Cutaneous metastasis of cholangiocarcinoma: report of two cases. Int J Organ Transplant Med. 2013;4(4):172–4. PMID: 25013671; PMCID: PMC4089326

Cutaneous Metastasis from Gastric Cancer

9

Dimitra Koumaki, Georgios Skoulas, Nikolaos Galanakis, and Eleni Lagoudaki

Abstract

Cutaneous metastasis from gastric cancer is an uncommon but clinically significant presentation of advanced disease, representing approximately 0.8% of gastric cancer patients. It presents in most cases in elderly adults and more often in men, with the most frequent association being with poorly differentiated adenocarcinoma, particularly the signet-ring cell type. Clinically, cutaneous metastases usually manifest as painless, hard nodules, which are multiple and located on the thoracoabdominal wall but may also take the form of benign dermatoses resulting in diagnostic delay. Inflammatory and scar-like manifestations have been reported, especially with signet-ring cell carcinoma. Diagnosis relies on high suspicion, histopathological analysis, and immunohistochemical characterization to distinguish metastatic lesions from primary cutaneous neoplasms. Dermoscopy may reveal nonspecific vascular and structureless patterns, helping in the selection of the biopsy site. Imaging, like PET-CT or CT, helps in staging and extracutaneous metastasis assessment. Synchronous visceral involvement is the mode of presentation in the majority of patients, and skin metastasis may be the initial sign of systemic spread in a very high percentage of cases. The prognosis is poor with a median overall survival of 6 months, but surgical resection of solitary lesions might provide long-term survival in some cases. Treatment is primarily systemic chemotherapy, and palliative surgical resection can be provided for symptomatic or solitary lesions. Early diagnosis and multidisciplinary management are sine qua non in optimizing the outcome in this rare but serious clinical presentation.

Keywords

Skin metastasis · Gastric cancer · Signet-ring cell carcinoma · Cutaneous metastasis · Prognosis · Histopathology · Diagnosis · Dermoscopy · Systemic chemotherapy · Multidisciplinary management

D. Koumaki (✉)
Dermatology Department, University Hospital of Heraklion, Heraklion, Greece

G. Skoulas
University of Crete Medical School, Voutes University Campus, Heraklion, Greece

N. Galanakis
Interventional Radiology Unit, Department of Medical Imaging, University Hospital of Heraklion, Heraklion, Greece

E. Lagoudaki
Pathology Department, University Hospital of Heraklion, Heraklion, Greece

D. Koumaki et al. (eds.), *Cutaneous Metastases*, https://doi.org/10.1007/978-3-032-26764-1_9

9.1 Introduction

Cutaneous metastasis of gastric cancer is a rare but significant presentation of advanced malignancy [1–3]. It typically presents as hard, nontender nodules, most often on the thoracoabdominal wall, and has a strong association with poorly differentiated adenocarcinoma, especially the signet-ring cell type [4–12]. Diagnosis is based on clinical suspicion, histopathology, and immunohistochemistry, and dermoscopy and imaging are assists. Therapy is primarily systemic chemotherapy, and surgery is reserved for exceptional cases. Prognosis is poor with a median survival of 6 months, though an isolated resectable lesion can confer longer survival.

9.2 Epidemiology

Cutaneous metastasis of gastric cancer occurs in approximately 0.8% of gastric cancers. A recent review by Yao GL et al. reported a male predominance in 72.2% (52/72) of cases and an average age of 60 ± SD 16 years [1]. The majority are associated with poorly differentiated adenocarcinoma (87.5%), and 66.1% contain signet-ring cell elements. The most frequent location is the thoracoabdominal wall (56.9%), but lesions may be found on the scalp, face, and limbs. The majority of patients have multiple nodular lesions (61.1%), and 64.7% present with synchronous extracutaneous metastases. Cutaneous metastasis can be the initial manifestation of metastatic dissemination in as many as 40.8% of cases.

9.3 Timing and Presentation

Cutaneous metastases may develop in patients with gastric cancer both synchronously and metachronously with respect to the original diagnosis. About 40% occur as the initial presentation of metastatic disease, i.e., the skin lesions can emerge prior to or concomitantly with the diagnosis of systemic relapse or progression, while the rest develop metachronously, usually months to years following primary tumor treatment [13–20].

The timing of skin metastasis in gastric cancer is highly variable: cutaneous metastases can occur within several months of the initial diagnosis, typically with widespread visceral disease, in a proportion of patients, while in others there is delayed cutaneous disease presenting years after curative gastrectomy, as has been reported in case series of signet-ring cell carcinoma where skin metastases have developed up to 7 years after surgery.

Synchronous cutaneous metastasis—when both skin and other metastasis sites are involved at the same time—generally represents aggressive tumor biology and is associated with a more rapid disease course and unfavorable prognosis. Metachronous cutaneous metastasis—when there is a period of disease-free status before cutaneous lesions occur—may also represent recurrence, but in either scenario, cutaneous involvement invariably represents advanced disseminated disease and is associated with a median survival of approximately 6 months from the time of diagnosis of skin metastasis.

In Yao et al.'s study, among 71 gastric cancer patients who were capable of specifying the time of cutaneous metastasis, 29 patients (40.8%) developed cutaneous metastases simultaneously with the diagnosis of their primary gastric cancer, while 42 patients (59.2%) developed cutaneous metastases after the diagnosis of their gastric cancer [1]. The median interval between the initial diagnosis of cancer and the occurrence of cutaneous metastasis was 53.6 months, with a very wide standard deviation (±63.4 months), indicating great variability in time.

In terms of the diagnostic process, among the 52 patients with available information, a pathological diagnosis of cutaneous metastasis was established in only 5 (9.6%) of them at initial presentation of the skin lesion. The remaining 47 patients (90.4%) developed delayed diagnosis with an average delay of 3.9 months (±4.2 months) from the initial presentation of the skin lesion to pathological confirmation. This highlights that delayed diagnosis and awareness of cutaneous metastasis are common in gastric cancer, and often, there is a delay between clinical presentation and definitive diagnosis.

Cutaneous metastases from gastric cancer may arise at any stage of the disease, either as an initial sign of dissemination or as a late development, and their appearance is a sign of aggressive disease with poor prognosis.

9.4 Clinical Appearance

The clinical presentation of skin metastasis from gastric cancer is heterogeneous, and various morphologic patterns have been described in the literature [4–20]. Most commonly, the nodular form is observed, manifesting as firm, painless, flesh-colored to erythematous nodules (Fig. 9.1a). They are often numerous, ranging from several millimeters to several centimeters, and most frequently appear on the thoracoabdominal wall but can also appear on the head, neck, groin, or extremities. Nodular lesions were present in approximately 45.8% of cases in a recent series, and the majority of patients had multiple lesions.

The erysipelas-like (inflammatory) type is less common but clinically significant due to its resemblance to inflammatory or infectious dermatoses. The lesions are erythematous, edematous, warm plaques with sometimes ill-defined borders, mimicking cellulitis or erysipelas. It may be incorrectly diagnosed and treated, with a delay in the correct management. At times, the inflammatory presentation can mimic livedo reticularis or acute dermatitis, as noted in case reports, which further complicates the diagnosis.

Plaque-type metastases are seen as indurated, infiltrative, or sclerodermoid plaques. They may mimic morphea, lichen simplex, or other chronic

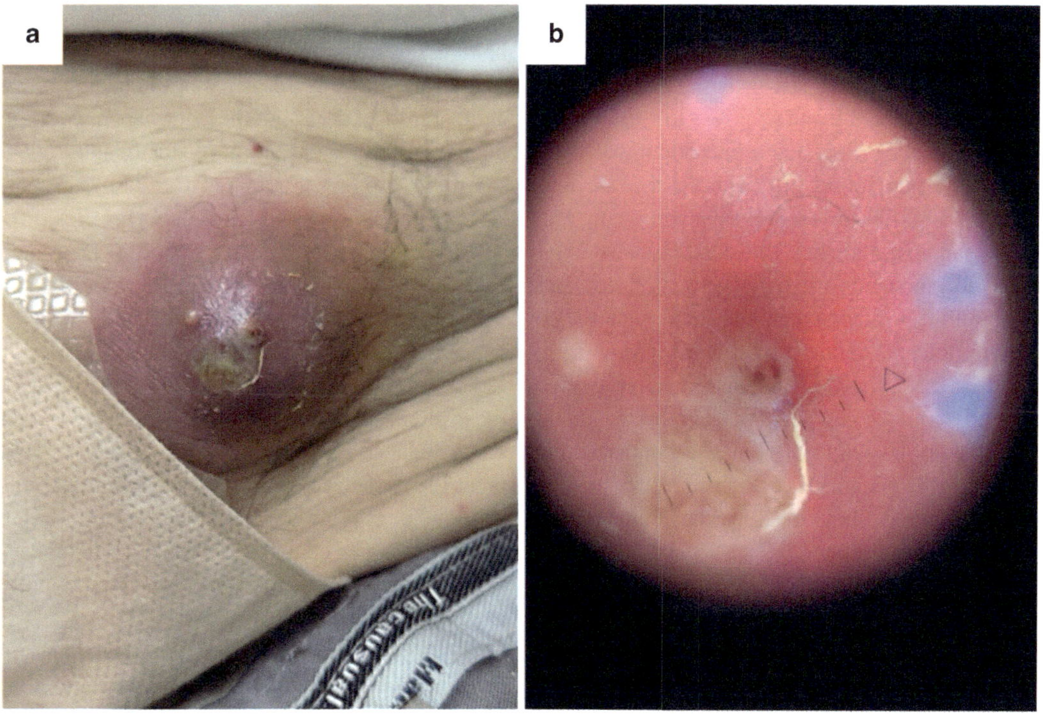

Fig. 9.1 (**a**) Clinical appearance of a violaceous, crateriform nodule measuring approximately 4 × 5 cm, showing central ulceration and necrotic crust, characteristic of cutaneous metastasis. The lesion is located on the lower left abdomen of an 80-year-old man with a prior history of poorly differentiated tubular-solid type gastric adenocarcinoma. (**b**) Polarized dermoscopy of the nodular lesion with a pink-violaceous structureless background and polymorphous vascular structures (linear, irregular, arborizing, and serpentine vessels), yellow-white necrotic central areas, whitish areas showing fibrosis, and ulceration with hemorrhagic crusts

dermatoses. The plaques are usually firm and non-tender and may be associated with overlying skin changes in the form of hyperpigmentation or ulceration. Scar-like or sclerotic lesions have also been reported, particularly in individuals with signet-ring cell histology.

Atypical presentations include ulcerated lesions, subcutaneous nodules, and livedoid or reticular patterns. Ulceration may occur in late stages, while subcutaneous metastases may mimic benign cysts or lipomas. Livedoid patterns are rare but have been described with signet-ring cell carcinoma and may present with reticulated, violaceous patches.

Diagnosis is difficult due to the nonspecificity of these lesions, their ability to mimic benign or inflammatory dermatologic conditions, and the frequently delayed biopsy and histopathologic diagnosis. Only a small percentage of cases are diagnosed at the time of lesion formation, whereas most require a high index of suspicion and early biopsy for diagnosis.

Ulcerated skin metastases from gastric carcinoma are typically fast-growing nodules or plaques that ulcerate and progress to form ulcers with irregular borders and a necrotic base. They are most often found in advanced disease and may be painful or secondarily infected. The ulceration distinguishes these metastases from more common non-ulcerated firm nodules and may mimic primary cutaneous malignancies or chronic ulcers, rendering clinical recognition less straightforward. Diagnosis is difficult since ulcerating metastatic lesions may be mistaken for infectious or inflammatory processes. Especially in patients without a previous history of malignancy, they need to have an urgent biopsy for diagnosis.

Subcutaneous nodules are firm, deep, sometimes mobile nodules beneath the skin surface. They may have no apparent epidermal changes and hence are less conspicuous than superficial plaques or nodules. They may be mistaken for benign lesions such as lipomas or epidermal cysts when they are painless and slowly enlarging. Subcutaneous metastases in gastric cancer are usually multiple and may be associated with other evidence of systemic disease. Their deep location and insidious onset may result in delayed diagnosis, particularly if they occur in atypical sites or in patients with a distant history of gastric cancer.

Reticular or livedoid patterns are unusual presentations, with violaceous or erythematous, net-like patches reminiscent of livedo reticularis. The lesions may be mistaken for vascular or inflammatory dermatoses, such as vasculitis or connective tissue disease. The literature describes cases where livedoid cutaneous metastasis of signet-ring cell gastric cancer mimicked benign vascularities, creating diagnostic confusion and postponing biopsy. Unlike nodular or ulcerated types, livedoid metastases are often non-tender and may be chronic or recalcitrant to standard dermatological treatments.

Each of these forms—ulcerated lesions, subcutaneous masses, and livedoid/reticular patterns—deviates from the more common nodular or erysipelas-like presentations by virtue of their atypical morphology and frequent mimicry of benign or inflammatory dermatoses. The main diagnostic challenge is the lack of specific clinical features, underlining the importance of a high degree of suspicion and early histopathological sampling in patients with a history of gastric carcinoma and new, unexplained cutaneous lesions.

9.5 Dermoscopic Findings

Dermoscopy is recognized as a useful adjunct for the evaluation of cutaneous metastases, including gastric cancer. Cutaneous metastases are rare, but their identification has significant ramifications in terms of staging and prognosis. Dermoscopic examination can enable early detection and expedited biopsy, especially in atypical clinically appearing lesions [21].

The most common dermoscopic characteristic of nonpigmented skin metastases is a vascular pattern, observed in almost all cases. Serpentine (linear irregular) vessels are the most frequent subtype, and they are typically accompanied by arborizing, dotted, or comma-shaped vessels (Fig. 9.1b). Such vascular elements are typically discrete and can be admixed within a single lesion. In some, a homogeneous pink or structureless white area is observed, without distinct vessels. The structureless white pattern is a very sensitive indicator for cutaneous metastasis, regardless of the primary tumor, in over 80% of cases in large series [22–28].

Pigmentation in gastric cancer metastasis is uncommon but can mimic other malignancies, such as melanoma or pigmented basal cell carcinoma, if present. Pigmented patterns are more typical of breast cancer or melanoma metastases, and identification in a patient without a history of melanoma should prompt the question of other primaries.

Dermoscopy does not give pathognomonic features of gastric cancer itself, but the detection of atypical vascular patterns, structureless white or pink pigmentation, and evolutionary change in a case of established gastric cancer must arouse suspicion of metastatic disease. Preliminary biopsy is still most important for definitive diagnosis, but dermoscopy may direct clinical suspicion and speed histopathological examination.

In conclusion, dermoscopy is a sensitive, non-invasive complement to the diagnosis of cutaneous metastases of gastric cancer, and the most informative features are vascular and structureless patterns. Its use may increase diagnostic precision and enable timely intervention in patients with oncology.

9.6 Diagnosis

Diagnosis of skin metastasis from gastric carcinoma depends heavily on clinical suspicion, particularly in individuals with a history of gastric carcinoma who develop new, persistent, or atypical cutaneous lesions. Clinical presentation alone is insufficient because these lesions disguise themselves as benign or inflammatory dermatological conditions. Confirmatory diagnosis is by histopathologic examination of a skin biopsy, which is required to exclude primary cutaneous neoplasms and metastatic deposits [29–31].

Immunohistochemistry is essential to establish gastric derivation and rule out other primary skin carcinomas, melanoma, and metastasis of different origins. Cytokeratin 7 (CK7), cytokeratin 20 (CK20), and CDX2 are markers characteristically expressed in metastatic gastric adenocarcinoma and clinch the diagnosis. Comparative immunoprofiling of the primary tumor and the skin lesion may be necessary in doubtful cases.

Dermoscopy is also a useful non-invasive modality for the preliminary assessment of suspicious skin lesions, often demonstrating atypical vascular patterns and structureless white or pink areas, which can guide biopsy decision-making [21–25]. PET-CT and CT imaging modalities are useful for staging and determining the extent of systemic involvement but do not eliminate the need for histopathological diagnosis.

Early detection and prompt biopsy, followed by immunohistochemical profiling, are important for accurate diagnosis and appropriate management of skin metastasis from gastric cancer.

9.7 Histopathology Findings

The histopathological features of skin metastasis of gastric carcinoma are typically infiltration of the dermis and, at times, the subcutis by neoplastic epithelial cells, most often in nodular, infiltrative, or diffuse patterns. Metastatic deposits are almost always dermal-centered, underneath a usually intact epidermis. Histologically, metastatic tumor deposits can assimilate the primary tumor's characteristics and consist of tubular or glandular structures of neoplastic cells usually containing apical mucin vacuoles, as in the intestinal type of gastric adenocarcinoma, or consist of diffusely infiltrating signet-ring cells when the primary tumor is of the diffuse type but are usually less differentiated compared to the primary tumor. In metastases of diffuse-type gastric carcinoma (Fig. 9.2), cells typically exhibit signet-ring morphology, in which a large intracellular mucin-containing vacuole displaces the nucleus to the periphery. Since neither glandular structures nor signet-ring formation is specific for cel-

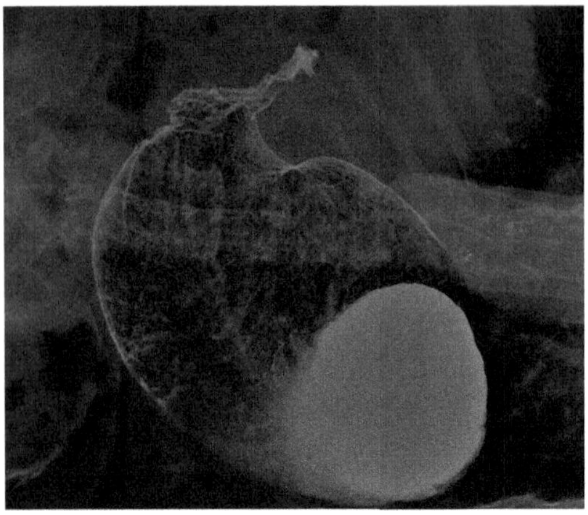

Fig. 9.2 Barium meal examination in a 76-year-old female patient with a history of poorly differentiated gastric adenocarcinoma reveals significant luminal narrowing in the prepyloric region of the antrum, measuring approximately 6 cm in length. The lesion demonstrates relative asymmetry, a micronodular contour, and microerosions, findings consistent with an infiltrative-type neoplastic process

lular lineage but can manifest in a variety of neoplasms, immunohistochemical evaluation is mandatory to confirm gastric origin. The differential diagnosis mainly involves primary adnexal skin carcinomas, and when signet-ring morphology is present, it encompasses undifferentiated primary skin carcinomas, most commonly, among others, squamous and basal cell skin carcinomas, but also malignant melanoma, and, importantly, metastasis from other organs. The latter mainly comprises metastatic lobular breast carcinoma and metastatic prostatic adenocarcinoma. An immunohistochemical study is mandatory to confirm gastric origin. An immunophenotype consisting of the combination of CK7 and CK20, CDX2, and MUC-5 AC expression supports the diagnosis of metastatic gastric adenocarcinoma. Histochemical staining with mucin stains such as Alcian blue (Fig. 9.2) can highlight the presence of intracellular mucin in the cytoplasm of the metastatic tumor cells [4–20].

Clinicopathologic correlation with strong clinical suspicion is the most important consideration in the patient with established gastric cancer presenting with new, persistent, or atypical cutaneous lesions.

9.8 Other Noninvasive Diagnostic Techniques

Confocal microscopy—reflectance confocal microscopy (RCM)—is an advanced, non-invasive imaging technique that allows visualization of the skin in vivo at nearly histological resolution, allowing real-time visualization of micro-anatomic structures and cellular morphology within cutaneous lesions. The majority of the published clinical experience has been with melanoma and non-melanoma skin cancers, but RCM has proved to be useful in indeterminate skin tumor analysis, including cutaneous metastases, by providing high-resolution morphologic detail and reducing unnecessary biopsies. RCM can identify atypical clusters of tumor cells, architectural disorder, increased vascularity, and alteration of collagen, which can suggest metastatic disease. Multimodal devices that combine RCM and optical coherence tomography (OCT) have allowed for simultaneous horizontal and vertical imaging in recent series of cases, improving the detection and characterization of cutaneous metastases, including their differentiation from benign mimics.

RCM is complementary to other non-invasive modalities. Dermoscopy is becoming more commonly used for initial assessment, reflecting vascular and structureless patterns which might guide suspicion of metastasis. Skin ultrasound provides information on the depth of lesions, vascularity, and subclinical spread and is complementary to surgical planning.

High-frequency skin ultrasound is a non-invasive imaging technique that can delineate cutaneous and subcutaneous lesions and evaluate depth, vascularity, and involvement of contiguous structures. It can be used to distinguish metastatic nodules from benign or inflammatory conditions and as a biopsy guide.

Gastroscopy is required for direct visualization and biopsy of the primary gastric lesion, especially when cutaneous metastasis is the initial symptom.

Advanced radiologic imaging—with and without contrast, PET-CT, and magnetic resonance imaging (MRI)—continues to be important in staging, extracutaneous disease detection, and guidance for management.

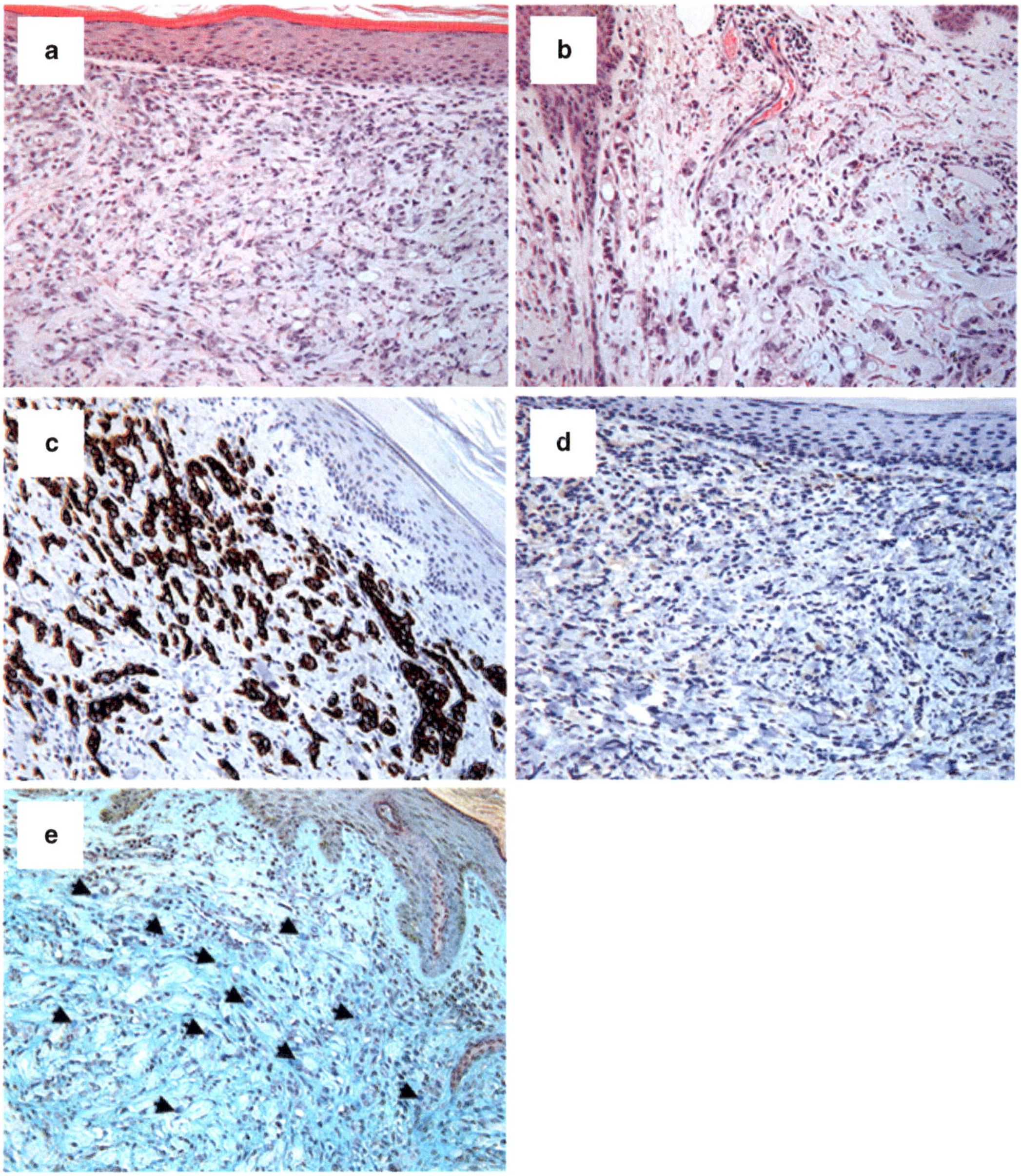

Fig. 9.3 Microscopic examination of the excised nodule of the scapula of a 76-year-old female patient with a past medical history of a poorly differentiated gastric adenocarcinoma shows extensive infiltration of the dermis by small clusters, scattered individual cells, and poorly formed glandular and cribriform structures of neoplastic cells showing no connection with the epidermis (**a**) or with skin adnexa (**b**), compatible with cutaneous metastasis showing no diagnostic morphologic traits of the primary origin tumor. Immunohistochemical staining was positive for CK7 (**c**) and CDX2 (not shown) and negative for CK20 (**d**). Furthermore, histochemical staining with Alcian blue stain highlighted the presence of globoid droplets of cytoplasmic mucin in the cytoplasm of scattered neoplastic cells (**e**)—*arrowheads*. While morphology was not specific, the immunophenotype was compatible with metastatic poorly differentiated adenocarcinoma of gastric origin. **a** & **b**: H/E ×40 magnification, **c**: CK7 ×100 magnification, **d**: CK20 ×100 magnification, **e**: *Alcian blue stain* ×100 magnification

High-frequency skin ultrasound can assess the depth, vascularity, and subclinical spread of lesions, distinguish between metastatic nodules and inflammatory or benign processes, and aid in biopsy and surgical planning guidance.

Contrast-enhanced computed tomography (CT) is the first imaging method for gastric cancer staging and surgical or neoadjuvant planning. It can be used to assess tumor extension, regional nodal involvement, and distant metastases. It can also depict mural thickening, ulceration, and nodularity of the gastric wall and highlight complications such as obstruction or bleeding. Fasting, gastric distention, and intravenous contrast are requirements in CT protocols to allow for the best evaluation [32–34]. Positron emission tomography-computed tomography (PET-CT) offers sensitivity for the detection of metabolically active lesions, including occult cutaneous and systemic metastasis, and is particularly useful in the detection of hypermetabolic nodules not visible on CT alone.

Magnetic resonance imaging (MRI) using diffusion-weighted and dynamic contrast-enhanced techniques is not routinely used to evaluate gastric cancer. However, it has particular value in assessing peritoneal and hepatic metastases (especially with liver-specific contrast agents and diffusion-weighted imaging).

Upper GI series with barium or water-soluble contrast historically played a major role in detecting gastric cancer by outlining mass lesions, mucosal irregularities, or obstructive patterns, but its use has declined significantly with the advent of endoscopy. They are now used as adjunctive studies, reserved for cases where endoscopy is contraindicated or incomplete, for evaluating gastric outlet obstruction, or for assessing postoperative anatomy and anastomotic integrity after gastrectomy. (Fig. 9.3).

9.9 Dissemination Patterns

Gastric carcinoma metastasizes by lymphatic, hematogenous, and transperitoneal routes, most typically involving the thoracoabdominal wall but also reported in distant sites such as the head, groin, and extremities. Imaging needs to be context-dependent, with high suspicion of atypical or unresponsive skin lesions in those with a past medical history of gastric carcinoma.

Multidisciplinary management: Radiologic findings must be correlated with clinical, dermatologic, and histopathologic information for accurate diagnosis and staging. Early detection and complete imaging evaluation are essential to determine management and enhance prognosis, considering the dismal prognosis of cutaneous metastasis of gastric cancer.

9.10 Disease Course

The disease course is typically aggressive, with cutaneous metastases occurring late in the disease or, in a minority, as an initial manifestation of metastatic dissemination. Most patients present with synchronous visceral metastases, and cutaneous metastasis is associated with more rapid progression and with poor prognosis.

9.11 Prognosis

The prognosis is poor, with a median survival of 6 months after cutaneous metastasis diagnosis. A single resectable lesion can give longer survival (median 48 months in a rare case), but most patients have extensive disease and limited therapy [35–40].

9.12 Management

The treatment is mostly systemic chemotherapy, modified according to the gastric cancer histology and prior treatment. Systemic chemotherapy is the most common treatment modality (65.6%), in the form of regimens containing platinum-based agents and fluoropyrimidines. Palliative surgical excision can be provided in isolated or symptomatic lesions, potentially improving quality of life and, very rarely, survival. Multidisciplinary treatment, involving oncologists, dermatologists, and surgeons, is vital for the best management. Isolated lesions can be managed with local excision and disseminated disease with systemic therapy. Radiotherapy is a palliative option for symptomatic lesions, but evidence is scarce.

In summary, skin metastasis of gastric cancer is an uncommon but clinically important one, most often seen in the context of extensive disease and high-grade histologic tumor types. Prompt recognition, timely biopsy, and multidisciplinary care are needed to optimize outcomes. Prognosis, despite systemic improvement, remains poor, and additional research and improved diagnostic methods are needed [41–48].

References

1. Yao GL, Tao YJ, Fan YG. Cutaneous metastasis from gastric cancer: manifestation, diagnosis, treatment and prognosis. Eur J Surg Oncol. 2024;50(2):107939. https://doi.org/10.1016/j.ejso.2023.107939. Epub 2023 Dec 28. PMID: 38219697.
2. Kawai S, Nishida T, Hayashi Y, Ezaki H, Yamada T, Shinzaki S, Miyazaki M, Nakai K, Yakushijin T, Watabe K, Iijima H, Tsujii M, Nishida K, Takehara T. Choroidal and cutaneous metastasis from gastric adenocarcinoma. World J Gastroenterol. 2013;19(9):1485–8. https://doi.org/10.3748/wjg.v19.i9.1485. PMID: 23538460.
3. Vernemmen AIP, Li X, Roemen GMJM, Speel EM, Kubat B, Hausen AZ, Winnepenninckx VJL, Samarska IV. Cutaneous metastases of internal malignancies: a single-institution experience. Histopathology. 2022;81(3):329–41. https://doi.org/10.1111/his.14705. Epub 2022 Jul 20. PMID: 35758186.
4. Demircioğlu D, Öztürk Durmaz E, Demirkesen C, Şahin S. Livedoid cutaneous metastasis of signet-ring cell gastric carcinoma. J Cutan Pathol. 2021;48(6):785–8. https://doi.org/10.1111/cup.13969. Epub 2021 Feb 8. PMID: 33476049.
5. Yao S, Zhou P, Li Y, Li Q. Case report: a case of delayed cutaneous metastases from signet-ring cell mixed-type gastric cancer. Front Oncol. 2023;13:1105080. https://doi.org/10.3389/fonc.2023.1105080. eCollection 2023. PMID: 36923441.
6. Kobayashi O, Murakami H, Yoshida T, Cho H, Yoshikawa T, Tsuburaya A, Sairenji M, Motohashi H, Sugiyama Y, Kameda Y. Clinical diagnosis of metastatic gastric tumors: clinicopathologic findings and prognosis of nine patients in a single cancer center. World J Surg. 2004;28(6):548–51. https://doi.org/10.1007/s00268-004-7216-8. PMID: 15366743.
7. Eckardt AM, Back W. Facial cutaneous metastases of gastric signet-ring cell carcinoma: resection and reconstruction as a palliative surgical treatment option. In Vivo. 2022;36(3):1508–12. https://doi.org/10.21873/invivo.12859. PMID: 35478122.
8. Frey L, Vetter-Kauczok C, Gesierich A, Bröcker EB, Ugurel S. Cutaneous metastases as the first clinical sign of metastatic gastric carcinoma. J Dtsch Dermatol Ges. 2009;7(10):893–5. https://doi.org/10.1111/j.1610-0387.2009.07102.x. PMID: 19538484.
9. Koo DH, Chang HM, Jung JY, Song JH, Lee JL, Ryu MH, Kim TW, Yook JH, Song JS, Lee JS, Kang YK. Cutaneous metastasis resembling acute dermatitis in patient with advanced gastric cancer. Clin Exp Dermatol. 2007;32(3):284–6. https://doi.org/10.1111/j.1365-2230.2007.02361.x. Epub 2007 Jan 30. PMID: 17263831.
10. De Giorgi V, Scarfì F, Trane L, Silvestri F, Maida P, Gori A, Covarelli P. Appearance of cutaneous melanoma and subcutaneous metastases in metastatic gastric carcinoma undergoing chemotherapy with oral 5-fluorouracil prodrug. Anti-Cancer Drugs. 2019;30(10):1055–7. https://doi.org/10.1097/CAD.0000000000000828. PMID: 31609761.
11. Schadt CR. The cutaneous manifestations of gastrointestinal malignancy. Semin Oncol. 2016;43(3):341–6. https://doi.org/10.1053/j.seminoncol.2016.02.028. Epub 2016 Feb 23. PMID: 27178686.
12. Yang S, Liu XL, Guo XL, Song B, Li SZ, Sun XF, Feng Y. Solitary metastasis to the skin and colon from gastric cancer after curative gastrectomy and chemotherapy: a case report. Medicine (Baltimore). 2020;99(31):e21532. https://doi.org/10.1097/MD.0000000000021532. PMID: 32756202
13. Sakhri S, Zemni I, Mansouri H, Boujelbene N, BenDhiab T. Cutaneous metastasis from gastrointestinal cancer: a rare presentation: case series. Int J Surg Case Rep. 2025;129:111158. https://doi.org/10.1016/j.ijscr.2025.111158. Epub 2025 Mar 14. PMID: 40106942.
14. Silva A, Monteiro N, Mateia E, Santos I, Correia M. Cutaneous metastasis in advanced gastric cancer. Acta Medica Port. 2025;38(3):202–3. https://doi.org/10.20344/amp.22555. Epub 2025 Jan 30. PMID: 39882740.
15. Kurmus GI, Canpolat F, Gönül M, Gökçe A, Kartal SP. Cutaneous metastases of signet-ring cell gastric carcinoma: a case report. Curr Health Sci J. 2024;50(3):444–7. https://doi.org/10.12865/CHSJ.50.03.12. Epub 2024 Sep 30. PMID: 39574817.
16. Hao W, Chang R, Liu J, Wang Y, Ren M, Xin K, Liu B, Xie J, Yang Y. Case report: a case of advanced gastric cancer with multiple skin metastases, with significant relief from immunotherapy. Front Immunol. 2024;15:1356350. https://doi.org/10.3389/fimmu.2024.1356350. eCollection 2024. PMID: 38500887.
17. Navarro V, Ramón D, Calduch L, Llombart B, Monteagudo C, Jordá E. Cutaneous metastasis of gastric adenocarcinoma: an unusual clinical presentation. Eur J Dermatol. 2002;12(1):85–7. PMID: 11809606.

18. Koyama R, Maeda Y, Minagawa N, Shinohara T, Hamada T. Late cutaneous metastasis originating from gastric cancer with synchronous metastasis. Case Rep Gastroenterol. 2019;13(1):95–101. https://doi.org/10.1159/000497099. eCollection 2019 Jan-Apr. PMID: 31043935.
19. Gündüz Ö, Emeksiz MC, Atasoy P, Kidir M, Yalçin S, Demirkan S. Signet-ring cells in the skin: a case of late-onset cutaneous metastasis of gastric carcinoma and a brief review of histological approach. Dermatol Reports. 2017;8(1):6819. https://doi.org/10.4081/dr.2016.6819. eCollection 2016 Jun 15. PMID: 28326183.
20. Ghosh J, Arun I, Ganguly A, Ganguly S. Cutaneous metastases in a patient with adenocarcinoma of the stomach. Indian J Dermatol Venereol Leprol. 2021;87(5):699–701. https://doi.org/10.25259/IJDVL_657_20. PMID: 34114411.
21. Ho PA, Shi RY, Oh CC. Dermatoscopic features of cutaneous metastasis in advanced gastric cancer. JAAD Case Rep. 2022;23:174–5. https://doi.org/10.1016/j.jdcr.2022.02.029. eCollection 2022 May. PMID: 35519795.
22. Chernoff KA, Marghoob AA, Lacouture ME, Deng L, Busam KJ, Myskowski PL. Dermoscopic findings in cutaneous metastases. JAMA Dermatol. 2014;150(4):429–33. https://doi.org/10.1001/jamadermatol.2013.8502. PMID: 24430974
23. Wang J, Liu J. Dermoscopy and high-frequency ultrasound provide diagnostic clues in a gastric adenocarcinoma with cutaneous metastasis as the initial presentation: a case report. Skin Res Technol. 2023;29(6):e13380. https://doi.org/10.1111/srt.13380. PMID: 37357645.
24. Tiodorovic D, Stojkovic-Filipovic J, Marghoob A, Argenziano G, Puig S, Malvehy J, Tognetti L, Pietro R, Akay BN, Zalaudek I, Haenssle HA, Müller-Christmann C, Cinotti E, Perrot JL, Zaballos P, Bakos RM, Thomas L, Peris K, Lallas A, Apalla Z, Kreusch JF, Tromme I, Stratigos AJ, Pizzichetta MA, Kandolf L, Longo C, Blum A, Tanaka M, Hofmann-Wellenhof R, Jovic A, Paoli J, Buljan M, Espasandín-Arias M, Cabo H, Saa SR, Salerni G, Nazzaro G, Kaminska-Winciorek G, Damiani G, Geszti F, Kittler H, IDS study group. Dermatoscopic patterns of cutaneous metastases: a multicentre cross-sectional study of the International Dermoscopy Society. J Eur Acad Dermatol Venereol. 2024;38(7):1432–8. https://doi.org/10.1111/jdv.19962. Epub 2024 Mar 14. PMID: 38483241.
25. Kamińska-Winciorek G, Pilśniak A, Piskorski W, Wydmański J. Skin metastases in the clinical and dermoscopic aspects. Semin Oncol. 2022;49(2):160–9. https://doi.org/10.1053/j.seminoncol.2022.04.005. Epub 2022 May 3. PMID: 35589424.
26. Ertop Doğan P, Akay BN, Hazinedar E, Koca R. Clinical and dermoscopic findings of cutaneous metastases: a case series. Int J Dermatol. 2022;61(9):e351–3. https://doi.org/10.1111/ijd.16177. Epub 2022 Mar 29. PMID: 35348215.
27. Grander LC, Cabral F, Lisboa AP, Vale G, Barcaui CB, Maceira JM. Multiple cutaneous melanomas associated with gastric and brain metastases. An Bras Dermatol. 2016;91(5 suppl 1):98–100. https://doi.org/10.1590/abd1806-4841.20164374. PMID: 28300909.
28. Morelli U, Cirocchi R, Mecarelli V, Farinella E, La Mura F, Ronca P, Giustozzi G, Sciannameo F. Gastric adenocarcinoma cutaneous metastasis arising at a previous surgical drain site: a case report. J Med Case Rep. 2009;3:65. https://doi.org/10.1186/1752-1947-3-65. PMID: 19220898.
29. Zadeh VB, Kadyan R, Al-Abdulrazzaq A, Al-Otaibi S, Sarhan A, Najem N. Sister Mary Joseph's nodule: a case of umbilical cutaneous metastasis with signet ring cell histology. Indian J Dermatol Venereol Leprol. 2009;75(5):503–5. https://doi.org/10.4103/0378-6323.55396. PMID: 19736432.
30. Young JJ, Pahwa A, Patel M, Jude CM, Nguyen M, Deshmukh M, Huang L, Mohammad SF. Ligaments and lymphatic pathways in gastric adenocarcinoma. Radiographics. 2019;39(3):668–89. https://doi.org/10.1148/rg.2019180113. Epub 2019 Apr 5. PMID: 30951438.
31. Juan YH, Saboo SS, Tirumani SH, Khandelwal A, Shinagare AB, Ramaiya N, Krajewski KM. Malignant skin and subcutaneous neoplasms in adults: multimodality imaging with CT, MRI, and 18F-FDG PET/CT. AJR Am J Roentgenol. 2014;202(5):W422–38. https://doi.org/10.2214/AJR.13.11424. PMID: 24758677
32. Di Gregorio F, Polici M, Pilozzi E, Giallorenzi MA, Ciolina M, Oedegaard PEK, Zerunian M, Caruso D, Iannicelli E, Laghi A. Staging of gastric cancer: CT patterns and correlation with pathologic findings. Radiographics. 2025;45(8):e240186. https://doi.org/10.1148/rg.240186. PMID: 40608556.
33. Kwee RM, Kwee TC. Modern imaging techniques for preoperative detection of distant metastases in gastric cancer. World J Gastroenterol. 2015;21(37):10502–9. https://doi.org/10.3748/wjg.v21.i37.10502. PMID: 26457011.
34. Pathak P, Wondimu B, Jalilianhasanpour R, Pooyan A, Matesan MC, Mansoori B. Skin malignancies: imaging review with radiologic-histopathologic correlationn. Radiographics. 2023;43(12):e230093. https://doi.org/10.1148/rg.230093. PMID: 38032822.
35. Hu HM, Tsai HJ, Ku HY, Lo SS, Shan YS, Chang HC, Chao Y, Chen JS, Chen SC, Chiang CJ, Li AF, Wang HP, Wang TE, Bai LY, Wu MS, Chen LT, Liu TW, Yang YH. Survival outcomes of management in metastatic gastric adenocarcinoma patients. Sci Rep. 2021;11(1):23142. https://doi.org/10.1038/s41598-021-02391-z. PMID: 34848751.
36. Mohri Y, Tanaka K, Ohi M, Saigusa S, Yasuda H, Toiyama Y, Araki T, Inoue Y, Kusunoki M. Identification of prognostic factors and surgical indications for metastatic gastric cancer. BMC Cancer. 2014;(14):409. https://doi.org/10.1186/1471-2407-14-409. PMID: 24906485

37. Luan X, Han X, Wang Z, Zhao L, Zhang X, Wang W, Niu P, Wang D, Zhao D, Zhu M, Chen Y. Heterogeneity of metastatic gastric cancer: solitary non-regional lymph node metastasis and solitary lung metastasis showed better survival outcomes than other metastatic patterns. BMC Cancer. 2025;25(1):1287. https://doi.org/10.1186/s12885-025-14748-y. PMID: 40781666
38. Biondi A, D'Ugo D, Cananzi F, Rausei S, Sicoli F, Santullo F, Laurino A, Ruspi L, Belia F, Quagliuolo V, Persiani R. Prognostic indicators in stage IV surgically treated gastric cancer patients: a retrospective multi-institutional study. Dig Surg. 2019;36(4):331–9. https://doi.org/10.1159/000488775. Epub 2018 Jun 26. PMID: 29945145.
39. Selcukbiricik F, Buyukunal E, Tural D, Ozguroglu M, Demirelli F, Serdengecti S. Clinicopathological features and outcomes of patients with gastric cancer: a single-center experience. World J Gastroenterol. 2013;19(14):2154–61. https://doi.org/10.3748/wjg.v19.i14.2154. PMID: 23599641
40. Xiaobin C, Zhaojun X, Tao L, Tianzeng D, Xuemei H, Fan Z, Chunyin H, Jianqiang H, Chen L. Analysis of related risk factors and prognostic factors of gastric cancer with bone metastasis: a SEER-based study. J Immunol Res. 2022;2022:3251051. https://doi.org/10.1155/2022/3251051. eCollection 2022. PMID: 35211630.
41. Oh BH, Kim KH, Chung KY. Skin imaging using ultrasound imaging, optical coherence tomography, confocal microscopy, and two-photon microscopy in cutaneous oncology. Front Med (Lausanne). 2019;6:274. https://doi.org/10.3389/fmed.2019.00274. eCollection 2019. PMID: 31824956.
42. Borsari S, Pampena R, Lallas A, Kyrgidis A, Moscarella E, Benati E, Raucci M, Pellacani G, Zalaudek I, Argenziano G, Longo C. Clinical indications for use of reflectance confocal microscopy for skin cancer diagnosis. JAMA Dermatol. 2016;152(10):1093–8. https://doi.org/10.1001/jamadermatol.2016.1188. PMID: 27580185
43. Eichert S, Möhrle M, Breuninger H, Röcken M, Garbe C, Bauer J. Diagnosis of cutaneous tumors with in vivo confocal laser scanning microscopy. J Dtsch Dermatol Ges. 2010;8(6):400–10. https://doi.org/10.1111/j.1610-0387.2010.07333.x. Epub 2010 Feb 5. PMID: 20141551.
44. Bakos RM, Blumetti TP, Roldán-Marín R, Salerni G. Noninvasive imaging tools in the diagnosis and treatment of skin cancers. Am J Clin Dermatol. 2018;19(Suppl 1):3–14. https://doi.org/10.1007/s40257-018-0367-4. PMID: 30374899
45. Soglia S, Pérez-Anker J, Lobos Guede N, Giavedoni P, Puig S, Malvehy J. Diagnostics using non-invasive technologies in dermatological oncology. Cancers (Basel). 2022;14(23):5886. https://doi.org/10.3390/cancers14235886. PMID: 36497368
46. Han W, Kong R, Wang N, Bao W, Mao X, Lu J. Confocal laser Endomicroscopy for detection of early upper gastrointestinal cancer. Cancers (Basel). 2023;15(3):776. https://doi.org/10.3390/cancers15030776. PMID: 36765734
47. Goetz M, Kiesslich R. Confocal endomicroscopy: in vivo diagnosis of neoplastic lesions of the gastrointestinal tract. Anticancer Res. 2008;28(1B):353–60. PMID: 18383869.
48. Bang AS, Monnier J, Harris U, Garfinkel J, Rubinstein G, Iftimia N, Pulitzer M, Murray M, Lacouture ME, Jain M. Non-invasive, in vivo, characterization of cutaneous metastases using a novel multimodal RCM-OCT imaging device: a case-series. J Eur Acad Dermatol Venereol. 2022;36(11):2051–4. https://doi.org/10.1111/jdv.18344. Epub 2022 Jul 4. PMID: 35729732.

Cutaneous Metastases of Colon Adenocarcinoma

10

Aikaterini Zacharopoulou, Dimitra Koumaki, and Stamatios Gregoriou

Abstract

Cutaneous metastases from internal malignancies are uncommon, with colorectal cancer accounting for a significant portion of these rare presentations due to its high incidence. These skin metastases typically indicate advanced disease and are associated with poor prognosis, as the majority of patients die within 6 months of diagnosis. Metastatic spread may occur via hematogenous, lymphatic, or direct extension, with the abdominal wall being the most common site, especially around surgical scars. Clinically, cutaneous metastases manifest in diverse forms, often mimicking benign or inflammatory skin conditions. Histologically, they vary in differentiation and appearance but frequently display glandular or signet-ring cell morphology. Immunohistochemical markers such as CK20, CDX2, and SATB2 play critical roles in confirming diagnosis, especially when tumors are poorly differentiated. Treatment is largely palliative, with surgical resection considered for solitary lesions and systemic therapy for widespread disease. Despite their rarity, early identification of cutaneous metastases can significantly influence management and improve patient outcomes. Physicians should maintain a high index of suspicion in patients with known colorectal cancer presenting with new or unusual skin lesions.

Keywords

Cutaneous metastasis · Colorectal cancer · Skin involvement · Abdominal wall metastasis · Histomorphology · Immunohistochemistry · CK20 · CDX2 · SATB2 · Palliative treatment

10.1 Epidemiology

Cutaneous metastases from internal malignant tumors are relatively rare, occurring in approximately 4–6.5% of cases [1]. Among these, colorectal adenocarcinoma is a significant source due to its high prevalence in the general population [2]. The pattern of cutaneous metastasis may differ between sexes, with a higher incidence reported in males [3, 4]. The presence of skin metastases generally indicates advanced disease and is associated with a poor prognosis; more than two-thirds of patients die within 6 months of diagnosis [5].

A. Zacharopoulou · S. Gregoriou (✉)
National and Kapodistrian University of Athens, First Department of Dermatology-Venereology, Andreas Sygros Hospital, Athens, Greece

D. Koumaki
Dermatology Department, University Hospital of Heraklion, Heraklion, Greece

D. Koumaki et al. (eds.), *Cutaneous Metastases*, https://doi.org/10.1007/978-3-032-26764-1_10

10.2 Pathogenesis and Routes of Spread

Cutaneous metastases may occur via hematogenous or lymphatic dissemination, direct extension from the primary tumor, or iatrogenic implantation, particularly during surgical procedures [5]. In rare instances, embryonic remnants such as the urachus may serve as pathways for tumor spread. Lesions commonly arise near the site of the primary tumor, with the abdominal wall being the most frequent location in colorectal cancer [2, 3, 6]. Although uncommon, a cutaneous lesion may occasionally represent the first manifestation of an internal malignancy.

10.3 Anatomical Distribution and Timing

The abdominal region, particularly areas adjacent to surgical scars, is the most common site of skin metastases from colorectal cancer. Other reported sites include the extremities, pelvis, perineum, penis, torso, thorax, head, neck, and upper lip [6–8]. These metastases typically appear within 2 years following surgical resection of the primary tumor and may coincide with metastases to the liver, lungs, or peritoneum [3].

10.4 Clinical Features

Skin metastases usually resemble the primary tumors; however, they tend to be more anaplastic [9, 10] and typically spread deeply into the dermis and subcutaneous tissue without maintaining continuity with the overlying epidermis [5, 7].

Cutaneous metastases occasionally display a non-specific appearance, exhibiting a range of clinical manifestations [11]. They may appear as rapidly growing, painless dermal or subcutaneous nodules with intact overlying epidermis. They can also mimic inflammatory conditions, such as cellulitis. Common presentations include ulceration, nodules, bullae, and fibrotic changes [12]. Additionally, blisters, alopecia plaques, and lesions resembling herpes zoster; epidermal cysts; neurofibromas; lymphomas; annular erythema; condylomas; and elephantiasis nostras verrucosa have been reported in the literature [2, 3].

The most typical form of cutaneous metastases is a single lesion, accounting for 70% of cases, while multiple lesions occur less frequently, representing around 30% [8]. The primary manifestation of cutaneous or subcutaneous nodules can range from small conchoidal changes to larger tumors. These nodules may be single or multiple, typically solid, and mobile, and often appear slightly papillose. Their coloration varies, generally showing hues of flesh-colored, rose-colored, or reddish-brown, and they may sometimes be ulcerated (Fig. 10.1).

Skin metastases can manifest as inflammatory plaques known as erysipelas carcinoma. These typically present as erythematous plaques with well-defined, flexible borders, resembling the condition called erysipelas. Depending on their size, skin metastases can also mimic localized or systemic scleroderma, or the skin may feel firm and have a texture similar to that of an orange peel [13].

Additionally, skin metastases may present as pink to tan papules near the umbilicus or periumbilical area, referred to as Sister Mary Joseph's nodule [9].

10.5 Histopathology and Immunohistochemistry

In most cases of metastasis, the diagnosis relies on visual morphological characteristics, histomorphology, and immunohistochemistry of the cutaneous lesion, along with a comparison to the morphology of the primary tumor when available [2, 14, 15]. The histological appearance can vary based on the clinical presentation.

When metastases appear as nodules, the tumor can exhibit variable small glandular formations or signet-ring cells, particularly if the tumor is well-differentiated. Key histological features include pleomorphism, hyperchromatism, and increased mitotic activity. Typically, it is difficult to determine the primary site of the tumor based

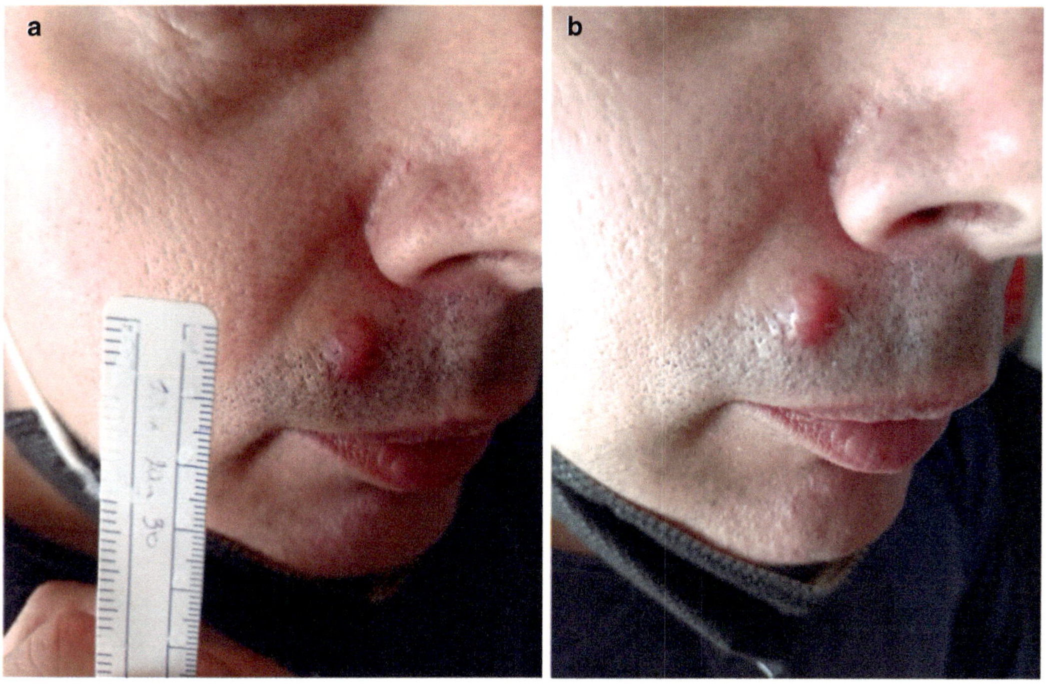

Fig. 10.1 (**a** and **b**) Colon cutaneous metastasis on the upper lip

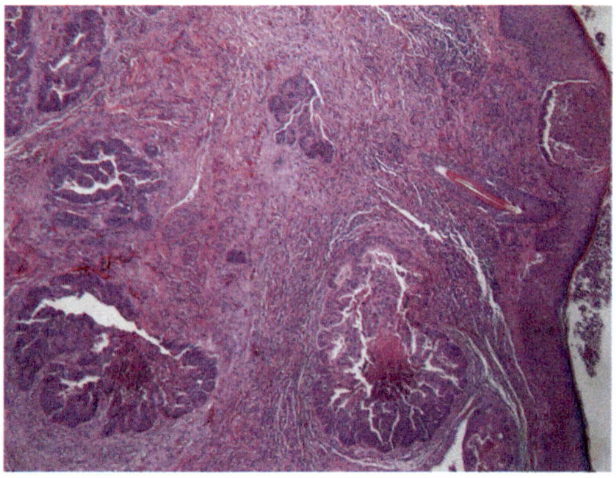

Fig. 10.2 H&E × 10: Neoplastic infiltration of the dermis by large, atypical blasts of adenocarcinoma with morphology similar to colonic adenocarcinoma

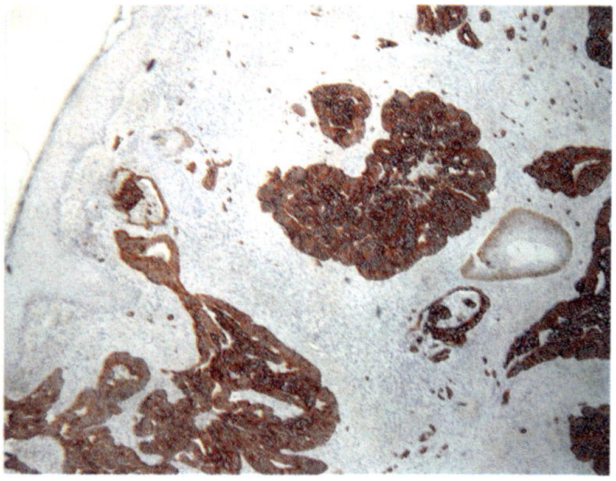

Fig. 10.3 CK 8-18 × 10: Expression of cytokeratin 8/18 by the blasts

solely on histological characteristics, although there are some exceptions. Mucin stains, such as mucicarmine, are often used to stain mucin within the tumor cells. Positive staining for pan-keratin can be helpful in challenging cases (Figs. 10.2, 10.3, and 10.4).

In instances where the lesions present as erysipelatoid carcinoma, histological examination reveals cells within distended lymphatic vessels. In contrast, if the appearance resembles scleroderma, the histological findings are consistent with fibrosis accompanied by infiltrating cancer cells.

Although metastatic cells may be more poorly differentiated than the primary tumor, a careful microscopic examination often reveals important clues. Immunohistochemical studies are valuable

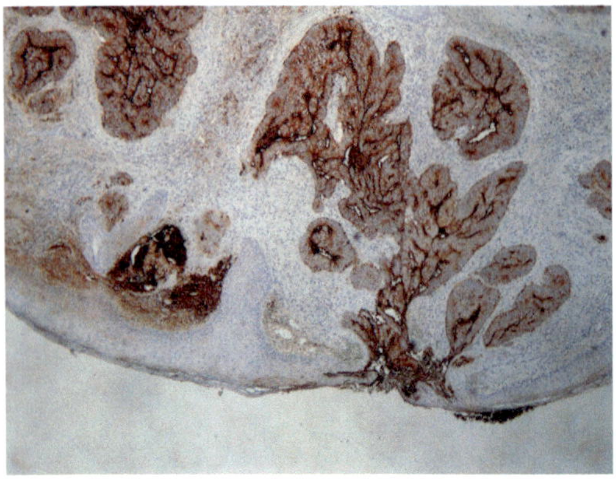

Fig. 10.4 CEA × 20: Expression of CEA by the blasts

complementary tools for histopathological analyses. When tumors are poorly differentiated or anaplastic, immunohistochemical studies—particularly those using markers such as CK7, CK20, CDX2, and SATB2—are essential for diagnosing cutaneous metastases originating from colorectal cancer [10].

A CK7-negative and CK20-positive pattern is commonly observed in these metastases, with CDX2 demonstrating high sensitivity and specificity. SATB2 is another sensitive and highly specific marker for colorectal cancer, with a significant proportion of cases testing positive. In fact, the combination of SATB2 and/or CK20 is positive in the vast majority of colorectal cancer cases. For cutaneous metastases originating from colorectal cancer, the CK7-negative and CK20-positive pattern is present in more than 70% of lesions [15].

10.6 Management Strategies

The treatment options for metastatic carcinoma of the skin are limited and lack standardized strategies. The management of cutaneous metastases primarily focuses on palliative care, with surgical resection typically reserved for solitary lesions. For a single cutaneous metastasis, surgical removal is recommended along with a 1-cm margin of healthy skin. In areas of high cosmetic importance or when the goal is solely palliation,

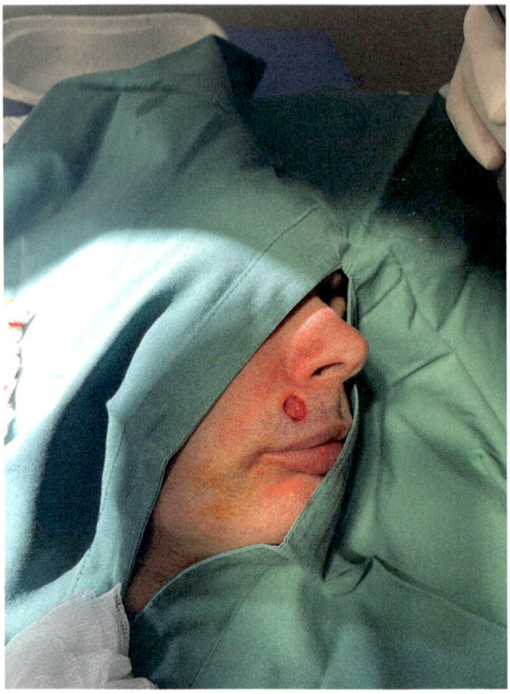

Fig. 10.5 Surgical removal of skin metastasis

excisions may be performed with much smaller margins [16] (Fig. 10.5).

For patients with widespread cutaneous metastases, treatment is exclusively palliative, as these cases are associated with significantly higher rates of distant metastases, uncontrolled local disease, and decreased survival rates. For those with multiple cutaneous metastases or unresectable lesions, systemic chemotherapy may be considered. In managing metastatic colorectal cancer, systemic chemotherapy has been the standard; however, surgical resection in selected patients offers the only chance for long-term survival [17].

In addition, radiotherapy and chemotherapy may be utilized to alleviate local symptoms. The occurrence of cutaneous metastases generally indicates a poor prognosis. Therefore, physicians treating patients with internal carcinomas should actively monitor for signs of skin involvement, even after prolonged periods without symptoms. It is critical to pay attention to any nodules, non-healing ulcers, or persistent erythema and induration. Early detection and recognition of metastatic disease on the skin can significantly influence treatment options and overall prognosis.

Other treatments mentioned in various studies include radiotherapy, polychemotherapy, isolated limb perfusion, interferon alpha injections, cryotherapy, laser ablation, radiofrequency ablation, imiquimod 5% cream, and targeted oncogene therapy [18–22].

References

1. Hashimi Y, Dholakia S. Facial cutaneous metastasis of colorectal adenocarcinoma. BMJ Case Rep. 2013;2013:bcr2013009875.
2. Cidon EU. Cutaneous metastases in 42 patients with cancer. Indian J Dermatol Venereol Leprol. 2010;76:409–12.
3. Aravind B, Kumar R, Basnyat P. Cutaneous metastases secondary to colorectal carcinoma may not be as ominous as previously thought: a case report and review of the literature. BMJ Case Rep. 2013;2013:bcr2013008556.
4. Fong SH, Narasimha N, Thakkar R, Misra S, Thakkar D. A rare isolated cutaneous metastatic mass after colon cancer resection. J Surg Case Rep. 2021;2021:rjab571.
5. Lookingbill DP, Spangler N, Helm KF. Cutaneous metastases in patients with metastatic carcinoma: a retrospective study of 4020 patients. J Am Acad Dermatol. 1993;29:228–36.
6. Bittencourt M, de Semblano J, et al. Cutaneous metastasis of colorectal cancer. An Bras Dermatol. 2018;93:884–6.
7. Wang DY, et al. Cutaneous metastasis: a rare phenomenon of colorectal cancer. Ann Surg Treat Res. 2017;93:277–80.
8. Stavrianos SD, McLean NR, Kelly CG, Fellows S. Cutaneous metastasis to the head and neck from colonic carcinoma. Eur J Surg Oncol. 2000;26:518.
9. Krathen RA, Orengo IF, Rosen T. Cutaneous metastasis: a meta-analysis of data. South Med J. 2003;96:164–7.
10. Nesseris I, Tsamakis C, Gregoriou S, Ditsos I, Christofidou E, Rigopoulos D. Cutaneous metastasis of colon adenocarcinoma: case report and review of the literature. An Bras Dermatol. 2013;88:56–8.
11. Faenza M, Del Torto G, Di Costanzo P, Pieretti G, Lamberti R, Franco R, et al. Large single cutaneous metastasis of colon adenocarcinoma mimicking a squamous cell carcinoma of the skin: a case report. Int J Surg Case Rep. 2019;56:96–100.
12. Parente P, Ciardiello D, Reggiani Bonetti L, Famiglietti V, Cazzato G, Caramaschi S, et al. Cutaneous metastasis from colorectal cancer: making light on an unusual and misdiagnosed event. Life (Basel). 2021;11
13. Oh SY, Kim DY, Suh KW. Oncologic outcomes following metastasectomy in colorectal cancer patients developing distant metastases after initial treatment. Ann Surg Treat Res. 2015;88:253–9.
14. Moonda A, Fatteh S. Metastatic colorectal carcinoma: an unusual presentation. J Cutan Pathol. 2009;36:64–6.
15. Saeed S, Keehn CA, Morgan MB. Cutaneous metastasis: a clinical, pathological, and immunohistochemical appraisal. J Cutan Pathol. 2004;31:419–30.
16. Wong NS, Chang BM, Toh HC, Koo WH. Inflammatory metastatic carcinoma of the colon: a case report and review of the literature. Tumori. 2004;90:253–5.
17. Leong SP, Gershenwald JE, Soong SJ, Schadendorf D, Tarhini AA, Agarwala S, et al. Cutaneous melanoma: a model to study cancer metastasis. J Surg Oncol. 2011;103:538–49.
18. Flaherty KT, Puzanov I, Kim KB, Ribas A, McArthur GA, Sosman JA, et al. Inhibition of mutated, activated BRAF in metastatic melanoma. N Engl J Med. 2010;363:809–19.
19. Góes HF, Lima C d S, Souza MB, Estrella RR, Faria MA, Rochael MC. Single cutaneous metastasis of colon adenocarcinoma: case report. An Bras Dermatol. 2016;91:517–9.
20. Attili VS, Rama Chandra C, Dadhich HK, Sahoo TP, Anupama G, Bapsy PP. Unusual metastasis in colorectal cancer. Indian J Cancer. 2006;43:93–5.
21. Tokarski E, Conan PL, Picchi H, Malgras B, Peroux E, Ezanno AC. Prognostic implications of cutaneous metastases in colorectal cancer: a comprehensive systematic review and meta-analysis. Cancer Med. 2025;14(18):e71197. https://doi.org/10.1002/cam4.71197. PMID: 40937814.
22. Tan KY, Ho KS, Lai JH, Lim JF, Ooi BS, Tang CL, Eu KW. Cutaneous and subcutaneous metastases of adenocarcinoma of the colon and rectum. Ann Acad Med Singap. 2006;35(8):585–7. PMID: 17006588

Cutaneous Metastases in Pancreatic Cancer

11

Anna Tagka and Ioannis Vathiotis

Abstract

Cutaneous metastases originating from pancreatic cancer (PC) are rare, affecting approximately 1% of patients. Although uncommon, they hold significant clinical importance as they may represent the first sign of an otherwise undiagnosed malignancy. The most well-known form is the Sister Mary Joseph nodule located at the umbilicus, but increasingly, metastases are being detected in non-umbilical areas such as surgical scars and distant skin regions. The presence of skin lesions often indicates widespread disease and is associated with poor prognosis, with a median overall survival of months. This article provides an overview of the frequency, underlying mechanisms, clinical presentation, diagnostic strategies, treatment approaches, and ongoing research regarding skin involvement in pancreatic cancer, aiming to support healthcare providers in early identification and appropriate management.

Keywords

Pancreatic cancer · Cutaneous · Metastasis · Biomarkers

11.1 Introduction

Pancreatic cancer (PC) is an aggressive malignancy characterized by subtle onset, swift progression, and limited treatment options [1]. Risk factors comprise age, smoking, type 2 diabetes mellitus, chronic pancreatitis, *Helicobacter pylori* infection, obesity, and dietary habits (increased red meat and alcohol intake and decreased fruit and vegetable intake) [2, 3]. Less than 20% of cases are due to germline mutations (most commonly in *BRCA2*); familial cases are defined by the accumulation of at least two first-degree relatives with the disease [4]. PC encompasses several histologic subtypes, with pancreatic ductal adenocarcinoma (PDAC), orig-

A. Tagka (✉)
First Department of Dermatology, School of Medicine, National and Kapodistrian University of Athens, Athens, Greece

I. Vathiotis
Third Pathology Department, National and Kapodistrian University of Athens, "Sotiria" General Hospital, Athens, Greece

D. Koumaki et al. (eds.), *Cutaneous Metastases*, https://doi.org/10.1007/978-3-032-26764-1_11

inating from the ductal epithelium, accounting for approximately 80% of the cases [5, 6].

Less frequently, neuroendocrine tumors develop from hormone-secreting pancreatic cells, displaying a wide range of malignant potential. Rare variants include acinar cell carcinoma, which resembles normal acinar cells, adenosquamous carcinoma, defined by the presence of both glandular and squamous components, anaplastic carcinoma, and undifferentiated carcinoma with osteoclast-like giant cells, which represent aggressive disease subtypes. In the US, PC represents the tenth most common cancer among males and the seventh most common among females, with an estimated 34,950 and 32,490 new cases in 2025, respectively [7].

Most patients with PC present with either locally advanced or metastatic disease. The five-year survival rate of PC is approximately 10%; PC is the fourth most common cause of cancer-related death among males and third most common among females, with an estimated 27,050 and 24,930 deaths in 2025, respectively [7]. The most common sites of metastatic dissemination include the liver, peritoneum, lungs, and bones. Cutaneous involvement is quite rare; nonetheless, recognizing skin metastases is crucial, since a superficial nodule may represent the sole clinical sign of an otherwise subtle disease [8]. In patients diagnosed with pancreatic cancer, the emergence of skin lesions may mark progression from localized or locally advanced to metastatic disease. The earliest report of a case of pancreatic cancer metastasis to the umbilicus [9] dates back to over a century ago, but comprehensive characterization has been limited by the low incidence of anecdotal cases [10–12]. Routine use of immunohistochemistry along with spatial transcriptomics has uncovered separate driver clones of PDAC with implications for the incidence, timing, and molecular identifiers of skin metastases [13, 14]. All the above will enable clinicians to develop rational diagnostic frameworks, balance promptness with resource allocation, and formulate patient-centered clinical practice guidelines.

11.2 Epidemiology

Autopsy studies have estimated that cutaneous metastases develop in approximately 0.3–0.7% of patients with PDAC [8]. Prospective registries report rates up to 1.1%, likely reflecting improved survival of patients with metastatic disease [15]. The median age at presentation is 63 years, with nearly equal sex distribution [16]. Roughly 40% of cutaneous metastases appear either before or concurrently with the diagnosis; the remainder arise later in the disease course with a median latency period of about 11 months [11, 12]. Sister Mary Joseph nodules constitute 23–50% of reported lesions, while recent studies show an increasing proportion of non-umbilical sites, including endoscopic ultrasound-guided fine-needle aspiration (EUS-FNA) tracts [8, 17–19]. The incidence of cutaneous metastases does not appear to be increased in patients with familial pancreatic cancer syndromes [8].

11.3 Pathophysiology

Several mechanisms have been implicated in cutaneous seeding of PC. Direct extension to the umbilicus via the ligamentum teres or remnant periumbilical veins possibly represents the preferred route for cutaneous seeding for gastrointestinal tumors [20, 21]. Hematogenous dissemination through systemic circulation appears to account for distant cutaneous deposits, involving the scalp or lower extremities [22]. In addition, lymphatic spread through para-aortic, inguinal, axillary, or internal mammary drainage pathways has been implicated in chest or abdominal wall lesions [23]. As stated above, iatrogenic seeding represents an additional concern, as biopsy needles may carry malignant cells superficially, especially in the context of larger caliber instruments or multiple diagnostic passes. 3-dimensional (3-D) lymphatic network imaging studies suggest an active role of lymphatic vessels in mediating metastatic spread of PC through extracellular matrix remodeling and tissue invasion [24].

Cutaneous metastases were predominantly non-umbilical (77% of cases, $n = 44$), with localized umbilical metastases being less common (23% of cases, $n = 13$). Among non-umbilical metastases, the most frequent sites were the head and neck (33%, $n = 19$).

11.4 Clinical Presentation

Cutaneous metastases clinically present as nodules, masses, or plaques associated with topical edema and/or ulceration. In some cases, lesions may be asymptomatic. Isolated skin metastases are more common than multiple lesions [8]. Skin metastases typically manifest as firm, painless nodules ranging from a few millimeters to several centimeters in diameter. The color may vary from flesh-toned to erythematous or violaceous lesions, with superficial telangiectasia or ulceration. Umbilical lesions often appear as raised, indurated plaques (Fig. 11.1) that may crust or be associated with serosanguinous discharge [10, 23]. Non-umbilical lesions (Fig. 11.2) can mimic epidermal cysts, dermatofibromas, or pyogenic granulomas, leading to potential misdiagnosis. While cutaneous metastases are solitary in two-thirds of cases, multiple synchronous nodules have been documented in the remainder. The presence of cutaneous metastases is not associated with the location of the primary tumor (head versus body or tail) [8, 18, 19].

A recent systematic review included 57 patients from different publications [8]. The majority of cutaneous metastases occurred outside the umbilical region, accounting for 77% of cases ($n = 44$), whereas those involving the umbilicus were less frequent, seen in 23% of cases ($n = 13$). Among the non-umbilical lesions, the head and neck were the most commonly affected areas (33%, $n = 19$), followed by the trunk (21%, $n = 12$), multiple body sites (12%, $n = 7$), lower extremities (7%, $n = 4$), upper extremities (4%, $n = 2$), and genital skin (2%, $n = 1$). Clinically, the skin lesions typically appeared as nodules, masses, or plaques in 89% of patients ($n = 51$), with swelling reported in 7% ($n = 4$) and ulceration in 4% ($n = 2$). In terms of symptoms, 34% of cases ($n = 21$) were asymptomatic, while 34% ($n = 14$) reported pain, and 19% ($n = 10$) exhibited ulceration or bleeding. Most lesions exceeded 1 cm in diameter (78%, $n = 39$), whereas 22% ($n = 11$) were smaller than 1 cm. Solitary skin metastases were more prevalent (68%, $n = 39$) compared to multiple lesions (32%, $n = 18$).

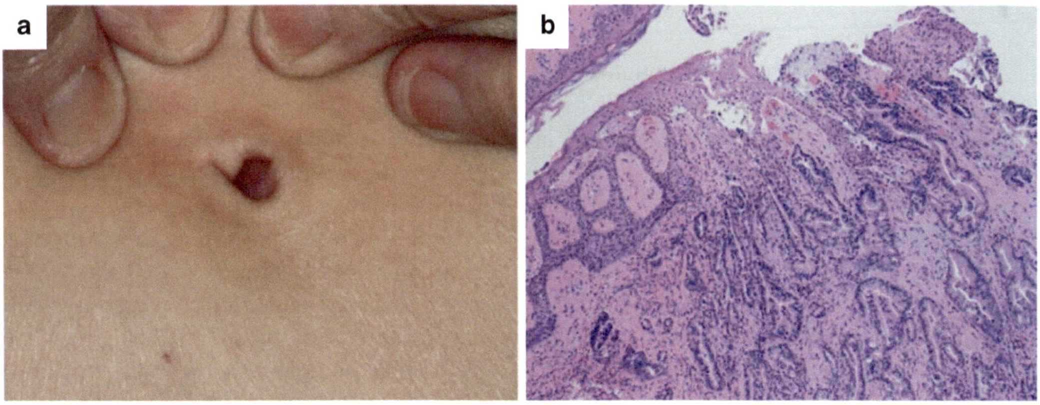

Fig. 11.1 Cutaneous umbilical metastasis from pancreatic cancer. (**a**) Clinical appearance of a cutaneous umbilical metastasis, described as a violaceous to red umbilical papulonodule. (**b**) The microscopic findings of the skin biopsy show infiltration of the dermis by a ductal adenocarcinoma. Its microscopic features are consistent with a pancreatic origin. (Reproduced from Gu et al. (2023) under the Creative Commons CC BY-SA 4.0 License https://creativecommons.org/licenses/by/4.0/ [18])

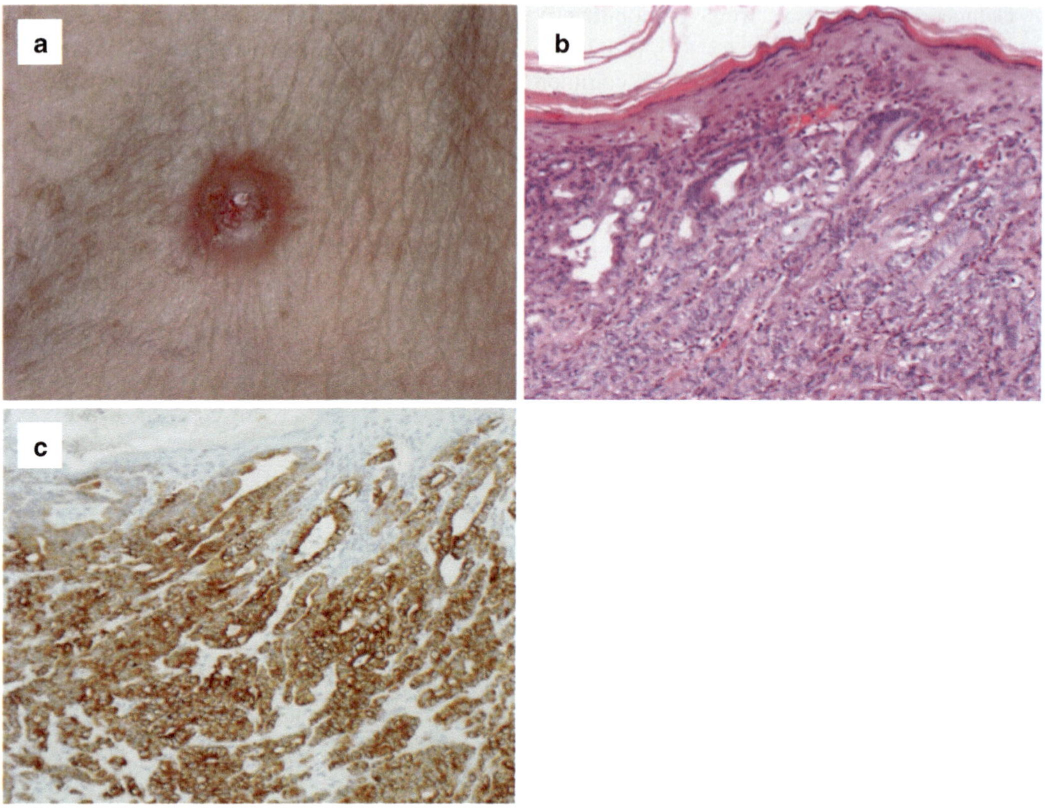

Fig. 11.2 Cutaneous non-umbilical metastasis from pancreatic cancer. (**a**) Clinical appearance of a cutaneous neck metastasis, described as a pink, scaly, eroded papulonodule. (**b**) Histopathologically, there is a moderately to poorly differentiated adenocarcinoma in the dermis. (**c**) The tumor cells are immunoreactive for cytokeratin 7. (Reproduced from Gu et al. (2023) under the Creative Commons CC BY-SA 4.0 License https://creativecommons.org/licenses/by/4.0/ [18])

The main findings of the aforementioned systematic review are summarized in Table 11.1 [8]. In addition, the main locations are depicted in Fig. 11.3, in ascending order.

Another clinical study including 40 patients found that the majority of cutaneous metastases were located in the umbilical region, accounting for 58% of cases (n = 23), followed by other abdominal sites accounting for 43% (n = 17). Similar to the previous report, among the non-umbilical lesions, the back and scalp were the most commonly affected areas, accounting for 13% (n = 5) and 10% (n = 4), respectively. The main findings of the aforementioned systematic review are summarized in Table 11.2 [18]. In addition, the main locations are depicted in Fig. 11.4, in ascending order.

Overall, there are not many studies concerning the cutaneous metastases in PC. Most works concern the presentation of case reports, while there is one retrospective clinical study on this topic. We have summarized those works in Table 11.3.

Table 11.1 Summary of 57 pancreatic cancer cases, with respect to the cutaneous metastases

Location	Count	Percentage
Umbilicus	13	23%
Other sites	44	77%
Head and neck	19	33%
Trunk	12	21%
Multiple sites	7	12%
Lower limbs	4	7%
Upper limbs	2	4%
Genital skin	1	2%
Clinical appearance		
Nodule/mass/plaque	51	89%
Swelling	4	7%
Ulceration	2	4%
Associated symptoms		
No symptoms	21	34%
Pain	14	34%
Bleeding	10	19%
Dimension		
>1 cm	39	78%
<1 cm	11	22%
Number		
Isolated metastases	39	68%
Multiple metastases	18	32%
Diagnosis		
Before pancreatic cancer	33	58%
After pancreatic cancer	23	40%
Concomitant to pancreatic cancer	1	2%

11.5 Diagnosis

Tissue biopsy remains essential for diagnosis. A 4-mm punch biopsy encompassing deep dermis and subcutaneous tissue is generally sufficient for histopathological and immunohistochemical assessment. On hematoxylin and eosin staining, metastatic PDAC is characterized by infiltrative glandular structures or solid nests surrounded by desmoplastic stroma. Immunohistochemistry is typically positive for CK7 and CK19, with variable CK20 expression. Loss of *SMAD4* expression occurs in about half of primary PDACs and, when present, supports pancreatic origin. Although serum CA19-9 levels are elevated in approximately 80% of patients, normal CA19-9 levels do not exclude the diagnosis [29]. Multiphasic contrast-enhanced thoracic, abdominal, and pelvic computed tomography (CT), including late arterial phase and portal venous phase, are the preferred imaging modalities for PC staging; abdominal magnetic resonance imaging (MRI) may help in the characterization of cystic lesions, while 18F-FDG PET/CT may be useful for staging localized tumors or detecting distant metastases [30]. The molecular landscape of PC comprises activation of oncogenes (*KRAS* mutations are found in >90% of PCs), inactivation of tumor suppressor genes (*TP53*,

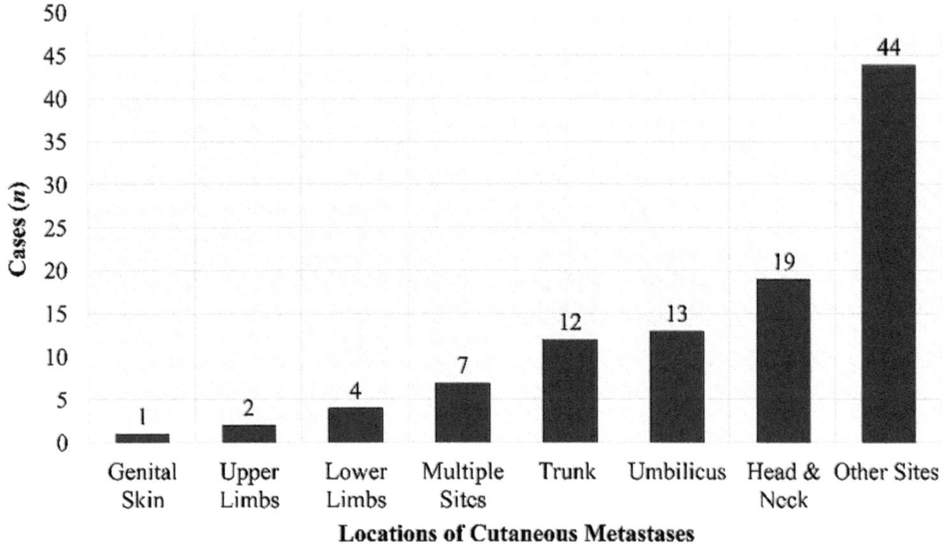

Fig. 11.3 Diagrammatic representation of the main cutaneous metastasis locations in ascending order. The most prevalent sites concerned various locations, followed by head and neck locations. (Data were derived from Table 11.1)

Table. 11.2 Summary of 40 pancreatic cancer cases, with respect to the cutaneous metastases

Location	Count	Percentage
Umbilicus	23	58%
Other abdomen	17	43%
Pelvis	1	3%
Scalp	4	10%
Face	2	5%
Neck	2	5%
Chest	1	3%
Breast	1	3%
Back	5	13%
Axilla	2	3
Upper extremity	1	5%
Lower extremity	2	3%
Onset of cutaneous metastasis relative to chemotherapy ($n = 40$)		
Before	20	50%
During	11	28%
Break	9	23%
First-line chemotherapy regimen		
Stage IV cancer	*26*	*65%*
Before	20	
Gemcitabine based	12	60%
5-FU based	5	25%
Other	1	5%
No chemotherapy	2	10%
During	6	
Gemcitabine based	1	17%
5-FU based	5	83%
Non-metastatic cancer	*14*	*35%*
During	5	
Gemcitabine based	3	60%
5-FU based	1	20%
Other	1	20%
Break	9	
Gemcitabine based	7	78%
5-FU based	1	11%
Other	1	11%
Number of chemotherapy lines before cutaneous metastasis ($n = 40$)		
0	20	50%
1	13	33%
2	3	8%
3	3	8%
4	1	3%
Number of chemotherapy lines after cutaneous metastasis ($n = 40$)		
0	6	15%
1	16	40%
2	8	20%
3	8	20%
4	2	5%
First-line chemotherapy regimen for stage IV cancer ($n = 24$)		
Gemcitabine based	13	54%
5-FU based	10	42%
Other	1	4%
First-line chemotherapy regimen for non-metastatic cancer ($n = 14$)		
Gemcitabine based	10	71%
5-FU based	2	14%
Other	2	14%
Skin biopsy ($n = 40$)		
Yes	35	88%
No	5	13%
Treatment of cutaneous metastasis ($n = 40$)		
Excision	11	28%
Local radiation	1	3%
Excision and radiation	2	5%
None	26	65%
Time from the development of pancreatic cancer and occurrence of cutaneous metastasis		
0–1 month	19	48%
1–6 months	4	10%
6–12 months	5	13%
>12 months	12	30%

p16/*CDKN2A,* and *SMAD4*), and inactivation of genome maintenance genes, which control DNA damage repair (DDR; *hMLH1* and *MSH2*). Most of these mutations are somatic. In addition, germline alterations in genes specifically involved in the homologous recombination repair (HRR) pathway are also found in PC (*BRCA1*, *BRCA2*, etc.). Multigene sequencing is a useful tool to screen for rare, potentially actionable alterations, especially in *KRAS*-wild type, metastatic PC.

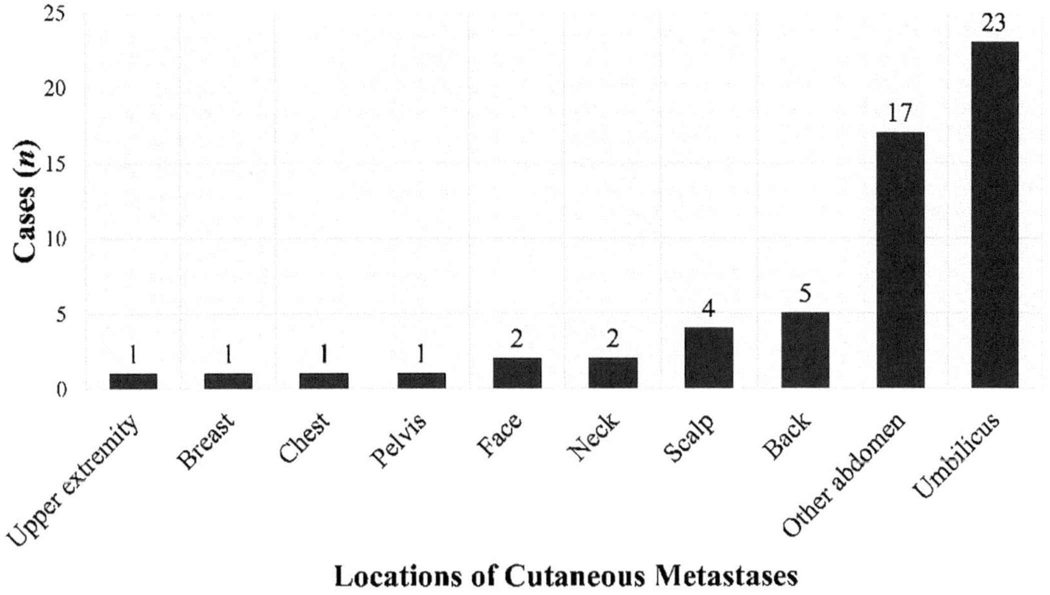

Fig. 11.4 Diagrammatic representation of the main cutaneous metastases' locations in ascending order. The most prevalent sites concerned umbilical locations, followed by abdominal and back lesions. (Data were derived from Table 11.2)

Table 11.3 Summary of the majority of works concerning pancreatic cancer cases with respect to the cutaneous metastases

Ref.	Type of Study	Total cases	Histological type	Anatomical site of skin lesion	Anatomical site & Description of skin lesion
Gu et al. (2023) [18]	Clinical study	40	98% Adenocarcinoma 3% Neuroendocrine	Umbilicus Abdominal Scalp Back	Abdominal wall or thorax: Nodules, firm plaques, ulcerations
Cassalia et al. (2023) [8]	Systematic review	57	77% Adenocarcinoma 7% Neuroendocrine carcinoma 4% Sarcoma 2% PDAC	Umbilicus Abdominal wall Thorax	Umbilicus: Sister Mary Joseph nodule, abdominal wall or thorax: Nodules, firm plaques, ulcerations
Zhou et al. (2014) [16]	Case series and review	63	84% Adenocarcinoma Other neuroendocrine or other types	Mainly umbilicus Various other sites	Umbilicus: Firm nodules, often painful, stable
Miyahara et al. (1996) [25]	Case series	5	Adenocarcinoma (probable)	Umbilicus	Umbilicus: Sister Mary Joseph nodule
Jung et al. (2005) [26]	Case report	1	Adenocarcinoma (probable, not histologically confirmed)	Anterior thorax and back	Anterior thorax and back: Firm nodules, approx. 1 cm, painful, erythematous

(continued)

Table 11.3 (continued)

Ref.	Type of Study	Total cases	Histological type	Anatomical site of skin lesion	Anatomical site & Description of skin lesion
Shi et al. (2020) [27]	Case report	1	Adenocarcinoma, moderate/high differentiation	Labia majora	Labia majora: Lesions up to slightly painful, swollen papules, 2 mm–1 cm
Takeuchi et al. (2003) [28]	Case report	1	Adenocarcinoma, CK-7/19 positive	Chest wall	Chest wall: Firm, painful, clearly ulcerated nodule (~1 cm)
Hafez et al. (2008)	Case report	1	Adenocarcinoma	Trapezius	Trapezius: Firm (indurated) plaque and nodule
Roptimer et al. (2010)	Case report	1	Adenocarcinoma of the pancreas	Surgical wound (abdominal wall)	Surgical wound (abdominal wall): Ulcerated metastatic nodule (~1–2 cm)

11.6 Treatment

Management focuses on systemic disease control, symptom palliation, and quality of life preservation. FOLFIRINOX represents the standard of care for fit patients (Eastern Cooperative Oncology Group Performance Status [ECOG PS] 0 or 1, bilirubin level <1.5 times the upper limit of normal [ULN], and no major comorbidities), offering a median progression-free survival (PFS) of 6.4 months and median overall survival (OS) of 11.1 months [31]. Gemcitabine combined with nab-paclitaxel (GN) serves as an alternative for patients with ECOG PS 2, Karnofsky Performance Status (KPS) ≥70, and bilirubin level ≤1.5 times the ULN, while less fit patients (ECOG PS 2, KPS <70, and bilirubin level >1.5 times the ULN) are treated with gemcitabine monotherapy [32]. Recently, NALIRIFOX (liposomal irinotecan/5-fluorouracil/leucovorin/oxaliplatin) showed superiority over GN in the randomized NAPOLI-3 phase III study, including 770 patients; both PFS and OS were significantly improved in the NALIRIFOX arm (median OS, 11.1 versus 9.2 months in the GN arm [Hazard ratio, 0.83; 95% confidence intervals [0.70–0.99; $P = 0.04$]]) [22]. Maintenance therapy with olaparib provided significant PFS benefit in patients with metastatic PC, harboring germline *BRCA1* or *BRCA2* mutations, who had not progressed during first-line platinum-based chemotherapy [33]. Symptomatic cutaneous lesions may also benefit from local treatment; simple excision provides rapid symptomatic relief, while external beam radiotherapy (20–30 Gy over 5–10 fractions) may help achieve hemostasis and pain control. Early referral to palliative care reduces emergency admissions and improves symptom management.

11.7 Prognosis

In general, the presence of cutaneous metastases signifiespoor prognosis. Contemporary real-world cohorts report a median OS of approximately 5 months, following cutaneous seeding of PC [5, 30, 34]. Sister Mary Joseph nodules are associated with somewhat poorer outcomes compared with non-umbilical skin metastases, likely reflecting concurrent peritoneal spread [3, 13]. Reported cumulative 1- and 2-year survival rates are 17.5% and 3.5%, respectively; typically, solitary skin lesions, low baseline CA19-9, and good ECOG PS represent good prognostic factors [31, 32].

11.8 Future Perspectives

Ongoing research prioritizes liquid biopsy techniques for minimal residual disease detection and spatial transcriptomics to elucidate epidermotropic mechanisms, as well as stromal-targeted therapies. Tract ablation techniques aim to reduce iatrogenic seeding following fine-needle biopsy.

Oncolytic viruses, adoptive cell transfer therapy, tumor-infiltrating lymphocyte (TIL) therapy, T-cell receptor (TCR)-engineered and chimeric antigen receptor (CAR) T-cell therapy, CAR natural killer (NK)-cell therapy, cytokine-induced killer cells, immune checkpoint inhibitors, immunomodulators, and personalized cancer vaccines and strategies targeting myeloid cells are also under investigation in PC [35].

11.9 Patient Counseling and Quality of Life

Cutaneous metastases represent an external revelation of metastatic dissemination of PC. Clinicians should employ open, empathic communication, assessing patient understanding, and aligning treatment with individual values. Addressing body image concerns through specialist nursing support, camouflage techniques, and peer support groups substantially empowers patients. Early goals-of-care discussions, using frameworks such as the SPIKES protocol, facilitate mutual understanding and shared decision-making. Routine distress screening and timely psycho-oncology referral are vital parts of patient care.

11.10 Conclusions

Cutaneous spread is present in approximately 1% of patients with PC and is associated with poor prognosis, with a median OS of less than 6 months. Sister Mary Joseph nodules represent the well-recognized form of disease; however, the prevalence of non-umbilical skin metastases has been increasing recently. Tissue biopsy remains the gold standard for diagnosis. Appropriate first-line treatment is chemotherapy; regimen selection is based on ECOG PS and serum bilirubin levels. Local treatment may be added for symptomatic relief, while early referral to palliative care is associated with improved outcomes.

References

1. Gyawali B, Booth CM. Treatment of metastatic pancreatic cancer: 25 years of innovation with little progress for patients. Lancet Oncol. 2024;25(2):167–70. https://doi.org/10.1016/S1470-2045(23)00516-8.
2. Collaborators GBDPC. The global, regional, and national burden of pancreatic cancer and its attributable risk factors in 195 countries and territories, 1990–2017: a systematic analysis for the global burden of disease study 2017. Lancet Gastroenterol Hepatol. 2019;4(12):934–47. https://doi.org/10.1016/S2468-1253(19)30347-4.
3. Maisonneuve P, Lowenfels AB. Risk factors for pancreatic cancer: a summary review of meta-analytical studies. Int J Epidemiol. 2015;44(1):186–98. https://doi.org/10.1093/ije/dyu240.
4. Pereira SP, Oldfield L, Ney A, Hart PA, Keane MG, Pandol SJ, et al. Early detection of pancreatic cancer. Lancet Gastroenterol Hepatol. 2020;5(7):698–710. https://doi.org/10.1016/S2468-1253(19)30416-9.
5. Stoop TF, Javed AA, Oba A, Koerkamp BG, Seufferlein T, Wilmink JW, et al. Pancreatic cancer. Lancet. 2025;405(10485):1182–202. https://doi.org/10.1016/S0140-6736(25)00261-2.
6. Brown TJ, Reiss KA, O'Hara MH. Advancements in systemic therapy for pancreatic cancer. Am Soc Clin Oncol Educ Book. 2023;43(43):e397082. https://doi.org/10.1200/EDBK_397082.
7. Siegel RL, Kratzer TB, Giaquinto AN, Sung H, Jemal A. Cancer statistics, 2025. CA Cancer J Clin. 2025;75(1):10–45. https://doi.org/10.3322/caac.21871.
8. Cassalia F, Bolzon A, Ponzano M, Ventura L, Danese A, Del Fiore P, et al. The importance of reading the skin: cutaneous metastases of pancreatic cancer, a systematic review. J Clin Med. 2023;13(1) https://doi.org/10.3390/jcm13010104.
9. Yendluri V, Centeno B, Springett GM. Pancreatic cancer presenting as a Sister Mary Joseph's nodule: case report and update of the literature. Pancreas. 2007;34(1):161–4. https://doi.org/10.1097/01.mpa.0000240602.18688.43.
10. Bai XL, Zhang Q, Masood W, Masood N, Tang Y, Cao CH, et al. Sister Mary Joseph's nodule as a first sign of pancreatic cancer. World J Gastroenterol: WJG. 2012;18(45):6686–9. https://doi.org/10.3748/wjg.v18.i45.6686.
11. Powell FC, Cooper AJ, Massa MC, Goellner JR, Su WP. Sister Mary Joseph's nodule: a clinical and histologic study. J Am Acad Dermatol. 1984;10(4):610–5. https://doi.org/10.1016/s0190-9622(84)80265-0.
12. Heatley MK, Toner PG. Sister Mary Joseph's nodule: a study of the incidence of biopsied umbilical secondary tumours in a defined population. Br J Surg. 1989;76(7):728–9. https://doi.org/10.1002/bjs.1800760726.

13. Cui Zhou D, Jayasinghe RG, Chen S, Herndon JM, Iglesia MD, Navale P, et al. Spatially restricted drivers and transitional cell populations cooperate with the microenvironment in untreated and chemo-resistant pancreatic cancer. Nat Genet. 2022;54(9):1390–405. https://doi.org/10.1038/s41588-022-01157-1.
14. Li Y, Du Y, Li R, Zhong W, Zou X, Li L, et al. Spatial transcriptomics in pancreatic cancer: advances, prospects and challenges. Crit Rev Oncol Hematol. 2024;203:104430. https://doi.org/10.1016/j.critrevonc.2024.104430.
15. Paniccia A, Hosokawa P, Henderson W, Schulick RD, Edil BH, McCarter MD, et al. Characteristics of 10-year survivors of pancreatic ductal adenocarcinoma. JAMA Surg. 2015;150(8):701–10. https://doi.org/10.1001/jamasurg.2015.0668.
16. Zhou HY, Wang XB, Gao F, Bu B, Zhang S, Wang Z. Cutaneous metastasis from pancreatic cancer: a case report and systematic review of the literature. Oncol Lett. 2014;8(6):2654–60. https://doi.org/10.3892/ol.2014.2610.
17. Matsui T, Nishikawa K, Yukimoto H, Katsuta K, Nakamura Y, Tanaka S, et al. Needle tract seeding following endoscopic ultrasound-guided fine-needle aspiration for pancreatic cancer: a report of two cases. World J Surg Oncol. 2019;17(1):134. https://doi.org/10.1186/s12957-019-1681-x.
18. Gu L, Mehta PP, Rao D, Rotemberg V, Capanu M, Chou J, et al. Pancreatic cancer: cutaneous metastases, clinical descriptors and outcomes. Cancer Med. 2023;12(1):179–88. https://doi.org/10.1002/cam4.4916.
19. Wang X, ChangSheng Y, Yun L, Xiaodan G. Pancreatic adenocarcinoma with distant soft tissue metastases: a case report and literature review. Front Surg. 2025;12:1447865. https://doi.org/10.3389/fsurg.2025.1447865.
20. Nagai H, Kuroda A, Morioka Y. Lymphatic and local spread of T1 and T2 pancreatic cancer. A study of autopsy material. Ann Surg. 1986;204(1):65–71. https://doi.org/10.1097/00000658-198607000-00009.
21. Fink DM, Steele MM, Hollingsworth MA. The lymphatic system and pancreatic cancer. Cancer Lett. 2016;381(1):217–36. https://doi.org/10.1016/j.canlet.2015.11.048.
22. Wainberg ZA, Melisi D, Macarulla T, Pazo Cid R, Chandana SR, De La Fouchardiere C, et al. NALIRIFOX versus nab-paclitaxel and gemcitabine in treatment-naive patients with metastatic pancreatic ductal adenocarcinoma (NAPOLI 3): a randomised, open-label, phase 3 trial. Lancet. 2023;402(10409):1272–81. https://doi.org/10.1016/S0140-6736(23)01366-1.
23. Gabriele R, Conte M, Egidi F, Borghese M. Umbilical metastases: current viewpoint. World J Surg Oncol. 2005;3(1):13. https://doi.org/10.1186/1477-7819-3-13.
24. Shen CN, Goh KS, Huang CR, Chiang TC, Lee CY, Jeng YM, et al. Lymphatic vessel remodeling and invasion in pancreatic cancer progression. EBioMedicine. 2019;47:98–113. https://doi.org/10.1016/j.ebiom.2019.08.044.
25. Miyahara M, Hamanaka Y, Kawabata A, Sato Y, Tanaka A, Yamamoto A, et al. Cutaneous metastases from pancreatic cancer. Int J Pancreatol. 1996;20(2):127–30. https://doi.org/10.1007/BF02825511.
26. Jung H, Lee KU, Shin WY, Ahn H. Treatment outcomes of surgical resection for hepatocellular carcinoma with inferior vena cava invasion and/or thrombosis. Hepato-Gastroenterology. 2011;58(110–111):1694–9. https://doi.org/10.5754/hge10653.
27. Shi Y, Li SS, Liu DY, Yu Y. Cutaneous metastases of pancreatic carcinoma to the labia majora: a case report and review of literature. World J Gastrointest Oncol. 2020;12(11):1372–80. https://doi.org/10.4251/wjgo.v12.i11.1372.
28. Takeuchi H, Kawano T, Toda T, Minamisono Y, Nagasaki S, Yao T, et al. Cutaneous metastasis from pancreatic adenocarcinoma: a case report and a review of the literature. Hepato-Gastroenterology. 2003;50(49):275–7.
29. Luo G, Jin K, Deng S, Cheng H, Fan Z, Gong Y, et al. Roles of CA19-9 in pancreatic cancer: biomarker, predictor and promoter. Biochim Biophys Acta Rev Cancer. 2021;1875(2):188409. https://doi.org/10.1016/j.bbcan.2020.188409.
30. Conroy T, Pfeiffer P, Vilgrain V, Lamarca A, Seufferlein T, O'Reilly EM, et al. Pancreatic cancer: ESMO clinical practice guideline for diagnosis, treatment and follow-up. Ann Oncol. 2023;34(11):987–1002. https://doi.org/10.1016/j.annonc.2023.08.009.
31. Conroy T, Desseigne F, Ychou M, Bouche O, Guimbaud R, Becouarn Y, et al. FOLFIRINOX versus gemcitabine for metastatic pancreatic cancer. N Engl J Med. 2011;364(19):1817–25. https://doi.org/10.1056/NEJMoa1011923.
32. Von Hoff DD, Ervin T, Arena FP, Chiorean EG, Infante J, Moore M, et al. Increased survival in pancreatic cancer with nab-paclitaxel plus gemcitabine. N Engl J Med. 2013;369(18):1691–703. https://doi.org/10.1056/NEJMoa1304369.
33. Golan T, Hammel P, Reni M, Van Cutsem E, Macarulla T, Hall MJ, et al. Maintenance Olaparib for germline BRCA-mutated metastatic pancreatic cancer. N Engl J Med. 2019;381(4):317–27. https://doi.org/10.1056/NEJMoa1903387.
34. Horino K, Takamori H, Ikuta Y, Nakahara O, Chikamoto A, Ishiko T, et al. Cutaneous metastases secondary to pancreatic cancer. World J Gastrointest Oncol. 2012;4(7):176–80. https://doi.org/10.4251/wjgo.v4.i7.176.
35. Farhangnia P, Khorramdelazad H, Nickho H, Delbandi AA. Current and future immunotherapeutic approaches in pancreatic cancer treatment. J Hematol Oncol. 2024;17(1):40. https://doi.org/10.1186/s13045-024-01561-6.

12 Sister Mary Joseph's Nodule

Dubois Jeanne and Gaide Olivier

Abstract

The Sister Mary Joseph nodule is a metastatic umbilical lesion, indicative of advanced intra-abdominal malignancies, particularly gastric, ovarian, or pancreatic cancers. Its presence often signifies poor prognosis, reflecting widespread peritoneal dissemination. Sister Mary Joseph's nodule presents as an umbilical mass, frequently misdiagnosed as an umbilical hernia. Its occurrence results from tumor dissemination via lymphatic, hematogenous, or contiguous spread. This chapter provides an in-depth review of this entity, incorporating historical significance, clinical relevance, and diagnostic strategies.

Keywords

Umbilical nodule · Cutaneous metastasis · Clinical signs

12.1 Introduction

The Sister Mary Joseph nodule (SMJN) is a rare but significant clinical sign of metastatic cancer, presenting as an umbilical mass. It typically originates from advanced intra-abdominal malignancies, such as gastric, ovarian, or pancreatic cancer, via peritoneal dissemination [1, 2]. Its presence indicates extensive disease spread and thus poor prognosis [3, 4]. Early recognition is crucial for appropriate management.

Its history dates back to the late nineteenth / early twentieth centuries and is linked to Julia Dempsey (1856–1939), who, upon entering holy orders, abandoned her given name in favor of Sister Marie Joseph [5]. Her convent worked closely with St. Mary's Hospital, managed by Dr. William J. Mayo (founder of the Mayo Clinic). In a short period, she advanced from nun to superior general, from nurse to head nurse, and eventually became the hospital's chief administrator and surgeon assistant. Through her extensive work with patients, she identified a connection between the presence of a visible nodule at the umbilicus and the occurrence of advanced intra-abdominal cancers and pointed Mayo's attention to the worsened prognosis of these patients [6, 7]. He was the first to document this observation in 1928 [8]. This discovery has since been confirmed as an indicator of peritoneal carcinomatosis and umbilical metastases from intra-abdominal malignant tumors.

D. Jeanne · G. Olivier (✉)
Department of Dermatology and Venereology,
Lausanne University Hospital, Lausanne, Switzerland
e-mail: jeanne.dubois@chuv.ch;
olivier.gaide@chuv.ch

D. Koumaki et al. (eds.), *Cutaneous Metastases*, https://doi.org/10.1007/978-3-032-26764-1_12

12.2 Clinical Features and Differential Diagnosis

SMJN typically presents as a firm, non-tender, irregular umbilical mass, often with associated skin ulceration, erythema, or serosanguinous discharge (Fig. 12.1). In some cases, the nodule may be the first sign of an underlying malignancy, emphasizing its diagnostic significance. Every health practitioner should thus be aware of the existence of this clinical entity.

The differential diagnosis of an umbilical cutaneous nodule is broad, and the following diagnoses must be considered and ruled out [9, 10]. Infectious causes include bacterial omphalitis caused by *Staphylococcus aureus*, Streptococcus species, or *Pseudomonas aeruginosa*, as well as fungal omphalitis due to *Candida*

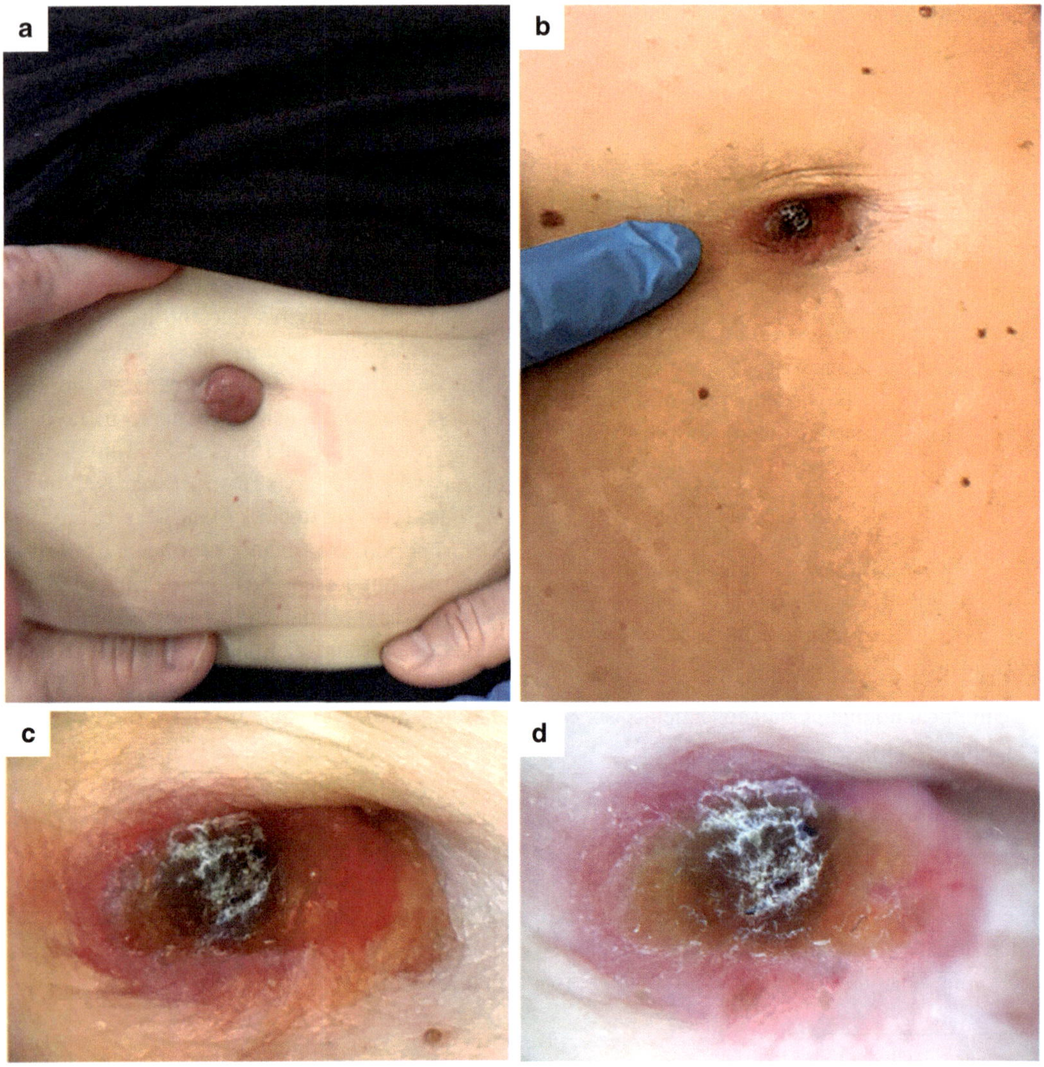

Fig. 12.1 Clinical appearance (**a/b/c**) and dermoscopy (**d**) of two SMJN diagnosed by the authors. In both panel **a** and **b/c**, there is the presence of a violaceous nodule in the umbilicus. Panel **a** shows the frequent violaceous appearance typical of highly vascularized metastasis, while panel **b/c/d** shows the typical erosion with crust and serous discharge often observed in SMJN

albicans. Inflammatory causes comprise inverse psoriasis, mixed intertrigo, pyoderma gangrenosum, and mechanical irritation by foreign objects. Neoplastic causes encompass primary cutaneous cancers such as basal cell or squamous cell carcinoma and melanoma, as well as endometriosis. In the latter case, the nodule is often painful. Other potential causes include an umbilical hernia. Given this broad spectrum, appropriate complementary examinations must be performed to guide the diagnostic process effectively.

Imaging techniques such as ultrasound, computed tomography (CT), or magnetic resonance imaging (MRI) may be necessary to assess the extent of the lesion and its potential connections to underlying structures. Laboratory tests, including microbial cultures, serologies, and tumor markers, can further aid in distinguishing between infectious, inflammatory, and neoplastic etiologies (Table 12.1).

Table 12.1 Causes of umbilical nodules and suggested investigations to perform

Causes	Suggested investigations
Infectious	
Staphylococci	Bacterial smear
Streptococci	Bacterial smear
Pseudomonas	Bacterial smear
Candida	Fungal smear
Inflammatory diseases	
Psoriasis	Clinical search for psoriasis on other body sites, biopsy
Pyoderma gangrenosum	Biopsy
Foreign body (in children mostly)	Clinical examination, foreign body removal, and ultrasound
Neoplasia (including benign lesions)	
Basal cell carcinoma	Biopsy
Squamous cell carcinoma	Biopsy
Melanoma	Biopsy (full lesion excision if possible)
SMJN	Biopsy and imaging (CT, PET-CT, or MRI)
Endometriosis	Biopsy, ultrasound
Keloid scars	History of piercing/laparoscopy, biopsy to exclude dermatofibrosacroma protuberans
Other	
Umbilical hernia	Ultrasound

In most cases, histopathological analysis is the cornerstone of diagnosis. A biopsy should be systematically undertaken to establish the histopathological nature of the lesion, thereby enabling precise classification. Histological examination provides essential information regarding cellular morphology and specific markers that can differentiate between benign and malignant conditions or between local tumors and metastasis. Moreover, it provides prognostic markers (proliferation indexes or specific mutations) and may help to guide treatment (providing tumor material allowing for testing for the presence of specific pathway mutations and establishing the tumor mutational burden).

Early and precise diagnosis is crucial for optimizing patient management and ensuring timely and effective treatment. Therefore, in the presence of an umbilical cutaneous nodule, a thorough diagnostic workup is warranted.

12.3 Pathophysiology of Metastatic Spread to the Umbilicus

The umbilical region represents a distinct zone of anatomical vulnerability within the abdominal wall [1, 2, 11]. It constitutes the site of confluence for several obliterated embryological structures, including the urachus, the umbilical arteries, and the vitelline duct, all of which traverse the linea alba. In contrast to other segments of the abdominal wall, the umbilicus is devoid of substantial muscular support and is primarily composed of dense connective tissue. This relative paucity of structural reinforcement predisposes the area to mechanical weakness and potential dehiscence. Consequently, the umbilical site serves as a common locus for the development of intestinal umbilical hernias. At this anatomical spot, the distance between the abdominal cavity and the skin is mere millimeters (Fig. 12.2).

In the context of peritoneal carcinomatosis, tumor cells disseminate within the peritoneal cavity, often via peritoneal fluid dynamics and direct seeding. The umbilicus, being a site of minimal resistance, facilitates the extraperitoneal extension of malignant cells.

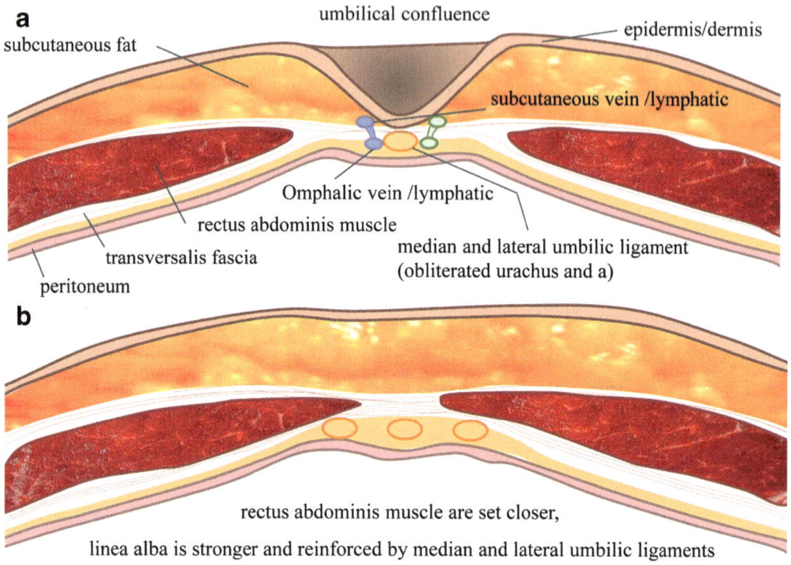

Fig. 12.2 Anatomy of the abdominal wall. Panel **a** illustrates a transverse section at the level of the umbilicus, while panel **b** illustrates a transverse section below that level. Panel **a** is based on a limited umbilical rectus diastasis, while the panel **b** would illustrate the normal linea alba in nulliparous young and non-obese patients

This process is further enhanced by the presence of lymphatic and venous connections between the umbilicus and the peritoneum, which can also serve as conduits for tumor spread. The venous drainage of the abdominal wall involves several anastomotic pathways, notably cranially via the axillary vein through the internal mammary vein and caudally via the femoral vein through the superficial epigastric vein. Additionally, the umbilicus may establish connections with the portal system through small paraumbilical veins. These venous routes are thought to play a crucial role in the cutaneous metastatic process, particularly in the development of umbilical metastases. Batson described a complex vertebral venous system composed of epidural, perivertebral, thoraco-abdominal, head and neck, and vertebral column veins [12]. These valveless vessels operate under low pressure and form a network that parallels and communicates with the portal, pulmonary, and caval venous systems, offering potential bypass pathways.

The lymphatic drainage of the umbilicus plays a critical role in the dissemination of malignant cells. This region is connected to both superficial and deep lymphatic networks, including the axillary, inguinal, para-aortic, internal mammary, and external iliac lymph nodes. Although anatomical variations are common, lymphoscintigraphic studies have demonstrated unusual drainage patterns, with approximately 20% of patients exhibiting lymphatic flow from the peri-umbilical skin to internal mammary nodes. Such variability may account for the occurrence of umbilical metastases and has significant implications for both prognosis and surgical strategy. The umbilicus serves as a pivotal crossroads within the lymphatic system, allowing not only anterograde but also retrograde dissemination of neoplastic cells. The deep lymphatic pathways often follow the falciform ligament, pierce the diaphragm, and extend into the anterior mediastinum or along the iliac vessels. These channels are presumed to represent the primary pathways for lymphatic dissemination to and from the umbilical region [11, 13].

The anatomical convergence of arterial, venous, and lymphatic networks at the umbilicus establishes it as a potential locus for metastatic seeding. While direct peritoneal extension is considered the predominant mechanism in gastrointestinal malignancies, the frequent co-occurrence of hepatic and umbilical metastases suggests a sequential spread—initially via the portal system to the liver, followed by secondary dissemination through lymphatic or venous routes to the umbilicus (Fig. 12.3).

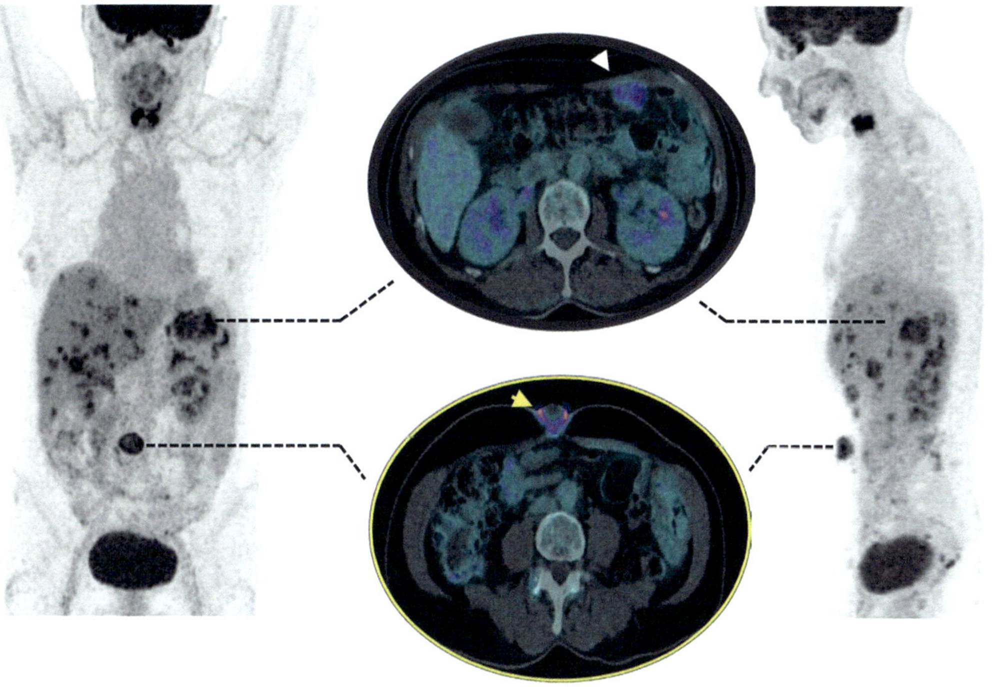

Fig. 12.3 PET-CT (frontal view of the scout/overlay sections at the splenic and umbilical stages/lateral view of the scout) displaying an SMJN (yellow arrowhead), several intra-abdominal, (hepatic) and at least one intraperitoneal metastasis (white arrowhead). Of relevance and interest are the diastasis recti (split occurring between the left and right rectus abdominis muscles) and the minimal distance between the epidermis and peritoneal cavity at the umbilical site

12.4 Tumoral Origins and Prognosis

We present here an analysis of the epidemiology findings, clinical significance, and statistical correlations of umbilical metastases in the context of cancer, drawing from clinicopathologic studies and retrospective reviews.

Although SMJN was described more than 100 years ago, the scientific literature is limited to case reports, with reviews or retrospective studies not available. A study published in 1998 analyzed a cohort of 407 patients, regardless of sex, and supported the hypothesis of a predominance of primary gastrointestinal cancers (52%, including 23% gastric), followed by gynecological cancers (28%, with 16.7% ovarian and 5.8% uterine primary cancers) [9]. Another study, which gathered 99 cases between 1994 and 2016, reported a gynecological origin in 49.1% of cases, followed by pancreatic and gastrointestinal tract cancers in 32.2% [14].

The most comprehensive and systematic review was published in 2024, analyzing data from 2003 to 2023, encompassing 550 articles and incorporating data from 1196 patients [15]. According to this review, the most common primary tumor associated with umbilical metastases was ovarian carcinoma (25.4%), followed by colorectal (17.9%), pancreatic (6.5%), and gastric cancers (5.9%). Gynecologic tumors (breast, ovary, tube, and endometrium) accounted for more than a third of all tumors (34.1%). These data, adapted and complemented by our own data, are presented in Table 12.2.

The majority of patients (73.4%) presented with SMJN as the initial sign of malignancy, while in 26.6% of cases, the metastasis was detected after primary tumor diagnosis or treatment.

Median survival after diagnosis is 7 months, with longer survival observed in ovarian

Table 12.2 Tumor of origin and frequency rates

Origin of the SMJN	Reported numbers	% of total
Gastrointestinal organs	*445*	*37.2*
Colon	214	17.9
Pancreas	78	6.5
Stomach	71	5.9
Gallbladder	22	1.8
Rectum	17	1.4
Appendix	15	1.3
Esophagus	11	0.9
Small intestine	8	0.7
Duodenum	2	0.2
Biliary system	5	0.4
Anus	2	0.2
Genitourinary organs	*407*	*34.0*
Ovary	304	25.4
Endometrium	55	4.6
Tuba	14	1.2
Prostate	14	1.2
Bladder	12	1.0
Kidney	5	0.4
Urachus	2	0.2
Penis	1	0.1
Other organs	*90*	*7.5*
Breast	35	2.9
Pulmonary	18	1.5
Peritoneum	17	1.4
Lymphoma	6	0.5
Neuroendocrine	4	0.3
Skin	4	0.3
DSRCT (desmoplastic small round cell tumor)	4	0.3
Liver	3	0.3
Unknown primary	*254*	*21.2*

(18 months) and endometrial cancers (9 months), while pancreatic primaries have the poorest prognosis (3 months).

Although the Sister Mary Joseph nodule (SMJN) typically indicates widespread metastatic disease, very rare cases may present as the sole metastatic site, warranting excisional surgery rather than mere biopsy. In such instances, meticulous surgical techniques are imperative to avoid breaching or injuring the peritoneal connection. Furthermore, it is well established that no universal treatment exists for SMJN; management must instead be tailored to the underlying malignancy, with therapeutic strategies ranging from curative interventions to palliative care.

12.5 Conclusions

Sister Mary Joseph nodules (SMJNs) are rare but clinically significant indicators of underlying malignancy, often representing the initial manifestation of an occult primary tumor. Hence, heightened clinical awareness of this condition is crucial.

The umbilicus is a convergence point for venous, lymphatic, and peritoneal pathways, making it a key anatomical site for secondary tumor spread from the abdominal cavity.

The presence of SMJN is highly indicative of advanced-stage malignancy and should prompt a thorough oncologic evaluation to determine the primary tumor and extent of disease dissemination. Histological assessment (through surgical biopsy) and imaging are essential for early diagnosis and staging, enabling timely therapeutic intervention.

The current understanding of the epidemiology of umbilical metastases is largely derived from isolated case reports and small series, instead of unbiased national or supra-national registries, thus painting a rather imprecise assessment of their incidence, tumor origin, and impact on survival. It nevertheless serves as a great reminder of the diversity of tumors that can present as SMJN.

References

1. Gabriele R, Conte M, Egidi F, Borghese M. Umbilical metastases: current viewpoint. World J Surg Oncol. 2005;3(1):13.
2. Dubreuil A, Dompmartin A, Barjot P, Louvet S, Leroy D. Umbilical metastasis or Sister Mary Joseph's nodule. Int J Dermatol. 1998;37(1):7–13.
3. Majdoubi A, Bouhout T, Harhar M, Mirry A, Badr S, Harroudi TE. Radical treatment of Sister Mary-Joseph nodule: case report and literature review. Pan Afr Med J [Internet] 2021 Nov 16 [cited 2025 Jun 18];40(161).

Available from: https://www.panafrican-med-journal.com//content/article/40/161/full.
4. Hugen N, Kanne H, Simmer F, van de Water C, Voorham QJ, Ho VK, et al. Umbilical metastases: real-world data shows abysmal outcome. Int J Cancer. 2021;149(6):1266–73.
5. Julia Dempsey. In: Wikipedia [Internet]. 2024 [cited 2025 Jun 17]. Available from: https://en.wikipedia.org/w/index.php?title=Julia_Dempsey&oldid=1206181175
6. Clements AB. Metastatic carcinoma of the umbilicus. JAMA J Am Med Assoc. 1952;150(6):556–9.
7. Segovis CM, Dyer RB. The "Sister Mary Joseph Nodule". Abdom Radiol. 2017;42(5):1610–1.
8. Mayo WJ. Metastasis in cancer. Proc Staff Meet Mayo Clin. 1928;3:327.
9. Galvan VG. Sister Mary Joseph's nodule. Ann Intern Med. 1998;128(5):410.
10. Tso S, Brockley J, Recica H, Ilchyshyn A. Sister Mary Joseph's nodule: an unusual but important physical finding characteristic of widespread internal malignancy. Br J Gen Pract. 2013;63(615):551–2.
11. Sasai K, Kawamura M, Okumura K, Kawai Y. Radiation therapy for Sister Mary Joseph's nodule: a review. Adv Radiat Oncol [Internet]. 2024 [cited 2025 Jun 18];9(2). Available from: https://www.advancesradonc.org/article/S2452-1094(23)00149-5/fulltext.
12. Batson OV. The function of the vertebral veins and their role in the spread of metastases. Ann Surg. 1940 Jul;112(1):138.
13. Nie X, Chen X, Jiang Y, Zhong Y, Chen T, Cheng W. Sister Mary Joseph nodule as cutaneous manifestations of metastatic ovarian cancer: a case report and review of the literature. Medicine. 2022;101(6):e28712.
14. Yan L, Sethi S, Bitterman P, Reddy V, Gattuso P. Umbilical lesions: Clinicopathologic features of 99 tumors. Int J Surg Pathol. 2018;26(5):417–22.
15. Gabriele R, Campagnol M, Borrelli V, Iannone I, Sapienza P, Sterpetti AV. Sister Mary Jospeh's nodule as metastasis of colorectal cancer. Systematic review of the literature and meta-analysis. Int J Surg Case Rep. 2024;123:110132.

Part IV

Cutaneous Metastases from Thoracic Cancer

13 Cutaneous Metastases from Lung Cancer

Alexandra Dobre and Ana-Maria Forsea

Abstract

Lung cancer remains the leading cause of cancer-related morbidity and mortality worldwide, with an estimated 2.5 million new cases in 2022. Although it frequently metastasizes to organs such as the liver, brain, and bones, cutaneous metastases (CM) from lung cancer are rare, occurring in approximately 1.7%–3.1% of cases, with an apparent predilection for male patients. CM often indicates advanced disease and poor prognosis, with a median survival of less than 9 months following diagnosis. Adenocarcinoma is the most common histological subtype associated with CM, although all lung cancer types can potentially metastasize to the skin. CM may present either after diagnosis or as the first clinical manifestation, appearing in various forms. This includes, most frequently, nodules and ulcerated lesions, but pseudo-inflammatory or sclerodermoid mimics are also possible. The supradiaphragmatic region and scalp are common sites, as CM favor the proximity of the primary tumor, but acral dissemination has been reported. Diagnosis relies on clinical suspicion, histopathological confirmation, and immunohistochemical markers such as cytokeratin-7 (CK7) and Thyroid transcription factor 1 (TTF-1). CM reflect an aggressive disease course but are not independently associated with worsened survival in multivariate analysis. Treatment is primarily palliative, including surgical excision, radiation, and systemic immune-chemo- or targeted therapies, depending on lesion number, symptoms and primary tumor type. Given their diverse clinical presentations and potential to mimic benign or infectious dermatoses, early recognition of CM is critical to avoid delays in diagnosis and appropriate management.

Keywords

Cutaneous metastases · Lung cancer · Metastatic cancer · Palliative oncology · Cancer outcomes · Skin

13.1 Introduction

Lung cancer currently has the highest incidence and mortality rates globally among human malignancies, with a reported 2.5 million new cases in

A. Dobre
Department of Pathophysiology, Carol Davila University of Medicine and Pharmacy, Bucharest, Romania

A.-M. Forsea (✉)
Department of Oncologic Dermatology, Elias University Hospital Bucharest, Carol Davila University of Medicine and Pharmacy, Bucharest, Romania

Dermatology Department, Health and Medical University Potsdam, Potsdam, Germany

D. Koumaki et al. (eds.), *Cutaneous Metastases*, https://doi.org/10.1007/978-3-032-26764-1_13

2022 alone [1]. These statistics underscore that the global burden of this disease has remained substantial, despite ongoing advancements in medical research and treatment strategies.

Lung cancer has a high metastatic potential, but dissemination to the skin is rather uncommon, and often signals advanced stages of the disease [2].

13.2 Epidemiology

Historically, the reported frequency of cutaneous metastases (CM) from lung cancer ranged between 1% and 12% [3, 4], but recent studies have narrowed this range to approximately 1.7%–3.1% [5, 6]. Notably, lung cancer metastasizing to the skin is more commonly observed in males, where it ranks as the second most frequent cause of CM after melanoma [7]. In contrast, this phenomenon is considerably rarer in females [5, 7], where lung cancer was the sixth cause of CM after breast (70.7%), melanoma (12%), ovary (3.3%), unknown site (3%), oral cavity (2.3%), and lung (2%) [5, 8].

Larger series studies suggested the skin is identified as the 13th most common site for lung cancer metastasis, after hilar nodes, liver, adrenal glands, bones, and brain [5, 8]. On the other hand, lung cancer appears to be the fastest among internal neoplasms to metastasize to the skin after initial diagnosis (mean time 5.75 months) [9].

13.3 Correlation with Lung Cancer Subtypes

Due to the limited number of comprehensive studies and the reliance on case reports, discrepancies exist in the literature regarding the frequency of CM from lung cancer across different populations. All histological subtypes of lung cancer can potentially metastasize to the skin [9, 10]. However, most studies that specifically analyze CM from lung cancer identify adenocarcinoma as the most common histological type to disseminate to the skin, and this is also the most frequent type of lung neoplasm, with a propensity to metastasize wide and early [9]. Large-cell carcinoma, although rarer, has been reported to have a particularly high incidence of CM compared to other histologic types [8]. Squamous cell carcinoma and small cell carcinoma disseminate less frequently to the skin, and when they do, it is late, as a sign of widespread disease and poor prognosis [9, 10]. Notably, CM originate more frequently from lesions in the upper lobes of the lungs [4, 8]. There is no clear link between CM from lung cancer and pleural involvement, indicating that the spread of cancer through the peritoneum or pleura does not necessarily promote cutaneous dissemination [2].

13.4 Clinical Appearance and Course

CM manifest during the progression of lung cancer and may appear either subsequent to the initial diagnosis or as the first clinical indication of the disease. In a large cohort study [5], involving 7316 oncological patients, metastatic disease was identified in 3839 individuals (52.5%). Among these, cutaneous involvement was observed in 367 patients, representing 5% of the total cohort and 9.6% of those with metastatic disease. Notably, in 59 cases (0.8% of the total cohort), CM was the initial presenting sign of cancer. Focusing specifically on lung cancer, among 1223 patients, 21 (1.7%) were found to have CM. Of these, only 4 patients (0.3%) presented with CM as the first manifestation of lung cancer [5] (Fig. 13.1).

CM from lung cancer can develop at any anatomical site, although they typically appear in close proximity to the primary tumor [9, 10], with the supradiaphragmatic region, including scalp, being the most commonly affected, followed by the abdomen. The extremities are rarely involved [2, 6, 10, 11]. Some studies found that CM most frequently occurs on the chest [2, 4], whereas others suggest that the scalp is the most common site, possibly due to its rich vascular supply [10, 12, 13]. Facial metastases have also been reported [14–16]. In most cases, the occurrence of CM is associated with dissemination to

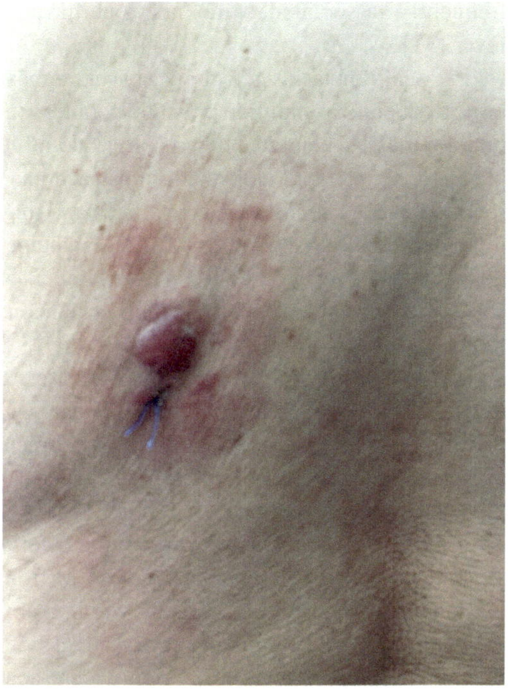

Fig. 13.1 *Nodular-infiltrative metastasis* of lung adenocarcinoma, presenting as single lesion on the left posterior thoracic wall

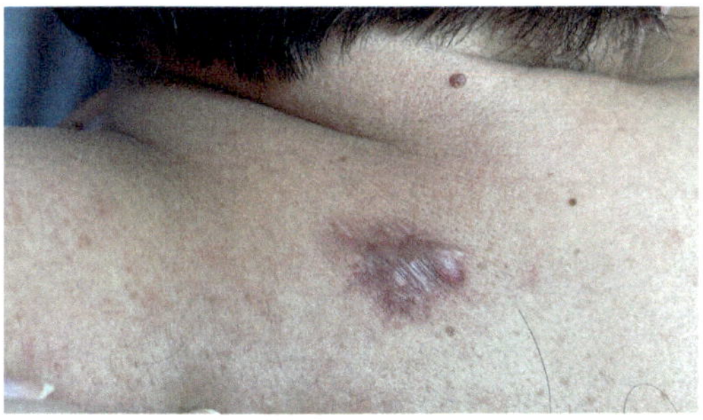

Fig. 13.2 *Infiltrative metastasis* of lung adenocarcinoma, presenting as a single cutaneous lesion in the posterior cervical area

other organs. Currently, no studies specifically assessed the distribution of CM from lung cancer based on sex or lung cancer subtype. However, some observations have been made: in small cell lung cancer, metastases may preferentially involve the back, while in mesothelioma, CM typically occurs through direct invasion or traumatic seeding of the thoracic wall, with distant cutaneous involvement being uncommon [8] (Fig. 13.2).

Table 13.1 Clinical aspects of cutaneous metastases from lung cancer

Solitary nodule [10, 19]
Multiple nodules [9, 15, 20, 21]
Tumor [17, 22]
Fungated ulcerated skin lesion/non-healing ulceration [23–25]
Zosteriform cutaneous metastases [26–29]
Morphea-like/ sclerodermoid type *"carcinoma en cuirasse"* [30]
Eczematiform rash [31]
Erysepelatoid rash- cutaneous lymphangitis carcinomatosa [31–33]
Keratoacanthoma-like [34, 35]
Rhinophyma-like [16]
Acral metastases: Oedema, erythematous- violaceous discoloration/ nodules/ fluctuating bullae of finger tips, subungual nodules [3, 11, 14, 24]
Cicatricial alopecia on the scalp [36]
Vasculitis-like lesions [14]

The clinical appearance of CM from lung cancer is not distinct or consistent, making them indistinguishable on mere skin examination from CM of other origins [8–10]. An overview of the various clinical aspects of CM from lung cancer is included in Table 13.1. Most frequently, skin metastases consist of a dense infiltrate of moderately or poorly differentiated neoplastic cells in the dermis or the hypodermis with no epidermal dysplasia and are described as painless, mobile or fixed indurated nodules, either solitary or more frequently multiple, often covered by normal skin [8, 10]. Although these lesions are often asymptomatic, potentially due to malignant invasion of the dermis and subcutaneous tissues, which could determine nerve damage/desensitization, they can sometimes, depending on location and extent, cause disfigurement, pain, bleeding, or drainage, which can markedly increase morbidity [17, 18]. The CM can vary significantly in color—ranging from flesh-toned to shades of red-purple or blue-black—and can differ in size [16].

CM are a great mimicker, therefore the differential diagnosis of lung cancer CM can be divided into the following categories: (1) primary malignant cutaneous tumors (e.g., squamous cell carcinoma, keratoacanthoma, basal cell carcinoma, amelanotic melanoma, and Merkel cell carcinoma); (2) benign cutaneous tumors (e.g., epidermoid/trichilemmal cyst and other adnexal tumors); (3) inflammatory disorders (e.g., morphea, vasculitis, and eczema); (4) infectious disorders (e.g., herpes zoster, cellulitis, erysipelas, and paronychia); (5) other conditions (e.g., superior vena cava syndrome) (Fig. 13.3).

Cutaneous lymphangitis carcinomatosa is a rare condition, accounting for less than 5% of CM [31, 37]. It is caused by the occlusion of the lymphatic channels in the dermis by neoplastic cells. Although described most often in breast cancer, adenocarcinoma is the most common subtype of lung cancer associated with this form of CM [31, 37]. Usually, patients present with a progressively erythematous, tender area, which may closely resemble other skin diseases such as morphea, erysipelas/cellulitis and particularly if located in the cervical region, it requires a differential diagnosis from superior vena cava syndrome [32]. When distinguishing cutaneous lymphangitis carcinomatosa from primary cutaneous infectious diseases, it is important to note that skin affected by the latter is usually warmer, more tender, responds to antibiotics, and is more frequently associated with neutrophilia and fever [31].

The scalp metastases of lung cancers appear most frequently as multiple or single nodules, but tumoral masses, ulcerated tumors, sclerodermoid plaques, or cicatricial alopecia lesions have been reported [12, 13, 15, 38]. When solitary, they must first be differentiated from primary cutaneous neoplasms, as well as from trichilemmal or sebaceous cysts or other benign cutaneous tumors.

It is estimated that in 40%–82% of cases, a diagnosis of CM is suspected before biopsy, but this rate is significantly lower when the clinical presentation is atypical or when lung cancer has not been previously suspected or diagnosed [6, 8, 39]. Adding to the diagnostic difficulty are collision tumors, such as a reported case of CM from pulmonary adenocarcinoma arising within a preexisting basal cell carcinoma in a patient with undiagnosed lung cancer [40]. Prompt identification of these lesions as malignant is essential to avoid unnecessary empirical treatments with anti-inflammatory or antimicrobial agents, which can delay accurate diagnosis and management.

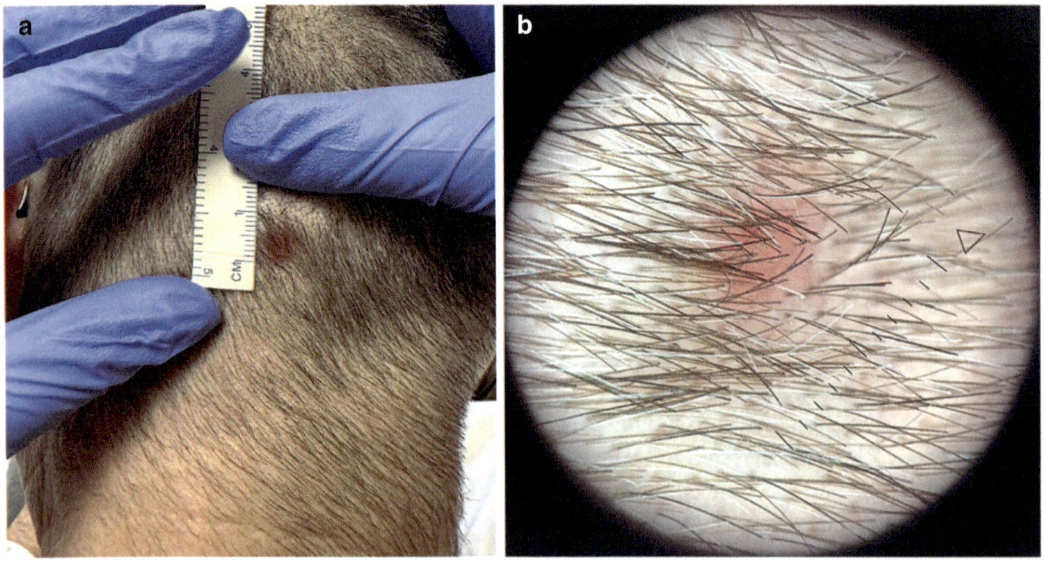

Fig. 13.3 *Scalp nodular metastases* from lung adenocarcinoma. (**a**) Clinical aspectş; (**b**) Dermoscopy. (Courtesy of Dr. Cristina Beiu)

13.5 Diagnosis

The diagnosis of CM relies on clinical suspicion and histopathological examination, with immunohistochemistry adding valuable insights. Given that CM can closely mimic other dermatological conditions, it is crucial to maintain a high level of clinical suspicion, especially when a new skin lesion appears in a chronic smoker, even in the absence of respiratory symptoms [23], and particularly if the patient has a known history of lung cancer. The definitive diagnosis is established through histopathological analysis.

CM from the lung are frequently moderately or poorly differentiated. When the histological features of the primary and metastatic lesions are identical, the diagnosis is confirmed. In the absence of a known primary tumor, it is essential to ascertain whether the lesion is primary or secondary. For identifying a primary site, a comprehensive evaluation needs to be undertaken, including patient history, physical examination, and cross-imaging techniques such as chest X-ray, mammography, ultrasound, computed tomography, and magnetic resonance imaging [8]. Immunohistochemistry remains the gold standard in differentiating the origin: the presence of cytokeratin 7 and antithyroid transcription factor, combined with the absence of cytokeratin 20, strongly suggests a primary lung carcinoma [6, 10].

13.6 Prognosis

CM of lung cancer are indicative of advanced disease [6, 8, 9, 13], often correlating with reduced progression-free survival [41]. The mean time from cancer diagnosis to the development of CM is estimated to be as short as 5–6 months [6, 9, 42], as in 20%–60% of cases, the CM are present at the moment of diagnosis [8, 9, 20, 21, 42, 43], usually along metastases in other organs. Most affected patients survive less than 9 months afterwards, with an average survival ranging from 3 to 5 months [6, 8, 10, 16, 42]. Studies have suggested a significantly shorter overall survival in patients with CM compared to those without (3.9 vs. 10.0 months, $P = 0.0001$) [44]. Furthermore, survival outcomes between patients with only CM and those with multiple metastases are comparable (4.0 vs. 3.0 months, $P = 0.36$) [38, 44]. Although patients with CM often have additional metastatic sites, multivariate analysis has not identified skin metastasis as an independent prognostic factor, possibly due to the limited sample size in studies [41].

13.7 Management

Although spontaneous regression of CM from lung cancer has been reported [13], their treatment remains primarily palliative. Surgical excision combined with radiotherapy may be considered for solitary lesions [18]. In contrast, when multiple CM are present, or other organs are concomitently involved, systemic therapy, according to the type of primary tumor is administered. This includes immunotherapy, chemo-immunotherapy, targeted therapy, or chemotherapy alone [45–47], with radiation reserved for managing symptoms such as pain or bleeding. Notably, the presence of skin or muscle metastases has been associated with a lower response rate to first-line therapy compared to cases without these metastases [41].

13.8 Conclusions

Lung cancers are an important source of CM. CM from lung cancer, although rare, represent a significant clinical finding that typically indicates advanced and aggressive disease. Most commonly arising from adenocarcinoma and upper lobe primaries, especially in men, CM often presents within months of initial cancer diagnosis or, in some cases, as the first clinical sign, underscoring the need for diagnostic evaluation. CM are associated with poor prognosis, with survival rarely exceeding a few months post-diagnosis.

Management remains largely palliative, guided by the extent of disease and tumor histology, highlighting the importance of early detection and diagnosis to optimize care and provide prompt oncologic treatment.

References

1. Luo G, et al. Estimated worldwide variation and trends in incidence of lung cancer by histological subtype in 2022 and over time: a population-based study. Lancet Respir Med. 2025;13:348–63.
2. Kovács KA, et al. Tumor type-specific and skin region-selective metastasis of human cancers: another example of the "seed and soil" hypothesis. Cancer Metastasis Rev. 2013:493–9.
3. Sweldens K, et al. Lung cancer with skin metastases. Dermatology. 1992:305–6.
4. Perng DW, et al. Cutaneous metastasis of lung cancer: an ominous prognostic sign. Chin Med J. 1996:343–7.
5. Lookingbill DP, Spangler N, Sexton FM. Skin involvement as the presenting sign of internal carcinoma: a retrospective study of 7316 cancer patients. J Am Acad Dermatol. 1990;22:19–26.
6. Queirós CS, Filipe PL, Soares de Almeida L. Cutaneous metastases from solid neoplasms in the 21st century: a retrospective study from a Portuguese tertiary care center. J Eur Acad Dermatol Venereol. 2020:1218–24.
7. Todisco A, et al. Cutaneous metastasis as a primary presentation of a pulmonary enteric adenocarcinoma. Int J Biol Markers. 2019:421–6.
8. Mollet TW, Garcia CA, Koester G. Skin metastases from lung cancer. Dermatol Online J. 2009;15
9. Marcoval J, et al. Cutaneous metastasis from lung cancer: retrospective analysis of 30 patients. Australas J Dermatol. 2012:288–90.
10. Sakhri S, et al. Cutaneous metastasis as a first presentation of lung carcinoma: a case series. J Med Case Rep. 2023;17:315.
11. Cohen PR. Metastatic tumors to the nail unit: subungual metastases. Dermatologic Surg. 2001;27(3):280–93.
12. Chiu CS, et al. Malignant cutaneous tumors of the scalp: a study of demographic characteristics and histologic distributions of 398 Taiwanese patients. J Am Acad Dermatol. 2007;56(3):448–52.
13. Salemis NS, et al. Scalp metastasis as the first sign of small-cell lung cancer: management and literature review. Int Surg. 2014:325.
14. Babacan NA, et al. A case of multifocal skin metastases from lung cancer presenting with vasculitic-type cutaneous nodule. Indian J Dermatol. 2015:213.
15. Iliescu CA, et al. Atypical presentation of rapidly progressive cutaneous metastases of clear cell renal carcinoma: a case report. Medicina (Kaunas). 2024;60(11)
16. Chun SM, et al. Nasal tip cutaneous metastases secondary to lung carcinoma: three case reports and a review of the literature. Acta Derm Venereol. 2013:569–72.
17. Ting W, Wang HC. Skin metastasis: rare first manifestation of lung cancer. In: Facial plastic surgery. Thieme Medical Publishers, Inc; 2022. p. 436–8.
18. Wang F, Tong ZH. Cutaneous metastasis as the first symptom: An uncommon presentation of squamous cell lung cancer. Chin Med J. 2017;130:115–6.
19. Vouchara A, et al. Cutaneous lesions: an unusual clinical presentation of small cell lung cancer. Am J Case Rep. 2022;
20. Garg A, et al. Not just skin deep: multiple cutaneous nodules as the first presenting sign of small cell cancer. Adv Resp Med. 2021;89:221–2.
21. Dhambri S, et al. Cutaneous metastasis of lung carcinoma: a retrospective study of 12 cases. J Eur Acad Dermatol Venereol. 2011;25:722–6.
22. Kerrouch H, et al. Metastatic adenocarcinoma of the lung presenting as a Presternal cutaneous mass: case report and brief literature review. Anticancer Res. 2023;43(5):2367–70.
23. Chisenga R, et al. Squamous cell carcinoma of the lung presenting as a fungating ulcerated skin lesion: a case report. J Med Case Rep. 2022;
24. Alkhayat H, Hong CH. Cutaneous metastases from non-small cell lung cancer. J Cutan Med Surg. 2006:304–7.
25. Pircher A, Gastl G, Heidegger I. Ulcerative skin metastases of primary lung cancer. Jpn J Clin Oncol. 2015;45:135.
26. Li WH, et al. Zosteriform skin metastasis of lung cancer. Chest. 2012;142:1652–4.
27. Maki Y, et al. Zosteriform skin metastasis caused by retrograde lymphatic migration of metastatic squamous cell lung carcinoma. BMC Pulmonary Medicine. 2021;21
28. Snow K, et al. Metastatic lung cancer mimicking varicella-zoster virus. Dermatol Online J. 2025;31(1)
29. Tsai PY, Lo Y. Rare cutaneous manifestation of zosteriform cutaneous metastases of lung cancer: two cases and literature review. Kaohsiung J Med Sci. 2024;40:768–9.
30. Lin Y, Zhou S, He W. Clinicopathological diagnosis of morphea-like carcinoma en cuirasse in the neck: a rare presentation of lung cancer. Diagn Pathol. 2025;20(1):16.
31. Prat L, et al. Cutaneous lymphangitis carcinomatosa in a patient with lung adenocarcinoma: case report and literature review. Lung Cancer. 2013:91–3.
32. Kashihara E, et al. Cutaneous lymphangitis carcinomatosa made cervicofacial oedema intractable in a patient with superior vena cava syndrome. BMJ Case Rep. 2018;
33. Homler HJ, Goetz CS, Weisenburger DD. Lymphangitic cutaneous metastases from lung cancer mimicking cellulitis. Carcinoma erysipeloides. West J Med. 1986;144:610.

34. Reich A, et al. Keratoacanthoma-like cutaneous metastasis of lung cancer: a learning point [8]. Acta Derm Venereol. 2006:459–60.
35. Sławińska M, et al. Keratoacanthoma-like cutaneous metastases as the frst presentation of lung cancer. Pol Arch Inter Med. 2017:66–7.
36. Elfatoiki FZ, Hali F. Cutaneous metastasis reveling lung cancer. Pan Afr Med J. 2015;20:19.
37. Peterson H, et al. Cutaneous lymphangitis carcinomatosa: a unique presentation of a rare disease. Dermatol Online J. 2023;29(2)
38. Lambertini M, et al. Scalp cutaneous metastases: a warning bell. In: Curr Probl Cancer, vol. 45; 2021.
39. Strickley JD, Jenson AB, Jung JY. Cutaneous Metastasis. Hematol Oncol Clin North Am. 2019;33(1):173–97.
40. Carey E, et al. Metastatic pulmonary adenocarcinoma deposit arising within a cutaneous basal cell carcinoma: a case report. Head Neck Pathol. 2011:410.
41. Kanaji N, et al. Association of specific metastatic organs with the prognosis and chemotherapeutic response in patients with advanced lung cancer. Respir Investig. 2019;57(5):472–80.
42. Betlloch-Mas I, et al. Cutaneous metastases of solid tumors: demographic, clinical, and survival characteristics. Cureus. 2021;13(11):e19970.
43. Irvine J, McKenna L, Wylie G. Cutaneous metastases as the presenting feature of lung cancer. BMJ Case Rep. 2023;16(12)
44. Song Z, et al. Cutaneous metastasis as a initial presentation in advanced non-small cell lung cancer and its poor survival prognosis. J Cancer Res Clin Oncol. 2012:1613–7.
45. Dingemans AC, et al. Small-cell lung cancer: ESMO clinical practice guidelines for diagnosis, treatment and follow-up(☆). Ann Oncol. 2021;32(7):839–53.
46. Hendriks LE, et al. ESMO Oncogene-Addicted Non-Small Cell Lung Cancer Living Guideline v1.2. 2025.
47. Hendriks LE, et al. ESMO Non-Oncogene-Addicted Non-Small Cell Lung Cancer Living Guideline v1.2. 2025.

Cutaneous Metastases Derived from Mesothelioma

14

Emmanouil Karampinis and Dimitra Koumaki

Abstract

Mesothelioma is a malignancy originating from mesothelial cells that line the body's internal cavities, most commonly affecting the pleura and less frequently the peritoneum, pericardium, or tunica vaginalis. Although distant spread is rare, cutaneous metastases can occasionally occur and present diagnostic challenges. These skin metastases may appear as non-tender nodules or papules, often on the face, or mimic carcinoma erysipelatoides or be zosteriform in case they appear on the trunk. In cases of peritoneal or tunica vaginalis mesothelioma, cutaneous metastases may appear as nodules in the genital area or present as Sister Mary Joseph nodules, respectively. Typically, cutaneous metastases are identified after the diagnosis of primary mesothelioma. A medical history of mesothelioma, along with pulmonary symptoms and abnormal imaging findings, may help guide suspicion for an advanced mesothelioma stage when skin lesions are present. Definitive diagnosis relies on histopathology and immunohistochemistry, with markers like calretinin and cytokeratin 5/6 playing a key role in confirming mesothelioma and distinguishing it from other malignancies such as adenocarcinoma.

Keywords

Mesothelioma · Cutaneous metastasis · Immunocytochemistry · Differential diagnosis · Peritoneal mesothelioma · Sister Mary Joseph's nodule · Malignant mesothelioma of the tunica vaginalis testis

E. Karampinis (✉)
Second Dermatology Department, School of Health Sciences, Aristotle University of Thessaloniki, Thessaloniki, Greece

Department of Dermatology, Faculty of Medicine, School of Health Sciences, University General Hospital of Larissa, University of Thessaly, Larissa, Greece

D. Koumaki
Dermatology Department, University Hospital of Heraklion, Heraklion, Greece

14.1 Basic Principles of Mesothelioma and Mesothelioma Cutaneous Metastases

Mesothelioma is a type of cancer that begins in mesothelial cells, which line the body's internal cavities. It most often affects the pleura and less commonly the peritoneum with rare cases involving the pericardium or the tunica vaginalis of the testes. Around 70%–80% of mesotheliomas develop in the pleura. This form of cancer is strongly linked to asbestos exposure and, less commonly, to radiation therapy [1].

There are three main types of mesotheliomas:

D. Koumaki et al. (eds.), *Cutaneous Metastases*, https://doi.org/10.1007/978-3-032-26764-1_14

(i) Epithelioid—the most common type, making up about 70% of cases.
(ii) Sarcomatoid—less common and generally more aggressive.
(iii) Biphasic—a mix of epithelioid and sarcomatoid features, seen in about 25% of cases [2].

Reports indicate that malignant mesothelioma most commonly arises in the pleura (85.5%), followed by the peritoneum (13.2%). Much rarer sites include the pericardium (0.8%) and the tunica vaginalis of the testis (0.5%) [3]. Data from the SEER database show that median survival after surgery for pleural mesothelioma varies by histologic subtype—19 months for epithelioid, 12 months for biphasic, and just 4 months for sarcomatoid types. Treatment decisions are also based on subtype, with surgery generally reserved for patients with epithelioid mesothelioma [4].

Malignant pleural mesothelioma usually appears 20–40 years usually followed by exposure to asbestos. It typically grows and spreads locally, often affecting nearby structures such as the lungs, heart and pericardium, chest wall, and spine. While it is uncommon for that type of mesothelioma to spread far from the chest, distant metastases can occur and have been found in sites such as brain, cerebellum, spleen, bone marrow, prostate, thyroid, uterus, pelvis, tonsils, tongue, and jawbone (mandibular alveolus) [5].

However, the majority of the reported cases were considered local invasion of the disease. Mesothelioma usually spreads to the skin by directly growing from the original tumor [6]. For example, pleural mesotheliomas can invade the chest wall and eventually reach the skin, while those in the abdomen (peritoneal mesotheliomas) may grow into the abdominal wall and present as Sister Mary Joseph's nodule [7]. Similarly, tumors from the tunica vaginalis can extend into the groin area. The cancer can also reach the skin by penetrating tissues along scars or sites of previous surgical procedures. In contrast, true distant skin metastases, where the cancer spreads to skin far from the original tumor site, are very rare. Cutaneous metastases can appear in a variety of presentations [8]. Most often, they present as firm, painless tumors, reddish or purplish in color, either solitary or multiple, and with progressive growth [6, 8].

Skin involvement from pleural mesothelioma usually appears after the primary cancer has already been diagnosed. Due to how rare mesothelioma is and how much it can resemble other tumors under the microscope, immunohistochemistry plays a critical role in confirming the diagnosis.

14.2 Presentation of Cases Reported in Medical Literature- Facial Cutaneous Metastases from Mesothelioma

We reported 12 cases in the medical literature that included patients with cutaneous metastases derived from pleural mesotheliomas to facial lesions (Table 14.1) and four cases with cutaneous metastases to non-facial areas such as the trunk or flank. As indicated by the cases presented, the most cases that developed mesothelioma with cutaneous metastases were men. This observation can be interpreted by the fact that men more likely work in occupations that involve exposure to asbestos. Asbestos-induced chronic inflammation is the key factor in how asbestos and similar carcinogenic mineral fibers cause cancer such as mesothelioma. When these fibers settle in the lungs or pleura, they have the potential to trigger a persistent inflammatory response involving mesothelial cells and macrophages. This micro-environment, along with the fact that many fibers remain in the body for a long time (biopersistence), makes mesothelial cells resistant to damage, and eventually they transform into cancer cells. About 5% of people with long-term occupational exposure (like miners or shipyard workers) develop mesothelioma [9]. However, regarding pleural mesothelioma with cutaneous facial metastases, the age range is from 47 to 77, which represents a wide range and the occupational exposure to asbestos seems not

Table 14.1 Cases describing patients with facial cutaneous metastases from mesothelioma

	Clinical presentation of cutaneous metastasis	Immunocytochemistry of the cutaneous metastasis	Mesothelioma presented as:	Immunocytochemistry of the mesothelioma
[10]	Discrete, firm, non-tender mass on the right upper lip-	Positive for cytokeratin 5/6 and calretinin, while being negative for carcinoembryonic antigen (CEA)	Pleural and peritoneal-mass lesion	Positive for Cam 5.2, calretinin, cytokeratin 5/6, and Wilms tumor 1 (WT-1) and negative for CD15, CEA, MOC31, Ber-Ep4, TTF-1, and B72.3
[10]	Firm, mobile subcutaneous nodule measuring on the right lateral forehead	Positive for calretinin, mesothelin, cytokeratin 5/6, WT1, and D2-40, while being negative for p40, ERG, and SOX10	Pleural mass	NM
[11]	Firm, smooth, fixed, and slightly tender nodule in the infraorbital area	NM	Confluent tumor nodules on the surface of the parietal pleura as well as on the opposing visceral pleura and subjacent pulmonary parenchyma	NM
[12]	Cutaneous and subcutaneous papules and nodules on the posterior cervical and right posterior lateral thoracic areas, right flank, and left abdominal wall-abdominal metastasis was also detected before cutaneous metastasis occur	NM	Diffuse malignant abdominal mesothelioma along with moderate right pleural effusion, with thickening along the posterior aspect of the pleura	NM
[11]	Cutaneous nodule on the right cheek	Positive for cytokeratin (CK) orthoceratid, and epithelial membrane antigen (EMA) and negative for Leu ML, CEA, S-100 protein factor VI11 related antigen, or Ulex europaeus lectin	Right pleural effusion	NM
[11]	Multiple cutaneous nodules involving the lip, leg, and groin. The first cutaneous metastasis was presented as a tender, bleeding, keratotic nodule on his right upper lip	Positive for antibodies directed against cytokeratins (AE1/3, CK19), anti-calretinin, and human body mesothelial epithelium antibody. (HBME-1) and for adenocarcinoma markers, monoclonal anti-CEA, Ber-Ep4, B72.3, and Leu-M1 antibodies	Pleural mesothelioma (not additional data regarding its characteristics)	NM

(continued)

Table 14.1 (continued)

	Clinical presentation of cutaneous metastasis	Immunocytochemistry of the cutaneous metastasis	Mesothelioma presented as:	Immunocytochemistry of the mesothelioma
[13]	Cutaneous nodules on lips and scalp	Positive staining for CK 5/6, epithelial membrane antigen (EMA), HBME1, calretinin (and CK7 in the tumors. Thyroid transcription factor 1 (TTF1) staining was negative	Lung mass-pleural mesothelioma	NM
[13]	Asymptomatic nodules on the inner and outer lip	Positive staining for cytokeratin marker AE1/AE3, Cam 5.2 and CK7 and calretinin (calcium-binding protein, mesothelial marker) positivity, with negative staining for Ber-EP4 (epithelial cell adhesion molecule, commonly positive in adenocarcinomas)	Lung mass -pleural mesothelioma	NM
[14]	Painful nodule on the left parieto-occipital scalp as well as nodule on the second finger	Positive staining for calretinin, vimentin, and creatine 5/6	Diffuse irregular pleural thickening on the right pleura with nodular masses at the posterior right and invasion of the chest wall	NM
[15]	Multiple facial skin lesion (an annular raised red area with eroded central area a small erythematous plaque posterior to the right ear and a 1 cm very firm subcutaneous lesion on the frontal area)	Positive staining for vimentin, CAM 5.2, and CD10 and focally with SMA and Calretinin	Right pleural effusion and a large right simple pleural effusion with no pleural thickening or masses	Staining were positive for mesothelial markers CK5/6 and Calretinin and negative for lung cancer markers TTF-1 and CEA
[16]	Soft tissue swelling on the scalp	Positive staining for calretinin and CK5/6	An extensive pleural-based tumor, encasing the left lung	Positive staining for calretinin, BerEp4, and CEA with occasional cells showing weak staining for CK5/6
[17]	Eruptive erythematous asymptomatic indurated nodules localized at the face, capillitium and right trunk	Positive staining to pan-cytokeratin antibodies (MNF116) and vimentin Staining for S100, CD31, and CD34 as well as carcinoembryonic antigen (CEA) was negative.	Intermittent pleural effusions on the right site	NM

For the acronyms of certain immunocytochemistry markers please see Table 14.6
NM not mentioned

to impact the occurrence of cutaneous metastases, as the data are scattered (Table 14.1).

In published cases of pleural mesothelioma presenting with cutaneous metastases, several common features seem to emerge, regarding the presentation of the pleural mesothelioma. Clinically, the primary tumor often manifests as a pleural-based mass accompanied by moderate to large pleural effusions, pleural thickening—particularly nodular or involving the posterior pleura—and, in some cases, extension into the adjacent pulmonary parenchyma or chest wall. Imaging frequently reveals diffuse pleural involvement, sometimes encasing the lung, while a few cases present with effusions in the absence of detectable pleural thickening or mass. Immunohistochemically, these tumors consistently express mesothelial markers, such as calretinin, cytokeratin 5/6 (CK5/6), Cam 5.2, and WT-1, while lacking expression of markers typical of adenocarcinomas or other non-mesothelial neoplasms, including CEA, TTF-1, BerEp4, CD15, B72.3, and MOC31. Immunohistochemistry plays a key role in identifying the origin of lung cancer and its associated skin metastasis. A CK7-positive/CK20-negative profile typically indicates lung adenocarcinoma, while a CK20-positive/CK7-negative pattern suggests a colorectal origin. Additionally, markers like TTF-1 and napsin A are both highly sensitive and specific for confirming lung adenocarcinoma. Skin metastases with glandular features often test positive for CK7, TTF-1, Ber-EP4, CEA, and surfactant apoprotein A and are usually negative for CK5/6 and CK20 [18]. Regarding the type of mesothelioma reported were epithelioid and were in terms of the general epidemiology of the mesothelioma subtypes. Two cases of cutaneous metastases to face from sarcomatoid subtypes were found. In that case, the metastases were presented also with ulcerative lesions [15].

Regarding the cutaneous metastases' appearance, they can be presented with a range of clinical manifestations from indurated or subcutaneous nodules to swelling. However, the appearance of the non-tender nodules seems to be the most frequent manifestation of the cutaneous metastasis. The presence of a new non-tender nodule in the facial area in a patient with a medical history of pleural mesothelioma or simultaneous presence of respiratory symptoms should raise suspicion of a skin metastasis. As in the case of the primary mesothelioma, immunohistochemistry provides important diagnostic information. Cytokeratins were the most common immunohistochemistry markers used for cutaneous metastasis diagnosis. Cytokeratins alone cannot definitively distinguish between mesothelioma and adenocarcinoma and their associated metastases, but the pattern of staining can aid the diagnosis—more precisely mesothelioma typically shows a membranous pattern, while adenocarcinoma tends to show cytoplasmic staining. Additionally, cytokeratins 5/6 are more commonly expressed in mesothelioma, making them more useful in differentiating the origin of the metastasis [19]. Calretinin (with both cytoplasmic and nuclear staining) and HBME-1 (which shows membranous staining) are considered specific markers for mesothelioma, and they are rarely encountered in adenocarcinomas [20].

Regarding the treatment status of the patients that developed cutaneous metastases, most of the patients presented were under chemotherapy treatment for their primary mesothelioma cancer. This observation indicates the aggressive nature of the mesothelioma. Also, the time period between primary mesothelioma diagnosis and cutaneous metastasis was calculated from the time of the primary cancer diagnosis to 12 years, but in most cases, the time period was a few months following the pleural mesothelioma diagnosis. Most of the patients died months following the cutaneous metastasis diagnosis.

14.3 Presentation of Cases Reported in Medical Literature—Non-facial Cutaneous Metastases from Mesothelioma

The cases focusing on the cutaneous metastases of mesothelioma were limited. We could find mainly five cases with the most cases appearing on the trunk or back, again in most cases appearing as non-tender nodules or papules. As previously mentioned, immunochemistry was again the most important diagnostic method used to assess the origin of the metastasis as well as the pleural cancer subtype (Table 14.2).

Also, there were special appearances when metastasis occurred in the back or chest, for example, the presence of an inflammatory carcinoma with erythematous plaques that could

Table 14.2 Cases describing patients with non-facial cutaneous metastases from mesothelioma

	Clinical presentation of cutaneous metastasis	Immunocytochemistry of the cutaneous metastasis	Mesothelioma presented as	Immunocytochemistry of the mesothelioma
[21]	A single, firm, pink cutaneous nodule measuring 6 × 8 mm on his upper back	Immunohistochemical stains showed immunoreactivity for CK5/6, CK7, calretinin, and D2-40 and negative staining for TTF-1, CK20, GLUT-1, and prostate-specific antigen (PSA)	Large left-sided pleural effusion	Immunohistochemical stains were positive for cytokeratin (CK) 5/6, CK7, calretinin, D2-40 (podoplanin), p53, GLUT-1, with focal positivity of MOC-31, and negative for thyroid transcription factor (TTF)-1, CK20, caudal-related homeobox gene 2 (CDX2), BerEP4, and napsin A
[22]	Nontender, indurated, erythematous plaques on the chest-inflammatory carcinoma appearance	Immunochemical stains revealed tumor cells were labeled with anticytokeratin antibodies (AE1-AE3, MNF 116, and CAM 5.2) and anti-EMA and were negative with UE and for CEA, LeuM1 antigen, CD34, and FVIIIra	NM	NM
[23]	Several confluent plaques on the right flank	Immunochemical stains revealed neoplastic cells strongly immunoreactive for cytokeratins (MoAb MNF116; Dako, Denmark), CK7, and calretinin and weakly positive for CK5/6; reactivities for CK20, CEA, S100 protein, CD34, and CD31 were negative	Right pleural effusion with marked thickening of the parietal and visceral pleura	NM
[24]	Right latero-thoracic subcutaneous nodule	NM	Pleural mass	NM
[25]	Multiple poorly defined erythematous papules and plaque	Immunohistochemical staining showed the tumor cells were positive for AE1/AE3 cytokeratins, cytokeratins 5/6, epithelial membrane antigen, vimentin, and calretinin. They were negative for thyroid transcription factor-1 (TTF-1), carcinoembryonic antigen (CEA), and Ber-EP4		

For the acronyms of certain immunocytochemistry markers please see Table 14.6
NM not mentioned

mimic skin infection. This type of clinical appearance is called also carcinoma erysipelatoides. While the most skin metastases from internal tumors typically appear as nodules, in certain cases the metastasis may mimic an inflammatory condition, presenting with redness and swelling. This presentation is most commonly associated with breast cancer but has also been observed in cancers of the lung, stomach, pancreas, and rectum. In reported cases of malignant mesothelioma spreading to the skin or metastases in the face, the disease usually manifests as nodules or plaques of varying sizes [22].

Zosteriform metastases were also reported as non-facial metastases of mesothelioma. They are a rare cutaneous sign of tumor spread in which lesions appear in a dermatomal distribution, mimicking herpes zoster. The primary tumor location varies but is most often the breast or lung. These cutaneous eruptions typically occur on the trunk. Their dermatomal pattern and associated pain lead most patients to initially be diagnosed with shingles and treated with antiviral therapy. The mechanism behind this distinct pattern is unknown. Some proposed explanations include spread of tumor cells along perineural lymphatic vessels, via fenestrated vessels near the dorsal root ganglion, surgical cell implantation, or an isomorphic phenomenon at the site of a previous herpes zoster infection. The time period between primary cancer diagnosis and cutaneous metastasis finding were from 4 months to 1 year while in one case the metastasis was found prior to mesothelioma [26].

Also worth mentioning is the differentiation between true cutaneous metastasis of the pleural mesothelioma to the trunk, etc., with direct extension of the primary mesothelioma to those tissues. The differentiation is important as it can impact the staging evaluation of the mesothelioma as well as the treatment approach. In case of direct extension, surgical removal or local radiation may be preferred to systemic chemotherapy or immunotherapy.

14.4 Presentation of Cases Reported in Medical Literature- Cutaneous Metastases from Peritoneal Mesothelioma

Metastasis to the site of the umbilical region is referred to as a Sister Mary Joseph's nodule. The umbilical region possesses a rich network of blood vessels and lymphatics, forming an arteriovenous loop that connects to the round ligament of the liver. Tumor spread to the umbilicus can occur through various pathways, including lymphatic or bloodborne (hematogenous) routes, direct extension from nearby tumors, or along the round ligament of the liver. Also, the umbilicus is one of the weakest regions in the abdominal wall, where the umbilical cord was previously penetrated and aponeurosis and subcutaneous fat are lacking. Sister Mary Joseph's nodule refers to a metastatic lesion at the umbilicus that originates from an underlying intra-abdominal malignancy. In some cases, it may be the first visible sign of advanced cancers such as fallopian tube carcinoma, ovarian cancer, cecal cancer, pancreatic, endometrial, and breast cancer or peritoneal mesothelioma [27].

The most cases were male individuals, while the asbestos exposure was not associated with mesothelioma with cutaneous metastasis. In all the cases of Sister joseph metastasis, peritoneal mesotheliomas were detected in almost all the cases at the time of the cancer diagnosis (Table 14.3).

Table 14.3 Cases describing patients with cutaneous metastases from peritoneal mesothelioma and more specifically Sister Mary Joseph's nodule

Study	Clinical presentation of cutaneous metastasis	Immunocytochemistry of the cutaneous metastasis	Mesothelioma presented as:	Immunocytochemistry of the mesothelioma
[7]	Sister joseph metastasis-nodule	NM	Peritoneal mass	Immunohistochemical stainings of calretinin, D2-40, and CK5/6, which are markers for mesothelial cells, were all positive, while Ber-EP4 and MOC31, which are markers for adenocarcinomas, were negative
[28]	Sister Joseph metastasis-nodule-as a firm nodule distorting the normal appearance of the umbilicus	NM	Peritoneal mass	The tumor was positive for calretinin, Cytokeratin5/6 and negative for CEA, CD34, and P53 protein
[29]	Sister joseph metastasis-nodule	NM	Peritoneal and pleural mesothelioma findings	NM
[30]	Sister Joseph metastasis-nodule	NM	Peritoneal mass	Immunocytochemistry showed positive staining of tumor cells for cytokeratin (CK)5// 6, calretinin, and thrombomodulin. Carcinoembryonic antigen and BerEP4 were

For the acronyms of certain immunocytochemistry markers, please see Table 14.6
NM not mentioned

14.5 Presentation of Cases Reported in Medical Literature—Cutaneous Metastases from Testicular Mesothelioma

Additionally, there were cases that included the presence of cutaneous nodules as metastases on the genital area by mesothelioma of the tunica vaginalis testis. This type of mesothelioma is an uncommon and aggressive form of cancer. While it can affect individuals of any age, it most often occurs in people between 55 and 75 years old (Table 14.4). The condition is frequently linked to exposure to asbestos or materials containing asbestos. Hydrocele (29%) and testicular mass (19%) are the most common initial signs of malignant mesothelioma of the tunica vaginalis testis (MMTVT), though diagnosis can be difficult since many patients show no symptoms. The retroperitoneal lymph nodes are the most frequent location where the cancer tends to spread. Hydrocele (in most cases) or hemoscrotum can be the first diagnosis while in case a palpable mass is detected teratoma diagnosis is on the differential diagnosis [31]. Worth mentioning was that immunochemistry was not used and distant cutaneous metastases were not observed as the cutaneous lesions were mainly observed in the genital area ranging from small papules to lesions that were organized into a large ulcerative mass disfiguring the genital area. All the mesothelioma types were epithelioid. Worth mentioning that immunochemistry assessment was performed less frequently in case of mesothelioma of the tunica vaginalis testis compared to pleural mesothelioma. Also, the cutaneous metastases seem to appear from mesothelioma of the tunica vaginalis testis appear later (2 years) compared to the cutaneous metastases from pleural mesothelioma [32].

Palliative chemotherapy for mesothelioma of the tunica vaginalis testis (MMTVT) generally follows the approach used for malignant pleural mesothelioma. The standard first-line treatment includes a combination of pemetrexed and cisplatin. For patients who cannot receive pemetrexed, alternative first-line chemotherapy options are recommended. One such option is vinorelbine, used alone or with navelbine [33]. Other second-line regimens include raltitrexed with oxaliplatin, or a combination of irinotecan, cisplatin, and mitomycin. Despite these treatment strategies, the prognosis for localized mesothelioma of the tunica vaginalis remains poor [34].

Table 14.4 Cases describing patients with cutaneous metastases from testicular mesothelioma

Case	Clinical presentation of cutaneous metastasis	Immunocytochemistry of the cutaneous metastasis	Mesothelioma presented as:	Immunocytochemistry of the mesothelioma
[35]	Skin-colored painful nodules	Immunohistochemical study showed strong nuclear and cytoplasmic positivity for calretinin, epithelial membrane antigen (cytoplasmic), cytokeratin-7 (CK-7) (cytoplasmic), and nuclear positivity for Wilms tumor-1 (WT-1)	Firm palpable testicular mass	NM
[22]	Several nontender, firm, waxy papules were noted on the penis and scrotum as well as a tender indurated plaque on the ventral aspect of the penis	NM	Nontender mass of the upper pole of the patient's right testis	NM
[36]	Firm, indurated plaques and nodules on the scrotum and lower abdominal skin with surrounding erythema	Immunohistochemical study showed that the neoplastic cells were positive for WT1, D2-40, and AE1/AE3, with rare positivity for calretinin. There was weak patchy staining for EMA, glypican 3, desmin, and MyoD1. The neoplastic cells were negative for CEA, claudin-4, MOC31, CK7, CK20, SOX10, S100, MelanA, ERG, CK5/6, myogenin, CD99, arginase, Hep-Par1, CDX2, TTF1, CD45, chromogranin, synaptophysin, NKX3.1, SALL4, OCT-4, and p40. BAP1 showed retained nuclear expression (normal) by immunohistochemistry	Enlarged left testicle	NM
[37]	Hard, painless thickening of the skin extending from the perineum and scrotum into both inguinal areas and the lower abdomen	NM	Painless swelling of the right scrotum	NM
[40]	Progressive induration of the skin of the scrotum developed, spreading in due course to the penis and perineal and pre-pubial skin. The skin lesions were organized into an ulcerating tumor mass	NM	Haematoscrotum	NM
[38]	Cutaneous metastases to the perineum -not further descriptions	NM	Scrotal swelling and solid mass	The tumor had a positive immunohistochemical reaction with cytokeratins, WT-1, and calretinin, while CD138, CK7, S-100, and CK 5/6 markers were negative

For the acronyms of certain immunocytochemistry markers, please see Table 14.6
NM not mentioned

14.6 Differentiating the Cutaneous Metastases of Mesothelioma from Other Lesions—Clinical, Histopathological, and Immunocytochemistry Parameters

Cutaneous metastases from mesothelioma, as previously noted, can present in many different ways. They most commonly appear as firm, non-painful nodules or plaques with a reddish or purplish hue, either solitary or in clusters, and tend to grow progressively. However, they can sometimes resemble benign skin conditions. For example:

1. Inflammatory presentations of metastases may mimic erysipelas (erysipeloid metastases), inflammatory carcinoma, or even herpes zoster.
2. Multiple non-tender nodules can resemble keratoacanthomas, lipomas, lymphangiomas, pyogenic granulomas, skin adnexal tumors like cylindromas, Kaposi's sarcoma, or hidradenitis suppurativa.
3. Swelling-type lesions may be mistaken for trichilemmal cysts or epidermoid cysts.
4. In cases of cutaneous metastases from mesothelioma involving the tunica vaginalis testis, the lesions may mimic conditions like teratoma metastasis, chancres, and condyloma acuminatum.
5. Umbilical nodules may be misdiagnosed as umbilical hernias, umbilical endometriosis, or metastases from other primary cancers unrelated to peritoneal mesothelioma.
6. Ulcerated lesions in the facial areas presented in case of sarcomatoid subtype of mesothelioma should be differentiated from ulcerated basal cell carcinoma or cutaneous TB.

Given this wide clinical spectrum, accurate diagnosis often requires histopathological confirmation to avoid misdiagnosis and ensure proper treatment. Medical history would aid the clinician when confronting tender nodules of uncertain origin. A prior medical history of pleural mesothelioma, abnormal CT findings as well as the presence of pulmonary symptoms with the simultaneous findings of cutaneous lesions that resemble the clinical images presented previously direct the diagnosis [39]. Additionally, the findings of a testicular swelling with skin lesions at the scrotum or perineum regions would also raise the suspicion for mesothelioma involving the tunica vaginalis testis. The simultaneous appearance of a hydrocele and skin lesions may raise clinical suspicion for underlying malignancy. While hydroceles are typically benign and present as painless scrotal swelling due to fluid accumulation, their co-occurrence with skin lesions—such as firm, non-tender nodules, or plaques—should prompt a thorough evaluation. These cutaneous lesions may represent metastatic spread, and when seen alongside a hydrocele, they could suggest that the hydrocele is not idiopathic but secondary to an occult neoplasm, such as malignant mesothelioma, testicular cancer, or other intra-abdominal malignancies. In such cases, further diagnostic work-up including scrotal ultrasound, imaging for intra-abdominal disease, and skin biopsies. Finally, when evaluating a patient with a suspicious umbilical lesion, key history points that may suggest mesothelioma include a prior or current diagnosis of mesothelioma, especially with evidence of disease progression or metastasis, and a history of asbestos exposure, often through occupations like shipyard work, construction, or mining. Patients may report abdominal distension, pain, or changes in bowel habits in case of peritoneal mesothelioma, or chest pain and dyspnea in pleural forms. Constitutional symptoms such as weight loss, fatigue, and loss of appetite are also common. In females, gynecologic complaints may need to be evaluated to rule out ovarian carcinoma, which is a more frequent cause of Sister Joseph's nodule [40, 41].

Dermoscopy can be a valuable tool in this context, primarily by helping to exclude cutaneous metastases rather than confirm them. While dermoscopic features of skin metastases are not specific as limited and scattered data describe nonspecific vascular patterns and colorations, it remains useful in the differential diagnosis.

Classic dermoscopic traits seen in other conditions can guide clinicians toward more likely benign or alternate malignant diagnoses. For instance, the rainbow pattern is characteristic of Kaposi sarcoma [42], while fingerlike or knob-like projections are often seen in large condylomas [43]. Identifying such patterns can support or rule out certain conditions, directing clinicians away from a presumptive diagnosis of metastasis and toward a more accurate workup and targeted biopsy when needed [44, 45].

The most important tool to assess such lesions is histopathology and immunocytochemistry evaluation, especially for the recognition between mesothelioma and adenocarcinoma cutaneous metastasis. The malignant mesothelioma appears as a dermal tumor, often with overlying ulceration with a glandular and tubulopapillary appearance, while metastatic adenocarcinoma appears as a poorly circumscribed tumor centered in the dermis. In the case of mesothelioma, a variable cell shape (epithelioid, spindled, or biphasic) can be observed in histopathology, while in adenocarcinoma the tissue can be moderately to poorly differentiated with solid nests, sheets, and cords of cells with possible mucinous or glandular differentiation [46]. Immunohistochemical markers [10, 47] for distinguishing malignant mesothelioma from other primary cutaneous tumors and metastatic adenocarcinomas to skin are presented in Tables 14.5 and 14.6.

Table 14.5 Presentation of positive and negatives immunohistochemical markers depended on the cancer type

Cancers	Positive markers	Negative markers
Breast cancer	CK7, ER, PR, GATA3, GCDFP15, mammaglobin	CK20
Ovary cancer	CK7, PAX8, ER, WT1	CK20, TTF1, GATA3
Lung cancer	CK7, TTF1, napsin A, CEA, B72.3, MOC31, BerEp4	CK20, Calretinin, WT1, CK 5/6, HMBE-1, Thrombomodulin, D2-40
Stomach cancer	CK7, CK20, CEA, CDX2 (±), MUC1 (±), MUC5AC (±)	SATB2
Bladder cancer	CK7, CK20, GATA3, p63, CK5/6, p40, uroplakin	
Malignant mesothelioma	Calretinin, WT1, CK 5/6, HMBE-1, thrombomodulin, D2–40	TTF1, CEA, BerEp4, B72.3

Table 14.6 Presentation of immunohistochemical markers, its function and their associated tumor

Markers	Full Name	Function/Role	Associated Tumors
CK7	Cytokeratin 7	Protein type, which is component of the cytoskeleton of epithelial cells	Breast, ovary, lung, stomach, bladder
CK20	Cytokeratin 20	Protein type, which is component of the cytoskeleton of epithelial cells	Stomach, bladder
ER	Estrogen receptor	Ligand-activated transcription factor	Breast, ovary
PR	Progesterone receptor	Hormone receptor with roles in development, physiologic processes and reproduction	Breast
GATA3	GATA binding protein 3	Transcriptional activator in the processes of growth and differentiation, which is highly expressed by the luminal epithelial cells in the breast.	Breast, bladder
GCDFP15	Gross cystic disease fluid protein 15	Marker of apocrine differentiation	Breast
Mammaglobin		Biomarker expressed in both primary and metastatic breast carcinomas, with greater expression in primary tumors	Breast
PAX8	Paired box gene 8	Member of the paired-box family of genes that plays a crucial role in the development of the kidney, thyroid gland, and Müllerian organs	Ovary
WT1	Wilms tumor 1	a transcription factor and plays an important role in cell growth and differentiation	Ovary, mesothelioma
TTF1	Thyroid transcription factor 1	a tissue specific transcription factor expressed in epithelial cells of the thyroid and lung	Lung
Napsin A		Aspartic protease	Lung
CEA	Carcinoembryonic antigen	Cell surface glycoproteins that function as a ligand for various selectins	Lung, stomach
B72.3		Tumor-associated glycoprotein	Lung
MOC31		Epithelial cell adhesion marker	Lung
BerEp4		Epithelial cell adhesion marker	Lung
Calretinin		Calcium-binding protein	Mesothelioma
CK5/6	Cytokeratin 5/6	Protein type, which is component of the cytoskeleton of epithelial cells	Mesothelioma, bladder
HMBE-1	Hector Battifora and mesothelioma	Marker of mesothelial cells	Mesothelioma
Thrombomodulin		Endothelial glycoprotein	Mesothelioma
D2–40		Podoplanin antibody. Podoplanin is a transmembrane, glycoprotein (mucin type) found on lymphatic endothelium, mesothelium, and fetal testis	Mesothelioma
CDX2	Caudal type homeobox 2	Protein that acts as major regulator of intestine-specific genes.	Stomach, colorectal
MUC1, MUC5AC	Mucin 1/mucin 5 AC	a type of mucin that is produced by surface goblet cells	Stomach
SATB2	Special AT-rich sequence-binding protein 2	Nuclear marker normally expressed by epithelium of the lower gastrointestinal tract, ductal epithelium of the testis and epididymis, etc.	Colorectal
p63		p53-related transcription factor	Bladder
p40		Antibody that identifies ΔNp63- which is an isoform lacks the N-terminal transactivation domain	Bladder
Uroplakin		Urothelial differentiation marker	Bladder
Vimentin	–	Antibody used as a specific marker of mesenchymal derivation or differentiation	Mesothelioma

References

1. Carbone M, Adusumilli PS, Alexander HR, et al. Mesothelioma: scientific clues for prevention, diagnosis, and therapy. CA Cancer J Clin. 2019;69:402–29.
2. Saddozai UAK, Wang F, Khattak S, et al. Define the two molecular subtypes of epithelioid malignant pleural mesothelioma. Cells. 2022;11:2924.
3. Qasim A, Allu SVV, Schmidt P, Parikh HR, Moore S, Yapor L, Soliman M. Comprehensive review of mesothelioma cases: from diagnosis to therapeutic strategies. Cureus. 2024; https://doi.org/10.7759/cureus.52859.
4. Schumann SO, Kocher G, Minervini F. Epidemiology, diagnosis and treatment of the malignant pleural mesothelioma, a narrative review of literature. J Thorac Dis. 2021;13:2510–23.
5. Jain M, Crites MK, Rich P, Bajantri B. Malignant pleural mesothelioma: a comprehensive review. J Clin Med. 2024;13:5837.
6. Dagogo-Jack I, Yeap BY, Mino-Kenudson M, Digumarthy SR. Extrathoracic metastases in pleural mesothelioma. JTO Clin Res Rep. 2023;4:100557.
7. Tsuruya K. Malignant peritoneal mesothelioma presenting umbilical hernia and Sister Mary Joseph's nodule. World J Gastrointest Endosc. 2013;5:407.
8. Mori T, Yamamoto T. Skin metastasis of malignant mesothelioma. An Bras Dermatol. 2021;96:642–3.
9. Gaudino G, Xue J, Yang H. How asbestos and other fibers cause mesothelioma. Transl Lung Cancer Res. 2020;9:S39–46.
10. Collins K, Nagarajan P, Aung PP. Distant cutaneous metastasis of malignant epithelioid mesothelioma. J Cutan Pathol. 2021;48:902–7.
11. Edstrom LE, Dawson PJ, Kohler J, Demeester TR. Malignant mesothelioma: a metastasis to the face. J Surg Oncol. 1980;14:251–4.
12. Ordóñez NG. Peritoneal malignant mesothelioma with multiple distant skin metastases. Arch Dermatol. 1983;119:827.
13. Beer TW, Heenan PJ. Malignant mesothelioma presenting as a lip tumor: report of two cases with one unrecognized by 166 pathologists. Am J Dermatopathol. 2007;29:388–91.
14. Kanbay A, Oguzulgen KI, Ozturk C, Memis L, Demircan S, Kurkcuoglu C, Akyurek N, Kurul C. Malignant pleural mesothelioma with scalp, cerebellar, and finger metastases: a rare case. South Med J. 2007;100:63–5.
15. Elbahaie AM, Kamel DE, Lawrence J, Davidson NG. Late cutaneous metastases to the face from malignant pleural mesothelioma: a case report and review of the literature. World J Surg Oncol. 2009;7:84.
16. Fletcher SV, Laws DE, McCutcheon J, Perkins P. Mesothelioma – a change in the natural history? Respir Med CME. 2009;2:25–6.
17. Müller C, Reichrath J, Tilgen W. Disseminated cutaneous metastasis of a biphasic pleural mesothelioma. J Eur Acad Dermatol Venereol. 2009;23:226–7.
18. Ye J, Findeis-Hosey JJ, Yang Q, McMahon LA, Yao JL, Li F, Xu H. Combination of Napsin A and TTF-1 immunohistochemistry helps in differentiating primary lung adenocarcinoma from metastatic carcinoma in the lung. Appl Immunohistochem Mol Morphol. 2011;19:313–7.
19. Barak V, Goike H, Panaretakis KW, Einarsson R. Clinical utility of cytokeratins as tumor markers. Clin Biochem. 2004;37:529–40.
20. Lugli A, Forster Y, Haas P, Nocito A, Bucher C, Bissig H, Mirlacher M, Storz M, Mihatsch MJ, Sauter G. Calretinin expression in human normal and neoplastic tissues: a tissue microarray analysis on 5233 tissue samples. Hum Pathol. 2003;34:994–1000.
21. Ward RE, Ali SA, Kuhar M. Epithelioid malignant mesothelioma metastatic to the skin: a case report and review of the literature. J Cutan Pathol. 2017;44:1057–63.
22. Prieto VG, Kenet BJ, Varghese M. Malignant mesothelioma metastatic to the skin, presenting as inflammatory carcinoma. Am J Dermatopathol. 1997;19:261–5.
23. Maiorana A, Giusti F, Cesinaro AM, Conti A, Rossi G. Cutaneous metastases as the first manifestation of pleural malignant mesothelioma. J Am Acad Dermatol. 2006;54:363–5.
24. Gaudy-Marqueste C, Dales J-P, Collet-Villette A-M, Grob J-J, Astoul P, Richard M-A. Cutaneous metastasis of pleural mesothelioma: two cases. Ann Dermatol Venereol. 2003;130:455–9.
25. Monteagudo Sánchez B, Cabanillas González M, Pérez Fernández A, de la Cámara Gómez J, Campo Cerecedo F. Metástasis cutáneas zosteriformes de mesotelioma pleural maligno. Rev Clin Esp. 2009;209:262–3.
26. Savoia P, Fava P, Deboli T, Quaglino P, Bernengo MG. Zosteriform cutaneous metastases. Dermatologic Surg. 2009;35:1355–63.
27. Tso S, Brockley J, Recica H, Ilchyshyn A. Sister Mary Joseph's nodule: an unusual but important physical finding characteristic of widespread internal malignancy. Br J Gen Pract. 2013;63:551–2.
28. Papalambros A, Sigala F, Vouza E, Hepp W, Antonakis P. Sister Mary Joseph's nodule as primary localized malignant mesothelioma. Report of a case. Zentralbl Chir. 2011;136:172–4.
29. Heatley MK. Sister Mary Joseph's nodule in malignant mesothelioma. Histopathology. 2004;45:299–300.
30. Boyde AM, Attanoos RL. Sister Mary Joseph's nodule in malignant peritoneal mesothelioma. Histopathology. 2003;43:303–4.
31. Arda E, Arıkan MG, Cetin G, Kuyumcuoğlu U, Usta U. Malignant mesothelioma of tunica vaginalis testis: macroscopic and microscopic features of a very rare malignancy. Cureus. 2017; https://doi.org/10.7759/cureus.1860.
32. Gilbert A, Wieland R, Zacher N, Rieger K, Berry GJ, Novoa R. Metastatic mesothelioma of the tunica vaginalis presenting as scrotal and abdominal nodules: a case report and review of the literature. Am J Dermatopathol. 2025;47:e6–e11.

33. Stebbing J, Powles T, McPherson K, Shamash J, Wells P, Sheaff MT, Slater S, Rudd RM, Fennell D, Steele JPC. The efficacy and safety of weekly vinorelbine in relapsed malignant pleural mesothelioma. Lung Cancer. 2009;63:94–7.
34. Radovanovic M, Kojic U, Zubelic A, Jakulic D, Filipovic Z. Timely surgical resection achieved prolonged remission in patients with malignant mesothelioma of the tunica vaginalis testis and retroperitoneal recurrence. Cureus. 2024; https://doi.org/10.7759/cureus.59052.
35. Hispán P, Pascual JC, González I, Bravo D, Peiró G. Cutaneous metastases from malignant mesothelioma of the tunica vaginalis testis. Am J Dermatopathol. 2016;38:222–5.
36. Cartwright LE, Steinman HK. Malignant papillary mesothelioma of the tunica vaginalis testes: cutaneous metastases showing pagetoid epidermal invasion. J Am Acad Dermatol. 1987;17:887–90.
37. Plas E, Riedl CR, Pflüger H. Malignant mesothelioma of the tunica vaginalis testis. Cancer. 1998;83:2437–46.
38. Van Der Rhee HJ, van Vloten WA, Scheffer E, Zwartendijk J. Cutaneous manifestations of malignant mesothelioma of the tunica vaginalis testis. J Cutan Pathol. 1983;10:213–6.
39. Chhabra S, Samra S, Thami G, Punia RS, Mohan H, Chopra R. Cutaneous metastases of internal malignancies: a clinicopathologic study. Indian J Dermatol Venereol Leprol. 2010;76:125.
40. Leonard N. Cutaneous metastases: where do they come from and what can they mimic? Curr Diagn Pathol. 2007;13:320–30.
41. Padden S, Abraham E, Viscosi E, Habin K, Lundquist D. Cutaneous metastases: a case study on clinical care for patients. Clin J Oncol Nurs. 2020;24:320–3.
42. Karampinis E, Toli O, Pappa G, et al. "Chasing rainbows" beyond Kaposi Sarcoma's dermoscopy: a mini-review. Dermatopathology. 2024;11:333–41.
43. Veasey JV, Framil VM d S, Nadal SR, Marta AC, Lellis RF. Genital warts: comparing clinical findings to dermatoscopic aspects, in vivo reflectance confocal features and histopathologic exam. An Bras Dermatol. 2014;89:137–40.
44. Tiodorovic D, Stojkovic-Filipovic J, Marghoob A, et al. Dermatoscopic patterns of cutaneous metastases: a multicentre cross-sectional study of the international dermoscopy society. J Eur Acad Dermatol Venereol. 2024;38:1432–8.
45. Simionescu O, Petrică M, Avram AM, Costache M, Scurtu LG, Tudorache SI, Iorga PG, Grigore M. Dermoscopy of skin metastases in advanced cancer—systemic (visceral, hematologic) and cutaneous. Front Med (Lausanne). 2024; https://doi.org/10.3389/fmed.2024.1445811.
46. Yılmaz U. A localized malignant mesothelioma of the visceral pleura treated with minimal resection of the lung. Turk J Thorac Cardiovasc Surg. 2012;20:155–7.
47. Chapel DB, Schulte JJ, Husain AN, Krausz T. Application of immunohistochemistry in diagnosis and management of malignant mesothelioma. Transl Lung Cancer Res. 2020;9:S3–S27.

Part V

Cutaneous Metastases from Breast Cancer

15 Cutaneous Metastases from Breast Cancer

Danica Tiodorovic

Abstract

Breast carcinoma is the leading malignancy associated with cutaneous metastases (CM), accounting for over 20% of all CM. While skin involvement may occasionally be the first sign of internal malignancy, it more often indicates advanced disease. These metastases most frequently appear on the chest and abdomen but may also involve the head and neck region, back, upper arms, and other regions. The incidence of CM in breast cancer patients is approximately 24%. Clinically, CM display diverse features, ranging from asymptomatic, firm papules, nodules, or indurated plaques. Lacking specific clinical criteria, diagnosis can be challenging. Dermoscopy aids in distinguishing these lesions from other dermatologic conditions. Vascular patterns are the most frequent dermoscopic features, with linear serpentine vessels being the most prevalent ones, followed by arborising vessels. The combination of a structureless white pattern with linear serpentine vessels is the most characteristic dermoscopic feature in breast CM. Recognising these features early in breast cancer patients is essential for prompt diagnosis and timely treatment.

Keywords

Cutaneous metastases · Breast cancer · Dermoscopy

15.1 Introduction

Breast cancer is the most common internal malignancy in women to metastasise to the skin, accounting for approximately 20–24% of all cutaneous metastases (CM) [1–3]. These lesions usually indicate advanced systemic disease and are associated with a poor prognosis. Cutaneous metastases (CM) most often present as nodules but may mimic other dermatological conditions, showing varied clinical and morphological features. Ductal carcinoma is the most frequent histological type linked to cutaneous spread, particularly in patients aged 50–70 [4]. Skin involvement typically develops within 3 years of the primary diagnosis and often follows metastasis to internal organs. The mean survival for patients with only CM is around 57 months, while the median survival for metastatic breast cancer overall is approximately 36 months [3, 4].

Cutaneous metastasis is defined as the spread of malignant cells from a primary cancer to the skin via direct invasion or lymphatic or haematogenous routes. They often appear after the diagnosis of the primary malignancy, typically within 6 months to 4 years, even up to 10 years

D. Tiodorovic (✉)
Clinic of Dermatology, University Clinical Centre of Nis, Medical Faculty of Nis, University of Nis, Niš, Serbia

D. Koumaki et al. (eds.), *Cutaneous Metastases*, https://doi.org/10.1007/978-3-032-26764-1_15

after [5, 6]. In a study by Lookingbill et al., 6.3% of breast cancer patients exhibited cutaneous involvement at the time of diagnosis, with 3.5% presenting with skin symptoms as the initial sign [1].

Metastases are classified by timing: *synchronous* when identified at the same time as the primary tumour, *metachronous* when diagnosed months or years later, and *late* if they appear more than 10 years after the initial diagnosis [5, 6]. Cutaneous metastases from breast cancer are categorised as either locoregional or distant. Locoregional metastases are defined as lesions on the same side as the primary tumour, while distant ones occur elsewhere. Locoregional lesions are more common and often arise in surgical scars. A Latin American study of 914 breast cancer patients identified cutaneous metastases in 3.4% of all patients [7]. The most common presentation was metachronous, asymptomatic nodular lesions, primarily locoregional. Immunohistochemical discrepancies between primary and metastatic sites were observed in 24% of evaluated cases. Median survival postdiagnosis of primary tumour was similar for locoregional and distant metastases (4.7 vs. 4.8 years), but patients with synchronous cutaneous and visceral metastases had the poorest prognosis [7]. Ronen et al. reviewed 232 cutaneous metastasis cases in 199 breast cancer patients, comparing ipsilateral anterior chest wall lesions (126 cases) with distant metastases (106 cases) [4]. Twelve patients had both. Distant metastases commonly involved the contralateral chest wall (11.2%) and head and neck region (6.4%), especially the scalp and neck. Other sites included the back, abdomen, mid-chest, shoulders, axilla, and arms. Most tumours were infiltrating ductal carcinomas. Distant metastases showed poorer differentiation than local lesions. Mean survival was slightly longer for localised chest wall involvement (23 months) than for distant metastases (20.6 months), suggesting differing biological behaviours between local and distant cutaneous spread [4]. In a study of 164 patients by Mordenti et al., the trunk was the most commonly affected site, followed by the head/neck and extremities [8].

In a recent multicentre study conducted by the International Dermoscopy Society (IDS), 42.9% of cutaneous metastases) were found in the head and neck region. However, the thoracic area, particularly the anterior chest wall, remains the most frequent site due to proximity to the primary tumour [9].

CM can occur many years after the initial diagnosis of breast cancer, posing diagnostic challenges, particularly when they mimic other dermatoses. Consequently, distinguishing features on histopathology and immunohistochemistry are essential [4]. From a research and clinical perspective, identifying molecular markers that predict the development of CM and elucidating the molecular distinctions between primary tumours and their cutaneous metastases is of great importance. Such investigations may inform the design of novel therapeutic strategies and improve disease monitoring [5, 7].

Hence, the early recognition of dubious lesions at an early stage is crucial for the treatment plan, as surgical excision of limited lesions may be feasible only in the case of early detection but may be unresectable in advanced stages. Apart from surgical excisions, there are other treatments including local application of imiquimod, cryotherapy, radiotherapy, photosensitisers, oxygen flow-assisted topical administration of methotrexate, aromatase inhibitors, immunomodulators, systemic chemotherapy, as well as targeted therapies and small-molecule tyrosine kinase inhibitors.

15.2 Clinical Presentations

The most common presentations of breast CM are erythematous nodules and plaques, although black, flesh-coloured lesions, and ulcerations have also been reported. Sometimes, breast skin oedema occurs, producing the characteristic 'orange peel' appearance [2, 10]. Additional symptoms may include ulceration, bleeding, pain, odour, secretion, and secondary infection. However, CM may resemble benign conditions like contact dermatitis, radiation recall, cellulitis, or lymphoedema, complicating diagnosing and making distinguishing metastatic lesions challenging. Cutaneous metastases) from breast cancer exhibit diverse clinical morphologies, with the nodular form being the most frequent. Other less common variants include erysipeloid (Fig. 15.1), telangiectatic, alopecia neoplastica, en cuirasse, sclerodermiform, bullous, zosteriform, and erythema-annulare-centrifugum-like patterns. Zosteriform metastases may mimic herpes zoster, complicating diagnosis [3]. Based on retrospective reports, the most common clinic-pathological presentations of breast cancer skin metastasis are skin papules or nodules, which occur in 80% of cases, followed by telangiectatic (11%), erysipeloid and en cuirasse (3% each), alopecia neoplastica (2%), and zosteriform (0.8%) [2, 7]. Misdiagnosis is common, especially in rapidly progressing types like carcinoma erysipeloides, stressing the need for early recognition and treatment [8]. In a study of 164 patients by Mordenti et al., 80% presented with papules or nodules, followed by telangiectatic carcinoma (11.2%), erysipeloid and en cuirasse (3% each), alopecia neoplastica (2%), and zosteriform lesions (0.8%) [8].

The clinical appearance of CM is influenced by the mode of tumour spread. Lymphatic obstruction by tumour cells may lead to peau d'orange or erythematous plaques, as seen in carcinoma erysipeloides. Carcinoma en cuirasse results from diffuse dermal infiltration, often with breast volume reduction [3].

15.3 Clinical Aspects

15.3.1 Nodules

Nodules represent the most common clinical presentation of CM, occurring in approximately 80% of cases (Fig. 15.2). These firm lesions, typically 1–3 cm in size, may appear singly or in clusters and are located in the dermis or subcutaneous tissue. Their colour often matches the surrounding skin but may range from pink to red-brown, bluish-black, or flesh-toned. While

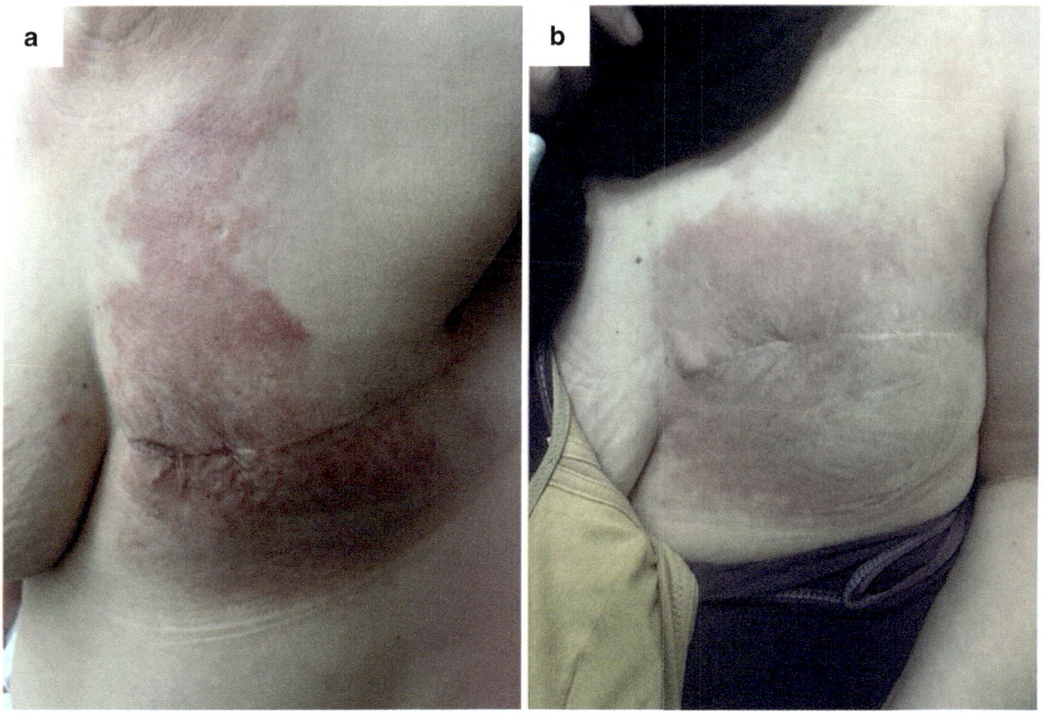

Fig. 15.1 Clinical presentation of erysipeloid breast CM. (**a**, **b**) Two female patients with erythematous patches over the mastectomy area

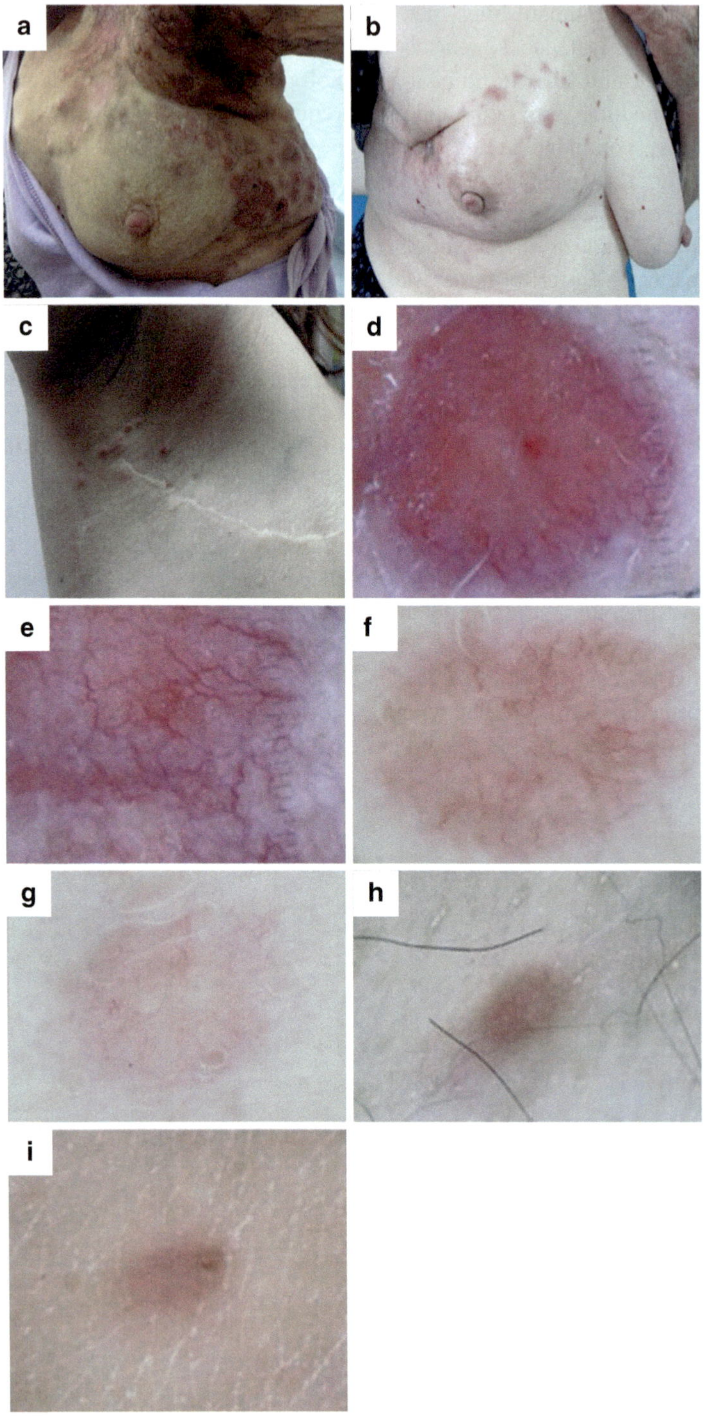

Fig. 15.2 Clinical and dermoscopical presentation of multiple macular, papular, and nodular breast CM. (**a**) Clinical presentation of multiple nodular breast CM. (**b**) Clinical presentation of multiple macular and papular breast CM. (**c**) Clinical presentation of papular breast CM. (**d**, **e**) Dermoscopy of nodular breast CM showing linear irregular vessels over the structureless red background; (**f**, **g**) dermoscopy revealing structureless white pattern with serpentine vessels; (**h**, **i**) dermoscopy revealing structureless red pattern

usually asymptomatic, nodules can ulcerate, become secondarily infected, or cause localised pain or tension. Histopathologically, they show dense clusters of tumour cells within fibrotic stroma. Neoplastic cells often form gland-like structures or align in an 'Indian file' pattern between dermal collagen bundles. Some specimens reveal diffuse interstitial infiltration by tumour cells [3, 8].

15.3.2 Carcinoma Erysipelatoides

Carcinoma erysipelatoides is a rare form of cutaneous metastasis), most commonly associated with breast cancer. However, it may also arise from malignancies of the pancreas, rectum, lung, ovary, prostate, and parotid gland. Clinically, it presents as sharply demarcated, erythematous, warm, and tender patches or plaques on the breast and surrounding skin, mimicking erysipelas. Lesions often lack systemic signs such as fever or leukocytosis and are unresponsive to antibiotics, helping distinguish them from infections like mastitis or cellulitis [3].

Histologically, malignant cells are densely packed within dilated dermal lymphatic vessels, often accompanied by mild perivascular lymphoplasmacytic infiltration. Lymphatic obstruction by tumour emboli may lead to localised lymphoedema and a ***peau d'orange*** (orange peel) appearance [3].

15.3.3 Telangiectatic Carcinoma

First described by Parkes Weber in 1933, telangiectatic carcinoma is a rare form of cutaneous breast cancer metastasis, occurring in 8–11% of cases [3, 11]. It typically presents as erythematous patches, purpuric papules, plaques, or pseudovesicular lesions, often near surgical scars on the chest wall. Lesions may resemble *lymphangioma circumscriptum* and are frequently pruritic. Histologically, the dermis shows dilated blood vessels filled with erythrocytes and clusters of atypical tumour cells, particularly in the papillary dermis [3].

15.3.4 Carcinoma en Cuirasse

Carcinoma en cuirasse, also known as scirrhous carcinoma, is a rare clinicopathologic variant of cutaneous metastatic breast cancer, seen in 3–4% of cases. It may represent either a metastatic manifestation, often from lobular carcinoma, or, more rarely, a primary tumour presentation. It has also been reported in metastases from nonbreast cancers such as prostate carcinoma. Clinically, it presents as indurated, erythematous plaques on the chest wall, sometimes with a fibrotic or yellowish appearance (Fig. 15.3). Histologically, it shows dense dermal fibrosis with sparse tumour cells, often arranged in a single-file (Indian file) pattern between collagen bundles [3].

15.3.5 Alopecia Neoplastica

It is a rare form of secondary cicatricial alopecia resulting from metastasis of a primary tumour, most commonly breast cancer (84% of cases), to the scalp, a frequent site of cutaneous metastases). This condition likely results from haematogenous rather than lymphatic spread. Clinically, it presents as single or multiple well-demarcated, painless, and nonpruritic areas of scarring alopecia, often in the parietal or frontal regions. The plaques are typically oval with a red-pink tone and smooth surface, potentially mimicking alopecia areata, discoid lupus erythematosus, lichen planopilaris, pseudopelade, or morpheiform basal cell carcinoma (BCC). Histopathologically, neoplastic cells destroy hair follicles by inducing fibroplasia, recruiting inflammatory cells, or directly replacing follicular structures. Infiltration may be subtle or clinically unapparent, complicating early diagnosis. The incidence of alopecia neoplastica in breast cancer patients ranges from 2% to 12% [3, 12].

15.3.6 Zosteriform Metastases

Zosteriform metastases are a rare clinical manifestation of cutaneous metastatic breast cancer. They may present in nodular, papulovesicular, or

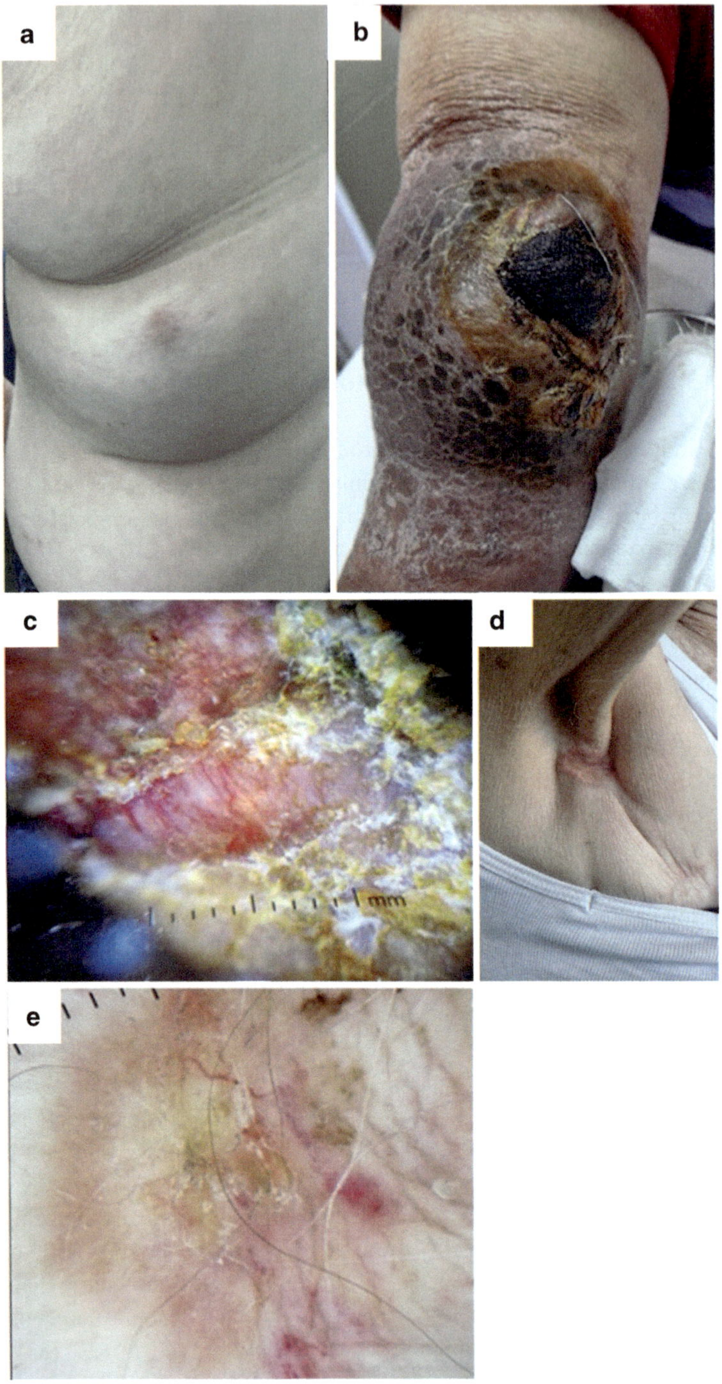

Fig. 15.3 Different clinical presentation of solitary breast CM. (**a**) Indurated erythematosus plaque on the trunk; (**b**) giant ulcerated lesion on the right leg; (**c**) dermoscopy revealing vascular pattern made of fine linear irregular vessels over the red structureless background, scales, and yellow crusts. (**d**) Solitary plaque in the right axilla resembling carcinoma en cuirasse; (**e**) dermoscopy examination showing structureless white with linear serpentine vessels with pigmentation on the periphery

vesiculobullous patterns and often follow a dermatomal distribution, most commonly affecting the chest wall and abdomen (Fig. 15.4). These lesions are frequently misdiagnosed as herpes zoster due to their similar appearance. Histologically, they show prominent infiltration of the epidermis by neoplastic cells arranged in nesting or linear patterns, with focal intraepidermal and subepidermal vesicle formation resulting from tumour cell discohesion and dermal oedema [3, 13].

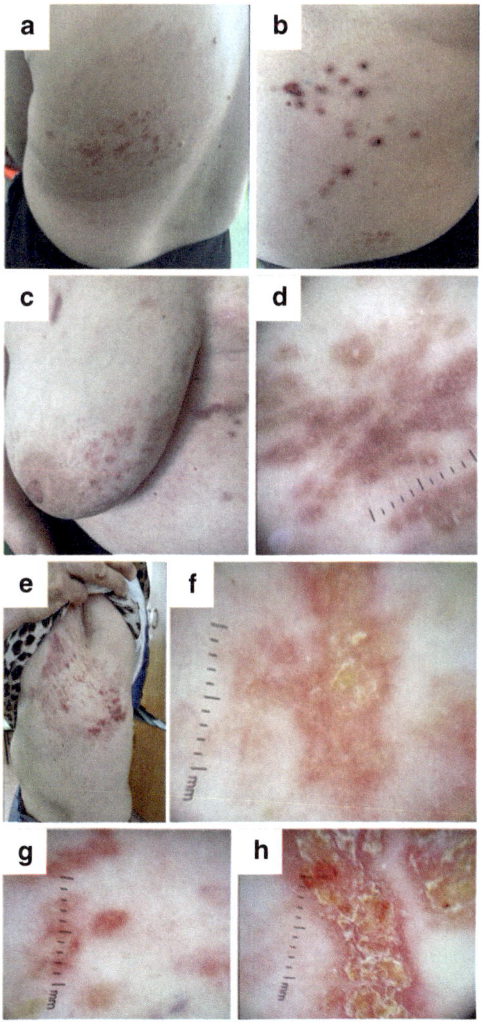

Fig. 15.4 Different clinical forms of breast CM in single patient. (**a–c**) Zosteriform, macular, and papular breast CM; (**d**) dermoscopy examination showing structureless red areas; (**e**) zosteriform, erysipeloid, and papular breast CM. (**f–h**) Dermoscopy revealing structureless red background with serpentine vessels and yellowish crusts

Multiple pathogenetic mechanisms have been proposed to explain this distribution, including perineural lymphatic dissemination, spread via lymphatic or haematogenous routes, koebnerisation following a prior zoster infection, and accidental surgical implantation of tumour cells. However, none of these theories has been definitively proven. Although rare, zosteriform metastases have been reported in malignancies such as breast, gastrointestinal, urothelial, and squamous cell carcinomas, as well as lymphomas. The presence of CM in a zosteriform distribution is an indicator of poor prognosis. It should prompt a thorough investigation in any patient with a dermatomal rash and a history of malignancy [13].

15.4 Rare Clinical Presentations of Cutaneous Metastatic Breast Carcinoma

Among the rare variants of cutaneous metastatic breast carcinoma, erythema annulare centrifugum-like lesions are exceptionally uncommon. To date, only two cases have been reported in the literature. These lesions clinically mimic erythema annulare centrifugum, a benign inflammatory dermatosis, and may be easily misdiagnosed without histopathological confirmation [3].

Another rare presentation is the targetoid pattern of cutaneous metastases). In one reported case, metastatic breast carcinoma manifested as papulonodular lesions and annular plaques attached to the skin but not fixed to underlying structures [3]. Some lesions displayed a depressed, hyperpigmented centre, resulting in a target-like appearance. These lesions can be confused with inflammatory or infectious dermatoses, further complicating diagnosis.

An unusual and striking clinical variant is the so-called 'clown nose' presentation, characterised by a reddish nodule located at the tip of the nose. Soyer et al. described this form as a unique manifestation of breast carcinoma metastasis to an acral location, reflecting the potential for breast cancer to metastasise to distal areas of the skin [3, 14].

Metastases to the eyelids are extremely rare, representing less than 1% of all malignant eyelid lesions [15]. However, breast carcinoma is the most common primary source for such metastases. Clinical appearances may vary and include diffuse swelling, violaceous infiltrated plaques, nodular ulcerations, or asymptomatic progressive enlargement of all four eyelids. Some cases present with erythematous rashes due to infiltration of the orbicularis oculi muscle. Other manifestations can simulate benign conditions such as xanthomatosis or cysts. Histologically, the presence of tumour cells arranged in an Indian file pattern aids in the diagnosis [16].

An exceptionally rare presentation is a metastatic breast adenocarcinoma arising within a benign intradermal nevus. Only a single case has been reported to date, underscoring the importance of careful histologic assessment of any new lesion in a patient with a history of breast cancer [17].

Subungual metastases are another unusual manifestation and can present as painful nail unit lesions that are frequently misdiagnosed as acute infections, such as paronychia [18]. A case has been described in which metastatic breast cancer mimicked an acute paronychia of the first toe. These lesions may represent either direct cutaneous involvement or metastasis and often require biopsy for definitive diagnosis [18].

Finally, umbilical metastasis, also known as Sister Mary Joseph's nodule, is a rare manifestation of underlying malignancy and is only infrequently associated with breast cancer [19]. Brunelli et al. documented a rare case of umbilical metastasis originating from breast carcinoma, highlighting the need to consider this possibility in patients presenting with periumbilical nodules and a relevant cancer history [20].

15.5 Dermoscopy of Cutaneous Metastases from Breast Cancer

Dermatologists are often the first to identify cutaneous metastases through clinical evaluation and dermoscopy. This noninvasive technique plays a valuable role in distinguishing metastatic lesions from benign dermatologic conditions or other malignancies, as well as in the surveillance of mastectomy scars. Additionally, dermoscopic features can aid in differentiating breast cancer metastases from cutaneous metastases of other primary tumours [9].

Several studies have outlined characteristic dermoscopic findings associated with cutaneous breast cancer metastases [9]. Kitamura et al. highlighted polymorphous and atypical vascular patterns, including linear fissure-like structures with small lateral depressions, as pathognomonic features, while Kelati et al. emphasised the prognostic relevance of polymorphic vessels [21, 22]. In another series, Alfaro et al. described dermoscopic findings in three Filipino women with CM of breast origin, reporting distinct vascular, structureless, and melanocytic patterns [23]. Observed features included linear, irregular, arborising, and polymorphic vessels, bright white lines at the lesion periphery, homogenous yellow to orange structureless areas, linear fissure-like structures, irregular diffuse blue-black pigmentation, brown globules, and pink homogeneous zones [23].

A review of case reports identified three predominant dermoscopic patterns in cutaneous breast cancer metastases: vascular, structureless, and melanocytic. Among these, vascular patterns are the most frequent, with serpentine or irregular linear vessels followed by arborising vessels. These findings reflect tumour angiogenesis and are supported by dynamic optical coherence tomography studies, which show dots, coiled, serpiginous, and branched vessels with size and distribution disarray [23]. The structureless dermoscopic pattern includes yellow-orange, white, and erythematous areas corresponding to fibrotic regions, scarring, or tumour proliferation. Confocal optical coherence tomography studies also describe hyporeflective dermal zones with clusters of tumour cells, bordered by connective tissue bundles, correlating with the white or yellow areas seen on dermoscopy [24]. Chernoff et al. evaluated 20 cases of cutaneous metastases) with underlying visceral malignancy [25]. Among these, three lesions from breast cancer demonstrated brown streaks, blue-grey globules, and vascular or melanocytic patterns. In one case, a bluish hue mimicked a blue-white veil, typically seen in melanocytic lesions. Histopathology confirmed melanocyte and melanophage presence within tumour nodules, supporting the theory of melanocyte colonisation, first noted in 1977. Melanocytic patterns have been documented in cases where tumour cells invade the epidermal basal layer, interacting with resident melanocytes. This interaction can result in irregular pigmentation, brown globules, streaks, and even pigment networks. These findings are attributed to processes such as epidermotropism, melanocyte colonisation, and melanin phagocytosis by melanophages [25]. Simionescu et al. found that 41.48% of breast cancer metastases showed blue colour, 34.32% red, 13.58% had irregular vessels, and 22.22% demonstrated a blue nevus-like pattern. The structureless white pattern appeared in over 95% of cases [26].

Despite these distinctive patterns, similar dermoscopic features may be seen in benign lesions and other malignancies. Keloids, hypertrophic scars, melanoma, pigmented basal cell carcinoma (BCC), dermatofibrosarcoma protuberans (DFSP), and mammary Paget's disease can all present overlapping features. Melanoma often displays a blue-white veil, atypical dots, streaks, and radial projections. Pigmented BCC may exhibit leaf-like structures, arborising vessels, and shiny white blotches, while DFSP can show a central white area, peripheral pigment network, and linear or comma-shaped vessels. Dermoscopy of mammary Paget's disease may reveal white scales, pink structureless areas, brown and grey dots, and erosions [21–25].

Dermoscopy is also helpful in diagnosing neoplastic alopecia (NA), which may be the first clinical manifestation of internal malignancy [3]. In such cases, the absence of classic dermoscopic criteria of other alopecias combined with the presence of vascular patterns seen in cutaneous metastases), such as arborising or polymorphic vessels, should prompt suspicion. Vezzoni et al. reported a case of NA secondary to breast cancer with prominent arborising vessels, telangiectasias, and milky-red and orange areas, surrounded by yellowish-white scales [27].

Kaminska-Winciorek et al. described two cases of peau d'orange-type metastases from breast cancer [10]. Both cases demonstrated linear serpentine and arborising vessels, densely aligned red dots, and irregularly branched vascular networks resembling a cobweb. Dermoscopy revealed multiple umbilicated pits measuring approximately 1 mm, a prominent feature of the orange peel sign. These pits were associated with linear fissures and small lateral depressions near metastatic nodules. These vascular findings reflect the infiltration or obstruction of lymphatic drainage, and dermoscopic features often mirror the underlying pathology [10].

Dash et al. documented a zosteriform cutaneous metastasis from breast adenocarcinoma in which dermoscopy showed reddish-white lacunae separated by pale septae, likely a result of lymphovascular tumour invasion [28].

A landmark multicentre study by the International Dermoscopy Society (IDS) provides the most extensive data set to date [9]. The study included 632 histologically confirmed lesions in 583 patients from countries across Europe, Asia, the Americas, and Oceania. Among these, 59 patients had cutaneous metastases) from breast cancer, the largest such cohort to date. Prominent vascular structures were seen in 96.6% of these cases. The combination of a structureless white pattern with serpentine vessels was present in 90.7% of cases, suggesting a dermoscopic signature pattern for breast cancer metastases. This consistent pattern may serve as a useful diagnostic clue in differentiating metastatic lesions from other cutaneous proliferations [9].

A skin biopsy is mandatory for the definitive diagnosis of CM. Histopathological examination, supported by immunohistochemistry, is crucial in confirming the metastatic nature of the lesion and determining its breast origin, especially in cases where clinical presentation overlaps with conditions such as cellulitis or lymphoedema.

15.6 Conclusion

Metastatic breast cancer can initially present as cutaneous lesions, which often have subtle and misleading appearances, making diagnosis challenging. A high degree of clinical suspicion is essential for the timely identification of these lesions, especially in patients with no prior history of breast cancer. Dermatologists play a crucial role in recognising these metastases through careful clinical and dermoscopic evaluation. Familiarity with the characteristic dermoscopic patterns improves diagnostic accuracy, aids in differentiating cutaneous metastases) from benign conditions, and supports monitoring of mastectomy scars.

Early recognition of cutaneous metastases allows for prompt diagnosis, appropriate staging, and timely multidisciplinary management involving oncology, surgery, dermatology, and supportive care. While cutaneous metastases generally indicate a poor prognosis, especially in metastatic breast cancer, outcomes can vary, and management should balance treatment efficacy with quality of life considerations, particularly in elderly patients.

Therefore, clinicians should remain suspicious of breast cancer metastasis when evaluating new erythematous or nodular lesions located on the chest, but also on the abdomen and head and neck region, facilitating early intervention and improving patient outcomes.

References

1. Lookingbill DP, Spangler N, Helm KF. Cutaneous metastases in patients with metastatic carcinoma: a retrospective study of 4020 patients. J Am Acad Dermatol. 1993;29(2 Pt 1):228–36.
2. Johnson C, Friedmann DP, Gade A, et al. Cutaneous manifestation as initial presentation of metastatic breast cancer: a systematic review. Cutis. 2021;107(3):E29–36.
3. De Giorgi V, Grazzini M, Alfaioli B, et al. Cutaneous manifestations of breast carcinoma. Dermatol Ther. 2010;23(6):581–9.
4. Ronen S, Suster D, Chen WS, et al. Histologic patterns of cutaneous metastases of breast carcinoma: a clinicopathologic study of 232 cases. Am J Dermatopathol. 2021;43(6):401–11.
5. Weinmann S, Leo MC, Francisco M, et al. Validation of a ductal carcinoma *in situ* biomarker profile for risk of recurrence after breast-conserving surgery with and without radiotherapy. Clin Cancer Res. 2020;26(15):4054–63.
6. Flindris S, Margioula-Siarkou C, Margioula-Siarkou G, et al. Cutaneous metastasis of triple negative breast cancer: a case report and review of literature. Cureus. 2025;17(3):e79926.
7. Bastard DP, Bollea-Garlatti ML, Belatti A, et al. Cutaneous metastases from breast cancer: an 8-year review of cases at a tertiary care hospital. Actas Dermosifiliogr (Engl Ed). 2019;110(3):206–11.
8. Mordenti C, Peris KM, Fargnoli C, et al. Cutaneous metastatic breast carcinoma. Acta dermatovenerologica. 2000;9:143–8.
9. Tiodorovic D, Stojkovic-Filipovic J, Marghoob A, et al. Dermatoscopic patterns of cutaneous metastases: a multicentre cross-sectional study of the International Dermoscopy Society. J Eur Acad Dermatol Venereol. 2024;38(7):1432–8.
10. Kamińska-Winciorek G, Wydmański J. Dermoscopy of skin metastases from breast cancer and of the orange peel type ("peau d'orange"): a report of two cases. Int J Dermatol. 2015;54(3):343–6.
11. Weber FP. Bilateral thoracic zosteroid spreading marginate telangiectasia—probably a variety of "carcinoma erysipelatodes"(C. Rasch)—associated with unilateral mammary carcinoma, and better termed "carcinoma telangiectaticum". Proc R Soc Med. 1933 Oct;26(12):1549–51.
12. Mallon E, Dawber RP. Alopecia neoplastica without alopecia: a unique presentation of breast carcinoma scalp metastasis. J Am Acad Dermatol. 1994;31(2 Pt 2):319–21.
13. Hernández-Coronado M, Rivera-Alonso IA, Cuellar-Barboza A, Ocampo-Candiani J. Zosteriform cutaneous metastases of HER-2 positive breast carcinoma resolved after treatment with lapatinib. An Bras Dermatol. 2025;100(2):403–6. https://doi.org/10.1016/j.abd.2024.07.012. Epub 2025 Jan 30. PMID: 39890533; PMCID: PMC11963095.
14. Soyer HP, Cerroni L, Smolle J, Kerl H. "Clown-Nase"--Hautmetastase eines Mammakarzinoms ["Clown nose"--skin metastasis of breast cancer]. Z Hautkr. 1990;65(10):929–31. German.
15. da Fonseca NL Jr, Lucci LM, Cha SB, et al. Metastatic eyelid disease associated with primary breast carcinoma: case report. Arq Bras Oftalmol. 2009;72(3):390–3.
16. Dabski K, Milgrom H, Stoll HL Jr. Breast carcinoma metastatic to eyelids: case report and review of the literature. J Surg Oncol. 1985;29(4):233–6.
17. Hayes AG, Chesney TM. Metastatic adenocarcinoma of the breast located within a benign intradermal nevus. Am J Dermatopathol. 1993;15(3):280–2.
18. Cohen PR, Buzdar AU. Metastatic breast carcinoma mimicking an acute paronychia of the great toe: case report and review of subungual metastases. Am J Clin Oncol. 1993;16(1):86–91.

19. Shen Z, Yang X, Chen L, et al. Sister Mary Joseph's nodule as a diagnostic clue to metastatic colon carcinoma. J Clin Oncol. 2009;27(19):e1–2. https://doi.org/10.1200/JCO.2009.22.1515. Epub 2009 May 11. PMID: 19433679.
20. Brunelli M, Manfrin E, Miller K, et al. Her-2/neu evaluation in Sister Mary Joseph's nodule from breast carcinoma: a case report and review of the literature. J Cutan Pathol. 2009;36(6):702–5.
21. Kitamura S, Hata H, Homma E, et al. Pigmented skin metastasis of breast cancer showing dermoscopic features of malignant melanoma. J Eur Acad Dermatol Venereol. 2015;29(5):1034–6.
22. Kelati A, Gallouj S. Dermoscopy of skin metastases from breast cancer: two case reports. J Med Case Rep. 2018;12(1):273.
23. Alfaro RQ, Siripunvarapon AH, Quinio MF, et al. A dermoscopy case series of cutaneous metastases from breast cancer in Filipino females. JEADV Clin Pract. 2024;3(5):1631–7.
24. Hobelsberger S, Gellrich FF, Laske J, Meier F, Beissert S, Steininger J. Immediate diagnosis of cutaneous metastases with optical coherence tomography, line-field confocal optical coherence tomography and dermoscopy: a case series. JEADV Clin Pract. 2024;3(2):622–8.
25. Chernoff KA, Marghoob AA, Lacouture ME, Deng L, Busam KJ, Myskowski PL. Dermoscopic findings in cutaneous metastases. JAMA Dermatol. 2014;150(4):429–33. https://doi.org/10.1001/jamadermatol.2013.8502. PMID: 24430974.
26. Simionescu O, Petrică M, Avram AM, Costache M, Scurtu LG, Tudorache SI, Iorga PG, Grigore M. Dermoscopy of skin metastases in advanced cancer-systemic (visceral, hematologic) and cutaneous. Front Med (Lausanne). 2024;11:1445811. https://doi.org/10.3389/fmed.2024.1445811. PMID: 39139791; PMCID: PMC11319161.
27. Vezzoni R, Toffoli L, Conforti C. Breast cancer-related neoplastic alopecia: a case report and review of the literature. Skin Appendage Disord. 2021;7(5):339–45. https://doi.org/10.1159/000514566. Epub 2021 May 4. PMID: 34604320; PMCID: PMC8436715.
28. Dash A, Kathuria S, Yadav AK. Dermoscopy of zosteriform cutaneous metastasis from breast adenocarcinoma. Am J Dermatopathol. 2025;47(3):248–9. https://doi.org/10.1097/DAD.0000000000002891. Epub 2024 Dec 31. PMID: 39787335.

Part VI

Cutaneous Metastases from Other Primary Tumours

16 Cutaneous Metastases from Other Primary Tumors

Michela Starace, Stephano Cedirian, and Luca Rapparini

Abstract

Cutaneous metastases are rare clinical manifestations of internal neoplasms, often indicative of advanced or terminal disease. Although rare, skin involvement can occur in prostate, kidney, and thyroid tumors. These lesions often present diagnostic challenges due to their variable morphology and ability to mimic benign dermatological conditions. Early identification is crucial for appropriate management and prognostic assessment. This chapter reviews the epidemiology, clinical features, diagnosis, and treatment options for skin metastases arising from prostate, kidney, and thyroid tumors, emphasizing the role of dermatologists in the multidisciplinary care of oncology patients.

Keywords

Cutaneous metastases · Prostate cancer · Kidney cancer · Thyroid cancer · Skin lesions · Oncology dermatology · Metastatic cancer

M. Starace (✉) · S. Cedirian · L. Rapparini
Dermatology Unit, IRCCS Azienda Ospedaliero-Universitaria di Bologna, Bologna, Italy

Department of Medical and Surgical Sciences, Alma Mater Studiorum University of Bologna, Bologna, Italy
e-mail: michela.starace2@unibo.it; luca.rapparini2@studio.unibo.it

16.1 Prostate Cancer

16.1.1 Introduction

Prostate cancer is one of the principal malignant tumors in males, with an increasing prevalence, especially in Western countries [1, 2]. Prostate cancer is often asymptomatic in its early stages and is diagnosed incidentally through prostate-specific antigen (PSA) testing or during a digital rectal examination [3]. When symptomatic, it can manifest itself with urinary disorders such as difficulty in urinating, nocturia, reduced flow, and urinary urgency, often similar to those of benign prostatic hypertrophy [3]. In more advanced cases, it can cause hematuria, pelvic pain, and symptoms related to obstruction of the lower urinary tract [2].

It is the second most frequently diagnosed solid tumor after lung cancer. According to GLOBOCAN estimates for 2022, there were over 1.4 million new cases of prostate cancer worldwide and around 397,000 related deaths.

In the majority of cases the prognosis is favorable. Five-year survival in patients with localized or locoregional disease can reach 98–100%, thanks to the combined use of screening (PSA dosage), advanced imaging, and effective treatments [4]. However, the situation changes radically for patients with metastatic disease, and in particular, in cases of castration-resistant prostate cancer (mCRPC). In these patients, median sur-

D. Koumaki et al. (eds.), *Cutaneous Metastases*, https://doi.org/10.1007/978-3-032-26764-1_16

vival is drastically reduced, ranging from 12 to 36 months [1]. Although rare, skin metastases are a particular manifestation, as they are a clinical sign of an advanced and often terminal phase of the disease. Their early identification can be an opportunity for the dermatologist to actively contribute to the diagnostic and therapeutic management of the cancer patient.

16.1.2 Epidemiology

Skin metastases from prostate cancer are an exceptional occurrence, with an estimated frequency of less than 1% in cancer patients [2, 3, 5]. Recent studies summarize an incidence of cutaneous metastasis between 0.36% and 0.7% in patients with prostate cancer, placing the skin among the least common metastatic sites for this neoplasm [1, 6, 7].

When they occur, skin metastases tend to appear in an advanced stage of the disease, sometimes as a terminal manifestation. Their presence is associated with a severe prognosis and often reflects the ineffectiveness of the systemic treatments adopted up to that point [8].

The hypotheses on the mechanism of prostate cancer spreading to the skin include direct invasion of contiguous tissues, dissemination via the lymphatic or hematogenous route, or a combination of these pathways [4, 9]. Also, cases of seeding from a surgical instrument are reported [4, 7].

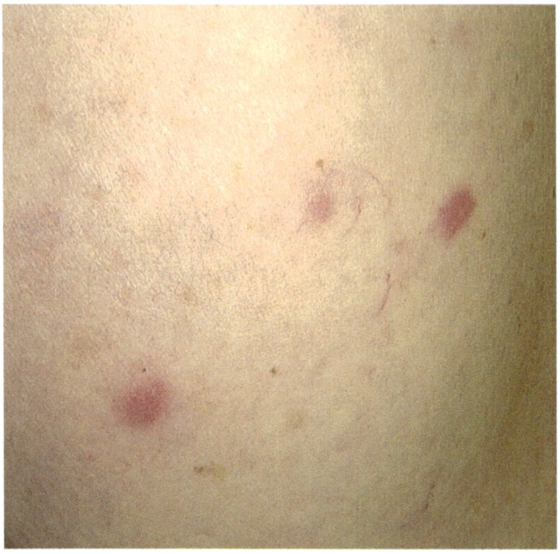

Fig. 16.1 Prostate cancer metastases presenting as pruritic erythematous nodules

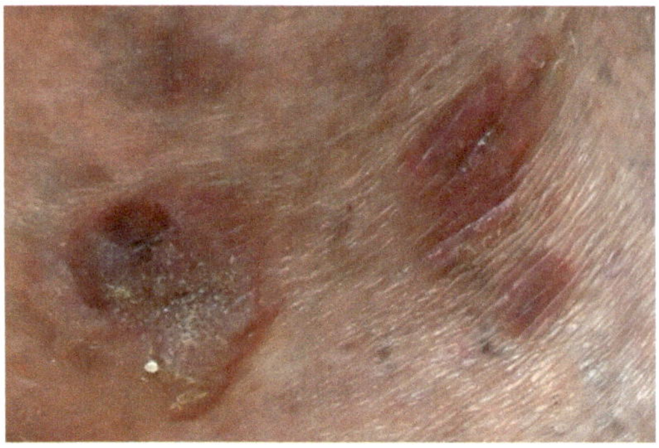

Fig. 16.2 Infiltrated plaques histologically confirmed as metastasis from prostate cancer

16.1.3 Clinical Features

The clinical presentation is heterogeneous and often deceptive. The lesions can appear as erythematous or purplish cutaneous or subcutaneous nodules, with a smooth or vegetating surface, and an elastic or hard consistency (Fig. 16.1). In some cases, they present as infiltrated plaques similar to scleroderma, or as ulcerated, painful or itchy lesions (Fig. 16.2). Zosteriform, polypoid, and condylomatous cases have also been described [3, 7–10]. They can be symptomatic for itching, ulceration, pain, or bleeding [7, 10]. The similarity to benign lesions such as sebaceous cysts, dermatofibromas, or keratoses can delay diagnosis, especially if the patient has no known oncological history.

From a topographical point of view, the most frequently affected sites include the suprapubic region, scrotum, penis, lower abdomen, chest, and back. Cases have also been reported in less typical sites such as the neck, the scalp, the breasts, and the submandibular region [1, 4, 5, 7–9]. A rare variant is subungual localization: the first documented case of nail metastasis from prostate adenocarcinoma was described in 2019, in a 66-year-old man, with a purplish and painful nodule on the distal phalanx of the fourth finger, which turned out to be a prostatic cancer metastasis [11].

It is interesting to note that, although the majority of cases occur in patients already diagnosed and treated for prostate cancer, skin metastases can also be the first clinical manifestation of the neoplasia.

16.1.4 Diagnostic Workup

Clinical suspicion is the first essential step, but it is not enough to diagnose skin metastases. The dermatologist plays a central role in the early recognition of suspicious lesions, in their clinical characterization and in the choice of the appropriate diagnostic procedure. Dermoscopic examination of cutaneous metastases from prostate cancer, as well as other cutaneous metastases, can show a variety of vascular patterns: arboriform, serpentine, irregular linear, and sometimes punctate vessels (Fig. 16.3). Homogeneous white areas, yellowish crusts, and, in rare cases, black dots suggestive of necrosis or pigment are also present [12, 13]. However, dermoscopy alone does not allow a definitive diagnosis, but can point toward a timely biopsy.

CT and MRI are well-established tools for the study of bone and visceral metastases [4]. However, PSMA PET/CT has revolutionized the staging of patients with prostate cancer, proving to be highly sensitive even in detecting PSMA-avid cutaneous and subcutaneous lesions [12, 14].

The definitive diagnosis is histological. Metastases usually present as infiltrates of poorly differentiated adenocarcinoma with a glandular pattern, localized in the dermis and subcutaneous tissues. The main immunohistochemical markers to confirm a prostatic origin are PSA, prostatic specific acid phosphatase (PSAP), and prostate-specific membrane antigen (PSMA) [7, 9, 14]. In cases where PSA is negative, the nuclear marker NKX3.1 can be used, as it is highly specific for prostate origin [1, 7, 9]. Synaptophysin, chromogranin A, and CD56 are useful immunohistochemical markers in the presence of suspected neuroendocrine differentiation [8].

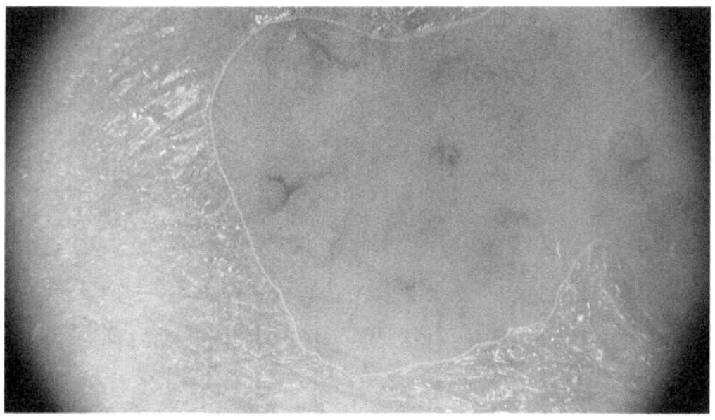

Fig. 16.3 Dermoscopy of prostate cancer metastasis showing arboriform, serpentine, and irregular vessels on a homogeneous white area (magnification 20×)

16.1.5 Management

The treatment of cutaneous metastases from prostate cancer depends on the patient's overall clinical situation and the presence of concomitant visceral metastases. In general, the appearance of skin lesions is a sign of systemic therapeutic failure and requires a multidisciplinary approach. Treatment options are mostly palliative and include surgery, radiotherapy, and intralesional chemotherapy [5, 7, 9]. Hormone therapy remains the cornerstone of treatment in mCRPC. Androgen synthesis inhibitors (e.g., abiraterone) and androgen receptor inhibitors (e.g., enzalutamide) have proven effective in prolonging survival even in patients with skin metastases [5, 10]. In cases of progression, chemotherapy with taxanes is used.

In patients with BRCA1 or BRCA2 mutations, the use of poly(ADP-ribose) polymerase (PARP) inhibitors such as olaparib has been shown to improve survival, and cases of regression of skin metastases have also been reported [10].

Local radiotherapy can be used to treat symptomatic, ulcerated, or hemorrhagic lesions. A therapeutic breakthrough is represented by radiotherapy with lutetium-177-labelled radioligands (177Lu-PSMA), particularly effective in patients with PSMA-avid disease, including cutaneous metastases [12, 15].

Surgical excision can have palliative, aesthetic, or diagnostic purposes. In some cases, excision alone has resulted in lasting local control of the disease [5].

The prognosis for patients with cutaneous metastases from prostate cancer is generally poor [2]. Average survival after diagnosis varies between 4 and 12 months [6, 8, 9]. Negative prognostic factors include advanced age, high PSA levels, presence of visceral metastases, neuroendocrine differentiation, and genetic mutations such as BRCA [10, 16, 17].

Skin metastases from prostate cancer, although rare, represent an important clinical challenge. Knowledge of the various clinical presentations, diagnostic techniques, and the latest treatment options allows for an integrated and timely approach, capable of improving the patient's quality of life and, in some cases, prolonging their survival.

16.2 Kidney Cancer

16.2.1 Introduction

Kidney cancer, or renal cell carcinoma (RCC), represents about 2–3% of all malignant neoplasms in adults. It is a heterogeneous disease, comprising different histological entities. The most frequent subtype (70–80% of cases) is clear cell renal cell carcinoma (ccRCC), followed by papillary carcinoma (10–15%) and chromophobe carcinoma (5%), while rarer forms include collecting duct carcinoma, medullary carcinoma, and tumors associated with translocations [18–21].

The classic clinical onset (macroscopic hematuria, lumbar pain, and palpable mass) is nowadays rare, occurring in less than 10% of patients [22]. Most renal tumors are diagnosed incidentally during radiological examinations performed for other reasons. However, up to 30% of patients already have metastases at the time of diagnosis [22]. The main sites of spread are the lungs, bones, liver, lymph nodes, and brain. The skin can also be rarely involved [19–21, 23].

Kidney cancer can also manifest itself as syndromes, which also present with cutaneous findings. Von Hippel-Lindau syndrome is a rare autosomal dominant syndrome caused by mutations in the oncosuppressor gene VHL. It predisposes affected individuals to highly vascular tumors, including ccRCCs, central nervous system tumors, retinal angiomas, and pheochromocytomas. Cutaneous manifestations are uncommon and nonspecific but may include hemangiomas and café au lait spots. Birt-Hogg-Dubé syndrome is a rare autosomal dominant disorder caused by germline mutations in the folliculin gene. It is associated with an increased risk of renal tumors and pulmonary cysts. Cutaneous manifestations are characteristic and include the triad of fibrofolliculomas, trichodiscomas, and fibromas. Other syndromes that associate renal tumors with cutaneous manifestations are Cowden syndrome, tuberous sclerosis, and hereditary leiomyomatosis and renal cell carcinoma syndrome [22].

16.2.2 Epidemiology

Skin metastases from kidney cancer are rare and generally indicate an advanced stage of the disease. The incidence varies between 1% and 6%, with an estimated average of 3.3% [19–23]. In about 10–20% of cases, skin lesions may be the first clinical manifestation of metastatic disease [18, 20, 24].

The most frequently associated histological subtype is ccRCC, probably concerning both its high frequency and its biological aggressiveness [25, 26]. However, cases of skin metastases from papillary carcinoma [23, 27], sarcomatoid variants [18, 25], and rare forms, such as biphasic squamoid alveolar RCC [28], have also been described.

16.2.3 Clinical Features

Cutaneous metastases from renal carcinoma present clinically as solitary or multiple, fast-growing nodules, of an elastic or hard-elastic consistency. They are often red-purple, or black, sometimes bluish, due to the high vasculariza-

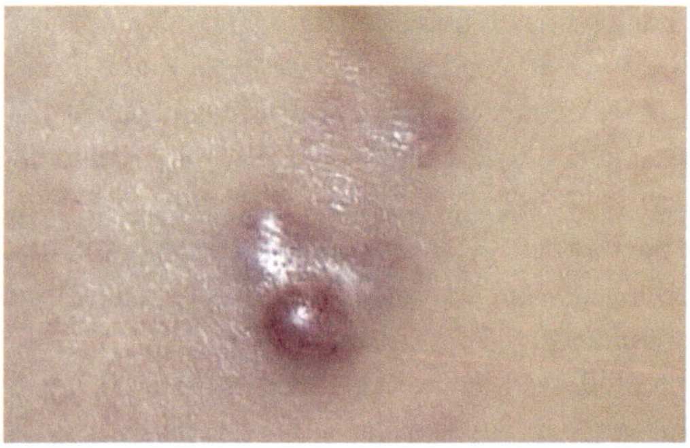

Fig. 16.4 Cutaneous metastases from kidney cancer presenting as a rapidly growing red-purple nodule

tion (Fig. 16.4). They can ulcerate or bleed easily and be painful on palpation. In some cases, they take on a pulsating appearance that makes them easily confused with angiomas, pyogenic granulomas, Kaposi sarcoma, hemangioma, hemangioendothelioma, or other vascular neoplasms [19–25, 27, 29, 30].

Presentations can be highly variable. In some patients, cutaneous metastases were initially mistaken for infections, adverse drug reactions, dermatitis, or benign lesions [20, 25, 29, 31]. There have been reports of ulcerated targetoid plaques, similar to erythema multiforme or fixed drug reactions [25], angiomatiform nodules on the face or gums, skin horn lesions [21], and even lingual metastases [26].

The scalp is the most frequently affected site, but the face, neck, chest, limbs, and mucous membranes can also be involved [20, 23–25]. Scalp involvement has been attributed to the rich vascularization and the presence of arteriovenous shunts in the cephalic region [12, 20, 29].

In transplanted or immunosuppressed patients, skin lesions can be the initial manifestation of neoplastic disease, as described in a case that appeared 12 years after kidney transplantation [32].

Sometimes, skin metastases can be found near the surgical scar or laparoscopic access site, suggesting iatrogenic inoculation [25]. Isolated lesions on the cheek, chin, fingers, or back have also been reported [18, 24, 30].

16.2.4 Diagnostic Workup

The diagnosis of cutaneous metastasis from RCC is based on a careful clinical examination, supported by imaging techniques and confirmed by biopsy.

Dermoscopy can highlight an atypical vascular morphology, with irregular linear patterns and radial vessels in a corona-like shape, on a pinkish-orange background lacking in structure. Although not pathognomonic, these aspects should orientate clinical suspicion [12, 25].

High-frequency skin ultrasound can show a solid lesion, hypoechoic or with mixed echogenicity, often well vascularized, useful for guiding the biopsy and distinguishing it from cysts or abscesses [20]. Computed tomography and magnetic resonance imaging are mandatory for systemic staging, identifying any synchronous metastases [20, 30].

Histological examination of clear cell carcinoma shows cells with large, clear cytoplasm, arranged in nests or cords, with rounded nuclei and evident nucleoli. Papillary forms have fibrovascular structures lined with cubic or columnar cells [20, 25, 27]. The sarcomatoid variants can simulate mesenchymal tumors, presenting spindle cell arranged in a storiform pattern, sometimes with necrosis and high mitotic activity [18, 31]. In these cases, diagnosis can be difficult without the support of immunohistochemistry. The most useful markers for confirming renal origin include PAX8, CAIX, CD10, and vimentin, with positivity for cytokeratins in epithelial subtypes. Sarcomatoid forms may also express EMA and MDM2, but with greater variability [18, 24, 25, 31].

16.2.5 Management

The treatment of RCC skin metastases depends on the number of lesions and the general condition of the patient. Individual lesions can be surgically excised, both for diagnostic and palliative purposes. Alternatively, radiotherapy can be used, particularly if the lesions are painful or ulcerated [30]. Systemic therapy is the mainstay of treatment in patients with disseminated disease. Tyrosine kinase inhibitors (TKIs), anti-VEGF inhibitors, mTOR inhibitors, and immune checkpoint inhibitors are all being utilized with varying degrees of success in RCC [22]. TKIs such as sunitinib, pazopanib, axitinib, or cabozantinib are effective in controlling even cutaneous localizations [19, 24, 26, 29]. In one case, axitinib led to a marked regression of nasal metastasis after only 8 weeks, with good tolerability [19]. Immunotherapy with checkpoint inhibitors (nivolumab and ipilimumab) is a well-established option in advanced forms, although responses at the skin level are variable. In some cases, skin metastases have appeared or progressed during immunotherapy [24, 26].

The prognosis remains unfavorable; in fact, the mean survival after the appearance of skin metastases is about 10 months [18, 23, 24].

16.3 Thyroid Cancer

16.3.1 Introduction

Thyroid carcinoma is the most common endocrine malignancy, with a rising incidence globally, largely due to papillary thyroid carcinoma (PTC), the predominant histologic subtype [33]. Although PTC and follicular thyroid carcinoma (FTC) are generally indolent and carry an excellent prognosis, distant metastases occur in up to 10% of cases and are associated with reduced survival [34]. The skin is a rare metastatic site, typically reflecting disseminated disease and poor prognosis [33, 35]. For dermatologists, recognition of these metastases is essential, as cutaneous lesions may represent the first clinical sign of internal malignancy [36, 37].

16.3.2 Epidemiology

Cutaneous metastases from thyroid carcinoma are rare, accounting for less than 0.1% of all skin metastases [38]. The actual incidence may be underestimated due to underdiagnosis or misclassification of skin lesions. Among thyroid cancers, PTC accounts for the majority of cutaneous metastases (~48%), followed by FTC (~30%), medullary (11%), and anaplastic (8%) carcinoma [33]. The average age at diagnosis of cutaneous metastasis is around 63 years, with a slight female predominance [33]. The scalp is the most common site, followed by the neck, face, and chest [33, 36, 37]. In rare cases, cutaneous metastases may be the first presentation of thyroid cancer, preceding the diagnosis of the primary tumor [39, 40].

16.3.3 Clinical Features

Clinically, cutaneous metastases of thyroid carcinoma typically appear as firm, erythematous or violaceous nodules or plaques, often localized on the scalp or near surgical scars [35, 37]. Lesions may ulcerate or bleed (mostly in late lesions or rapidly growing tumors) and are sometimes mistaken for entities such as epidermal cysts or basal cell carcinomas (Fig. 16.5) [37, 38]. They can also be asymptomatic or mildly pruritic [41]. In dermoscopy, a polymorphous vascular pattern may be observed [41]. The variability in appearance warrants a high index of suspicion, especially in patients with a history of thyroid cancer or unexplained skin lesions in typical locations.

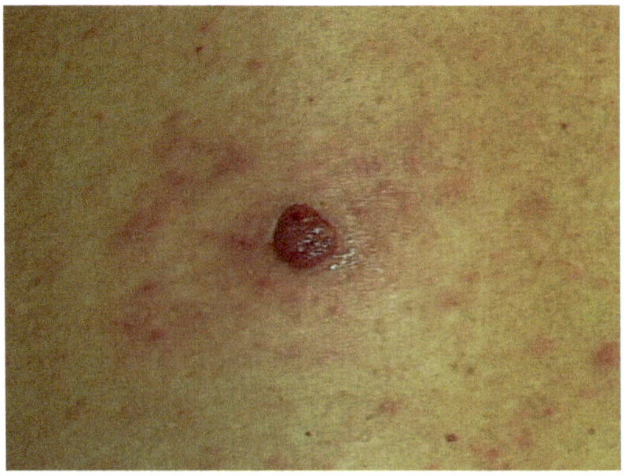

Fig. 16.5 Histologically confirmed thyroid carcinoma metastasis characterized by an erythematous ulcerated nodule, initially clinically diagnosed as basal cell carcinoma

16.3.4 Diagnostic Workup

Diagnosis relies on histopathological evaluation of a biopsy specimen. Histology reveals follicular or papillary structures, depending on the subtype, and immunohistochemical staining is critical for confirmation. Markers such as TTF-1, thyroglobulin, PAX8, and calcitonin (in medullary carcinoma) help establish thyroid origin [35, 36, 40, 42]. FTC metastases may present with angioinvasion and be positive for PAX8 and TTF-1, even when thyroglobulin is negative [36, 43]. Anaplastic carcinomas may lack classic markers and require a broad immunopanel [42, 43]. Molecular analyses, such as the detection of TERT promoter or BRAF mutations, can provide further diagnostic and prognostic information [39, 43]. Imaging studies (ultrasound, CT, and PET-CT) are essential for assessing the primary tumor and staging the disease. Fine-needle aspiration of suspicious nodules can aid in confirming systemic dissemination [33, 44].

16.3.5 Management

Cutaneous metastases indicate advanced disease and usually necessitate a multidisciplinary approach. Treatment depends on tumor type, disease burden, and patient performance status. Local management includes surgical excision or electrochemotherapy, which can alleviate symptoms like pain and bleeding [34, 45]. Mohs micrographic surgery has been successfully used for scalp lesions to ensure margin control and tissue conservation [45].

Systemic therapy may involve radioactive iodine (RAI) for differentiated and iodine-avid tumors, kinase inhibitors (e.g., sorafenib and vandetanib) for RAI-refractory or medullary tumors, RET inhibitors (e.g., selpercatinib/pralsetinib) for medullary/RET-altered tumors, and BRAF/MEK inhibitors for BRAF-mutated ATC (e.g., dabrafenib + trametinib) and cytotoxic chemotherapy for anaplastic variants [37, 38, 43]. Despite therapy, the prognosis remains poor, with

Table 16.1 Summary of cutaneous metastasis from prostate, kidney, and thyroid cancers

	Prostate cancer	Kidney cancer	Thyroid cancer
Epidemiology	Incidence <1%; rare, typically in advanced disease	Incidence 1–6%; may precede or signal advanced disease	Incidence <0.1%; rare manifestation of advanced disease
Clinical features	Cutaneous lesions may appear as nodules or plaques, often erythematous or violaceous. They can be ulcerated, painful, or pruritic and are frequently misdiagnosed as benign lesions. Commonly affect genital and lower abdominal areas, but can also involve the chest, back, scalp, or nails	Lesions typically present as red to purple vascular nodules that grow rapidly and may ulcerate or bleed. They often mimic vascular lesions, especially on the scalp, face, or mucosa. Can be solitary or multiple and mistaken for inflammatory or infectious dermatoses	Firm, erythematous or violaceous nodules or plaques, most often found on the scalp or near surgical scars. Lesions may ulcerate, bleed, or remain asymptomatic
Diagnostic workup	Clinical exam, dermoscopy, histology with PSA, PSMA, NKX3.1 stains; PSMA-PET/CT helpful	Clinical exam, dermoscopy, histology with PAX8, CD10, CAIX stains; ultrasound	Clinical exam, dermoscopy, histology with TTF-1, thyroglobulin, PAX8, calcitonine stains; imaging and mutation analysis supportive

(continued)

Table 16.1 (continued)

	Prostate cancer	Kidney cancer	Thyroid cancer
Management	Hormonal therapy, taxanes, PARP inhibitors, radiotherapy, 177Lu-PSMA	TKIs, immune checkpoint inhibitors, surgery, palliative radiotherapy	Surgery, electrochemotherapy, radioactive iodine, TKIs, chemotherapy
Prognosis	Poor (mean 4–12 months); worse with BRCA mutations, visceral disease	Poor (mean 10 months); highly variable depending on burden and histology	Poor (mean 6–13 months); prognosis varies by subtype and molecular profile

average survival after diagnosis of cutaneous metastasis ranging from 6 to 13 months [33, 37].

A summary of the approach to cutaneous metastases from prostate, kidney, and thyroid cancers is shown in Table 16.1.

References

1. Elsharawi I, Moss P, Wang C, Wood LA. Uncommon case of metastatic prostate cancer developing cutaneous metastasis. BMJ Case Rep. 2022;15(12):e251661. https://doi.org/10.1136/bcr-2022-251661.
2. Patel P, Patel J, Siddiqui S. Recurrence of prostate cancer with cutaneous metastasis after radical prostatectomy. Case Rep Urol. 2015;2015:825175. https://doi.org/10.1155/2015/825175.
3. Brito Y, Wilson BW, Bacchus KI, Mwaniki J, Jorge J, Tiesenga F. Cutaneous metastases in progressive prostate adenocarcinoma: a case report and literature review. Cureus. 2023;15(9):e46219. doi:https://doi.org/10.7759/cureus.46219.
4. Ziani I, Makhoukh ZEBE, Ibrahimi A, Bellouki O, Benahmed J, Laraqui Y, et al. Scrotal skin metastases revealing a prostatic adenocarcinoma. Case Rep Urol. 2020;2020:8826627. https://doi.org/10.1155/2020/8826627.
5. Marampon F, Parisi M, Cicco PR, Serpone M, Tomaciello M, Musio D, et al. Skin metastases from prostate cancer successfully treated with radiation therapy. BJR Case Rep. 2023;9(4):20200142. https://doi.org/10.1259/bjrcr.20200142.
6. Mueller TJ, Wu H, Greenberg RE, Hudes G, Topham N, Lessin SR, et al. Cutaneous metastases from genitourinary malignancies. Urology. 2004;63(6):1021–6. https://doi.org/10.1016/j.urology.2004.01.014.
7. Dills A, Obi O, Bustos K, Jiang J, Gupta S. Cutaneous metastasis of prostate adenocarcinoma: a rare presentation of a common disease. J Investig Med High Impact Case Rep. 2021;9:2324709621990769. https://doi.org/10.1177/2324709621990769.
8. Munera-Campos M, Bielsa I, Plana-Pla A, Posada R, Quer A, Ferrándiz C. Cutaneous metastases from prostate cancer revealing neuroendocrine differentiation. J Cutan Pathol. 2019;46(12):976–8. https://doi.org/10.1111/cup.13561.
9. Rodríguez-Lojo R, Castiñeiras I, Rey-Sanjurjo JL, Fernández-Díaz ML. Metástasis cutáneas a distancia de cáncer de próstata: 2 casos. Actas Dermosifiliogr. 2016;107(7):e52–6. https://doi.org/10.1016/j.ad.2015.09.021.
10. Jubran S, Basso U, Milani A, Erbetta E, Di Marco A, Pittarello C, et al. Skin metastasis of BRCA mutated prostate cancer: a case report and a brief review of literature. Medicine (Baltimore). 2024;103(41):e40016. https://doi.org/10.1097/MD.0000000000040016.
11. García-Galaviz R, Domínguez-Cherit J, Caro-Sánchez C, Salazar-Rojas E. Subungual metastasis of an adenocarcinoma of the prostate in a finger. Skin Appendage Disord. 2019;5(1):46–9. https://doi.org/10.1159/000489279.
12. Cedirian S, Rapparini L, Sechi A, Piraccini BM, Starace M. Diagnosis and management of scalp metastases: a review. Diagnostics (Basel). 2024;14(15):1638. https://doi.org/10.3390/diagnostics14151638.
13. Chernoff KA, Marghoob AA, Lacouture ME, Deng L, Busam KJ, Myskowski PL. Dermoscopic findings in cutaneous metastases. JAMA Dermatol. 2014;150(4):429–33. https://doi.org/10.1001/jamadermatol.2013.8502.
14. Piqué D, Patel P, Hui Y, Lee T, Amin B, Sarungbam J, et al. A case of prostatic adenocarcinoma with NKX3.1-positive cutaneous metastases. Int J Dermatol. 2020;59(12):e456–9. https://doi.org/10.1111/ijd.14965.
15. Rafiei Z, Saber Tanha A, Tayyebi Meibodi N, Zahed Anaraki S, Askari E. Cutaneous and subcutaneous prostate-specific membrane antigen–avid lesions. Clin Nucl Med. 2025;50(3):e164–5. https://doi.org/10.1097/RLU.0000000000005525.
16. Sarangi SS, Singh V, Bhirud DP. Cutaneous metastasis of castration-resistant prostate cancer: a rare case report and review of literature. Urol Ann. 2023;15(1):98–100. https://doi.org/10.4103/ua.ua_102_22.
17. Oh TH, Kim HS, Park SC. Scalp nodules as the first presentation of prostate cancer: a CARE-compliant article. Medicine (Baltimore). 2023;102(50):e36570. https://doi.org/10.1097/MD.0000000000036570.

18. Logunova V, Sokumbi O, Iczkowski KA. Metastatic sarcomatoid renal cell carcinoma manifesting as a subcutaneous soft tissue mass. J Cutan Pathol. 2017;44(10):874–7. https://doi.org/10.1111/cup.12998.
19. Cui P, Cong X, Yin J, Liu M, Wang X, Yang L, et al. Metastases to the nose from clear cell renal cell carcinoma: a case report. Medicine (Baltimore). 2019;98(4):e14012. https://doi.org/10.1097/MD.0000000000014012.
20. Wang W, Kang Y, Qu X, Li Y, Zhou H. A rare case report of renal clear cell carcinoma with multiple skin metastases and a review of the literature. Front Oncol. 2024;14:1461791. https://doi.org/10.3389/fonc.2024.1461791.
21. Georgy JT, Mathuram AJ, George AA, Chandramohan J. Renal cell carcinoma presenting as a cutaneous horn and nodules on the gingiva and scalp. BMJ Case Rep. 2017;2017:bcr-2017-220913. https://doi.org/10.1136/bcr-2017-220913.
22. Amin A, Burgess EF. Skin manifestations associated with kidney cancer. Semin Oncol. 2016;43(3):408–12. https://doi.org/10.1053/j.seminoncol.2016.02.016.
23. Ohlsson R, Geertsen L, Berge Stuveseth S, Lund L. Cutaneous metastases in renal cell carcinoma: a systematic review and a case report. Scand J Urol. 2019;53(1):9–13. https://doi.org/10.1080/21681805.2018.1557600.
24. Kesireddy M, Correa A, Correa R, Venkatesan R. A pedunculated skin lesion in a case of clear cell renal carcinoma. Cureus. 2019;11(6):e5021. https://doi.org/10.7759/cureus.5021.
25. Iliescu CA, Beiu C, Racoviță A, Olaru CM, Tudose I, Vrancianu A, et al. Atypical presentation of rapidly progressive cutaneous metastases of clear cell renal carcinoma: a case report. Medicina (Kaunas). 2024;60(11):1797. https://doi.org/10.3390/medicina60111797.
26. Abro C, Sedhom R, Soni A, Markowski M. Cutaneous finger and tongue metastases in renal cell carcinoma. BMJ Case Rep. 2019;12(6):e230516. https://doi.org/10.1136/bcr-2019-230516.
27. Cardwell LA, Bender NR, Sokumbi O. Cutaneous metastases of papillary renal cell carcinoma: a case report and review of the literature. J Cutan Pathol. 2019;46(12):960–4. https://doi.org/10.1111/cup.13546.
28. Sherin SB, Gunabooshanam B, Sundaram S, D'Cruze L. Biphasic squamoid alveolar renal cell carcinoma: a rare entity with an even rarer presentation as cutaneous metastases—a case report. Indian J Pathol Microbiol. 2023;66(1):174–6. https://doi.org/10.4103/ijpm.ijpm_837_21.
29. Lee HJ, Lee A, Tan D, Du J, Wang Y, Tang PY, et al. Cutaneous metastasis of renal cell carcinoma. Lancet Oncol. 2020;21(5):e292. https://doi.org/10.1016/S1470-2045(20)30143-1.
30. Silver E, Roudakova K, Bial N, Daniel D. Cutaneous metastasis of renal cell carcinoma to the cheek: a case report and literature review. Am J Case Rep. 2021;22:e928999. https://doi.org/10.12659/AJCR.928999.
31. Gradecki SE, Gru AA. An unusual case of sarcomatoid renal cell carcinoma presenting in the skin by direct extension at a laparoscopic port site. J Cutan Pathol. 2020;47(7):617–20. https://doi.org/10.1111/cup.13657.
32. Basic-Jukic N, Mesar I, Kirincich J. Cutaneous metastasis as a presenting feature of renal adenocarcinoma in a renal transplant recipient: a case report. Transplant Proc. 2019;51(9):3072–3. https://doi.org/10.1016/j.transproceed.2019.04.021.
33. Sciscent BY, Eberly HW, Goyal N, Goldenberg D. Thyroid cancer with cutaneous metastases. Ear Nose Throat J. 2024:01455613241239533. https://doi.org/10.1177/01455613241239533.
34. Cavaco D, Carvalhal S, Leite V. Palliative electrochemotherapy treatment of cutaneous metastases in a patient with advanced thyroid papillary carcinoma. Eur Thyroid J. 2020;9(4):221–4. https://doi.org/10.1159/000507888.
35. Kojima M, Ito S, Saikawa M, Kajino K, Ohtsuji N, Matsumoto F, et al. A rare case of scalp metastasis from encapsulated angioinvasive follicular thyroid carcinoma. Ear Nose Throat J. 2025;104(1_suppl):405S–9S. https://doi.org/10.1177/01455613231154063.
36. Lira MLA, Almeida MAD, Reis-Feroldi MM, Rocha JA. Follicular thyroid carcinoma metastatic to skin: a small papule and a big diagnostic change. An Bras Dermatol. 2019;94(1):76–8. https://doi.org/10.1590/abd1806-4841.20198299.
37. Cohen PR. Metastatic papillary thyroid carcinoma to the nose: report and review of cutaneous metastases of papillary thyroid cancer. Dermatol Pract Concept. 2015;5(4):7–11. https://doi.org/10.5826/dpc.0504a03.
38. Tanal M, Aygun N, Uludag M. Papillary thyroid cancer presenting with incidental skin lesion: critical management of distant metastasis. Sisli Etfal Hastan Tip Bul. 2021;55(1):112–5. https://doi.org/10.14744/SEMB.2021.70846.
39. Monti E, Dono M, Gonella E, Spina B, Pitto F, Petrogalli F, et al. An H-TERT mutated skin metastasis as first occurrence in a case of follicular thyroid carcinoma. Front Endocrinol (Lausanne). 2019;10:513. https://doi.org/10.3389/fendo.2019.00513.
40. Ferreres-Riera JR, Vinyals-Rioseco A, Penin-Mosquera RM, Servitje-Bedate O, Marcoval-Caus J, Mascaro-Galy JM, et al. A nodule on the scalp as the first sign of extranodal disease in medullary thyroid carcinoma. Dermatol Online J. 2017;23(5):13030/qt5r8475br.
41. Márquez García A, Ferrándiz Pulido L, Ríos-Martín JJ, Camacho Martínez FM. Metástasis cutáneas craneocervicales de un carcinoma papilar de tiroides variedad folicular. Actas Dermosifiliogr. 2016;107(1):83–5. https://doi.org/10.1016/j.ad.2015.06.008.
42. McKenzie GW, Callen JP, Haeberle MT. CK7 negative anaplastic thyroid carcinoma presenting as cuta-

neous metastases to the scalp. Dermatol Online J. 2018;24(11):13030/qt34h0w9j4.

43. Danialan R, Tetzlaff MT, Torres-Cabala CA, Mays SR, Prieto VG, Bell D, et al. Cutaneous metastasis from anaplastic thyroid carcinoma exhibiting exclusively a spindle cell morphology: a case report and review of literature. J Cutan Pathol. 2016;43(3):252–7. https://doi.org/10.1111/cup.12618.
44. Phelan PS, Mull JL, Rajput MZ, Musiek AC. Concurrent metastases of papillary thyroid carcinoma to the scalp and Meckel's cave. BMJ Case Rep. 2018;2018:bcr-2017-222552. https://doi.org/10.1136/bcr-2017-222552.
45. Aria A, Chen L, Rosenbaum LE, Migden MR. Mohs micrographic surgery for the treatment of cutaneous metastases in a patient with papillary thyroid carcinoma. Dermatologic Surg. 2018;44(11):1457–9. https://doi.org/10.1097/DSS.0000000000001459.

Part VII

Skin Infiltrations of Hematological Malignancies

Leukemia Cutis

17

Dimitra Koumaki, Eleni Lagoudaki,
Bouse Malkots, and Christoforos Roumpakis

Abstract

Skin infiltration by circulating leukemic cells is traditionally referred to as leukemia cutis (LC), although the term does not adequately indicate either the unique features of the underlying hematologic malignancy or its cutaneous manifestations. Skin involvement may result from a number of different acute and chronic myeloid neoplasms and, more rarely, lymphoid neoplasms. Such primary diseases include acute myeloid leukemia (AML), chronic myelomonocytic leukemia (CMML), myelodysplastic syndrome (MDS), acute lymphoblastic leukemia (ALL), and other circulating hematologic malignancies. Accurate classification requires morphologic, immunophenotypic, and sometimes genetic analyses; clinical correlation remains crucial in distinguishing LC from primary cutaneous neoplasms. Epidemiology, clinical manifestations, dermoscopic features, and histopathology of LC are summarized in this chapter. The reported incidence of LC is very variable, ranging from 2% to 30%. There is a predilection for AML, particularly the FAB M4 and M5 subtypes, with incidences of up to 50%. LC in CLL has been reported to occur with an incidence of 4–27%, but skin involvement by ALL or CML rarely occurs. LC can present before, simultaneously with, or after systemic leukemia onset. About 7% of patients have aleukemic LC at presentation. Clinically, LC presents as erythematous to violaceous papules, nodules, or plaques that may ulcerate and simulate several dermatoses. Molecular profiling exhibits recurrent mutations including NPM1, FLT3, and NRAS/KRAS, with variable expression of CD34 and CD117 between skin lesions and bone marrow samples. The prognosis remains guarded but is increasingly influenced by genetic factors. Allogeneic stem cell transplantation can improve survival outcomes for patients with high-risk features.

Keywords

Leukemia cutis · Acute myeloid leukemia · Aleukemic leukemia cutis · Dermoscopy · Extramedullary disease · Myeloid sarcoma · Cutaneous infiltration · Prognosis

D. Koumaki (✉)
Dermatology Department, University Hospital of Heraklion, Heraklion, Greece

E. Lagoudaki
Pathology Department, University Hospital of Heraklion, Heraklion, Greece

B. Malkots · C. Roumpakis
Department of Haematology, University Hospital of Alexandroupolis, Alexandroupoli, Greece

D. Koumaki et al. (eds.), *Cutaneous Metastases*, https://doi.org/10.1007/978-3-032-26764-1_17

17.1 Introduction

Leukemia cutis (LC) refers to the infiltration of the skin by neoplastic leukemic cells, typically occurring alongside systemic leukemia, and represents a specific form of extramedullary leukemic disease [1]. It most commonly affects patients with established leukemia but can also be present at the initial diagnosis and rarely precedes systemic disease. Aleukemic leukemia cutis, where skin involvement occurs without detectable leukemia in the blood or bone marrow, is uncommon, occurring in fewer than 10% of cases [2]. Distinct from leukemia cutis, myeloid sarcoma is a tumor mass of myeloid blasts occurring at any extramedullary site, including the skin, leading to the destruction of normal tissue architecture. It arises in the context of acute myeloid leukemia (AML), transformed myelodysplastic syndromes (MDS), or myeloproliferative neoplasms (MPNs). Extramedullary manifestations of AML are generally termed myeloid sarcoma, while leukemia cutis can also rarely appear in acute lymphoblastic leukemia (ALL) [3–6]. Myeloid sarcoma is characterized by a mass of myeloid blasts, with or without maturation, outside the bone marrow, causing tissue destruction at the affected site. Extramedullary involvement occurs in about 10% of AML cases, with the skin being the most commonly affected organ; leukemia cutis itself is estimated to occur in 3–5% of these cases. AML with monocytic differentiation, especially in patients with NPM1 mutations, shows a higher incidence of extramedullary disease, frequently affecting the gingiva, skin, and central nervous system. Leukemia cutis usually appears in advanced leukemia but can be concurrent with diagnosis (~30%), occasionally precede clinically detectable leukemia (<10%), or rarely be the initial or sole manifestation. The last two scenarios are termed aleukemic leukemia cutis. Similar leukemia cutis-like skin infiltrations may be seen in MPNs, including chronic myeloid leukemia (CML), MDS, and myelodysplastic/myeloproliferative neoplasms such as chronic myelomonocytic leukemia (CMML). In these cases, skin involvement often reflects an immature extramedullary component of the chronic myeloid disease, although mature extramedullary myeloid proliferations—such as sclerosing extramedullary hematopoietic tumor (SEMHT) or myelodysplasia cutis—can also occur.

17.2 Incidence and Epidemiology of Leukemia Cutis (LC)

Leukemia cutis (LC) is a specific extramedullary manifestation of leukemia in the skin and may occur with any leukemia subtype. The reported frequency of LC varies from 2% to 30%, depending on study design, population, and diagnostic criteria. Among all leukemias, LC is most frequently associated with acute

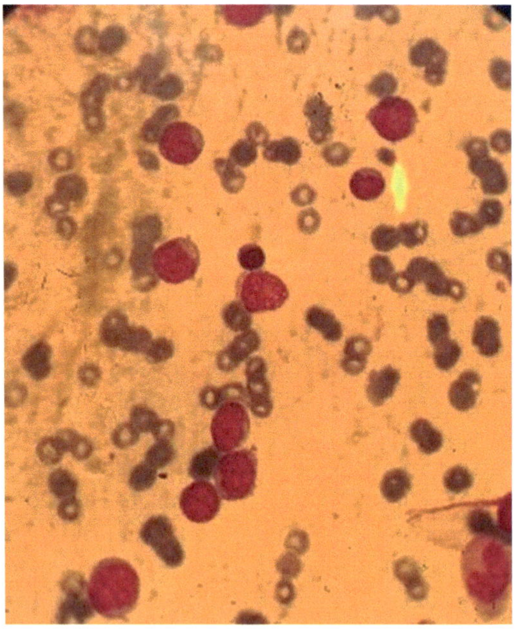

Fig. 17.1 Peripheral blood smear from a patient with acute myelomonocytic leukemia (AML-M4) who also developed leukemia cutis. The image demonstrates a predominance of large myeloblasts and monoblasts characterized by high nuclear-to-cytoplasmic ratios, fine chromatin, and conspicuous nucleoli. Cytoplasmic basophilia and occasional azurophilic granules are evident. Background cells include mature neutrophils and erythrocytes. The morphologic findings are consistent with AML-M4, a subtype showing dual granulocytic and monocytic differentiation. The patient exhibited concurrent leukemia cutis, reflecting extramedullary dissemination of leukemic blasts to the skin

myeloid leukemia (Fig. 17.1), particularly the FAB M4 (acute myelomonocytic) and M5 (acute monocytic) subtypes, with incidences reported as high as 10–50% in these groups. In contrast, the occurrence in acute lymphoblastic leukemia is rare (1–3%), while in chronic myeloid leukemia (CML), it is below 5%. Chronic lymphoblastic leukemia (CLL) also demonstrates a significant predilection for cutaneous involvement, with LC reported in 4–27% of patients [1]. While CLL represents the most common leukemia subtype in Western populations, the absolute number of LC cases remains higher in AML due to the latter's more aggressive biology and myelomonocytic tropism.

Epidemiologic studies have confirmed that LC may precede, accompany, or follow systemic leukemia. In most patients, LC occurs after the diagnosis of leukemia (55–77%); in 23–38%, it presents concurrently, and in about 7%, it precedes systemic disease, termed aleukemic leukemia cutis (ALC) or primary extramedullary leukemia (EML) [7–10]. The aleukemic form may precede hematologic evidence of leukemia by several months or even years, highlighting its diagnostic importance [11–20]. Age and sex distribution generally reflect that of the underlying leukemia, with a slight male preponderance (ratio 1.1:1) and a mean presentation age between 60 and 70 years in adults [21, 22]. In infants with congenital leukemia, LC has been reported in 25–30% of cases, most often in congenital myelogenous leukemia; interestingly, LC does not appear to worsen prognosis in this group [11]. A large Korean cohort of 75 patients by Kang et al. [12] also confirmed AML and CML as the most common associated subtypes, with extremities as the most frequently affected sites, along with a 2:1 male predominance. Despite therapeutic advances, the prognosis remained poor, with most patients dying within one year, comparable to earlier Western data. Although this traditionally has been a poor-prognosis marker, recent molecular and outcome studies reveal a nuanced picture. In the matched-cohort study presented by Zhao et al. in 2025 [7], which included AML patients, there were recurrent mutations, including NPM1, FLT3, NRAS/KRAS, and trisomy 8, with frequent discordance in CD34 and CD117 expression between skin and marrow samples. Although the median overall survival for patients with LC was shorter (14.6 vs. 23 months), this did not reach statistical significance, suggesting that prognosis depends more on the molecular profile than on cutaneous involvement alone. Complementing this, a meta-analysis by Lin et al. performed in 2025, including more than 3000 AML patients, reported the presence of extramedullary disease, including LC in 1–30% of patients [23]. It was independently associated with poorer overall survival, HR 1.49; 95% CI 1.34–1.67, although allogenic stem cell transplantation, allo-HSCT, mitigated this effect. Taken together, LC is most common, particularly in AML-M4, followed by CLL, and is rare in ALL or CML. In pediatric cases, especially congenital AML, the incidence is highest, but the outcome is different. Although many studies vary, LC remains a clinically relevant marker for extramedullary disease and warrants a comprehensive systemic workup and molecular profiling.

17.3 Clinical Appearance of Leukemia Cutis

LC is a specific extramedullary manifestation of leukemia, characterized by the infiltration of neoplastic leukocytes into the skin, leading to visible cutaneous lesions that may precede, coincide with, or develop after the diagnosis of systemic leukemia [24–28]. Clinical manifestations of LC are remarkably polymorphic and reflect differences related to the underlying leukemia subtype, disease phase, and depth of dermal infiltration.

17.4 Timing and Distribution

The temporal relationship between LC and systemic leukemia is variable [29, 30]. In 55–77% of patients, LC develops after the diagnosis of leukemia, while in 23–38%, it appears simultaneously, and in approximately 7%, it precedes systemic disease (aleukemic LC). There are no consistent predilection sites. The most affected body parts are the legs, followed by arms, back, chest, scalp, and face, while palmoplantar and oral mucosa involvement is rare. Sites of previous or concomitant inflammation tend to be preferentially involved. Lesions are typically multiple, less often single. A large Korean series by Kang et al. published in 2013 that involved 75 patients found the extremities (37%) and trunk (28%) to be the most commonly affected regions, particularly in AML and CML. Most patients had multiple lesions (84%), while solitary nodules accounted for 16%.

17.5 Morphologic Spectrum

The morphology of LC lesions is highly variable, ranging from subtle erythematous macules to large nodules or tumors. The most common presentations include:

- Papules, nodules, and plaques, which may be solitary, grouped, or disseminated (Figs. 17.2, 17.3, 17.4, and 17.5).
- Lesions are mostly dome-shaped, soft to rubbery, and may vary in color from red, brown, violaceous, yellowish, or even blue-gray,

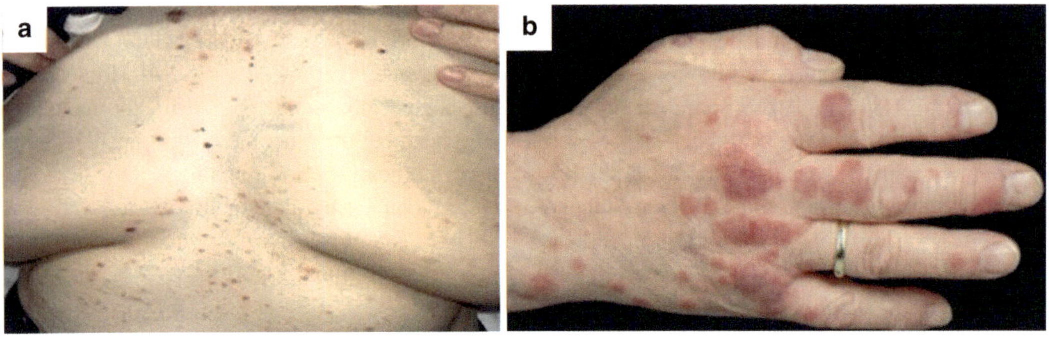

Fig. 17.2 Clinical presentation of leukemia cutis in a 65-year-old female patient with acute myelomonocytic leukemia (AML-M4). (**a**) Multiple erythematous to violaceous papules and nodules scattered over the trunk. (**b**) Similar infiltrated plaques and nodules on the dorsal surface of the hand

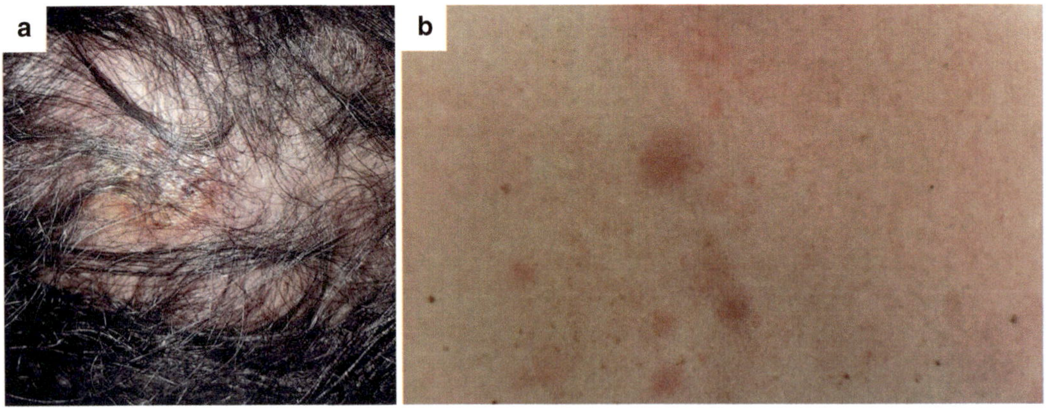

Fig. 17.3 Cutaneous involvement in a 64-year-old woman with acute myeloid leukemia (AML). (**a**) Infiltrated erythematous plaque with overlying crusting and erosion on the scalp. (**b**) Multiple erythematous to violaceous papules and nodules scattered over the back, consistent with leukemia cutis

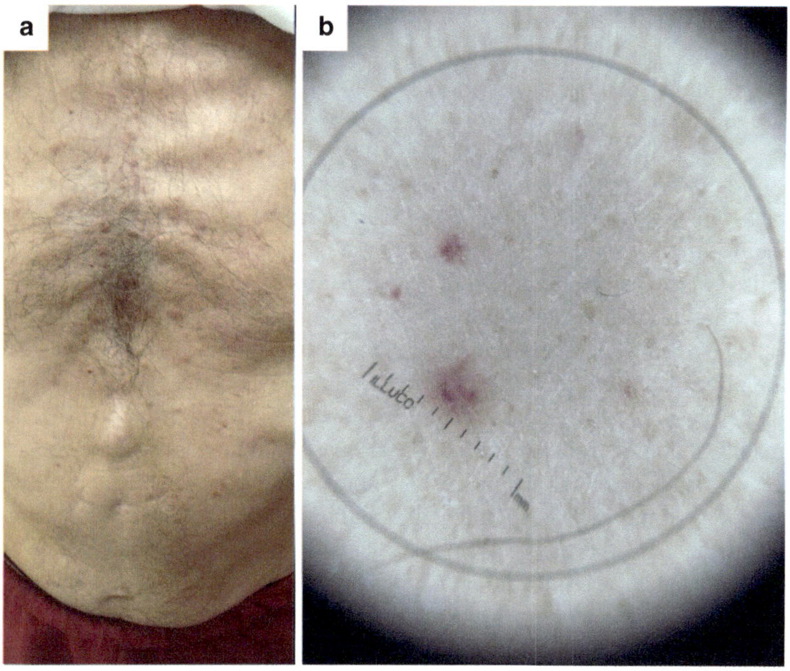

Fig. 17.4 (**a**) Clinical image of a 66-year-old male with acute monocytic leukemia (AMoL) demonstrating leukemic infiltration of the skin on the abdomen and limbs. Multiple erythematous papules and nodules are scattered over the abdomen (**b**) Dermoscopy of representative lesions demonstrates multiple nonspecific pink to red structureless areas, with occasional subtle vascular patterns consistent with dermal leukemic infiltration. These findings represent the often-subtle presentation of leukemia cutis and the value added by dermoscopy in demonstrating vascular and color changes

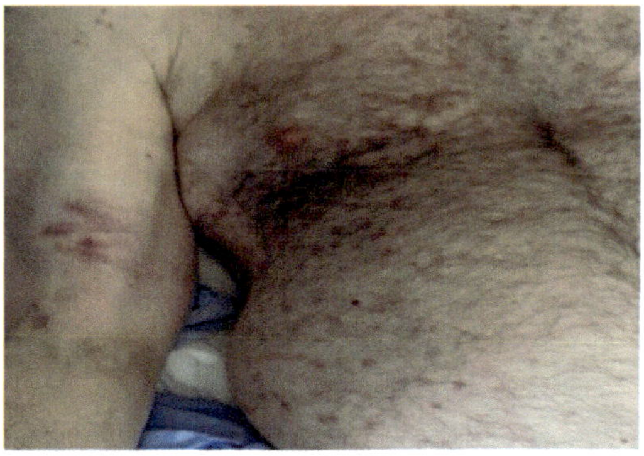

Fig. 17.5 Clinical presentation of leukemia cutis in a 60-year-old male with acute myelomonocytic leukemia (AML M4). Multiple erythematous-to-violaceous, firm papules and nodules are distributed on the trunk and proximal upper limbs. The skin lesions represent leukemic infiltration, with some demonstrating coalescence and overlying ecchymosis. Such infiltrates, often seen in AML M4, are indicative of cutaneous involvement by leukemic cells

occasionally with hemorrhagic discoloration or purpuric.

- Plaques and tumors may be up to several centimeters in diameter, with larger lesions often exhibiting ulceration or crusting.
- Rare presentations include blisters, erosions, and ulcers resistant to conventional therapy.

The color of the lesion will depend on the depth of infiltration and vascular involvement. Deeply seated infiltrates may appear skin-colored with a rubbery consistency, while superficial lesions are often erythematous or violaceous.

17.6 Special Clinical Patterns

Certain clinical patterns are characteristic and diagnostically significant:

- Chloroma or granulocytic/myeloid sarcoma may appear as green-tinged, firm nodules or plaques due to the peroxidase content of myeloid cells. It is most commonly linked with acute myeloid leukemia, especially M2–M5 types, and has also been reported in other myeloproliferative disorders.
- Gingival hyperplasia is the characteristic mucosal manifestation, especially in acute monocytic, M5, and myelomonocytic, M4 leukemias. The gingiva is enlarged, erythematous, friable, and partially covers the teeth; occasionally, necrosis or ulceration may also occur.

  Leonine facies due to the coalescing nodules and plaques on the face can be seen in advanced disease.
- Involvement of scars and erythrodermic forms has also been documented, though these are rare.
- Blistering bullous LC is a rare variant; in it, vesiculobullous lesions may sometimes contain serous or hemorrhagic fluid.

17.7 Dermoscopic Features of Leukemia Cutis

Although histopathologic examination remains the gold standard in diagnosing LC, dermoscopy has recently emerged as a useful noninvasive adjunctive tool that may aid in the clinical assessment of suspected lesions. The present literature is scarce in dermoscopic descriptions of LC, and the first systematic observations have been reported only within the last few years [31–33].

Sławińska et al. in 2021 reported a case series, representing the dermoscopic presentation of LC in five patients with various forms of leukemia: acute myeloid leukemia (AML), chronic lymphocytic leukemia (CLL), and chronic myelomonocytic leukemia (CMML) [34]. The most consistent finding, observed in four out of five cases, was a polymorphic vascular pattern, characterized by a mixture of dotted, linear curved, and branched linear vessels (Fig. 17.4b). These vascular structures were distributed on diffuse pink to red or pink-brown structureless backgrounds. Further dermoscopic features included white thick lines arranged in a network-like pattern, corresponding histologically to dermal fibrosis, and yellow-orange structureless areas in patchy distribution, likely indicating dermal infiltration by leukemic cells or necrotic foci. Nodular or ulcerated lesions demonstrated central yellow-red or black crusted areas in some cases, while the pigment network or other melanocytic structures were uniformly absent. The authors underlined that the polymorphous vascular pattern, that is, the coexistence of two or more vessel morphologies, is not specific to LC but is frequently associated with malignant non-melanocytic skin tumors, including amelanotic melanoma, squamous cell carcinoma, Merkel cell carcinoma, and cutaneous metastases. Thus, in the appropriate clinical context, this dermoscopic finding should raise suspicion for LC and warrant histopathologic confirmation. The presence of yellow-orange structureless areas, also described in granulomatous and xanthomatous dermatoses, may be an additional, though nonspecific, clue to dermal infiltration.

In a separate report, Calderón-Castrat et al. in 2019 described the dermoscopic findings in neonatal leukemia cutis, a condition that may present clinically as a "blueberry muffin" eruption. Dermoscopy showed fine arborizing telangiectatic vessels distributed within a homogeneous pink background without pigment or keratin-related structures. Such findings reflect superficial vascular proliferation and leukemic infiltration of the dermis, in keeping with the infiltrative but non-keratinizing nature of neonatal LC. Altogether, the literature indicates that LC dermoscopy most commonly shows a non-specific but suspicious vascular morphology, often polymorphous, in association with pink, red, or orange structureless backgrounds. Such features should be considered in the appropriate clinical setting, namely, in the context of a known hematologic malignancy or in the presence of unexplained violaceous, brownish, or erythematous nodules or plaques. Under these circumstances, dermoscopy may be useful in pointing out those lesions that warrant biopsy and histopathologic confirmation.

17.8 Clinical Differential Diagnosis of Leukemia Cutis

1. *Secondary cutaneous involvement by*: Skin infiltration by both B-cell and T-cell lymphomas can result in lesions similar to leukemia cutis. Clinical context, immunophenotyping, and molecular studies are necessary for differentiation (Fig. 17.6a, b) [35–48].
2. *Primary cutaneous T-cell lymphoma*, such as mycosis fungoides and Sézary syndrome: these present with patches, plaques, or tumors and can be difficult to distinguish from secondary involvement, especially in the more advanced stages. Epidermotropism and clinical history help differentiate these entities [35].
3. *Blastic plasmacytoid dendritic cell neoplasm (BPDCN)*: BPDCN commonly presents as cutaneous lesions with violaceous or bruise-like nodules or plaques. It may easily be confused with leukemia cutis. Diagnosis is by immunophenotyping for CD4, CD56, and CD123.
4. *Langerhans cell histiocytosis*: Presenting lesions may be papules or nodules, which can be ulcerated; this condition can resemble leukemia cutis, particularly in children. Diagnosis is by histopathology and immunohistochemistry.
5. *Cutaneous metastases from solid tumors*: Nodular or plaque-like lesions that may be similar to leukemia cutis, especially in patients with a previously diagnosed malignancy. Histopathology and clinical history are the prime discriminants.
6. *A disseminated opportunistic fungal infection* can include histoplasmosis, presenting with papules, nodules, or ulcers in the setting of immunocompromised states, which would include leukemia. Diagnosis is confirmed with fungal stains, cultures, or antigen testing, as recommended by the American Thoracic Society.
7. *Sweet's syndrome* (acute febrile neutrophilic dermatosis): Tender erythematous papules or plaques often with fever and neutrophilia. Histology discloses a dense neutrophilic infiltrate without leukemic cells. Because the disease responds quickly to corticosteroid treatment, it can easily be differentiated from leukemia cutis.

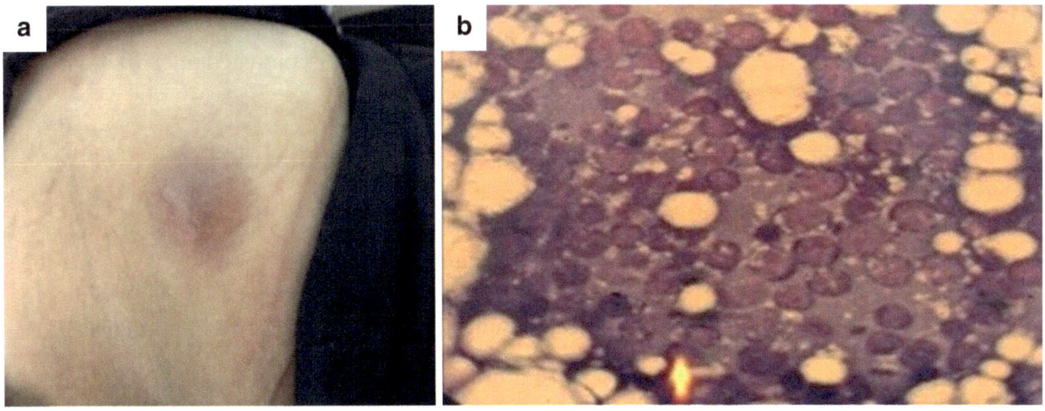

Fig. 17.6 (**a**) Left: Abdominal skin of a 57-year-old male with relapsed Burkitt lymphoma, showing a solitary, indurated, erythematous-violaceous nodule consistent with cutaneous infiltration by neoplastic lymphoid cells. (**b**) Right: Bone marrow aspirate smear from the same patient, demonstrating prominent abnormal lymphoid cells with round nuclei, coarse chromatin, and multiple cytoplasmic vacuoles, characteristic of Burkitt lymphoma involvement

17.9 Case Presentation 1: Cutaneous Infiltration in Late Relapse of NPM1-Positive Acute Myeloid Leukemia

17.9.1 Patient Background

A 70-year-old woman was diagnosed seven years earlier with acute myeloid leukemia (AML) harboring an NPM1 mutation. She achieved complete remission following induction and consolidation therapy but experienced relapse three months after completing treatment. Salvage therapy with fludarabine, cytarabine, granulocyte colony-stimulating factor (G-CSF), and idarubicin (FLAG-IDA) was administered, followed by an allogeneic hematopoietic stem cell transplantation (allo-HSCT) from a matched unrelated donor one year later.

17.9.2 Clinical Presentation

Approximately six years post-transplant, the patient presented with a crusted, honey-colored, infiltrated plaque on the left parietal scalp (Fig. 17.3a). One month later, she developed multiple large, hyperpigmented macules and patches on the trunk, mainly affecting the upper back (Fig. 17.3b).

17.9.3 Diagnostic Workup

Skin biopsies from the scalp and back demonstrated cutaneous infiltration by myeloid blasts, confirming leukemic cutis (Fig. 17.7a–e).

Bone marrow aspiration, biopsy, and flow cytometric analysis showed no evidence of systemic AML relapse.

Molecular testing showed:

- *NPM1*: negative
- *FLT3-ITD*: negative
- *FLT3-TKD*: positive

Next-generation sequencing (NGS) did not detect pathogenic variants in the analyzed exons or gene regions.

A Positron Emission Tomography (PET) scan demonstrated increased metabolic activity involving:

- Cervical lymph node regions (occipital, jugular, supraclavicular)
- Right parietal bone
- Right fifth rib
- Right clavicle
- Right tibia

These findings were consistent with extramedullary leukemic involvement.

17.9.4 Management

The patient initiated treatment with azacitidine in combination with venetoclax:

- Azacitidine was administered at a subcutaneous dose of 75 mg/m^2 daily for 7 days every 4 weeks.
- Venetoclax 400 mg orally once daily

She also received G-CSF as needed. Venetoclax was discontinued after 10 months.

17.9.5 Current Status

The patient remains on azacitidine monotherapy. Treatment is currently on hold due to neutropenia, and she is receiving daily G-CSF with ongoing clinical and laboratory monitoring.

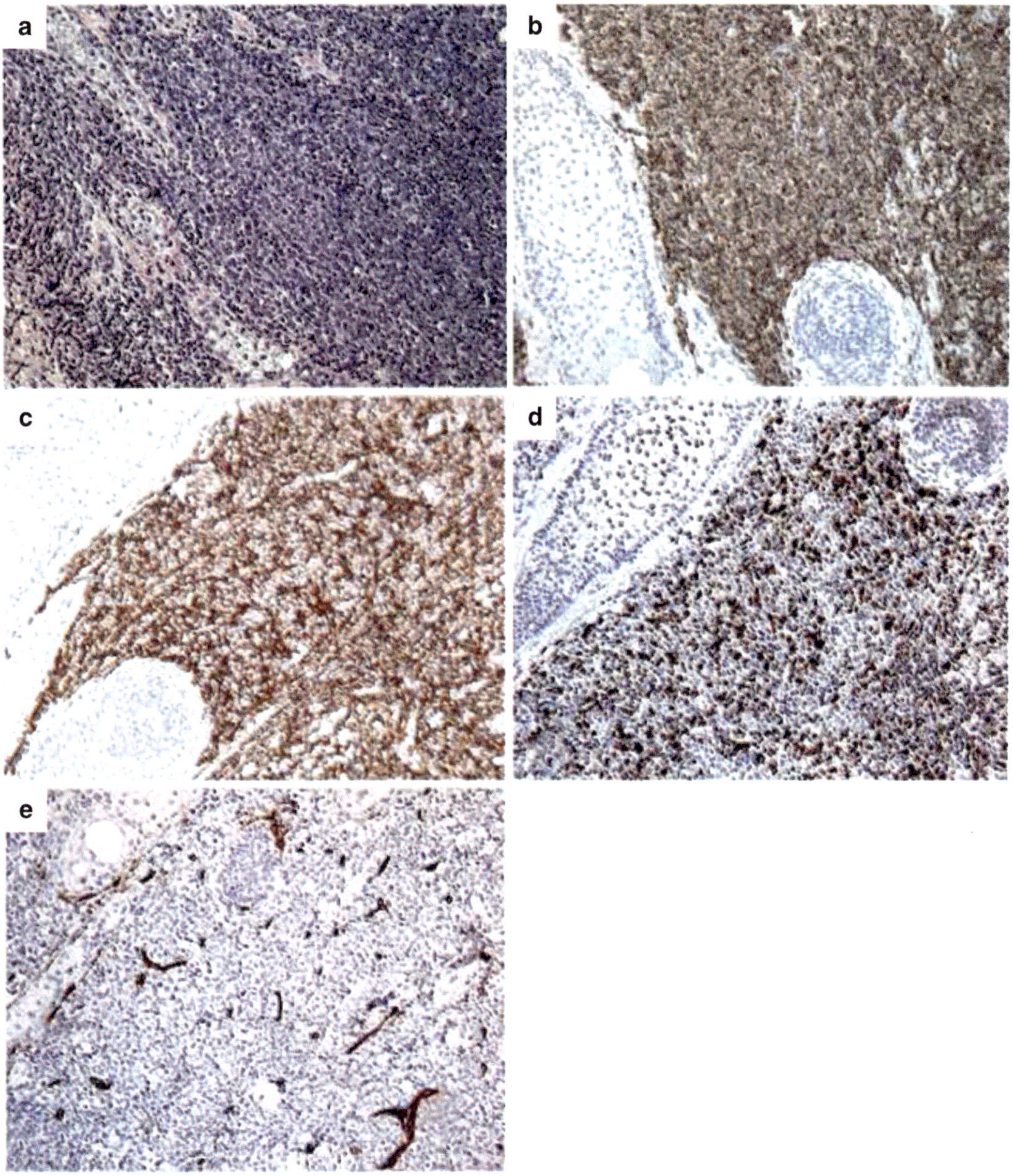

Fig. 17.7 The microscopic examination of the violaceous nodule on the scalp showed thorough infiltration of the dermis and superficial subcutaneous fat by a monotonous population of large cells with a high nuclear to cytoplasmic ratio, round to slightly irregular nuclear contours, finely dispersed chromatin, distinct nucleoli, and numerous mitoses (**a**). Immunohistochemical examination of the neoplastic cells was diffusely positive for MPO (**b**) and CD43 (**c**), locally positive for C-KIT (**d**) and TdT (not shown), while it was negative for CD34 (**e**), CD3, CD20, and CD30 (not shown), an immunophenotype consistent with leukemia cutis with >80% myeloid differentiation—AML. (**a**): H/E X 100 magnification, (**b–e**): × 100 magnification

17.10 Case Presentation 2: Acute Monocytic Leukemia Presenting with Rapid Progression and Leukemic Cutis

17.10.1 Patient Background

A 67-year-old man initially underwent a bone marrow biopsy at age 66 for evaluation of unexplained cytopenias. The biopsy revealed a myelodysplastic process without excess blasts and no evidence of increased monocytic populations, consistent with early-stage MDS. Eight months later, he developed progressive leukocytosis and worsening anemia, prompting a repeat bone marrow biopsy. At that time, his medical history was notable for a recently diagnosed myelodysplastic syndrome, which was now showing evolution toward acute leukemia.

17.10.2 Diagnostic Findings

The repeat bone marrow biopsy demonstrated acute monoblastic/monocytic leukemia. Immunohistochemistry revealed the following profile: PGM1+ >>MPO+, CD34–, c-KIT–, CD33–, PAX5–, LAT–, Glycophorin-C–, CD20–, CD79a–, TdT–, CD3–. The myeloid lineage showed complete maturation arrest with marked effacement of the remaining hematopoietic elements, consistent with acute myeloid leukemia arising from immature monocytic precursors.

17.10.3 Treatment Course

Initial therapy consisted of hydroxyurea for cytoreduction, followed by FLAG (fludarabine, cytarabine, and G-CSF) with G-CSF support. Additional treatment included Vyxeos (liposomal daunorubicin 44 mg/m^2 and cytarabine 100 mg/m^2). The patient subsequently began venetoclax 400 mg orally once daily after a 5-week dose ramp-up in combination with azacitidine (120 mg).

17.10.4 Cutaneous Manifestations

Four months later, the patient developed multiple infiltrated red–red-violaceous papules and nodules on the trunk and extremities (Fig. 17.4a). Dermoscopy showed nonspecific features with diffuse pink-brownish structureless areas (Fig. 17.4b). A skin biopsy from the trunk revealed cutaneous infiltration by acute myelomonocytic leukemia. Histopathology demonstrated a diffuse dermal infiltrate composed of large, markedly atypical cells with scant cytoplasm and blastoid nuclear chromatin (Fig. 17.8a, b).

Immunohistochemical staining showed that the neoplastic cells were CD45+, CD43+, CD34–, MPO–, c-KIT–, TdT–, PAX5–, CD14–, CD11c–, CD68–, CD3–, CD4+, CD56+, CD123–, with a very high proliferative index (Ki-67~95%) (Fig. 17.8c, d). These findings were compatible with leukemic cutis corresponding to the patient's known acute monocytic leukemia.

17.10.5 Outcome

Despite intensive treatment and supportive care, the patient experienced a rapid clinical decline and died three months later.

17.10.6 Histologic Diagnosis of Leukemia Cutis

Cutaneous involvement may antedate, occur simultaneously with, or postdate systemic leukemia and, rarely, may occur in the absence of detectable systemic disease, a condition termed aleukemic leukemia cutis. Approximately 3–5% of AML patients develop cutaneous involvement by acute myeloid leukemia (c-AML) (Fig. 17.9a–d), with the presence of destructive infiltrates of mostly immature myeloid cells in the skin and with a particular enrichment for those with monocytic features or *NPM1* mutations. CMML less often involves the skin and can display a broad spectrum of lesions that include both mature and immature monocytic cells. In cases where the

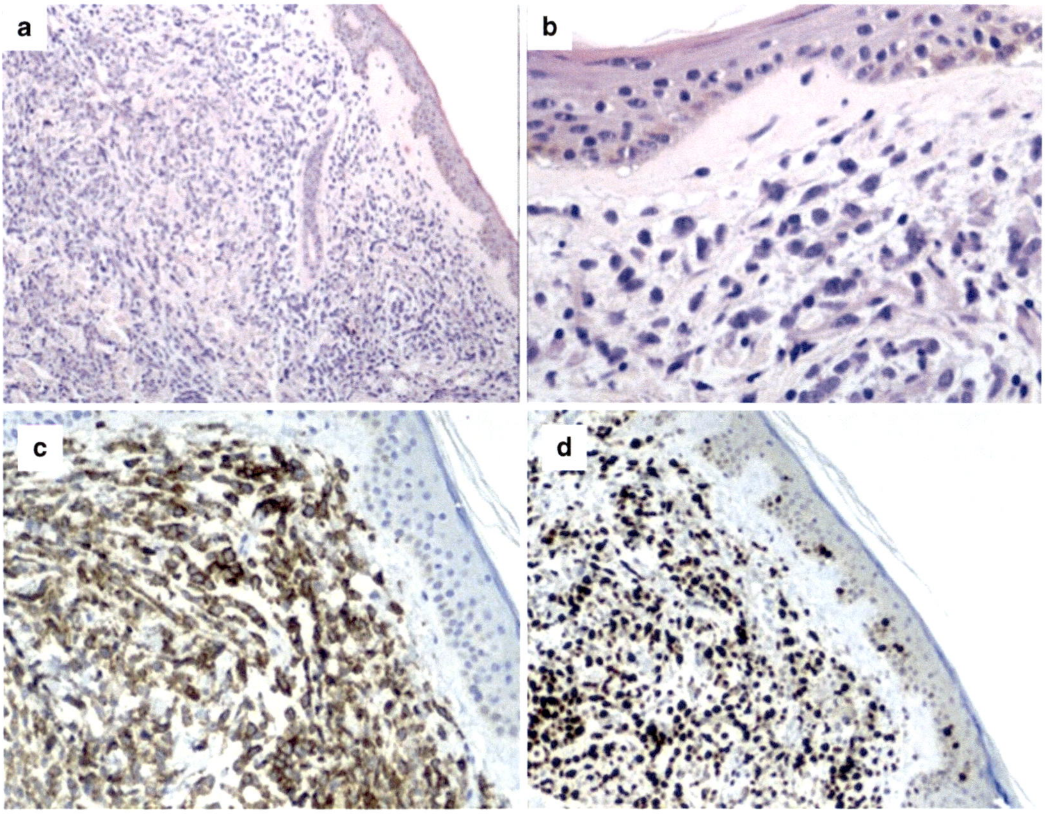

Fig. 17.8 Skin biopsy from a 66-year-old male with acute monocytic leukemia (AML-M5) presenting with leukemia cutis. (**a**) The dermis is diffusely infiltrated by blastic monocytic cells (H&E, ×100). (**b**) High-power view showing a very high proliferation rate (H&E, ×400). (**c**) LCA (Leukocyte Common Antigen) immunostaining confirming hematopoietic origin. (**d**) Ki-67 immunohistochemistry showing a proliferation index of approximately 95%, findings consistent with the reported hematologic neoplasm acute monocytic leukemia

predominant cells are immature, it is considered progression to AML.

More unusual manifestations of myeloid neoplasms include histiocytic, Langerhans cell, and other dendritic cell neoplasms. These latter lesions are often considered to be derived from mature histiocytic/dendritic cells, although technically derived from a common granulocyte–monocyte precursor progenitor cell.

Most leukemia cutis cases show a small blue round cell tumor morphology with a deeper than expected perivascular and/or periadnexal pattern or a dense interstitial or nodular infiltrate of dermis and subcutis (Fig. 17.7a, b) with sparing of the upper papillary dermis (Grenz zone) (Fig. 17.8a). Epidermotropism is typically absent (Fig. 17.8b). The infiltrate consists of medium to large blasts with round to oval nuclei and often detectable nucleoli. In monocytic differentiation, irregular, convoluted, and/or lobulated nuclei can be seen.

In AML, the infiltrate consists mostly of large or medium-sized, immature myeloid cells with blastic chromatin with nucleoli and abundant mitotic activity with scattered apoptotic cells (Fig. 17.7a, b). Eosinophilic myelocytes can also be seen. Immunophenotypically, CD68/KP1 is the most commonly expressed marker, followed by MPO, C-KIT (Fig. 17.7d, e), lysozyme, CD34, TdT, CD56, CD61, and CD99.

In cases of AMoL ≥80% of the leukemic cells are monocytes and their precursors (monoblasts and promonocytes), and the monocytic lineage can be determined by NSE staining or monocytic

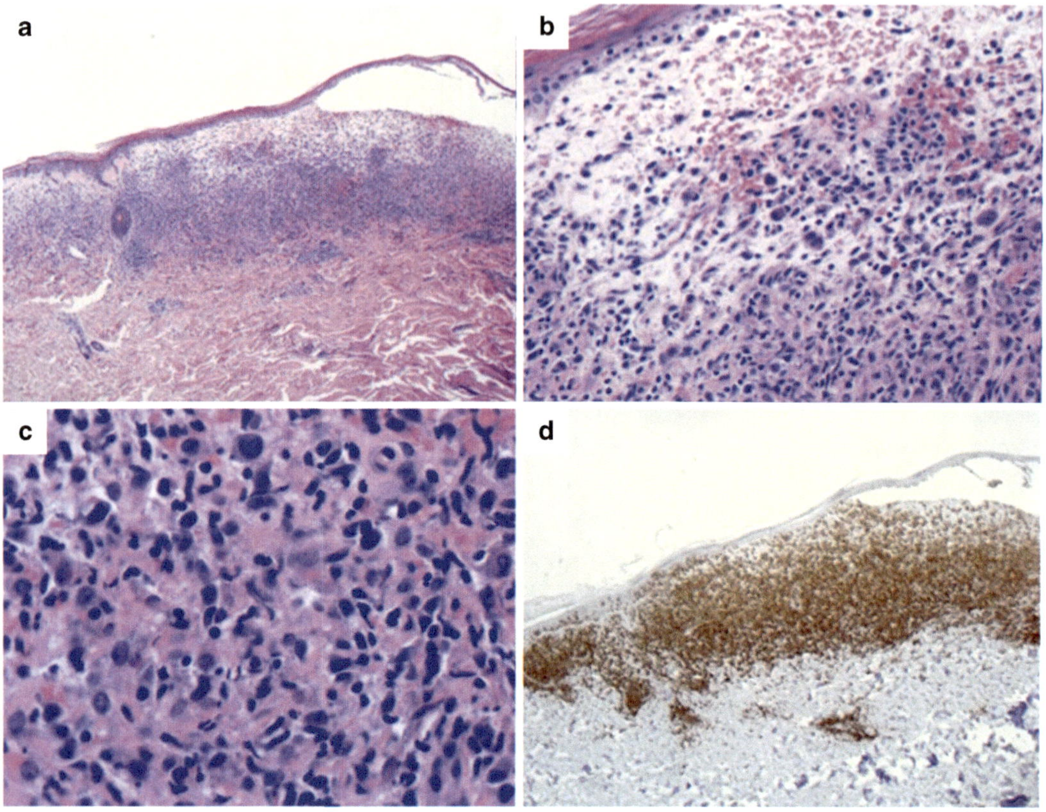

Fig. 17.9 Histopathology of a skin biopsy from an infiltrated plaque on the trunk in a 74-year-old male with acute monocytic leukemia (AML) receiving gilteritinib 120 mg daily. Immunohistochemistry showed the atypical cells to be MPO–, CD34–, CD117–, TdT–, CD3–, CD19–, and positive for CD43 and PGM1, findings consistent with cutaneous infiltration by acute monocytic leukemia. Correlation with clinical and hematologic data is recommended. (**a**) The biopsy demonstrates epidermal erosion with diffuse infiltration of the upper dermis by atypical monocytic leukemic cells arranged in a lichenoid pattern, accompanied by dermal edema and focal detachment of the overlying epidermis. Hematoxylin and eosin (H&E) stain; DAB chromogen with hematoxylin counterstain; original magnification ×40. (**b**) H&E stain; original magnification ×200. (**c**) H&E stain; original magnification ×400. (**d**) CD43 immunostain highlighting infiltration of the dermis by monocytic leukemic cells

immunophenotype (CD14+, CD11c+, CD163+, lysozyme+, CD64+, CD34-, C-KIT-). Monoblasts are medium to large cells with abundant basophilic cytoplasm round/ovoid nuclei with open chromatin, one or more nucleoli and promonocytes (blasts equivalent) with characteristic nuclei with delicate infoldings and inconspicuous nucleoli. Monocytes show morphologic abnormalities (convoluted nuclei with less clumped nuclear chromatin and occasional nucleoli). Monoblasts are typically MPO-, and promonocytes are typically MPO variable.

irregular, convoluted, and/or lobulated nuclei of immature morphology with dispersed nuclear chromatin (Fig. 17.8a, b).

The blasts of ALL are morphologically indistinguishable from myeloid blasts, yet they less often display nucleoli, and the infiltrate usually affects even deeper cutaneous structures.

The histologic diagnosis may be easy and/or unequivocal in the context of a known leukemic disease. In contrast, significant differential diagnostic difficulties in clinically contextless cases are expected, with extramedullary leukemia being among the most common misdiagnoses in surgical pathology. Ancillary techniques such as immunohistochemistry are crucial to accurate diagnosis.

Nevertheless in case of suspected LC, the discordant antigen expression /antigenic shift such as decreased/lacking expression of CD34 and/or CD117 and gain of CD56, lysozyme, and/or myeloperoxidase (MPO) compared to that observed in the bone marrow or the blood explicable by a distinct subgroup of blasts that preferentially occupy extramedullary sites should be taken into account to avoid diagnostic pitfalls.

In a clinical context, significant differential diagnostic difficulties are expected, with extramedullary leukemia being among the most common misdiagnoses in surgical pathology.

In case of suspected leukemia cutis, a first round of phenotypic examination with CD43, CD45, INSM1, lysozyme, MPO, pan-cytokeratin, and TdT is advisable and a characteristic phenotype with CD43+, CD45±, lysozyme±, MPO±, CK–, and TdT± should lead to next-step examinations to establish an entity-specific diagnosis.

If the above-described immunophenotype is observed, the suspect diagnosis of a hematolymphoid small round cell tumor can be rendered, and a second round of immunohistochemical markers should follow to establish a specific diagnosis. Discordant antigen expression/antigenic shift applying to the blast population affecting the skin, such as decreased/lacking expression of CD34 (Fig. 17.7e) and/or CD117 and gain of CD56, lysozyme, and/or myeloperoxidase (MPO) compared to that observed in the bone marrow or the blood, should be considered.

In myeloid marker-negative cases, the expression of CD2, CD3, CD5, CD7, TCRβF1, or δ for the T-cell lineage and CD19, CD20, CD22, CD79a, or PAX5 for the B-cell lineage indicates lymphoid origin. Additionally, in the background of CD3 and CD20 negativity, the expression of CD14, CD68, CD117, CD123, IRF8, lysozyme, or MPO indicates a myeloid origin. Provided that the myeloid origin of the immature infiltrate is determined, additional immunohistochemical stainings for p53 and NPM1 should be performed and interpreted along with the application of selected fluorescence in situ hybridization probes and next-generation sequencing (NGS) panels for subentity-defining genetic aberrations, such as AML with inv(16) (p13;q22), to establish a WHO-5/ICC 2024 diagnosis (World Health Organization Classification of Tumours Editorial Board. (2024). WHO classification of haematolymphoid tumours (5th ed., Vol. 11). International Agency for Research on Cancer. https://publications.iarc.fr/Book-And-Report-Series/Who-Classification-Of-Tumours/Haematolymphoid-Tumours-2024) .

17.10.7 Histological Differential Diagnosis

Various cutaneous neoplastic infiltrates, primary and not, as well as malignant non-hematolymphoid tumors (neuroendocrine and mesenchymal tumors), can overlap with LC in the spectrum of small blue round cell tumors involving the skin and should be unequivocally ruled out by immunohistochemistry.

The differential diagnosis should consider and exclude Myelodysplasia Cutis (MDS), a cutaneous infiltrate of immature but non-blastic myeloid cells showing a clonal relationship with the MDS clone in the bone marrow and/or peripheral blood. Cases of MDS cutis closely resemble the histiocytoid variant of Sweet syndrome, from which it cannot be distinguished based on histomorphology alone. NGS can be useful in separating MDS cutis from the latter.

Furthermore, mature lymphoid B and T cell neoplasms involving the skin, as well as primary high-grade cutaneous lymphomas, should also be considered in the differential diagnosis and excluded.

The plasmablastic variant of multiple myeloma enters the differential diagnosis and can be a challenge, but the expression of CD138, CD38, and MUM1, in addition to light chain restriction, can confirm its diagnosis. Cases of BPDCN should be excluded in any hematolymphoid small round cell tumor by applying markers to detect the characteristic constellation of negativity for CD3, CD20, CD34, lysozyme, and

MPO and the coexpression—along with CD43 and/or CD45—of CD4, CD56, CD68, CD123, CD303, IRF8, and TCL1 (and TdT) in various constellations.

Additionally, Blastic Plasmacytoid Dendritic Cell Neoplasm (BPDCN), a rare, aggressive hematopoietic neoplasm derived from plasmacytoid dendritic cells (PDCs) that mainly affects the elderly, is characterized by high skin tropism (skin involvement in 64–100% of cases) and should be excluded in the presence of any hematolymphoid small round cell tumor. Immunohistochemical examination aiming to detect the characteristic combined negativity for CD3, CD20, CD34, lysozyme, and MPO, and the coexpression—along with CD43 and/or CD45—of CD4, CD56, CD68, CD123, CD303, IRF8, and TCL1 (and TdT) expression is essential for the diagnosis.

In the non-hematolymphoid tumor setting, Merkel cell carcinoma (MCC) is a rare, aggressive cutaneous neuroendocrine tumor that often occurs in the head and neck area on sun-exposed skin of elderly individuals. This is due to the blue round morphology of the cells and the characteristic non-epidermotropic dermal/subcutis-based distribution of the infiltrates that enters into the differential diagnosis. Combined positivity for synaptophysin and dot-like positivity for CK20, which may be substantiated by positivity for Merkel cell polyomavirus (MCPyV) and PAX8, will lead to the diagnosis of Merkel cell carcinoma. A positivity of small blue round cell tumors involving the skin for CK7, synaptophysin, and TTF1 strongly suggests metastatic small cell (neuroendocrine) lung cancer; such cases will regularly express CD56 and can be PAX5 and/or TdT positive.

Ultimately, very few sarcomas, primary and metastatic, belong to the small blue round cell tumor group, and are very rare. These include tumors of the primitive neuroectodermal tumors/Ewing sarcomas group and synovial sarcoma. In cases that express CD99 and, in certain instances, CD30, CD56, CD117, PAX8, SOX9, and/or S100, a tumor of the primitive neuroectodermal tumors/Ewing sarcomas group should be suspected, and specific EWS fusion testing ought to be performed. A CD99±, CK7+/±, PAX8±, SS18-SSX+, S100± immunophenotype is diagnostic of synovial sarcoma, and such cases can express CD34, CD56, and CD57.

17.10.8 Management

The cornerstone of management for leukemia cutis is systemic therapy aimed at the underlying leukemia. This often includes aggressive induction chemotherapy and, when possible, allogeneic HSCT. Cutaneous lesions usually resolve with hematologic remission. In cases of refractory or relapsed skin involvement, local radiotherapy may serve as a useful adjunct. Due to its poor prognosis and propensity to be associated with extramedullary dissemination, patients with leukemia cutis should be followed closely and may benefit from more aggressive or innovative therapeutic regimens.

Recent advances have indeed extended the therapeutic options available for high-risk and relapsed AML, including those with leukemia cutis. Hypomethylating agents such as azacitidine and decitabine, often combined with venetoclax, have improved outcomes in older or unfit patients and those with adverse-risk features. Targeted therapies are now available for specific molecular subtypes, including IDH1/2 inhibitors such as ivosidenib and enasidenib, and FLT3 inhibitors, including midostaurin and gilteritinib, which are FDA-approved for AML harboring corresponding mutations. Finally, emerging agents such as menin inhibitors for NPM1-mutated or KMT2A-rearranged AML and CD47-SIRPα inhibitors—particularly in TP53-mutated disease—have also reported promising early results, including MRD-negative complete responses and improved survival in preliminary studies.

Immunotherapy and cellular approaches are rapidly evolving in the management of high-risk and relapsed AML, including leukemia cutis. Allogeneic HSCT and donor lymphocyte infusions remain standard for eligible patients, but novel strategies such as chimeric antigen receptor T-cell (CAR-T) therapy, bispecific T-cell engagers (BiTEs), dual antigen receptor targeting (DARTs), and immune checkpoint inhibitors are under active investigation. These approaches are particularly relevant in the post-transplant relapse setting and for patients with minimal residual disease. Early-phase trials have demonstrated feasibility, safety, and encouraging response rates, but challenges remain regarding antigen selection, toxicity, and durability of response.

Despite these advances, no novel or targeted therapy has thus far demonstrated a definitive improvement in survival or remission rates specifically for patients with leukemia cutis in large, prospectively designed clinical trials. Most data are extrapolated from studies in high-risk or extramedullary AML populations, and the optimal sequencing of novel agents, long-term outcomes, and LC-specific management strategies remain areas of active investigation. Inclusion in clinical trials and molecular profiling to guide therapy are strongly encouraged for this high-risk group. In summary, therapeutic strategies for leukemia cutis are centered on the systemic treatment of the underlying leukemia. Novel targeted agents and immunotherapies offer promising options for select molecular subtypes and for relapsed/refractory disease, but data specific to LC outcomes are limited, and further research is needed to define optimal management.

17.11 Clinical Correlations and Prognosis

The growth rate and distribution of LC lesions may also be indicative of the biological behavior of the underlying leukemia. The nodules that enlarge rapidly usually signify an acute leukemia, whereas chronic forms are characterized by slowly enlarging plaques. Because morphology is not a predictable determinant of the type of leukemia, nodular or tumorous lesions are seen more in myeloid leukemias, while papules or erythematous plaques tend to predominate in lymphoid variants.

Prognostic factors associated with leukemia cutis include:

AML subtype: The monocytic variant FAB M5 and the myelomonocytic variant FAB M4 carry the highest risk.

Cytogenetic and molecular features: Trisomy 8, NPM1, FLT3, and NRAS/KRAS mutations are more frequent among AML patients with LC, though these do not significantly affect survival.

Clinical features: Organomegaly, such as hepatomegaly or lymphadenopathy, is an independent predictor for LC, associated with poorer outcomes.

Extramedullary disease: LC often coexists with other extramedullary sites and further worsens the prognosis.

Overall, the development of cutaneous lesions in leukemia reflects advanced disease biology and is widely regarded as an indicator of poor prognosis. Median survival after the diagnosis of LC ranges from 5 to 14 months, with 5-year survival rates at about 8.6%, compared to 28.3% in AML without cutaneous involvement. In a Korean series with LC, 88% of patients died within one year following diagnosis. The presence of leukemia cutis should prompt consideration of more aggressive or alternative therapeutic strategies and close monitoring for disease progression.

References

1. World Health Organization Classification of Tumours Editorial Board. WHO classification of haematolymphoid tumours (5th ed., Vol. 11). International Agency for Research on Cancer; 2024. https://publications.iarc.fr/Book-And-Report-Series/Who-Classification-Of-Tumours/Haematolymphoid-Tumours-2024
2. Arber DA, Orazi A, Hasserjian R, Thiele J, Borowitz MJ, Le Beau MM, Bloomfield CD, Cazzola M, Vardiman JW. The 2016 revision to the World Health Organization classification of myeloid neoplasms and acute leukemia. Blood. 2016;127(20):2391–405. https://doi.org/10.1182/blood-2016-03-643544. Epub 2016 Apr 11. PMID: 27069254.
3. Kaddu S, Zenahlik P, Beham-Schmid C, Kerl H, Cerroni L. Specific cutaneous infiltrates in patients with myelogenous leukemia: a clinicopathologic

study of 26 patients with assessment of diagnostic criteria. J Am Acad Dermatol. 1999;40(6 Pt 1):966–78. https://doi.org/10.1016/s0190-9622(99)70086-1. PMID: 10365929
4. Yook HJ, Son JH, Kim YH, Han JH, Lee JH, Park YM, Chung NG, Kim HJ, Bang CH. Leukaemia cutis: clinical features and outcomes of 56 patients. Acta Derm Venereol. 2022;102:adv00647. https://doi.org/10.2340/actadv.v102.1123. PMID: 35088871.
5. Robak E, Braun M, Robak T. Leukemia cutis-the current view on pathogenesis, diagnosis, and treatment. Cancers (Basel). 2023;15(22):5393. https://doi.org/10.3390/cancers15225393. PMID: 38001655.
6. Wagner G, Fenchel K, Back W, Schulz A, Sachse MM. Leukemia cutis - epidemiology, clinical presentation, and differential diagnoses J Dtsch Dermatol Ges. 2012;10(1):27–36. https://doi.org/10.1111/j.1610-0387.2011.07842.x. Epub 2011 Nov 17. PMID: 22115500.
7. Zhao GZ, Guhan S, Liszewski WJ, Nguyen CV. Molecular and immunophenotypic profiling of leukemia cutis in acute myeloid leukemia: A retrospective matched-cohort study. J Am Acad Dermatol. 2025;93(4):988–92. https://doi.org/10.1016/j.jaad.2025.05.1414. Epub 2025 May 23. PMID: 40414606.
8. Valente M, Sanches JA, Nukui Y, Cury-Martins J, Souza BC, Pereira J, Miyashiro D. Characterization of adult T-cell leukemia/lymphoma patients with specific skin lesions in a tertiary dermatological service in Brazil. Front Med (Lausanne). 2025;12:1505865. https://doi.org/10.3389/fmed.2025.1505865. eCollection 2025. PMID: 39991055
9. Helm KF, Su WP, Muller SA, Kurtin PJ. Malignant lymphoma and leukemia with prominent ulceration: clinicopathologic correlation of 33 cases. J Am Acad Dermatol. 1992;27(4):553–9. https://doi.org/10.1016/0190-9622(92)70221-z. PMID: 1401306
10. Wang HQ, Li J. Clinicopathological features of myeloid sarcoma: report of 39 cases and literature review. Pathol Res Pract. 2016;212(9):817–24. https://doi.org/10.1016/j.prp.2016.06.014. Epub 2016 Jul 20. PMID: 27515547.
11. Rijlaarsdam JU, van der Putte SC, Berti E, Kerl H, Rieger E, Toonstra J, Geerts ML, Meijer CJ, Willemze R. Cutaneous immunocytomas: a clinicopathologic study of 26 cases. Histopathology. 1993;23(2):117–25. https://doi.org/10.1111/j.1365-2559.1993.tb00469.x. PMID: 8406383.
12. Kang YS, Kim HS, Park HJ, Lee JY, Kim HO, Cho BK, Park YM. Clinical characteristics of 75 patients with leukemia cutis. J Korean Med Sci. 2013;28(4):614–9. https://doi.org/10.3346/jkms.2013.28.4.614. Epub 2013 Mar 27. PMID: 23579733.
13. Cañueto J, Meseguer-Yebra C, Román-Curto C, Santos-Briz A, Fernández-López E, Fraile C, Unamuno P. Leukemic vasculitis: a rare pattern of leukemia cutis. J Cutan Pathol. 2011;38(4):360–4. https://doi.org/10.1111/j.1600-0560.2010.01623.x. Epub 2010 Sep 23. PMID: 20860730.
14. Schneider LA, Weber L, Viardot A, Schubert R, Hinrichs R, Scharffetter-Kochanek K. Cutaneous leukaemic infiltrations in a patient with previously undiagnosed myelodysplastic syndrome. Clin Exp Dermatol. 2004;29(5):468–70. https://doi.org/10.1111/j.1365-2230.2004.01550.x. PMID: 15347325.
15. Ratnam KV, Khor CJ, Su WP. Leukemia cutis. Dermatol Clin. 1994;12(2):419–31. PMID: 8045053.
16. Brazão C, Mancha D, Antunes-Duarte S, Kempf W, Soares-de-Almeida L. Chilblain-like eruption unveiling cutaneous Aleukemic relapse of acute myeloid leukemia. Am J Dermatopathol. 2023;45(12):847–51. https://doi.org/10.1097/DAD.0000000000002530. Epub 2023 Sep 13. PMID: 37703321.
17. Singh S, Taneja N, Kaul S, Arava S, Bhari N. Aleukemic leukemia cutis mimicking urticaria pigmentosa in a patient of T-cell acute lymphoblastic leukemia. Indian J Dermatol Venereol Leprol. 2020;86(1):105. https://doi.org/10.4103/ijdvl.IJDVL_355_18. PMID: 31397398.
18. Andriescu EC, Coughlin CC, Cheng CE, Prajapati VH, Huang JT, Schmidt BA, Degar BA, Aplenc R, Pillai V, Yan AC, Liang MG. Pediatric leukemia cutis: a case series. Pediatr Dermatol. 2019;36(5):658–63. https://doi.org/10.1111/pde.13864. Epub 2019 Jul 5. PMID: 31273836.
19. Elkeeb D, Hopkins Z, Miles RR, Halwani A, Wada D. Ominous cutaneous presentation of acute myeloid leukemia without peripheral blood involvement upon initial presentation and relapse: case report and literature review. Eur J Dermatol. 2018;28(6):809–17. https://doi.org/10.1684/ejd.2018.3463. PMID: 30698150.
20. Joshi K, Panchal H, Parikh S, Modi G, Talele A, Anand A, Uparkar U, Joshi N, Khatawani I. Aleukemic leukemia cutis presenting as a sole sign of relapsed paediatric acute lymphoblastic leukemia. Indian J Hematol Blood Transfus. 2016;32(Suppl 1):46–9. https://doi.org/10.1007/s12288-015-0597-z. Epub 2015 Sep 23. PMID: 27408353.
21. Gru AA, Coughlin CC, Schapiro ML, Lombardi M, Martin A, Bayliss SJ, Frater J, Dehner LP. Pediatric aleukemic leukemia cutis: report of 3 cases and review of the literature. Am J Dermatopathol. 2015;37(6):477–84. https://doi.org/10.1097/DAD.0000000000000190. PMID: 25148106.
22. Narváez-Moreno B, Pereyra-Rodríguez JJ, Pulpillo-Ruiz A, Cabrera-Pérez R, Espigado-Tocino I, Conejo-Mir J. Acute myeloid leukemia 7 years after aleukemic leukemia cutis. Int J Dermatol. 2015;54(4):459–61. https://doi.org/10.1111/ijd.12024. Epub 2013 Nov 21. PMID: 24261792.
23. Hejmadi RK, Thompson D, Shah F, Naresh KN. Cutaneous presentation of aleukemic monoblastic leukemia cutis - a case report and review of literature with focus on immunohistochemistry. J Cutan Pathol 2008;35 Suppl 1:46–9. https://doi.org/10.1111/j.1600-0560.2008.00982.x. Epub 2008 Jun 9. PMID: 18544052.

24. Lin Y, Liu P, Zhuang Q, Deng H, Liu X, Wang Y, Tong H, Liu A, Sun J. Prognostic impact of extramedullary disease in acute myeloid leukemia: A meta-analysis. Int J Cancer. 2025;157(11):2334–42. https://doi.org/10.1002/ijc.70024. Epub 2025 Jun 25. PMID: 40558061.
25. Dekio I, Anzai H, Ohyama M, Tanikawa A, Amagai M, Yokoyama K, Okamoto S, Tanaka M. Aleukaemic leukaemia cutis as an initial manifestation of myeloid/NK cell precursor acute leukaemia. J Eur Acad Dermatol Venereol. 2006;20(4):453–6. https://doi.org/10.1111/j.1468-3083.2006.01491.x. PMID: 16643148.
26. Onozawa M, Hashino S, Kanamori H, Izumiyama K, Yonezumi M, Chiba K, Kondo T, Fukuhara T, Tanaka J, Imamura M, Asaka M. Aleukemic leukemia cutis in a patient with Philadelphia chromosome-positive biphenotypic leukemia. Int J Hematol. 2004;80(3):278–80. https://doi.org/10.1532/ijh97.04010. PMID: 15540904.
27. Kawai K, Uchida Y, Kanekura T. Prognostic significance of TBX21 and GATA3 subtype classification in indolent adult T-cell leukemia-lymphoma with cutaneous lesions. J Dermatol. 2025;52(11):1674–81. https://doi.org/10.1111/1346-8138.17917. Epub 2025 Aug 20. PMID: 40833211.
28. Buzzatti E, Mauro C, Botti C, Presicci R, Paterno G, Palmieri R, Gurnari C, Mallegni F, Meddi E, Moretti F, Cardillo L, Mezzanotte V, Taka K, De Marchi L, Maurillo L, Buccisano F, Venditti A, Del Principe MI. Leukemia cutis in a patient with acute myeloid leukemia undergoing Azacitidine-Venetoclax: case presentation and review of the literature. Mediterr J Hematol Infect Dis 2025;17(1):e2025013. https://doi.org/10.4084/MJHID.2025.013. eCollection 2025. PMID: 40084096.
29. Bisschop MM, Révész T, Bierings M, van Weerden JF, van Wering ER, Hählen K, van der Does-van den Berg A. Extramedullary infiltrates at diagnosis have no prognostic significance in children with acute myeloid leukaemia. Leukemia. 2001;15(1):46–49. https://doi.org/10.1038/sj.leu.2401971. PMID: 11243398.
30. Lal A, Agrawal S, Gaurav V. Co-occurrence of pityriasis amiantacea and Cutis verticis gyrata secondary to Leukaemia cutis of the scalp. Skin Appendage Disord. 2024;10(2):144–7. https://doi.org/10.1159/000535081. Epub 2023 Nov 28. PMID: 38572192.
31. Calderón-Castrat X, Pomar R, Lipa-Chancolla RM, Apagüeño C, Castro R, Ballona R. Dermoscopic findings in neonatal leukemia cutis. Pediatr Dermatol. 2019;36(6):988–9. https://doi.org/10.1111/pde.13890. Epub 2019 Aug 29. PMID: 31468564.
32. Simionescu O, Petrică M, Avram AM, Costache M, Scurtu LG, Tudorache SI, Iorga PG, Grigore M. Dermoscopy of skin metastases in advanced cancer-systemic (visceral, hematologic) and cutaneous. Front Med (Lausanne). 2024;11:1445811. https://doi.org/10.3389/fmed.2024.1445811. eCollection 2024. PMID: 39139791.
33. Kiyohara T, Makimura K, Nakamaru S, Miyamoto M, Shijimaya T, Nagano N, Tanimura H. B-cell lymphoblastic leukemia/lymphoma in infants: report of two cases on the face. J Dermatol. 2019;46(7):e255–6. https://doi.org/10.1111/1346-8138.14799. Epub 2019 Feb 5. PMID: 30719747.
34. Sławińska M, Sokołowska-Wojdyło M, Biernat W, Zaryczańska A, Nowicki RJ, Sobjanek M. Dermoscopic features of leukemia cutis-case series. Indian J Dermatol. 2021;66(2):187–90. https://doi.org/10.4103/ijd.IJD_534_19. PMID: 34188276.
35. Cho-Vega JH, Medeiros LJ, Prieto VG, Vega F. Leukemia cutis. Am J Clin Pathol. 2008;129(1).130–42. https://doi.org/10.1309/WYACYWF6NGM3WBRT. PMID: 18089498.
36. Wankel B, Afzal M, Loo EY, LeBlanc RE, Carter JB, Lansigan E, Yerrabothala S. Acute myeloid leukemia cutis with KMT2A::MLLT3 fusion presenting with leonine facies. Leuk Res Rep. 2023;21:100400. https://doi.org/10.1016/j.lrr.2023.100400. eCollection 2024. PMID: 38162585.
37. Eckardt JN, Stölzel F, Kunadt D, Röllig C, Stasik S, Wagenführ L, Jöhrens K, Kuithan F, Krämer A, Scholl S, Hochhaus A, Crysandt M, Brümmendorf TH, Naumann R, Steffen B, Kunzmann V, Einsele H, Schaich M, Burchert A, Neubauer A, Schäfer-Eckart K, Schliemann C, Krause SW, Herbst R, Hänel M, Hanoun M, Kaiser U, Kaufmann M, Rácil Z, Mayer J, Kroschinsky F, Berdel WE, Ehninger G, Serve H, Müller-Tidow C, Platzbecker U, Baldus CD, Schetelig J, Bornhäuser M, Thiede C, Middeke JM. Molecular profiling and clinical implications of patients with acute myeloid leukemia and extramedullary manifestations. J Hematol Oncol. 2022;15(1):60. https://doi.org/10.1186/s13045-022-01267-7. PMID: 35562747.
38. Garcia Fasanella M, Mozos A, Briones J, Nomdedeu JF, Novelli S. Evaluation of clinical outcomes and treatment complications in hairy cell leukemia: a single-center retrospective analysis. Cancer Rep (Hoboken). 2025;8(10):e70356. https://doi.org/10.1002/cnr2.70356. PMID: 41031578.
39. Cibull TL, Thomas AB, O'Malley DP, Billings SD. Myeloid leukemia cutis: a histologic and immunohistochemical review. J Cutan Pathol. 2008;35(2):180–5. https://doi.org/10.1111/j.1600-0560.2007.00784.x. PMID: 18190442.
40. Chen L, Rodgers TR, Chaffins ML, Maeda K. Acute monocytic leukemia with cutaneous manifestation. Arch Pathol Lab Med. 2005;129(3):425–426. https://doi.org/10.5858/2005-129-425-AMLWCM. PMID: 15737049.
41. Maciá J, Gómez X, Parra R, Gallart MA, Casanovas A, Ortiz P, Araguás C. Cutaneous infiltration by histiocytic lymphoma in a patient with acute monocytic leukemia (M5a). Eur J Haematol. 1994;53(5):304–5. https://doi.org/10.1111/j.1600-0609.1994.tb01325.x. PMID: 7813712.

42. Solimani F, Dilling A, Heisterkamp K, Damm F, Penack O, Oberender C, Le-Coutre P, Rudelius M, Ghoreschi K, Nast A. Acute lymphoblastic B-cell leukemia or CAR-T cell related skin changes - a relevant diagnostic challenge. J Dtsch Dermatol Ges. 2025. https://doi.org/10.1111/ddg.15931. Online ahead of print. PMID: 41047857.
43. Kanitthamniyom C, Wannaphut C, Pattanaprichakul P, Kungwankiattichi S, Owattanapanich W. Organomegalies as a predictive indicator of leukemia cutis in patients with acute myeloid leukemia. PLoS One. 2024;19(2):e0297805. https://doi.org/10.1371/journal.pone.0297805. eCollection 2024. PMID: 38363781.
44. Watson KM, Mufti G, Salisbury JR, du Vivier AW, Creamer D. Spectrum of clinical presentation, treatment and prognosis in a series of eight patients with leukaemia cutis. Clin Exp Dermatol. 2006;31(2):218–21. https://doi.org/10.1111/j.1365-2230.2005.02022.x. PMID: 16487095.
45. Scherer LD, Rouce RH. Targeted cellular therapy for treatment of relapsed or refractory leukemia. Best Pract Res Clin Haematol. 2023;36(3):101481. https://doi.org/10.1016/j.beha.2023.101481. Epub 2023 May 25. PMID: 37612000.
46. Kinsella FAM, Maroto MAL, Loke J, Craddock C. Strategies to reduce relapse risk in patients undergoing allogeneic stem cell transplantation for acute myeloid leukaemia. Br J Haematol. 2024;204(6):2173–2183. https://doi.org/10.1111/bjh.19463. Epub 2024 Apr 11. PMID: 38602216.
47. O'Hagan Henderson S, Frietsch JJ, Hilgendorf I, Hochhaus A, Köhne CH, Casper J. Combination of treosulfan, fludarabine and cytarabine as conditioning in patients with acute myeloid leukemia, myelodysplastic syndrome and myeloproliferative neoplasms. J Cancer Res Clin Oncol. 2022;148(10):2599–609. https://doi.org/10.1007/s00432-021-03836-8. Epub 2021 Oct 21. PMID: 34674031.
48. Sadigh S, et al. Cutaneous manifestations of myeloid neoplasms exhibit broad and divergent morphologic and immunophenotypic features but share ancestral clonal mutations with bone marrow. 2024;37(1):100352. https://doi.org/10.1016/j.modpat.2023.100352. Epub 2023 Oct 13.

18 Cutaneous Metastases from Multiple Myeloma

Vasiliki Nikolaou and Alexander Stratigos

Abstract

Cutaneous involvement in multiple myeloma (MM) is rare, affecting approximately 1% of patients, and typically indicates hematogenous dissemination in advanced, high-risk disease. Clinically, lesions present as violaceous papules, nodules, or plaques, occasionally ulcerated. Histopathology reveals dermal or subcutaneous infiltrates of CD138-positive monoclonal plasma cells, and the immunoglobulin isotype and light-chain restriction usually parallel the systemic clone. Prognosis is poor, with survival commonly limited to a few months, particularly in patients with IgA isotype or plasmablastic variants.

Management follows principles established for extramedullary MM, with systemic therapy prioritized—using proteasome inhibitors, immunomodulatory drugs, CD38-directed antibodies, and increasingly BCMA-targeted therapies. Radiotherapy may provide local palliation for painful or ulcerated lesions but is not disease-modifying. Supportive care, including wound management and infection prevention, alongside close collaboration between dermatology and hematology, is essential. These observations are consistent with multi-institutional cohorts and align with broader frameworks of extramedullary MM biology and treatment.

Keywords

Multiple myeloma · Extramedullary myeloma · Cutaneous metastases · Skin neoplasms · Prognosis · Plasma cells/pathology

18.1 Introduction

Multiple myeloma (MM) is a plasma cell dyscrasia characterized by the clonal proliferation and accumulation of malignant plasma cells within the bone marrow, typically associated with the production of a monoclonal immunoglobulin. Cutaneous involvement is uncommon and may present in two broad categories: (i) disease-specific lesions related to abnormal protein deposition, such as AL amyloidosis and type I cryoglobulinemia; and (ii) non-specific dermatoses associated with an underlying monoclonal gammopathy, including necrobiotic xanthogranuloma, Schnitzler syndrome, and scleromyxedema [1]. True cutaneous metastases of MM are rare but well-documented. These may arise either through contiguous extension from adjacent neoplastic foci—most often osteolytic skull, rib, or

V. Nikolaou (✉) · A. Stratigos
First Department of Dermatology-Venereology, "Andreas Sygros" Hospital, National and Kapodistrian University of Athens, Athens, Greece
e-mail: alstrat@hol.gr

D. Koumaki et al. (eds.), *Cutaneous Metastases*, https://doi.org/10.1007/978-3-032-26764-1_18

other osseous plasmacytomas invading the overlying skin—or via hematogenous dissemination, where circulating malignant plasma cells infiltrate the dermis or subcutis. This chapter reviews the epidemiology, clinicopathologic features, differential diagnosis, and current evidence-based strategies for the management of cutaneous metastases of MM.

18.2 Epidemiology

Metastatic skin lesions in multiple myeloma (MM) without underlying bony involvement are exceedingly rare. Only a limited number of series have been reported, and contemporary data suggest that biopsy-confirmed cutaneous involvement occurs in approximately 1% of MM patients. Even less common are cases of multiple myeloma that are first recognized in the skin.

Metastatic skin lesions typically appear late in the disease course, usually in the context of high tumor burden and aggressive disease biology. The median time from initial myeloma diagnosis to the development of cutaneous involvement is about 2 years [3]. Once present, cutaneous metastases portend a poor prognosis, with median overall survival ranging from 8.5 to 12 months [2–4].

There is no consistent association between cutaneous involvement and a specific immunoglobulin class in multiple myeloma, and any class of myeloma protein is capable of producing cutaneous dissemination. Immunoglobulin G (IgG) is the most common subtype seen in cases with skin involvement, which reflects its overall predominance among myeloma subtypes rather than a specific predilection for cutaneous spread [4, 5]. However, some series have reported a relative overrepresentation of immunoglobulin A (IgA) and light-chain disease among patients with cutaneous metastases [3, 4]. The development of cutaneous metastases has not been correlated with a specific cytogenetic abnormality, but deletion of the rb-1 gene has been observed in some cases and may identify a high-risk subset of patients with aggressive disease biology [3].

18.3 Prognostic Features

Certain clinical and histopathologic characteristics are associated with poor outcomes in cutaneous metastases of multiple myeloma. The IgA isotype has been linked to shorter survival compared to other isotypes in some series [3, 4]. Plasmablastic cytology, characterized by immature plasma cells with prominent nucleoli and increased mitotic activity, is a recurrent adverse feature and indicates aggressive disease biology [3, 4]. Clinically, patients presenting with multiple cutaneous lesions, particularly erythematous nodules, have significantly worse outcomes than those with solitary or less extensive skin involvement [2]. From a histopathologic perspective, the absence of a Grenz zone has been associated with worse prognosis [2]. Overall, cutaneous metastases in multiple myeloma are a marker of advanced disease and confer a significantly reduced survival compared to patients without skin involvement.

18.4 Clinical Presentation

The clinical presentation of cutaneous metastases in MM is heterogeneous. The predominant phenotype consists of firm, pink-red to violaceous papules, nodules, or plaques with a smooth surface and firm consistency (Figs. 18.1 and 18.2). Lesions may occasionally ulcerate or become secondarily infected and can develop at any body site, with a relative predilection for the extremities, followed by the trunk and head. Notably, a Korean series reported that nearly 30% of cases presented as skin-colored nodules, underscoring the importance of considering multiple myeloma in the differential diagnosis of common cutaneous nodules such as lipomas, epidermal cysts, and panniculitis. In such patients, biopsy remains essential for accurate diagnosis [2, 6]. Rarely, lesions have been described at sites of prior trauma or surgical intervention, including venous catheter insertion sites, pacemaker implantation scars, and fracture locations [7]. These reports suggest a potential role of trauma-related plasma cell migration in lesion development. Cutaneous

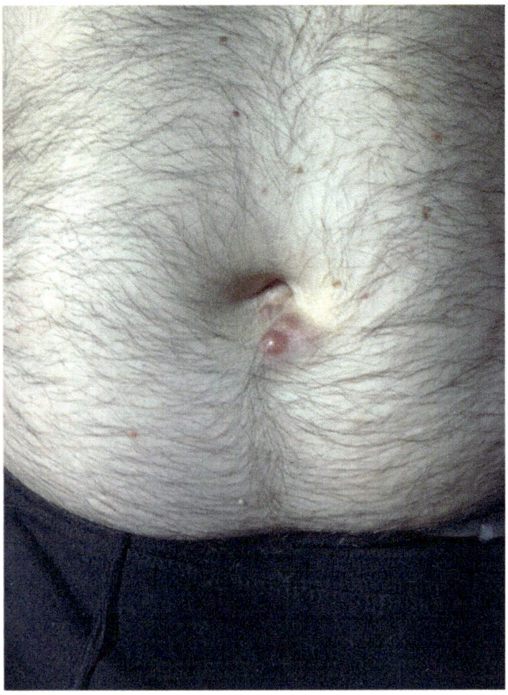

Fig. 18.1 Firm, erythematous nodule on the abdominal wall of a patient with multiple myeloma

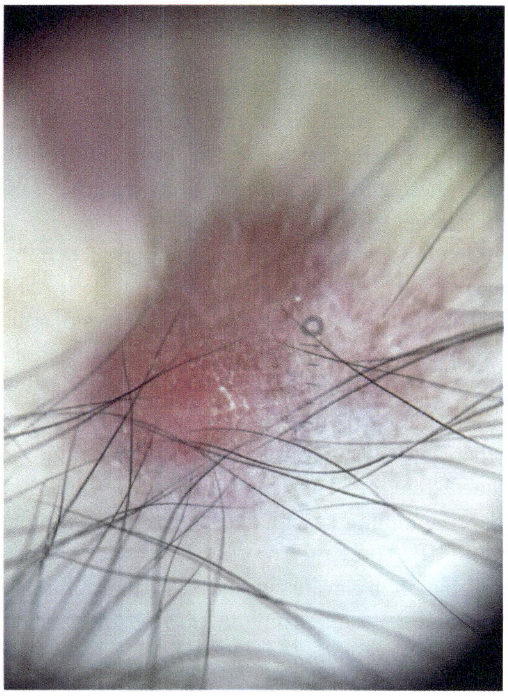

Fig. 18.2 Dermoscopy of cutaneous infiltration of multiple myeloma shows a structureless violaceous to pink area with diffuse and homogeneous pigmentation

metastases may appear at the time of initial myeloma diagnosis but are more frequently observed during disease relapse [2, 6].

The differential diagnosis includes primary cutaneous marginal zone lymphoma with plasmacytic differentiation; plasmablastic lymphoma [typically Epstein-Barr virus (EBV)-positive], with an oral cavity predilection in immunosuppressed patients, and secondary cutaneous involvement by other B-cell lymphomas with plasmacytoid morphology. Reactive plasmacytosis in the context of infections should also be considered, as well as amyloid-related skin changes in AL amyloidosis, which are common in MM but reflect protein deposition rather than neoplastic infiltration. Demonstration of monoclonal immunoglobulin restriction concordant with the systemic clone supports the diagnosis of MM, while EBV negativity and correlation with the overall clinical context help distinguish MM from plasmablastic lymphoma [4, 8, 9].

18.5 Diagnosis

Any suspicious new papulonodular lesion in a patient with known MM—particularly in relapse or with rising markers—should prompt punch or excisional biopsy. Standard evaluation includes hematoxylin and eosin (H&E) staining and immunohistochemistry for CD138, CD38, CD79a, EMA, and kappa/lambda in situ hybridization, interpreted in conjunction with serum and urine protein studies. In ambiguous cases, Epstein-Barr virus in situ hybridization (EBV-ISH) should be performed to exclude EBV-positive plasmablastic lymphoma, as EBV is typically negative in cutaneous MM. Imaging with PET-CT may assist in distinguishing contiguous extension from separate extramedullary disease foci and in assessing overall disease burden, in line with established MM evaluation frameworks.

Histopathological examination usually reveals clonal plasma cell infiltrates involving the dermis and/or subcutis, while the epidermis is generally spared [2, 6]. The infiltrates may display diffuse, nodular, or interstitial growth patterns. Cytologic appearances range from mature plasma cells to atypical plasmablastic or anaplastic morphologies, the latter correlating with aggressive clinical behavior [6].

Immunophenotyping confirms plasma cell lineage, with strong expression of CD138 and CD79a, frequent EMA positivity, and monoclonal cytoplasmic immunoglobulin showing light-chain restriction concordant with the systemic paraprotein [3]. CD56 is frequently expressed, whereas CD20 is consistently negative, aiding in the distinction from cutaneous involvement by B-cell lymphomas with plasmacytoid differentiation [10]. The Ki-67 proliferation index is variable but often elevated in cases with plasmablastic morphology, supporting their more aggressive biological potential [6, 10].

Molecular studies can provide additional confirmation, with IgH rearrangement analyses demonstrating clonality. Furthermore, deletions such as RB1 loss have been identified in plasma cells from cutaneous lesions, linking these findings to high-risk disease biology [3].

18.6 Management

There are no randomized clinical trials or evidence-based guidelines specific to cutaneous involvement in multiple myeloma (MM), and therefore no established standard of care. Management of cutaneous involvement in multiple myeloma requires a comprehensive approach integrating systemic therapy, local measures, and supportive management. Treatment follows the therapeutic principles applied to extramedullary and relapsed MM, with systemic therapy prioritized, as cutaneous lesions almost invariably signify disseminated disease. Modern treatment backbones include proteasome inhibitors (e.g., bortezomib and carfilzomib), immunomodulatory drugs (lenalidomide and pomalidomide), and anti-CD38 monoclonal antibodies (daratumumab and isatuximab) [2, 11–15]. More recently, B-cell maturation antigen (BCMA)–targeted therapies—including antibody–drug conjugates, bispecific antibodies, and CAR T-cell approaches—are increasingly incorporated into appropriate treatment lines. Importantly, extramedullary MM typically requires combination regimens and dose-intense strategies to achieve meaningful responses. Case-based reports describe transient regression of cutaneous lesions with systemic corticosteroids or chemotherapy; however, such remissions are usually short-lived, reflecting the aggressive nature of this disease phenotype [11].

Local measures may have a role in selected circumstances. Radiation therapy provides high local control owing to the intrinsic radiosensitivity of plasma cells and may be considered for painful, ulcerated, or infection-prone lesions or for palliation in oligofocal cutaneous disease [11, 16, 17]. Nevertheless, given the frequent multiplicity of lesions and the systemic nature of the disease, radiotherapy should be regarded as adjunctive rather than definitive therapy [18, 19].

Surgical excision is rarely indicated and may be considered only for isolated symptomatic nodules, without expectation of altering the overall disease course.

Supportive management is essential to optimize patient outcomes. Vigilant wound care and infection prevention are critical in immunocompromised hosts. Multidisciplinary collaboration between dermatology and hematology teams is strongly recommended, as cutaneous eruptions in MM patients may also represent drug-related or transplant-associated reactions. Input from dermatopathology is therefore crucial to avoid misattribution of skin lesions and to guide appropriate adjustments in oncologic therapy.

References

1. Claveau JS, Wetter DA, Kumar S. Cutaneous manifestations of monoclonal gammopathy. Blood Cancer J. 2022;12(4):58. https://doi.org/10.1038/s41408-022-00661-1.
2. Woo YR, Kim JS, Lim JH, et al. Prevalence and clinicopathologic characteristics of multiple myeloma with cutaneous involvement: a case series from Korea. J Am Acad Dermatol. 2018;78(3):471–478.e4. https://doi.org/10.1016/j.jaad.2017.08.054.

3. Jurczyszyn A, Olszewska-Szopa M, Hungria V, et al. Cutaneous involvement in multiple myeloma: a multi-institutional retrospective study of 53 patients. Leuk Lymphoma. 2016;57(9):2071–6. https://doi.org/10.3109/10428194.2015.1128542.
4. Requena L, Kutzner H, Palmedo G, et al. Cutaneous involvement in multiple MyelomaA Clinicopathologic, Immunohistochemical, and cytogenetic study of 8 cases. Arch Dermatol. 2003;139(4):475–86. https://doi.org/10.1001/archderm.139.4.475.
5. Kato N, Kimura K, Yasukawa K, Aikawa K. Metastatic cutaneous plasmacytoma: a case report associated with IgA lambda multiple myeloma and a review of the literature of metastatic cutaneous plasmacytomas associated with multiple myeloma and primary cutaneous plasmacytomas. J Dermatol. 1999;26(9):587–94. https://doi.org/10.1111/j.1346-8138.1999.tb02053.x.
6. Malysz J, Talamo G, Zhu J, et al. Cutaneous involvement in multiple myeloma (MM): a case series with clinicopathologic correlation. J Am Acad Dermatol. 2016;74(5):878–84. https://doi.org/10.1016/j.jaad.2015.12.028.
7. Rosenblum MD, Bredeson CN, Chang CC, Rizzo JD. Subcutaneous plasmacytomas with tropism to sites of previous trauma in a multiple myeloma patient treated with an autologous bone marrow transplant. 2003;72(4):274–277. doi:https://doi.org/10.1002/ajh.10296.
8. Cantu MD, Chen W. Differential diagnosis of multiple myeloma. Semin Diagn Pathol. 2025:150944. https://doi.org/10.1016/j.semdp.2025.150944.
9. Bhutani M, Shahid Z, Schnebelen A, Alapat D, Usmani SZ. Cutaneous manifestations of multiple myeloma and other plasma cell proliferative disorders. Semin Oncol. 2016;43(3):395–400.
10. Panse G, Subtil A, McNiff JM, et al. Cutaneous involvement in plasma cell myeloma. Am J Clin Pathol. 2021 Jan 4;155(1):106–16. https://doi.org/10.1093/ajcp/aqaa122.
11. Cowan AJ, Green DJ, Kwok M, et al. Diagnosis and management of multiple myeloma. A review. JAMA. 2022;327(5):464–77. https://doi.org/10.1001/jama.2022.0003.
12. Banerjee R, King T, Faiman B, Harding S, Rosenberg AS, Sanchorawala V, Mikhael JR, Cowan AJ. Past, present, and future of dexamethasone in multiple myeloma and AL amyloidosis. J Clin Oncol. 2026:JCO2501713. https://doi.org/10.1200/JCO-25-01713. Online ahead of print. PMID: 41592262.
13. Cohen YC, Magen H, Gatt M, Sebag M, Kim K, Min CK, Ocio EM, Yoon SS, Chu MP, Rodríguez-Otero P, Avivi I, Quijano Cardé NA, Kumar A, Krevvata M, Peterson MR, Di Scala L, Scott E, Hilder B, Vanak J, Banerjee A, Oriol A, Morillo D, Mateos MV, RedirecTT-1 investigators and study Group. Talquetamab plus Teclistamab in relapsed or refractory multiple myeloma. N Engl J Med. 2025;392(2):138–49. https://doi.org/10.1056/NEJMoa2406536. PMID: 39778168.
14. Chari A, Touzeau C, Schinke C, Minnema MC, Berdeja JG, Oriol A, van de Donk NWCJ, Rodríguez-Otero P, Morillo D, Martinez-Chamorro C, Mateos MV, Costa LJ, Caers J, Rasche L, Krishnan A, Ye JC, Karlin L, Lipe B, Vishwamitra D, Skerget S, Verona R, Ma X, Qin X, Ludlage H, Campagna M, Masterson T, Hilder B, Tolbert J, Renaud T, Goldberg JD, Kane C, Heuck C, San-Miguel J, Moreau P. Safety and activity of talquetamab in patients with relapsed or refractory multiple myeloma (MonumenTAL-1): a multicentre, open-label, phase 1-2 study. Lancet Haematol. 2025;12(4):e269–81. https://doi.org/10.1016/S2352-3026(24)00385-5. Epub 2025 Mar 13. PMID: 40090350.
15. Moore DC, Elsey G, McElwee J, Atrash S. Talquetamab for the treatment of relapsed/refractory multiple myeloma: a review of efficacy, safety, and real-world evidence. Expert Opin Biol Ther. 2025;25(11):1233–40. https://doi.org/10.1080/14712598.2025.2595122. Epub 2025 Nov 26. PMID: 41275395.
16. Timmerman RD, Bizekis CS, Pass HI, Fong Y, Dupuy DE, Dawson LA, Lu D. Local surgical, ablative, and radiation treatment of metastases. CA Cancer J Clin. 2009;59(3):145–70. https://doi.org/10.3322/caac.20013. Epub 2009 Apr 10. PMID: 19364702.
17. Willemze R, Assaf C, Bagot M, Beylot-Barry M, Berti E, Busschots AM, Cerroni L, Climent F, Diercks G, Geskin L, Gniadecki R, Gru AA, Guenova E, Guitart J, Jansen P, Kempf W, Kim E, Kim YH, Koldijk M, Marschalkó M, Mitteldorf C, Molgó M, Muniesa C, Neelis KJ, Olsen E, Ortiz-Romero PL, Papadavid E, Pimpinelli N, Pulitzer M, Quaglino P, Querfeld C, Quint K, Scarisbrick JJ, Schrader AMR, Stadler R, Vermeer M, Wehkamp U, Whittaker S, Wobser M. European Organisation for Research and Treatment of Cancer, United States Cutaneous Lymphoma Consortium and International Society for Cutaneous Lymphomas consensus recommendations for management and treatment of cutaneous lymphoproliferative disorders. Br J Dermatol. 2025;193(6):1090–100. https://doi.org/10.1093/bjd/ljaf312. PMID: 40795052
18. Adamietz IA, Schöber C, Schulte RW, Peest D, Renner K. Palliative radiotherapy in plasma cell myeloma. Radiother Oncol. 1991;20(2):111–6. https://doi.org/10.1016/0167-8140(91)90144-6. PMID: 1709508
19. Matuschek C, Ochtrop TA, Bölke E, Ganswindt U, Fenk R, Gripp S, Kröpil P, Gerber PA, Kammers K, Hamilton J, Orth K, Budach W. Effects of radiotherapy in the treatment of multiple myeloma: a retrospective analysis of a single institution. Radiat Oncol. 2015;10:71. https://doi.org/10.1186/s13014-015-0374-z. PMID: 25889851

19 Secondary Cutaneous Involvement by Lymphoma and Other Haematolymphoid Malignancies

Dimitra Koumaki, Georgios Anagnostakis, Ioannis Kokkinakis, and Leonidas Marinos

Abstract

Secondary cutaneous involvement by lymphoma and hematolymphoid malignancies presents complex diagnostic and clinical challenges. This chapter explores skin involvement patterns in systemic lymphomas of B-cell and T-/NK-cell lineages, focusing on their clinical, dermoscopic, and histopathological features alongside prognostic implications. Secondary cutaneous follicular lymphoma (SCFL), seen in 3–4% of systemic cases, manifests as erythematous to violaceous papules or plaques predominantly on sun-exposed areas during advanced stages. Diffuse large B-cell lymphoma (DLBCL) typically presents with erythematous nodules or plaques; dermoscopy may show salmon backgrounds with arborizing vessels, while intravascular large B-cell lymphoma (IVLBCL) demonstrates angiocentric intraluminal growth with clinically indurated erythema and telangiectasias. Primary cutaneous diffuse large B-cell lymphoma, leg type (PCDLBCL-LT), presents aggressively with nodules primarily on the legs. Secondary involvement by marginal zone, mantle cell, and other T-/NK-cell lymphomas exhibits variable morphologies, often ulcerated and painful, with poor prognosis. Blastic plasmacytoid dendritic cell neoplasm (BPDCN), with predilection for skin infiltration, shows dense dermal blasts positive for CD4, CD56, TCL-1, TCF4, and CD123 in skin and bone marrow. Diagnosis integrates clinical exam, dermoscopy, reflectance confocal microscopy, histopathology, and immunophenotyping to ensure timely biopsy and therapy. Dermoscopic patterns provide valuable non-invasive clues despite nonspecificity, aiding early suspicion. Histologically, lymphomas demonstrate distinct growth patterns and immunophenotypes critical for subclassification and prognostication. This comprehensive overview underscores the diagnostic complexity requiring multidisciplinary approaches for optimal management of cutaneous manifestations of systemic lymphomas.

D. Koumaki (✉)
Dermatology Department, University Hospital of Heraklion, Heraklion, Greece

G. Anagnostakis
Haematology Department, University Hospital of Heraklion, Heraklion, Greece

I. Kokkinakis
Pathology Department, University Hospital of Heraklion, Heraklion, Greece

L. Marinos
Haematopathology Department, Evangelismos General Hospital, Polyclinic, Athens, Greece

D. Koumaki et al. (eds.), *Cutaneous Metastases*, https://doi.org/10.1007/978-3-032-26764-1_19

Keywords

Cutaneous involvement · Systemic lymphoma · Follicular lymphoma · Diffuse large B-cell lymphoma · Mantle cell lymphoma · T-cell lymphoma · Dermoscopy · Histopathology · Blastic plasmacytoid dendritic cell neoplasm · Skin infiltration

19.1 Skin Involvement in the B-Cell Lineage

19.1.1 Skin Involvement in Mature B-Cell Lymphomas

19.1.1.1 Skin Infiltration by Systemic FollicularLymphomas(FL)

Introduction

Follicular lymphoma (FL) is the second most common subtype of non-Hodgkin B-cell lymphoma and typically arises within lymph nodes and consists of neoplastic germinal center B cells arranged in nodular or follicular patterns [1–4]. While predominantly nodal, FL can secondarily affect extranodal tissues, including the skin, as a manifestation of systemic disease, but not as a de novo cutaneous lymphoma. Skin involvement by systemic FL—secondary cutaneous follicular lymphoma (SCFL)—occurs in approximately 3–4% of patients and may represent the first clinical presentation of disseminated lymphoma.

Clinical Presentation of Skin Infiltration of Systemic Follicular Lymphomas

Secondary cutaneous follicular lymphoma (SCFL) is encountered primarily as cutaneous involvement by systemic follicular lymphoma, typically in advanced stages (III-IV). Although systemic follicular lymphoma (FL) typically manifests with lymphadenopathy, hepatosplenomegaly, and bone marrow involvement, the skin is involved in approximately 4% of cases, typically as a late or relapse phenomenon [5–10].

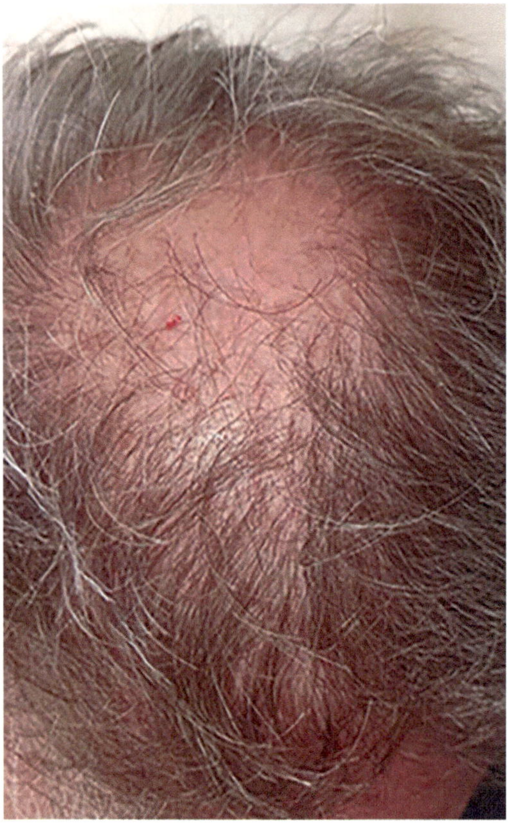

Fig. 19.1 Clinical features of follicular lymphoma with scalp involvement. A 54-year-old man presented with several erythematous, infiltrated alopecic plaques and nodules on the scalp, corresponding to cutaneous infiltration by follicular lymphoma

- Lesion Morphology: Skin lesions in SCFL are very heterogeneous but most commonly present as multiple, erythematous to violaceous, infiltrated papules, nodules, or plaques. They range from a few millimeters to a few centimeters in size. Lesions may be solitary but are more frequently multiple and disseminated (Fig. 19.1). Besides classical skin nodules and plaques, SCFL may also present atypically as ill-defined, partially hypopigmented, erythematous macules or diffuse pale patches or alopecia, and these can be mistaken for inflammatory dermatoses. Such clinical variability makes histopathological confirmation obligatory [6].
- Distribution: Lesions favor sun-exposed areas such as the scalp, forehead, face, and trunk, although any cutaneous surface can be involved. The scalp and facial areas are common solitary locations and may sometimes

present with alopecia secondary to follicular involvement [8, 10].

- Course: The clinical course can be indolent yet chronic, with a possibility of relapses confined to the skin only without systemic progression. Partial or spontaneous regression of skin lesions can be seen in a few patients, whereas others progress with persistent or progressive skin disease despite systemic therapy.
- Symptoms: Lesions are typically asymptomatic, painless, and non-ulcerating. B symptoms (fever, night sweats, weight loss) tend to correlate with the bulk of systemic disease but are not caused directly by the cutaneous lesions themselves.
- Differential Diagnosis: SCFL must be distinguished from primary cutaneous follicular lymphomas (PCFCL) and other cutaneous lymphomas, pseudolymphomas, and benign dermatoses. This is necessary because SCFL signifies systemic disease that requires systemic treatment, whereas PCFCL generally follows an indolent course that may be managed with local therapies.
- Patterns of Relapse: SCFL can also recur in the skin alone, as reported in clinical series. These cutaneous-only relapses underscore the importance of thorough skin examination in the follow-up of FL patients [11, 12].

Dermoscopic Findings of Skin Infiltrations of Systemic Follicular Lymphomas

Dermoscopy in secondary cutaneous follicular lymphoma (SCFL) shows typical but not specific vascular and pigmentary findings that match the dermal lymphoid infiltration and fibrosis [13–16]. The most common findings are a white pseudonetwork, which is secondary to confluent dermal lymphoid infiltrates and fibrosis that create a white, net-like appearance between follicular openings, and white, structureless areas, which represent dermal fibrosis and dense aggregates of lymphoid cells without recognizable structure or pigment. The vascular patterns are usually polymorphous and may include fine short linear vessels, curved linear vessels in a pattern that resembles "spermatozoa," and arborizing telangiectasias or branching vessels on the lesion surface. The background is salmon-pink to erythematous secondary to underlying lymphoid infiltration and vascular proliferation. Fine, inconspicuous scaling on the surface and yellow perifollicular circles or structures, representing perifollicular lymphoid infiltration, are other associated features.

These dermoscopic structures closely resemble those in primary cutaneous follicle center lymphoma (pcFCL) because they share the same histopathologic architecture. Recognition of these changes may contribute to the development of clinical suspicion for lymphoid infiltration, guide the selection of optimal sites for biopsy, and assist with distinguishing SCFL from other affected cutaneous neoplasms such as basal cell carcinoma or amelanotic melanoma. Unappreciable differences between SCFL and pcFCL can, nevertheless, be detected. SCFL lesions are also more likely to exhibit more widespread and more marked white pseudonetworks or structureless white zones due to deeper and denser dermal infiltrates. A more polymorphous vascular pattern with fine linear, curved linear ("spermatozoa-like"), and arborizing vessels may also be noted. Yellow perifollicular rings may be more noticeable in SCFL due to the perifollicular extension of systemic disease.

Reflectance Confocal Microscopy (RCM) Findings of Skin Infiltrations of Systemic Follicular Lymphomas

Reflectance confocal microscopy offers in vivo microscopic correlation of the) dermoscopic findings, permitting non-invasive visualization of the cutaneous architecture in SCFL [17]. The epidermis is generally intact, exhibiting a normal honeycomb pattern and lack of atypical melanocytes or pagetoid spread, features that help to exclude melanocytic neoplasms. In the dermis, RCM reveals dense, bright, nucleated cellular infiltrates consistent with lymphoid cells, typically periadnexal and perivascularly located around hair follicles and sweat glands. Pale collagen bundles are often seen to surround the infiltrates, which are the dermal fibroses. Even though the infiltrate is tight, the general dermal architecture is preserved, with no evidence of melanocytic nests or epidermal disruption.

These RCM findings are highly consistent with histopathologic evidence of dense dermal lymphoid infiltrate with perifollicular and perivascular distribution and associated fibrosis. With the assistance of dermoscopy, RCM enables enhanced diagnostic assurance by confirming the lymphoid nature of the infiltrate and distinguishing SCFL from its clinical mimics, such as amelanotic melanoma, basal cell carcinoma, or pseudolymphomatous infiltrates. These non-invasive methods combined are helpful, supportive diagnostics and may guide targeted biopsy and early diagnosis.

Histological Findings of Skin Infiltrations of Systemic Follicular Lymphomas

Histopathologic examination of secondary cutaneous follicular lymphoma (SCFL) reveals a nodular to diffuse), dense lymphoid infiltrate primarily in the deep and mid dermis and typically extending into the subcutaneous tissue but not involving the papillary dermis and epidermis and producing a characteristic Grenz zone (Fig. 19.2). Infiltrates contain germinal center B cells with variable numbers of small cleaved centrocytes and larger centroblasts that occur in confluent neoplastic follicles, which may coalesce or lack mantle zones. Reactive germinal centers are absent, and admixed reactive T cells may occur. Epidermotropism and reactive follicular hyper-

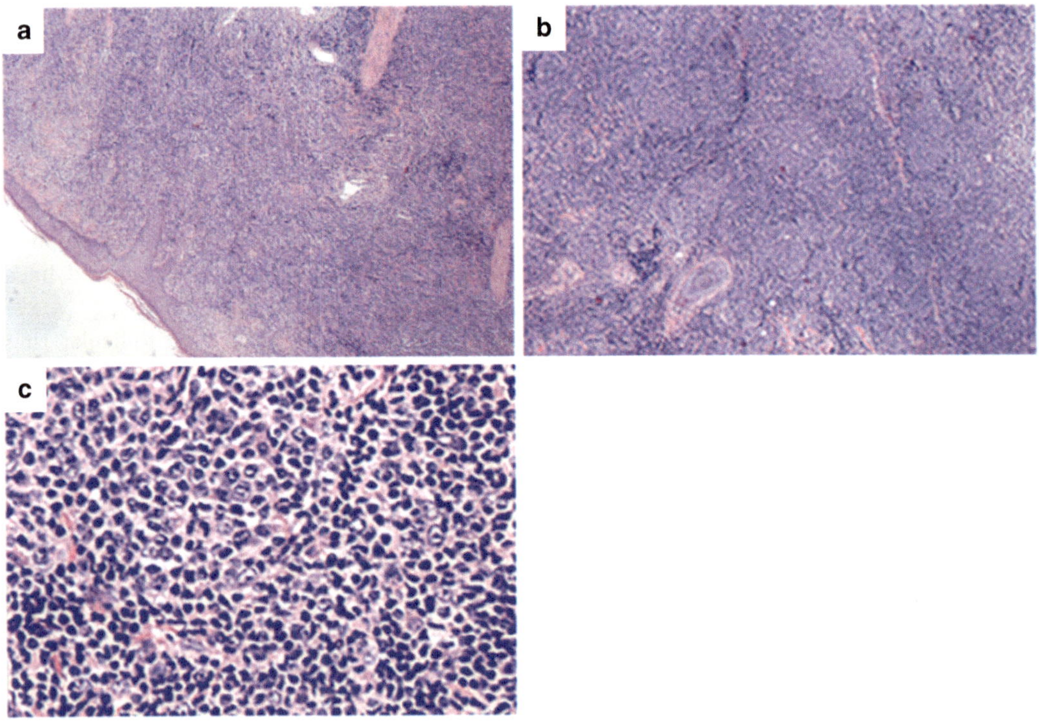

Fig. 19.2 Histopathology of scalp nodule consistent with follicular lymphoma biopsy (H&E). (**a**) Low-power view (H&E, 4×) showing diffuse and nodular infiltration of the dermis by a lymphoproliferative neoplasm. (**b**) Intermediate magnification (H&E, 10×) highlighting nodular aggregates composed of atypical lymphoid cells. (**c**) High-power view (H&E, 40×) demonstrating closely packed atypical lymphoid follicles with centrocyte-like cells and scattered centroblasts

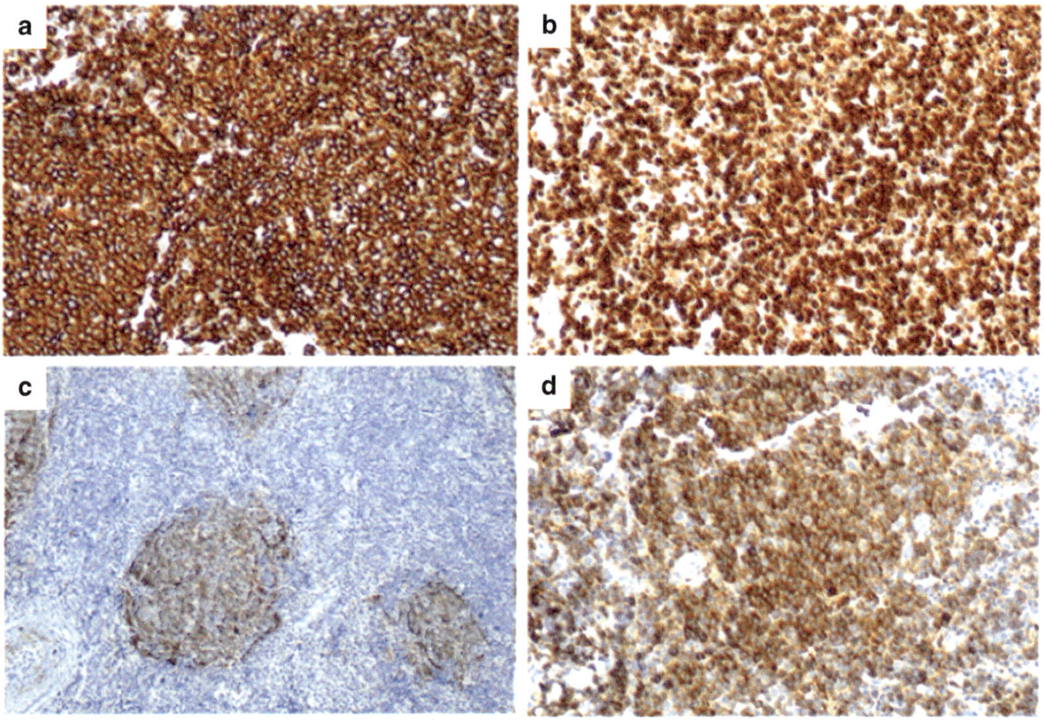

Fig. 19.3 Immunohistochemical profile of follicular lymphoma of a skin biopsy of a nodule on the scalp. (**a**) Strong positivity of neoplastic lymphoid cells for CD20 (20×). (**b**) Positivity for germinal center marker CD10 (20×). (**c**) BCL-2 positivity in neoplastic follicles (20×). (**d**) CD21 highlighting the disrupted follicular dendritic cell meshwork (20×)

plasia are not observed. Immunohistochemically, the neoplastic cells are CD20, CD79a, CD10, and BCL6 positive with a germinal center phenotype, and BCL2 is strongly positive in almost all the cases, suggesting the t(14;18)(q32;q21) IgH::BCL2 translocation. CD5 and cyclin D1 are negative, excluding mantle cell lymphoma (Fig. 19.3). Follicular dendritic networks are highlighted by CD21 or CD23, outlining neoplastic follicles. The proliferation index (Ki-67) is usually low to intermediate, mirroring the indolent behavior of systemic follicular lymphoma. Molecular analysis shows BCL2 rearrangements and shared loss-of-function mutations in chromatin-modifying genes such as CREBBP and KMT2D, confirming the systemic nature of the cutaneous) infiltrate. In contrast to primary cutaneous follicle center lymphoma (PCFCL), with its typical absence of BCL2 expression and t(14;18)) rearrangement, SCFL is an expression of disseminated follicular lymphoma and stage III–IV disease in many cases.

19.2 Skin Infiltrations of Diffuse Large B-Cell Lymphoma (DLBCL)

19.2.1 Clinical Features of Skin Infiltration Secondary to Systemic Diffuse Large B-Cell Lymphoma

Cutaneous involvement in systemic diffuse large B-cell lymphoma (DLBCL) generally) represents secondary infiltration from an extranodal primary site such as the testis, gastrointestinal tract, or lymph nodes. Clinically, these lesions display considerable heterogeneity depending on the depth and pattern of dermal or vascular invasion [18–23].

The majority of the patients present with erythematous to violaceous nodules, plaques, or indurated swellings that can be tender or symptom-free [24–28]. Lesions often appear on the lower extremities, thighs, face, or trunk, reflecting either hematogenous dissemination or local vascular tropism (Fig. 19.4). In the case of cutaneous *involvement by* testicular DLBCL, as reported by Mikami et al. [29], multiple small brown nodules were observed on the face, neck, and thigh within 1 month after orchiectomy. The presence of a coexisting erythematous plaque on the leg, initially suspected as Bowen disease, accentuated the variable morphology of the secondary lesions.

On the other hand, cutaneous intravascular large B-cell lymphoma (IVLBCL), a rare, aggressive type of non-Hodgkin's lymphoma, usually manifests *with* painful erythematous induration and telangiectatic patches, often on the lower limbs. These lesions may mimic features of erythema nodosum or thrombophlebitis, as in Koizumi et al. [24]. Histologically, they correspond to vascular occlusion by neoplastic B cells in small and medium-*sized* vessels of the dermis and subcutis, explaining the indurated texture and telangiectatic surface.

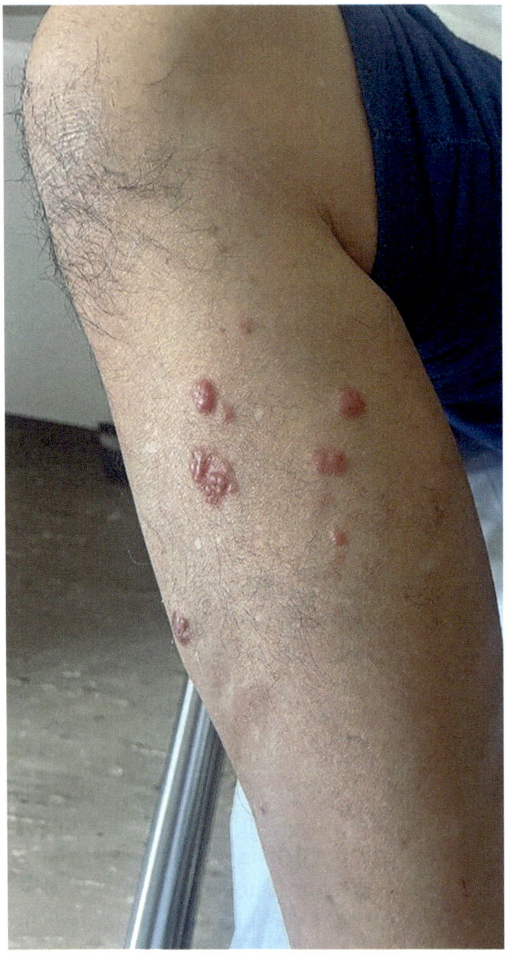

Fig. 19.4 Clinical images from a 64-year-old patient with a history of diffuse large B-cell lymphoma. He was treated with an anti-CD20 antibody and, after 1 year, developed secondary cutaneous infiltration of diffuse large B-cell lymphoma with multiple erythematous to violaceous nodules and plaques on the left knee

Primary Cutaneous Diffuse Large B-cell Lymphoma, Leg Type (PCDLBCL-LT) shares overlapping morphology with secondary lesions but usually arises de novo in the skin. Clinically, the tumor presents as rapidly enlarging, erythematous, or violaceous nodules and plaques on one or both legs. However, atypical locations, including the face or scalp, have been reported [28]. Infiltrative growth can extend to subcutaneous tissue or bone, as evidenced by scalp bone erosion in the reported case.

In all variants, the suspicion for cutaneous lymphoma should be raised by rapid onset, erythematous induration, and telangiectatic or nodular surface changes, particularly if systemic symptoms or known lymphoma history coexist. The absence of ulceration and the lack of epidermal change may provide clues that help differentiate these lesions from inflammatory dermatosis or cutaneous carcinoma in situ. Early biopsy is important not only to confirm the diagnosis but also to distinguish secondary cutaneous infiltration from a primary cutaneous lymphoma.

19.2.2 Dermoscopy of Secondary Cutaneous Diffuse Large B-Cell Lymphoma (DLBCL)

Dermoscopy has emerged as a useful non-invasive adjunct for identifying subtle vascular and structural changes in cutaneous lymphomas, aiding early detection and biopsy site selection.

In secondary skin involvement by diffuse large B-cell lymphoma (DLBCL), dermoscopy may include a pale yellowish or whitish background with scattered erythematous areas and polymorphous vascular structures (Fig. 19.5). The vascular structures often show fine and linear shapes,

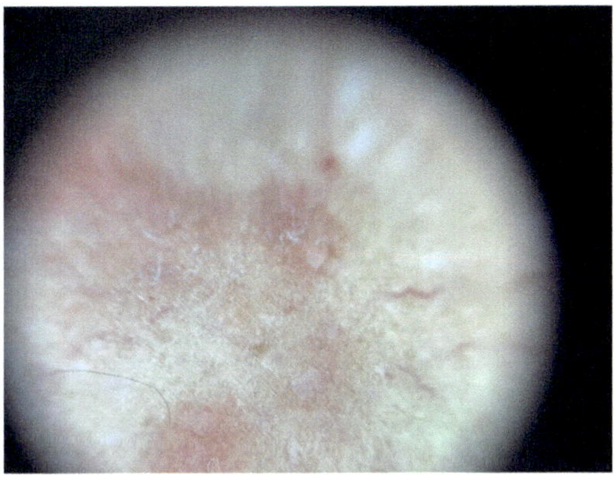

Fig. 19.5 Dermoscopic image of a cutaneous lesion in a 64-year-old male patient with secondary skin involvement by diffuse large B-cell lymphoma (DLBCL). The image demonstrates a pale yellowish-white background, scattered erythematous areas, polymorphous vessels including fine linear and curved forms, and subtle surface scaling. Red dots and irregular vascular structures are also present, consistent with dermoscopic findings in cutaneous lymphomatous infiltration

but some of them may appear curved or irregular. Surface scaling or crusting, tiny red dots, or pinpoint vessels may be seen within the lesion. Lack of typical melanocytic features, such as a pigment network, may help the differential diagnosis. These dermoscopic features put together correspond to the neoplastic proliferation and vascular changes associated with the secondary cutaneous dissemination of DLBCL [27].

Behera et al. [28] reported the following features on facial and scalp lesions of primary cutaneous diffuse large B-cell lymphoma, leg type (PCDLBCL-LT): arborizing vessels, white shiny structures, rosettes, brown peppering, and serpentine vessels. These vascular features are similar to those of other primary cutaneous B-cell lymphomas, such as PCFCL and PCMZL, but are usually more polymorphous and prominent in DLBCL. Koizumi et al. [24] demonstrated cutaneous intravascular large B-cell lymphoma-associated telangiectasias on erythematous indurated plaques, better noticeable by dermoscopy. These telangiectasias correspond to reactive and compensatory vascular dilation due to the luminal obstruction by lymphoma cells. The presence of such linear, irregular, or arborizing telangiectasias over a pale erythematous background may thus be an early diagnostic clue to IVLBCL and, consequently, prompt histologic confirmation, even without signs of systemic disease.

19.2.3 Histopathological and Immunophenotypic Correlation of Secondary Cutaneous Diffuse Large B-Cell Lymphoma (DLBCL)

Histopathologically, it is characterized by a dense, nonepidermotropic infiltrate of large atypical lymphoid cells within the dermis and subcutis with sparing of the epidermis, separated by a narrow Grenz zone in most cases (Fig. 19.6a and b). Large neoplastic cells are of centroblastic or immunoblastic appearance with vesicular nuclei, containing prominent nucleoli and scant cytoplasm; the cells may be arranged in sheets or in perivascular aggregates. Mitotic figures are frequent, reflecting high proliferative activity.

In cutaneous metastases from systemic DLBCL, including the testicular origin described by Mikami et al. [29], infiltration of the dermis and subcutaneous fat by CD20+ B cells is typical, with less frequent perivascular extension. Adnexal destruction or epidermotropism is lacking in most lesions, distinguishing these from inflammatory dermatoses. These neoplastic lymphomatous foci show strong Bcl-2 and Bcl-6 positivity, confirming their germinal center or activated B-cell phenotype. The proliferation index (Ki-67/MIB1) is usually high (>70%), reflecting the aggressive biologic behavior of systemic DLBCL (Fig. 19.6c). Both CD20 and CD19 are pan-B-cell markers, commonly expressed on the surface of neoplastic B cells in systemic cutaneous DLBCL. Their detection by either immunohistochemistry or flow cytometry confirms the B-cell nature of the tumor (Fig. 19.6d and e). Systemic DLBCL lymphoma cells typically coexpress CD20 and CD19, along with other markers such as CD22, CD79a, CD45, and sometimes CD10. Among these, CD20 expression is particularly significant when considering therapy, since this antigen may be targeted therapeutically with anti-CD20 monoclonal antibod-

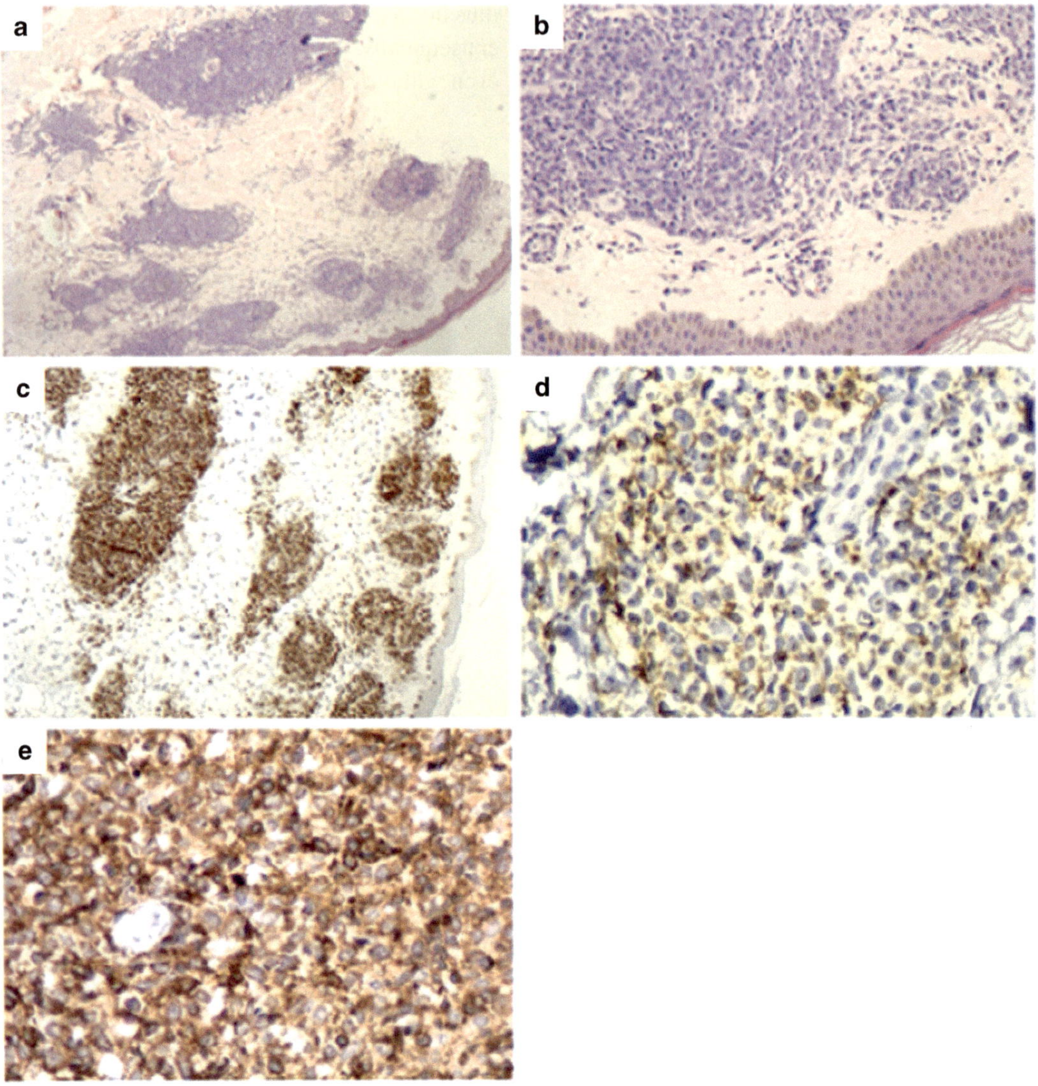

Fig. 19.6 Histopathological features of a cutaneous biopsy from a 64-year-old patient with secondary cutaneous involvement by diffuse large B-cell lymphoma. (**a**) Hematoxylin and eosin stain showing dermal infiltration in a nodular/solid pattern. (**b**) Hematoxylin and eosin stain highlighting large atypical lymphoid cells with centroblastic and immunoblastic morphology. (**c**) Ki-67 (MIB-1 antibody) immunostaining demonstrating a proliferation index approaching 100%. (**d**) CD20 immunostaining showing patchy positivity, consistent with prior anti-CD20 therapy. (**e**) CD19 immunostaining demonstrating diffuse positivity

ies such as rituximab. However, reduced or absent expression of CD20 can occur and is associated with a more aggressive disease course and worse prognosis.

According to Koizumi et al. [24] and Miyabe et al. [25], the IVLBCL variant characteristically manifests as an angiocentric and intraluminal growth pattern, with its atypical B cells confined within small- and medium-sized blood vessels of the dermis and subcutaneous tissue. This histologic feature accounts for the indurated erythema and telangiectasia seen clinically. The neoplastic cells in IVLBCL express CD20, CD79a, and MUM1 but are negative for CD3, CD5, and CD10, consistent with a non-germinal center (activated B-cell) phenotype [26]. Such endothelial proliferation and vascular dilatation, noted histologically, account for the telangiectasias visible dermoscopically [27, 28].

In PCDLBCL-LT, the histology consists of a monotonous diffuse infiltrate of large atypical lymphoid cells extending from the dermis to the subcutis, as elaborated by Behera et al. [28]. Immunohistochemistry typically demonstrates the expression of CD20+, Bcl-2+, and Bcl-6+, while MUM1 is variably positive and CD10 is negative, confirming its post-germinal center phenotype. The high MIB-1 proliferation index (>75%) further underlines the aggressive potential of the tumor. Bcl-2 expression in PCDLBCL-LT correlates with a worse prognosis than Bcl-2-negative PCDLBCL-NOS or PCFCL.

In general, these histopathological profiles reflect the biological continuum between primary and secondary cutaneous DLBCLs. The pattern of infiltration (diffuse vs. intravascular), immunophenotypic signature (Bcl-2/Bcl-6 expression), and site-specific features (subcutis or vascular confinement) are of value in subclassification and prognostication. Importantly, correlation with clinical history and dermoscopic findings—such as erythematous induration with telangiectasias or salmon-colored plaques with arborizing vessels—can guide targeted biopsy from representative sites for early and accurate diagnosis.

19.3 Skin Infiltration in Extranodal Marginal Zone MALT (Mucosa-Associated Lymphoid Tissue) Lymphoma

19.3.1 Incidence and Prevalence

Skin infiltration secondary to systemic extranodal MALT lymphoma is rare. Extranodal marginal zone lymphomas account for approximately 5–15% of all B-cell non-Hodgkin lymphomas, and the skin is a very uncommon secondary site compared with primary cutaneous MZL [29–36]. The majority of secondary cutaneous cases occur in the setting of disseminated disease, which at the time of diagnosis or at the time of relapse is found in 25–50% of patients with extranodal MZL. The exact prevalence of secondary skin involvement remains unclear because it is quite rare and can be difficult to distinguish from primary cutaneous presentations.

19.3.2 Clinical Findings

Secondary cutaneous involvement by systemic MALT lymphoma usually occurs in older adults with lesions favoring the head and neck region, in contrast to primary cutaneous MZL, which favors the trunk and extremities. The lesions can appear as reddish or violaceous papules, plaques, or nodules and may be solitary or multiple (Fig. 19.7). The clinical course is usually indolent, but relapses often involve multiple extranodal sites [37]. Systemic symptoms are uncommon except in cases of transformation to a more aggressive lymphoma.

19.3.3 Dermoscopic Findings

Dermoscopic features of secondary cutaneous MALT lymphoma are not well characterized in the literature. Available reports suggest that lesions may show nonspecific vascular patterns and structureless areas, but no pathognomonic dermoscopic findings have been established [27]. Dermoscopy of a cutaneous infiltration in a case of an elderly female patient with systemic non-Hodgkin B-cell marginal zone lymphoma shows a feature-poor, structureless pattern characterized by diffuse, faint purple-brown coloration and subtle erythema (Fig. 19.7b). No well-defined vascular structures, pigment networks, or surface scales are seen within the observed area. The lesion appears homogeneous and lacks the characteristic dermoscopic features of most of the primary cutaneous neoplasms or inflammatory dermatoses. Such absence of specific morphological features, especially the absence of dotted, linear, or serpentine vessels, reflects the underlying diffuse neoplastic infiltration of the dermis by lymphoma cells, a finding frequently reported in cases of secondary cutaneous involvement by hematologic malignan-

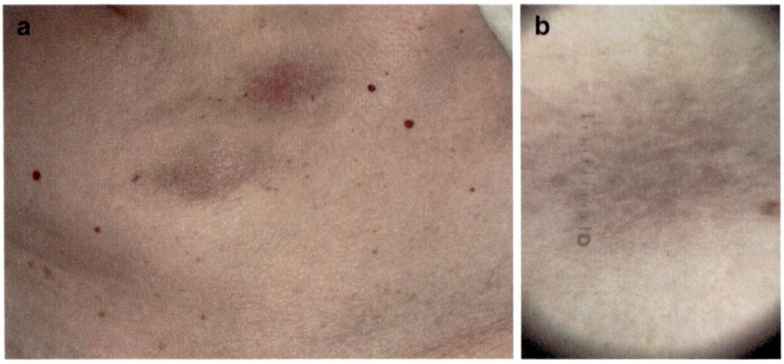

Fig. 19.7 (**a**) Clinical image of an 83-year-old female patient with cutaneous infiltration by systemic non-Hodgkin B-cell lymphoma of marginal zone origin. A few ill-defined, violaceous, non-ulcerated plaques are evident on the trunk. The lesions are slightly palpable, with a livedoid, bruise-like appearance and without surface scale or crust. (**b**) Dermoscopy of cutaneous infiltration by systemic non-Hodgkin B-cell lymphoma of marginal zone origin reveals a structureless pattern characterized by faint, diffusely distributed purplish-to-brown hues with subtle underlying erythema. Notably, specific vascular structures and scales are absent, or there is a pigment network. The image highlights the homogeneity of color and the lack of well-defined morphological clues.

cies. Dermoscopy may assist in identifying suspicious lesions for biopsy but cannot reliably distinguish secondary from primary cutaneous MZL or other cutaneous lymphomas [28].

19.3.4 Histopathology

Skin biopsies show a dense, non-epidermotropic lymphoid infiltrate, often with nodular or diffuse patterns. The infiltrate consists of small B cells with marginal zone and monocytoid features, admixed with plasma cells and reactive germinal centers. Immunophenotyping demonstrates the presence of CD20+, CD79a+, CD5–, and CD10– B cells with monotypic light chain expression. Molecular studies may show clonal IgH rearrangements and, less frequently, translocations like t(14;18)(q32;q21).

19.3.5 Prognosis

The prognosis in general is favorable for patients with secondary skin involvement by systemic MALT lymphoma, with a tendency toward long-term survival despite frequent recurrences. However, those with extracutaneous spread at presentation or transformation to large cell lymphoma have a worse prognosis. Treatment is tailored to disease extent and may include local therapies, rituximab-based regimens, or targeted therapy against underlying infectious or autoimmune drivers.

19.4 Skin Involvement in Mantle Cell Lymphoma MCL

19.4.1 Incidence

Cutaneous involvement by systemic mantle cell lymphoma is rare, occurring in about 1–1.4% of all cases of MCL. Initial diagnosis of systemic MCL in the skin is even more infrequent, accounting for 0.4% of all systemic B-cell lymphomas presenting in the skin. Most cases represent secondary dissemination rather than primary cutaneous disease [38–41].

19.4.2 Clinical Findings

Patients are usually older individuals (median age 66–70 years) with a male predominance. Skin lesions most often appear as nodules, tumors, or plaques, frequently on the extremities, trunk, or head and neck. Lesions may be solitary or multiple; multiple lesions are more common when skin involvement is the initial manifestation, while solitary lesions predominate in relapse/progression. The majority of patients have advanced (stage III/IV) disease at the time of skin involvement. Blastoid and pleomorphic variants are overrepresented in cutaneous cases and are associated with a higher proliferation index and worse prognosis. Rarely, skin involvement may mimic other entities, such as subcutaneous panniculitis-like T-cell lymphoma or primary cutaneous diffuse large B-cell lymphoma, leg type.

19.4.3 Dermoscopic Findings

Dermoscopic features of secondary cutaneous MCL are not well characterized in the literature. The available reports indicate that the lesions may exhibit nonspecific vascular patterns and structureless areas with no pathognomonic dermoscopic findings established. Dermoscopy may help identify suspicious lesions for biopsy but cannot reliably distinguish MCL from other cutaneous lymphomas.

19.4.4 Histopathology

Skin biopsies usually reveal a dense dermal and/or subcutaneous infiltrate, often sparing the epidermis, with a Grenz zone. The infiltrate consists of small to medium-sized lymphocytes with irregular nuclear contours; blastoid and pleomorphic cytology is common in cutaneous cases. Immunophenotyping shows CD20+, CD5+, and cyclin D1+ cells, and t(11;14) translocation is characteristic. SOX11 is positive in most cases. Rare cases may show surface IgM expression or coexist with other malignancies.

19.4.5 Prognosis

Poor prognosis is related to cutaneous involvement by MCL, especially in cases with a blastoid or pleomorphic morphology. The median survival was considerably shorter in the aggressive variants (median: 59 months) compared to classic MCL (median: 155.8 months). Most patients die from the disease within several months after cutaneous involvement, though rare indolent cases have also been reported.

19.5 Cutaneous Involvement Secondary to Hodgkin Lymphoma

The incidence of skin infiltration secondary to systemic Hodgkin lymphoma is 0.5–3.4% of all Hodgkin lymphoma cases. This manifestation is almost always secondary to nodal or visceral disease and is usually seen in advanced stages, most often stage IV [41–46].

Clinical findings include solitary or multiple nodules, tumors, infiltrative plaques, papules, or ulcerated lesions. Lesions are often erythematous, violaceous, or flesh-colored and may be indurated, necrotic, or present as draining sinuses or cellulitis-like eruptions. Distribution is often near involved lymph nodes, reflecting retrograde lymphatic spread, direct extension, or hematogenous dissemination. Skin involvement may rarely precede systemic diagnosis but usually develops months to years after initial diagnosis.

Dermoscopic findings are neither specific nor well described in the literature. Reported cases have described nonspecific features, including structureless areas, polymorphous vascular patterns, and focal ulceration, which do not distinguish Hodgkin lymphoma from other cutaneous lymphoma or metastatic processes.

Histopathological findings will reveal a relatively paucicellular neoplastic population of large atypical cells (Hodgkin and Reed-Sternberg forms) in a mixed inflammatory background, often with prominent necrosis. Immunohistochemically, it typically shows positivity for CD30 and CD15, variable expression of PAX5, and negativity for CD20 and CD3.

The prognosis is generally poor, since cutaneous involvement usually signifies disseminated, refractory, or relapsed disease. Rare cases with a good response to standard therapy have been described, however. Prognosis depends on overall disease burden and response to systemic treatment.

19.6 Skin Involvement in T-/NK-Cell Lineage

19.6.1 Skin Involvement Secondary to Mature T-Cell/Natural Killer-Cell (T/NK-Cell) Lymphoma

19.6.1.1 Incidence

Skin infiltration secondary to systemic mature T-cell or NK-cell lymphoma is relatively uncommon, with most published series and institutional reports documenting few cases over extended periods. The cases associated with aggressive subtypes most often include extranodal NK/T--cell lymphoma, nasal type, subcutaneous panniculitis-like T-cell lymphoma, and other cytotoxic T-cell lymphomas. Secondary cutaneous involvement is less common than primary cutaneous T-cell lymphomas and has a poor prognosis [47–50].

19.6.1.2 Clinical Findings

The usual presentation of secondary skin involvement is rapidly progressive, multiple erythematous to violaceous nodules, plaques, or tumors, often with ulceration, necrosis, and pain. The lesions may be disseminated or localized. The trunk and extremities are most commonly affected. Systemic symptoms like fever, weight loss, and night sweats are frequent, reflecting the aggressive nature and multiorgan involvement of these lymphomas. Fulminant progression and resistance to chemotherapy are common; overall survival is often measured in months [50].

19.6.1.3 Dermoscopic Features

Dermoscopic data for secondary cutaneous T/NK-cell lymphomas are limited; however, available studies and inferences made from primary cutaneous forms suggest nonspecific findings. These features include orange or salmon-colored structureless areas, polymorphous vascular patterns (dotted, linear, or serpentine vessels), and focal white structureless zones [27, 28]. These features are not pathognomonic, and there is an overlap with other cutaneous lymphomas and inflammatory dermatoses.

19.6.1.4 Histology

Histopathological characteristics include a dense, atypical lymphoid infiltrate in the dermis and/or subcutis, often with angiocentricity, necrosis, and cytotoxic features such as large pleomorphic cells, frequent mitoses, and apoptotic bodies. Angioinvasion and coagulative necrosis may be features of subtypes such as extranodal NK/T-cell lymphoma, nasal type. Immunophenotyping is essential, with most expressing the pan-T-cell markers (CD3, CD2, CD5) but with variable losses of CD5 and/or CD7. Cytotoxic markers that are positive include TIA-1, granzyme B, and perforin. NK-cell lymphomas are positive for CD56 and cytotoxic markers but are usually negative for surface CD3, while cytoplasmic CD3ε may be present. EBV-encoded RNA (EBER) is often positive in extranodal NK/T-cell lymphoma. Clonality and distinction of T cells from NK-cell origin can be confirmed by TCR gene rearrangement studies.

Accurate diagnosis requires the integration of clinical, histopathological, immunophenotypic, and molecular findings, as recommended in recent consensus and review articles.

19.6.1.5 Skin Infiltration Secondary to Peripheral T-Cell Lymphoma

Skin infiltration associated with PTCL, except for primary cutaneous T-cell lymphoma, is rare and clinically significant. Secondary cutaneous involvement is associated with several PTCL subtypes, but skin lesions in the context of advanced systemic disease most often occur in AITL and PTCL, unspecified. Cutaneous involvement typically occurs simultaneously with or after nodal/systemic disease and rarely precedes it [51–61].

Clinical findings are heterogeneous. Lesions may appear as erythematous to violaceous papules, nodules, plaques, or patches and may mimic benign dermatoses such as drug eruptions, folliculitis, or eczematous dermatitis. Morphologies include generalized morbilliform maculopatches, folliculitis-like papules, and eczematous papules/patches. AITL may present with evanescent rashes or persistent lesions, and granulomatous, panniculitic, vasculitic, and epidermotropic patterns have all been described. Lesions may be solitary or generalized; B symptoms are typically absent at cutaneous presentation [62–65]. The presence of skin lesions in PTCL is associated with a poor prognosis, especially when concurrent with extracutaneous disease.

The dermoscopic features of secondary cutaneous PTCL are nonspecific. Some of the possible findings that might be encountered include orange structureless areas, poorly focused linear vessels with branching, and white structureless areas, but these overlap with other conditions that are either infiltrative or inflammatory and, therefore, cannot be diagnostic. Dermoscopy might raise suspicion, but it cannot definitively distinguish between secondary PTCL and other cutaneous lymphomas or their look-alikes.

Histopathology typically demonstrates a dense dermal or subcutaneous infiltrate of atypical lymphoid cells with perivascular or periadnexal accentuation, having variable cell size and pleomorphism. In some cases, granulomatous inflammation, panniculitis-like changes, and sarcoid-like granulomas may be seen. Epidermotropism is generally absent, distinguishing this manifestation of secondary PTCL from mycosis fungoides.

Immunophenotype expression of pan-T-cell markers (CD2, CD3, and CD5) with variable CD4 and CD8 expression depending on subtype. The T-follicular helper phenotype (PD-1, CD10, BCL6, CXCL13, ICOS) is expressed in AITL and some PTCL. Loss of one or more pan-T-cell markers (CD2, CD5, or CD7) may be present; cytotoxic markers (TIA-1 and granzyme B) are variably expressed. Clonal T-cell receptor gene rearrangement is often demonstrable.

Overall prognosis is generally poor, with 5-year overall survival rates as low as 12% if skin involvement occurs with extracutaneous disease. More favorable outcome in localized skin-limited disease with a CD3+CD4+CD8 phenotype.

Accurate diagnosis and management of secondary cutaneous PTCL requires the integration of clinical, histopathologic, immunophenotypic, and molecular data.

19.7 Skin Infiltration Secondary to Systemic Anaplastic Large Cell Lymphoma (ALCL)

The incidence of skin infiltration secondary to systemic anaplastic large cell lymphoma, excluding primary cutaneous ALCL, is about 20–35% of systemic ALCL cases, higher in pediatric populations and in ALK-positive subtypes. Systemic ALCL often presents with advanced-stage disease and extranodal involvement, with cutaneous lesions being a well-recognized manifestation [58, 59].

Clinical findings consist of rapidly growing erythematous to violaceous nodules, plaques, or tumors that are often multiple and sometimes ulcerated or necrotic (Fig. 19.8a). B symptoms, such as fever, weight loss, and night sweats, are common, with generalized lymphadenopathy. The skin involvement may be associated with visceral and bone marrow disease.

Dermoscopic findings are nonspecific but may include orange structureless areas, vague linear vessels with branches, and focal white structureless zones, as described in nodular/plaque-type T-cell lymphomas (Fig. 19.8b). These findings are not pathognomonic and thus overlap with other cutaneous lymphomas and inflammatory dermatoses.

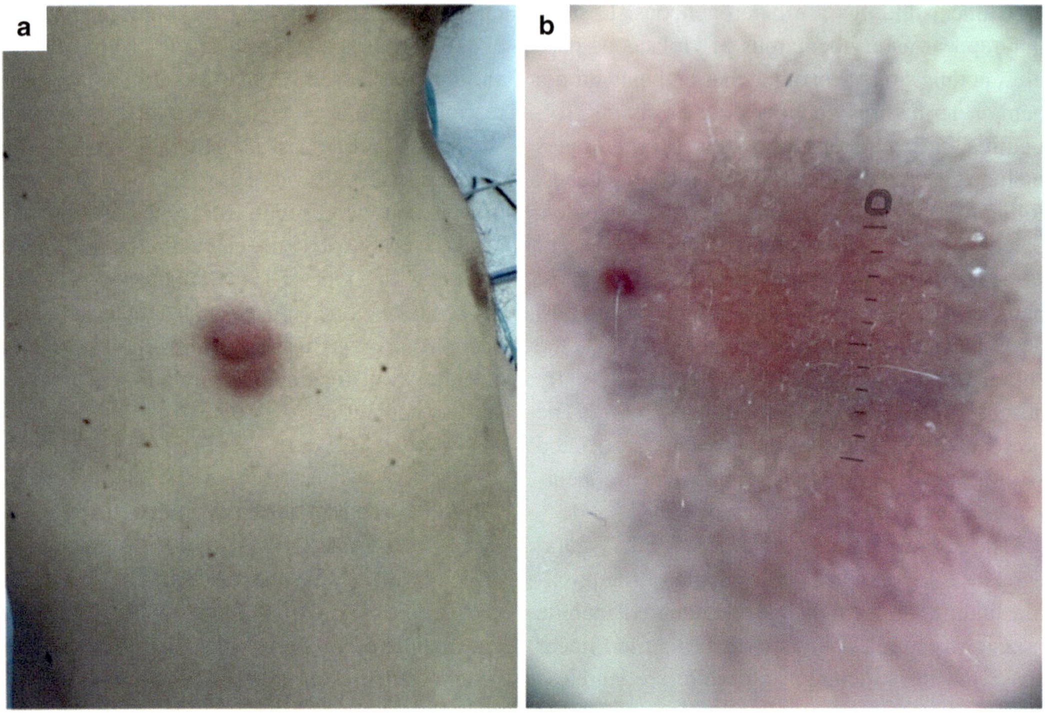

Fig. 19.8 Clinical and dermoscopic features of cutaneous infiltration by anaplastic large cell lymphoma (ALCL), ALK-negative subtype, in a 54-year-old male patient. (**a**) Clinical image showing a solitary, well-demarcated, erythematous to violaceous nodule on the trunk with central ulceration and surrounding erythema, reflecting dermal and subcutaneous infiltration. (**b**) Dermoscopic examination reveals a polymorphous vascular pattern characterized by irregular linear and dotted vessels over a pinkish-reddish background. This vascular pattern corresponds to the underlying dense lymphoproliferative infiltration

Histopathological features include a diffuse dermal and subcutaneous infiltrate of large, pleomorphic, anaplastic cells with abundant cytoplasm and horseshoe-shaped nuclei (Fig. 19.9a–c). Tumor cells are strongly CD30+, variably express EMA and ALK (depending on subtype), and may show angiocentricity and necrosis. Immunophenotyping is crucial in differentiating systemic ALCL from primary cutaneous ALCL and other CD30+ lymphoproliferative disorders (Fig. 19.10a–c).

The prognosis is overall less favorable than for primary cutaneous ALCL. The ALK-positive systemic ALCL, particularly in children, has a relatively good prognosis, with a high long-term survival rate when treated with anthracycline-based chemotherapy. Poorer outcomes are seen in ALK-negative cases and those with widespread extranodal disease. Skin involvement itself does not independently worsen the prognosis but reflects the advanced disease stage.

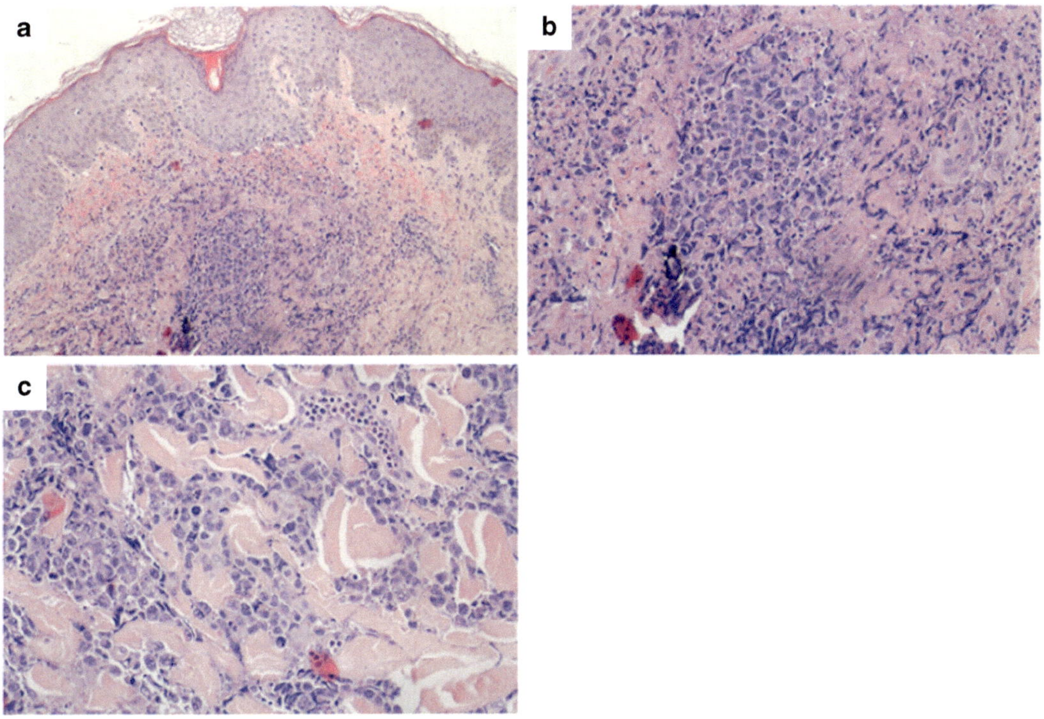

Fig. 19.9 Histology of a biopsy of the cutaneous infiltration of the patient with cutaneous ALCL, ALK-negative. (**a**) The subcutis and dermis are diffusely infiltrated by a lymphoproliferative disorder with clusters and sheets of abnormally enlarged neoplastic cells. The cells are variably multinucleated or mononucleated and exhibit extreme cytologic atypia with irregular nuclear borders and prominent nucleoli. The diffuse pattern highlights the aggressive infiltration typical of ALCL, ALK-negative subtype. (**b** & **c**) High-power views depict large neoplastic lymphoid cells that are multinucleated or mononucleated with overt cytological atypia and generous amphophilic cytoplasm. The majority of cells exhibit anaplastic features like pleomorphism, nuclear enlargement, and prominent nucleoli, supported by the presence of mitotic figures and apoptotic bodies

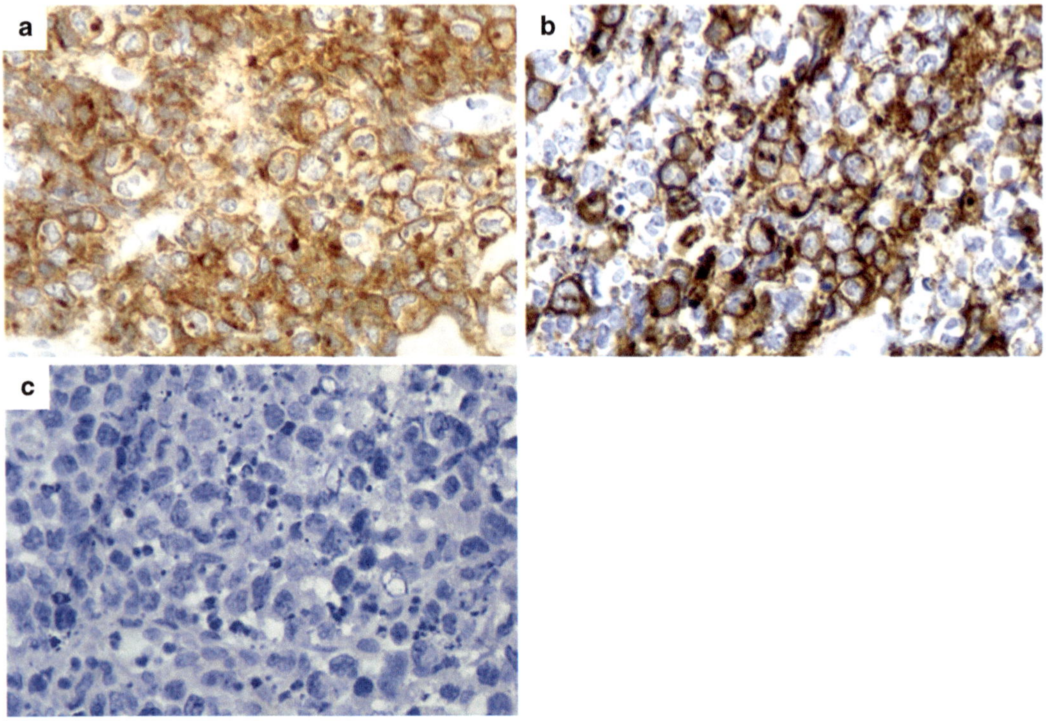

Fig. 19.10 Immunohistochemistry of a biopsy of the cutaneous infiltration of the patient with cutaneous ALCL, ALK-negative (**a**) CD30+: The tumor cells are diffusely and strongly membranous and paranuclear (Golgi) positive for CD30, the characteristic marker for ALCL. Staining is detectable in >75% of the neoplastic cells and aids in the distinction of ALCL from other lymphoproliferative malignancies. (**b**) CD2+: Immunostaining with CD2 is positive in tumor cells, confirming their T-cell origin despite the lack of pan-T-cell markers (e.g., CD3). (**c**) ALK: Negative immunohistochemistry for ALK confirms the diagnosis of ALK-negative ALCL and excludes the ALK-positive subtypes

19.8 Angioimmunoblastic Lymphoma (AITL) Skin Infiltration Overview

19.8.1 Incidence and Prevalence

Cutaneous involvement occurs in 21–50% of patients with systemic angioimmunoblastic T-cell lymphoma (AITL). Skin lesions are almost invariably secondary to nodal or systemic disease and rarely predate lymph node involvement. The prevalence of cutaneous findings at diagnosis varies by cohort, but generalized lymphadenopathy and advanced-stage disease are nearly uniform in affected patients [56].

19.8.2 Clinical Findings

Cutaneous infiltration by AITL is clinically heterogeneous. The most common features are evanescent morbilliform or urticarial rashes, persistent violaceous papules, nodules, plaques, and ulcers on the oral mucosa (Fig. 19.11a–c). In such cases, lesions can be both localized and generalized, frequently involving the trunk and extremities. Indeed, early eruptions may closely resemble drug or viral exanthems or connective tissue disorders, whereas later nodular phases are more suggestive of lymphomatous disease. Constitutional symptoms, including fever and weight loss, lymphadenopathy, and laboratory features of

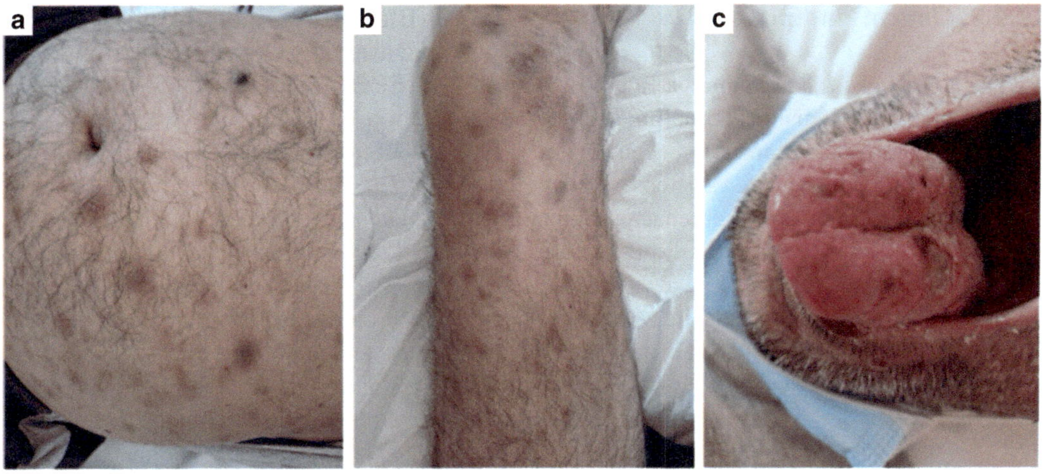

Fig. 19.11 Angioimmunoblastic T-cell lymphoma (AITL). Clinical images of a male patient with skin infiltrations of systemic angioimmunoblastic lymphoma (AITL) who developed multiple purple plaques mainly on the abdomen (**a**) and legs (**b**) and mouth ulcers (**c**)

hypergammaglobulinemia and anemia, are commonly found in the systemic context [57].

19.8.3 Dermoscopic Findings

Dermoscopic data in secondary cutaneous AITL are scant. Dermoscopy may help identify atypical vascularity or infiltrative patterns, but it has very limited value for distinguishing AITL from other entities.

19.8.4 Histopathology

Skin biopsies show various infiltrate patterns: perivascular, nodular, granulomatous, panniculitic, vasculitic, and rarely epidermotropic. 1–5, 9, 10 The infiltrate consists of small to medium-sized lymphocytes, usually with plasma cells, eosinophils, and conspicuous high endothelial venules. Follicular helper T-cell markers, such as PD-1, BCL6, and CD10, are commonly expressed. 3 EBV-positive B cells can be detected and are related to aggressive disease courses. 1, 4 Molecular *analysis often reveals* concordant skin and nodal lesions, including mutations involving RHOA and TET2 in a subset.

19.8.5 Prognosis

Cutaneous involvement in AITL represents advanced disease and portends a poor prognosis. The overall five-year survival rates of the patients with systemic AITL are 33–44%, in whom EBV positivity in the skin lesion is an independent negative prognostic factor. Early diagnosis and incorporation of clinical and histopathologic features and molecular data are crucial in diagnosing and managing.

19.9 Secondary Cutaneous Involvement by Lymphoblastic Lymphoma

19.9.1 Incidence and Prevalence

Secondary cutaneous involvement by lymphoblastic lymphoma is rare. T-lymphoblastic lymphoma shows cutaneous involvement in a minority of cases, with published literature indicating *that* less than 20% of systemic cases present with skin lesions; B-lymphoblastic lymphoma may reach up to 33% in some series but overall remains uncommon [59].

19.9.2 Clinical Findings

The skin lesions of lymphoblastic lymphoma often appear as erythematous to violaceous papules, nodules, or plaques and can be solitary or multifocal. Skin lesions can develop prior to, concurrently with, or even subsequent to the diagnosis of systemic disease. Distribution also varies by subtype in that B-LBL tends to involve the head and neck, whereas T-LBL tends to involve the trunk and extremities. Systemic symptoms include lymphadenopathy and constitutional complaints .

19.9.3 Dermoscopic Findings

Dermoscopic features are not specific for secondary cutaneous lymphoblastic lymphoma. One available report of two patients describes linear irregular or arborizing vessels, but these findings are not diagnostic. Most dermoscopic studies focus on primary cutaneous lymphomas, and extrapolation to secondary cases should be cautious [62–65].

19.9.4 Histopathology

Biopsies disclose a dense, diffuse dermal infiltrate of medium to large immature lymphoid cells (blasts), often sparing the epidermis. Immunophenotyping is essential and can be confirmed by markers for TdT, *CD34 (variable), CD10 (selectively),* CD3 (T-cell), or CD79a/CD19 (B-cell) lineage.

19.9.5 Prognosis

Cutaneous involvement generally indicates an aggressive, disseminated disease and is associated with a higher risk of relapse and reduced survival.

19.10 Blastic Plasmacytoid Dendritic Cell Neoplasm (BPDCN) Skin Infiltration

19.10.1 Incidence and Prevalence

Skin involvement is one of the defining features of BPDCN, with cutaneous infiltration present in about 80–85% of patients at some stage during the disease course. Most cases occur in older adults, median age 60–70 years, with a marked male predominance, male:female ratio up to 7:1 in some series. Though overall a rare disease, the strong skin tropism means dermatologic presentation is often the first clinical sign [66].

19.10.2 Clinical Findings

BPDCN commonly presents as asymptomatic, violaceous, or reddish-brown papules, plaques, or nodules, which may be solitary, localized, or generalized. The lesions may have a bruise-like appearance and may mimic lichen planus, lupus erythematosus, or other dermatoses (Fig. 19.12a and b). Flat solitary lesions are present in up to 30% of cases, and B symptoms are generally absent. Three patterns of presentation have been described: nodular, bruise-like, and disseminated, with frequent evolution into systemic disease [67–71].

19.10.3 Dermoscopic Findings

Dermoscopic features of BPDCN are nonspecific. Various findings have been reported, including homogeneous violaceous coloration, structureless areas, and linear vessels out of focus; however, these features overlap with other conditions characterized by cutaneous infiltration or vascular proliferation and do not provide a pathognomonic pattern (Fig. 19.12c–f). Dermoscopy can raise suspicion for the disease but cannot reliably distinguish BPDCN)from other cutaneous hematologic neoplasms [72, 73].

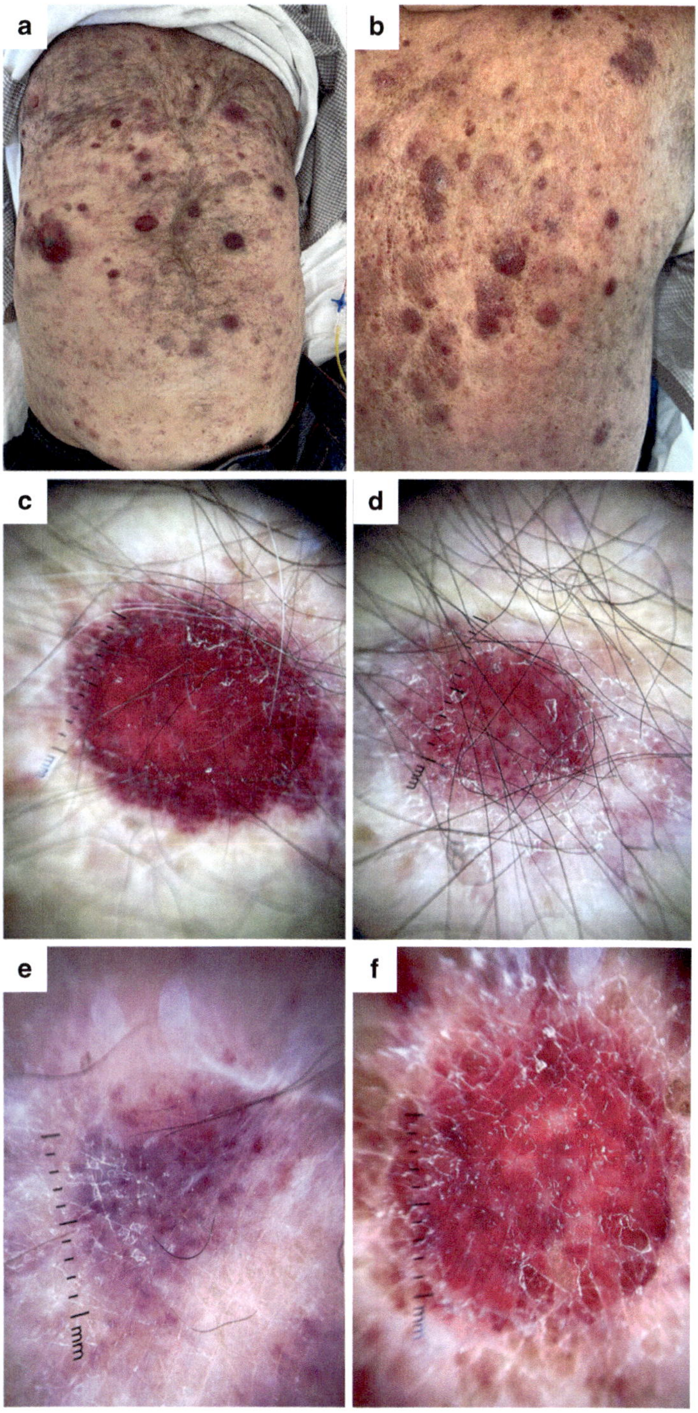

Fig. 19.12 Clinical and dermoscopic features in a 78-year-old patient with Blastic Plasmacytoid Dendritic Cell Neoplasm (BPDCN). (**a**, **b**) Multiple violaceous to purpuric infiltrated plaques and nodules involving the trunk in a 78-year-old man. (**c**–**f**) *Polarized dermoscopy* of representative lesions shows homogenous purplish-red, structureless areas with polymorphous vascular structures (including dotted and linear irregular vessels), white shiny lines, and fine superficial scaling

19.10.4 Histopathology

Skin biopsies show a nonepidermotropic, dense dermal infiltrate of monomorphic, medium-sized blastoid cells with irregular nuclei and scant cytoplasm (Figs. 19.13 and 19.14). Immunophenotyping is crucial, with neoplastic cells expressing CD4, CD56, and CD123 in the majority of cases, while markers like TCL-1, CD303, and BDCA2/CD2AP are *most specific and establish the diagnosis* (Figs. 19.15, 19.16, 19.17, 19.18, 19.19, 19.20 and 19.21). The absence of B-cell, T-cell, and myeloid lineage markers is characteristic.

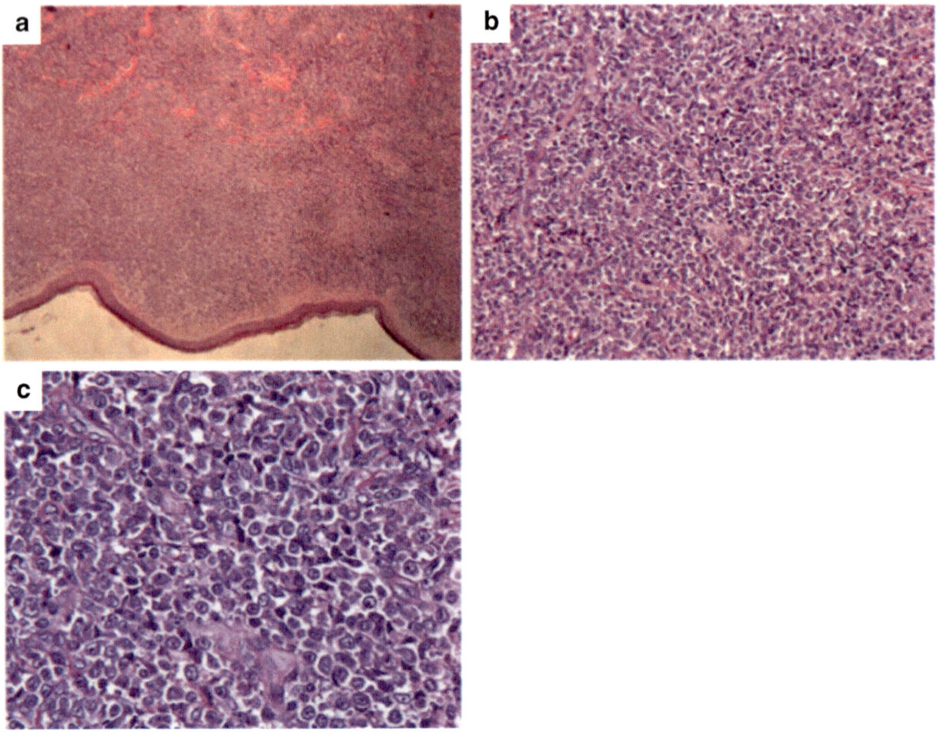

Fig. 19.13 Histopathological features of a skin biopsy in a 78-year-old patient with Blastic Plasmacytoid Dendritic Cell Neoplasm (BPDCN). (**a**–**c**) Hematoxylin and eosin (H&E) stained sections (10×, 40×, 60×) from an abdominal plaque demonstrating diffuse dermal infiltration by large mononuclear atypical cells with blastoid morphology and scant cytoplasm, sparing the epidermis

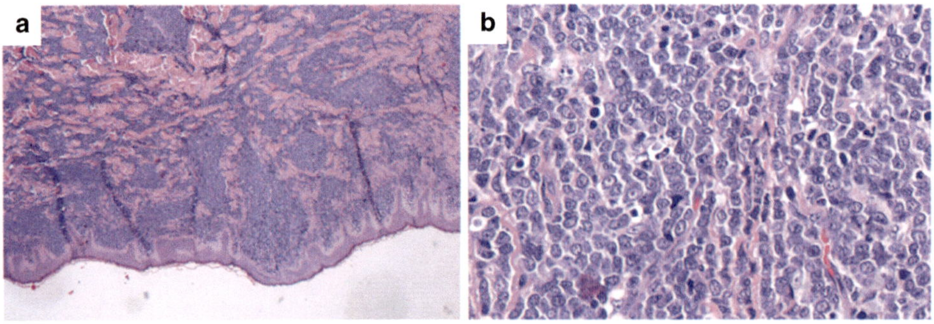

Fig. 19.14 Histopathological findings from the skin biopsy of a 64-year-old male with a history of acute myeloid leukemia, dendritic type, who developed blastic plasmacytoid dendritic cell neoplasm (BPDCN). (**a**) Diffuse dermal and subcutaneous infiltrate of blastic cells (Hematoxylin & Eosin stain). (**b**) Medium-sized blastic cells infiltrating the dermis and subcutis in a diffuse growth pattern (Hematoxylin & Eosin stain)

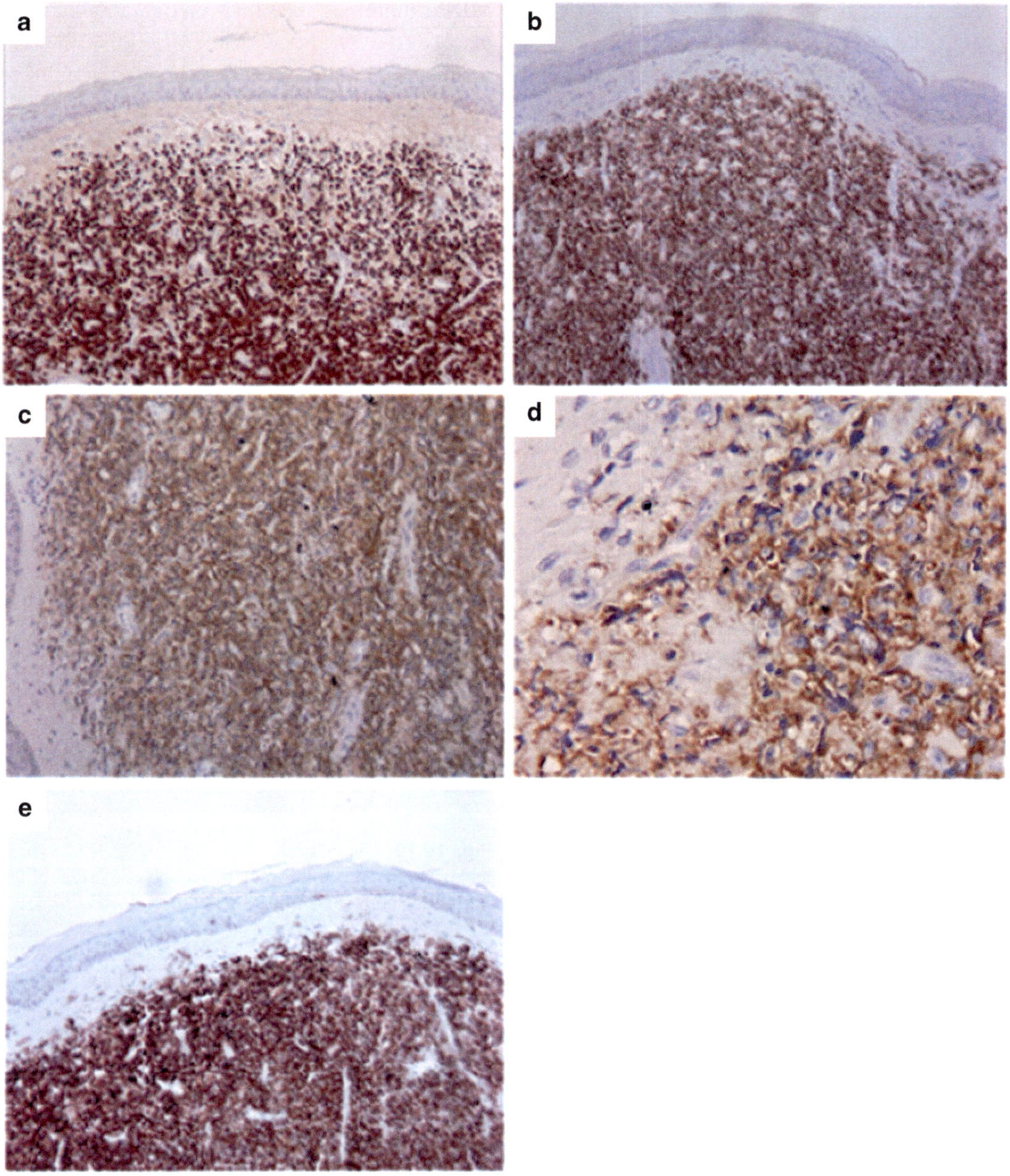

Fig. 19.15 Immunohistochemical profile of skin biopsy in a 78-year-old patient with Blastic Plasmacytoid Dendritic Cell Neoplasm (BPDCN). (**a**) Strong cytoplasmic positivity for TCL-1 (20×). (**b**) Membranous positivity for CD56 (20×). (**c**, **d**) Intense positivity for CD123 (20×, 60×). (**e**) Diffuse positivity for CD4 (20×). Findings confirm a plasmacytoid dendritic cell lineage

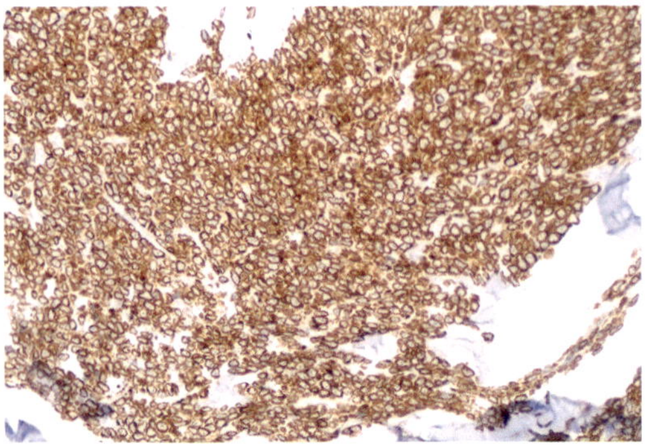

Fig. 19.16 Immunohistochemical findings from the skin biopsy of a 64-year-old male with a history of acute myeloid leukemia, dendritic type, who developed blastic plasmacytoid dendritic cell neoplasm (BPDCN). The tumor cells showed positivity for CD45, CD4, CD43, CD7, bcl2, and CD123, while they were negative for CD56, TdT, CD20, CD3, CD5, MPO, CD34, c-kit, PAX5, CyclinD1, CD68, CD8, CD2, CD30, CD11c, CD163, CD10, CD1a, Lysozyme, Perforin, Granzyme, s100, Langerin, CD21, CD138, MUM1, CD14, and CD23. The Ki-67 proliferation index assessed by the MIB1 antibody was approximately 70%. Immunohistochemistry demonstrating cytoplasmic positivity for BCL2 in neoplastic B cells, supporting the diagnosis of aggressive lymphoma (magnification ×200)

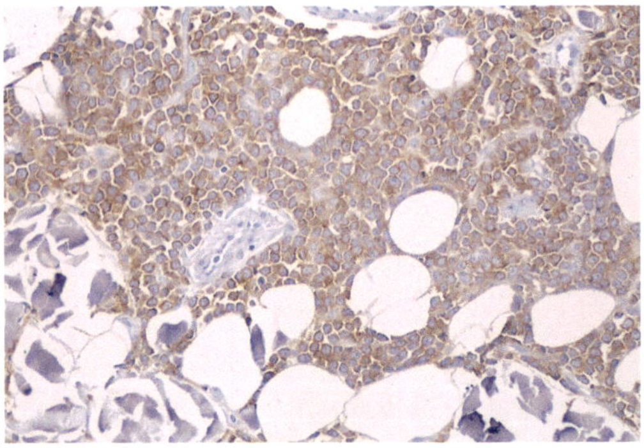

Fig. 19.17 Immunohistochemical staining positive for CD4 in lymphoma cells, indicating T-cell marker expression in this case (magnification ×200)

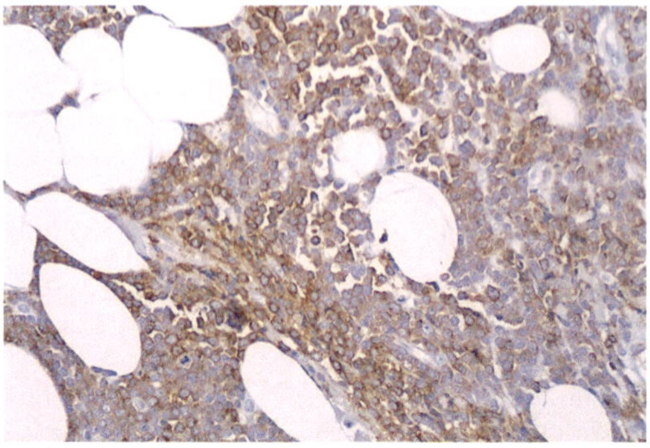

Fig. 19.18 Cytoplasmic positivity for CD7 observed in lymphoma cells, reflecting expression of this T-cell-associated antigen (magnification ×200)

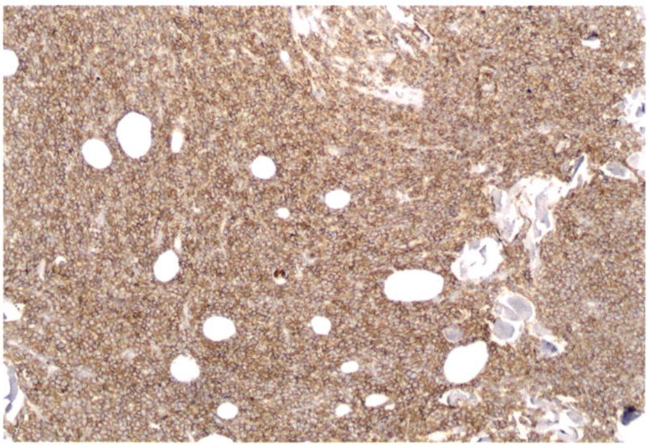

Fig. 19.19 Cytoplasmic positivity for CD45, a pan-leukocyte marker, confirming hematopoietic origin of the infiltrating cells (magnification ×200)

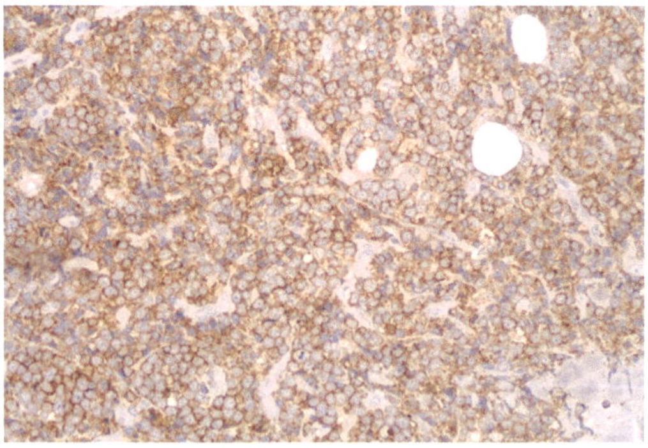

Fig. 19.20 Cytoplasmic positivity for CD43 in a patient who developed blastic plasmacytoid dendritic cell neoplasm (BPDCN) (magnification ×200)

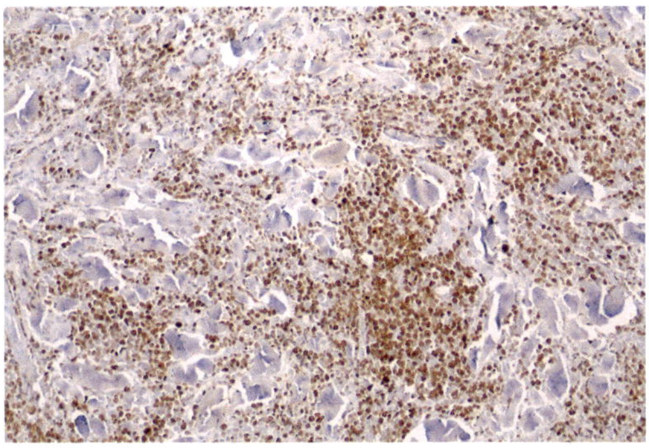

Fig. 19.21 High proliferation index (Ki-67, MIB-1) showing approximately 70% nuclear staining in BPDCN cells (magnification ×200)

Bone marrow findings in BPDCN)usually range from minimal infiltration to extensive marrow replacement by neoplastic cells. Morphologically, the hematoxylin and eosin (H&E) sections may appear unremarkable without overt signs of infiltration, especially in cases with minimal disease. However, immunohistochemical staining demonstrates characteristic interstitial and small aggregates of neoplastic blastic plasmacytoid dendritic cells that stain for markers such as TCL-1, CD56, and CD123, which is consistent with the immunophenotype noted in the cutaneous lesions. These usually appear as medium-sized cells with round to oval nuclei, fine chromatin, and scant basophilic cytoplasm. Bone marrow involvement is confirmed by strong positivity for CD4, CD56, CD123, and TCL-1 and negativity for CD34 and myeloperoxidase, thus distinguishing BPDCN from other hematologic malignancies. The proliferation index assessed by Ki-67 may be variably elevated (Fig. 19.22). Overall, the bone marrow infiltration by BPDCN may be subtle histologically but is identified by this immunophenotypic profile necessary for the correct diagnosis and to guide appropriate treatment strategies.

19.10.5 Outcome

BPDCN is an aggressive neoplasm, with a median overall survival ranging from 14 to 24 months. In its typical clinical course, cutaneous lesions are followed by a rapid systemic dissemination to the bone marrow, blood, and central nervous system. Initial responses to chemotherapy or radiotherapy may be frequent, but short-lived; allogeneic stem cell transplantation offers the only chance of sustained remission in eligible patients. Poor prognostic factors include older age, overt involvement of bone marrow, and adverse genetic features. The recent administration) of tagraxofusp, a fusion protein (diphtheria toxin + interleukin-3) targeting CD123 on the blast cells, offers promising results at the initial stages of the disease, with the goal of partial remission, which will allow for allogeneic stem cell transplantation [74–78].

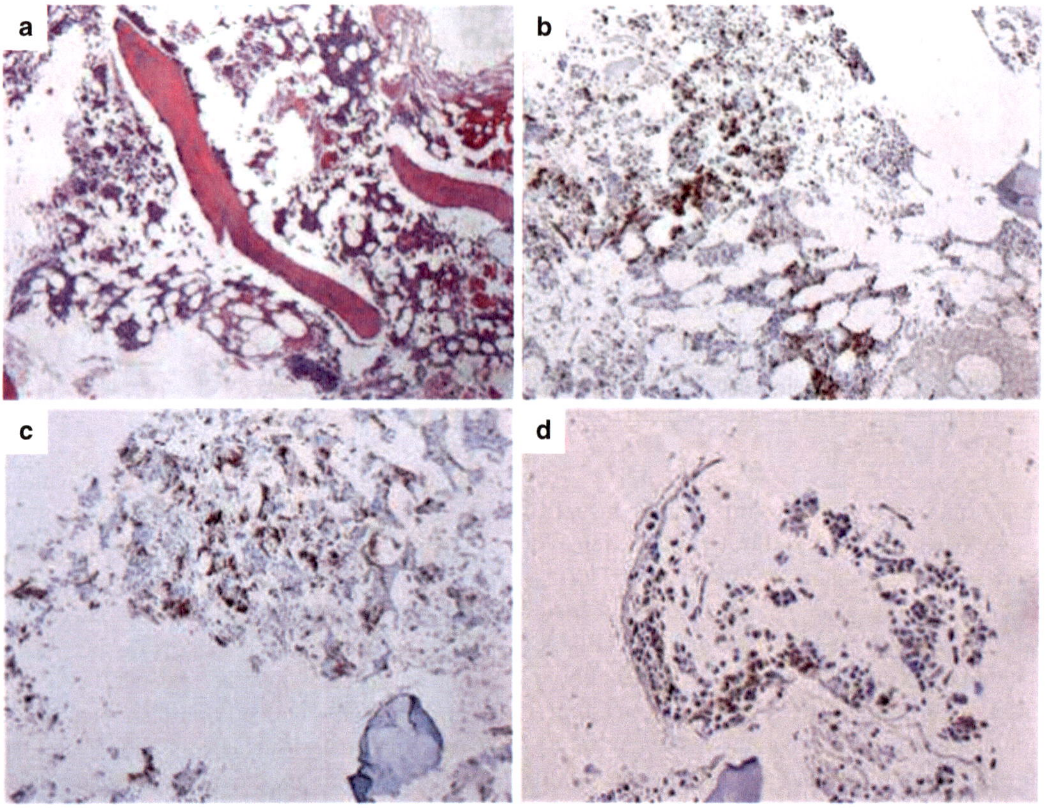

Fig. 19.22 Bone marrow biopsy findings in a 78-year-old patient with Blastic Plasmacytoid Dendritic Cell Neoplasm (BPDCN). (**a**) H&E section showing no overt morphologic evidence of neoplastic infiltration (magnification ×10). (**b**–**d**) Immunohistochemistry reveals interstitial and small aggregate positivity for TCL-1 (magnification ×10), CD56 (magnification ×10), and CD123 (magnification ×20), consistent with minimal bone marrow involvement by blastic plasmacytoid dendritic cells, similar to the cutaneous infiltrate

Acknowledgments The authors would like to thank Professor Elias Drakos, MD, PhD, Department of Pathology, Medical School, University of Crete, Heraklion, Greece, for providing the histological images and slides for some of the cases.

The authors would also like to thank Dr. Georgios Evangelou, Consultant Dermatologist-Venereologist, MD, PhD, Department of Dermatology, University Hospital of Heraklion, Heraklion, Greece, and Dr. Konstantinos Liapis, MD, PhD, Associate Professor of Haematology, at the Democritus University of Thrace Medical School, for providing clinical and dermoscopic images for some of the cases.

References

1. Willemze R, Jaffe ES, Burg G, Cerroni L, Berti E, Swerdlow SH, Ralfkiaer E, Chimenti S, Diaz-Perez JL, Duncan LM, Grange F, Harris NL, Kempf W, Kerl H, Kurrer M, Knobler R, Pimpinelli N, Sander C, Santucci M, Sterry W, Vermeer MH, Wechsler J, Whittaker S, Meijer CJ. WHO-EORTC classification for cutaneous lymphomas. Blood. 2005;105(10):3768–85. https://doi.org/10.1182/blood-2004-09-3502. Epub 2005 Feb 3. PMID: 15692063.
2. Wilcox RA. Cutaneous B-cell lymphomas: 2019 update on diagnosis, risk stratification, and management. Am J Hematol. 2018;93(11):1427–30. https://doi.org/10.1002/ajh.25224. PMID: 30039522.
3. Lee WJ, Won KH, Won CH, Chang SE, Choi JH, Moon KC, Park CS, Huh J, Suh C, Lee MW. Secondary cutaneous lymphoma: comparative clinical features and survival outcome analysis of 106 cases according to lymphoma cell lineage. Br J Dermatol. 2015;173(1):134–45. https://doi.org/10.1111/bjd.13582. Epub 2015 Apr 1. PMID: 25556641.
4. Rickaby RW, Calonje E. Cutaneous involvement from systemic lymphoma. Br J Dermatol. 2015;173(1):12–3. https://doi.org/10.1111/bjd.13904. PMID: 26174642.
5. Souza PK, Amorim RO, Sousa LS, Batista MD. Dermatological manifestations of hematologic

neoplasms. Part I: secondary specific skin lesions. An Bras Dermatol. 2023;98(1):5–12. https://doi.org/10.1016/j.abd.2022.06.002. Epub 2022 Nov 4. PMID: 36344350.

6. Dar AR, Jordan K, Yartsev S. Secondary cutaneous involvement in follicular diffuse lymphoma treated with helical tomotherapy. Cureus. 2017;9(7):e1471. https://doi.org/10.7759/cureus.1471. PMID: 28944110.
7. Zhou XA, Yang J, Ringbloom KG, Martinez-Escala ME, Stevenson KE, Wenzel AT, Fantini D, Martin HK, Moy AP, Morgan EA, Harkins S, Paxton CN, Hong B, Andersen EF, Guitart J, Weinstock DM, Cerroni L, Choi J, Louissaint A. Genomic landscape of cutaneous follicular lymphomas reveals 2 subgroups with clinically predictive molecular features. Blood Adv. 2021;5(3):649–61. https://doi.org/10.1182/bloodadvances.2020002469. PMID: 33560380.
8. Franco R, Fernandez-Vazquez A, Rodriguez-Peralto JL, Bellas C, López-Ríos F, Sáez A, Villuendas R, Navarrete M, Fernandez I, Zarco C, Piris MA. Cutaneous follicular B-cell lymphoma: description of a series of 18 cases. Am J Surg Pathol. 2001a;25(7):875–83. https://doi.org/10.1097/00000478-200107000-00005. PMID: 11420458.
9. Franco R, Fernández-Vázquez A, Mollejo M, Cruz MA, Camacho FI, García JF, Navarrete M, Piris MA. Cutaneous presentation of follicular lymphomas. Mod Pathol. 2001b;14(9):913–9. https://doi.org/10.1038/modpathol.3880411. PMID: 11557789.
10. Dabski K, Banks PM, Winkelmann RK. Clinicopathologic spectrum of cutaneous manifestations in systemic follicular lymphoma. A study of 11 patients. Cancer. 1989;64(7):1480–5. https://doi.org/10.1002/1097-0142(19891001)64:7<1480::aid-cncr2820640720>3.0.co;2-s. PMID: 2789095.
11. Palacios Abufón A, Acebo Mariñas E, Gardeazabal García J, García-Ruiz JC. Systemic follicular lymphoma with cutaneous manifestations and exclusively cutaneous recurrence. Actas Dermosifiliogr. 2012;103(3):253–5. https://doi.org/10.1016/j.ad.2011.06.008. Epub 2011 Nov 16. PMID: 22093542.
12. Servitje O, Climent F, Colomo L, Ruiz N, García-Herrera A, Gallardo F, Mercadal S, Pomares H, Muniesa C, Martin-Callizo C, Marcoval J, Rovira R, Estrach T, Pujol RM. Primary cutaneous vs secondary cutaneous follicular lymphomas: a comparative study focused on BCL2, CD10, and t(14;18) expression. J Cutan Pathol. 2019;46(3):182–9. https://doi.org/10.1111/cup.13399. Epub 2018 Dec 26. PMID: 30511443.
13. Laghi A, Lee C, Witkowski A, Hsu M, Pellacani G, Ludzik J. The role of dermatoscopy and reflectance confocal microscopy in the assessment of relapsing secondary cutaneous follicular B-cell lymphoma. JAAD Case Rep. 2022;24:91–3. https://doi.org/10.1016/j.jdcr.2022.03.035. eCollection 2022 Jun. PMID: 35647248.
14. Ghahramani GK, Goetz KE, Liu V. Dermoscopic characterization of cutaneous lymphomas: a pilot survey. Int J Dermatol. 2018;57(3):339–43. https://doi.org/10.1111/ijd.13860. Epub 2018 Jan 10. PMID: 29318585.
15. Errichetti E, Geller S, Zalaudek I, Longo C, Kyrgidis A, Akay BN, Piccolo V, Myskowski P, Vitiello P, Russo T, Argenziano G, Sławińska M, Sokołowska-Wojdyło M, Sobjanek M, Toncic RJ, Rados J, Drvar DL, Ceovic R, Kaminska-Winciorek G, Zaballos P, Reggiani C, Kremic Z, Lanssens S, Güleç AT, Lobato-Berezo A, Damiani G, Maione V, Calzavara-Pinton P, Sotiriou E, Stinco G, Apalla Z, Lallas A. Dermatoscopy of nodular/plaque-type primary cutaneous T- and B-cell lymphomas: a retrospective comparative study with pseudolymphomas and tumoral/inflammatory mimickers by the international dermoscopy society. J Am Acad Dermatol. 2022;86(4):774–81. https://doi.org/10.1016/j.jaad.2021.10.020. Epub 2021 Oct 23. PMID: 34695527.
16. Bombonato C, Pampena R, Lallas A, Giovanni P, Longo C. Dermoscopy of lymphomas and pseudolymphomas. Dermatol Clin. 2018;36(4):377–88. https://doi.org/10.1016/j.det.2018.05.005. Epub 2018 Aug 14. PMID: 30201147.
17. Melhoranse Gouveia B, Wells J, Kim J, Consuegra G, Longo C, Fernandez-Penas P. Systematic review and proposal of an in vivo reflectance confocal microscopy assessment tool for cutaneous lymphoma. J Cutan Pathol. 2020;47(3):295–304. https://doi.org/10.1111/cup.13598. Epub 2019 Nov 6. PMID: 31618473.
18. Winkler M, Albrecht JD, Sauer C, Kordaß T, Guenova E, Livingstone E, Wobser M, Mitteldorf C, Géraud C, Nicolay JP. Spontaneous regression of primary cutaneous diffuse large B-cell lymphoma, leg type: a case series and review of the literature. J Dermatol. 2024;51(9):1233–9. https://doi.org/10.1111/1346-8138.17339. Epub 2024 Jul 19. PMID: 39031169.
19. Goyal N, Rubin N, Goyal A. Differential survival of systemic B-cell lymphomas initially diagnosed in the skin: a population-based study of 883 patients. Arch Dermatol Res. 2023;315(2):259–63. https://doi.org/10.1007/s00403-021-02293-0. Epub 2021 Nov 15. PMID: 34779893.
20. Goyal N, O'Leary D, Rubin N, Bohjanen K, Goyal A. Localization patterns and survival of extranodal natural killer/T-cell lymphomas in the United States: a population-based study of 945 cases. J Am Acad Dermatol. 2021;85(5):1318–21. https://doi.org/10.1016/j.jaad.2020.08.109. Epub 2020 Sep 3. PMID: 32891786.
21. Shamsudin N, Chang CC. Diffuse large B-cell lymphoma presenting with extensive cutaneous infiltration. Singapore Med J. 2012;53(9):e198–200. PMID: 23023915.
22. Muniesa C, Pujol RM, Estrach MT, Gallardo F, García-Muret MP, Climent J, Salar A, Servitje O. Primary cutaneous diffuse large B-cell lymphoma, leg type and secondary cutaneous involvement by testicular B-cell lymphoma share identical clinicopathological and immunophenotypical features. J Am Acad Dermatol. 2012;66(4):650–4. https://doi.org/10.

1016/j.jaad.2011.03.031. Epub 2011 Aug 3. PMID: 21816504.
23. Berendsen MR, Bladel DAGV, Hesius E, de Groot FA, Kroeze LI, Rijntjes J, Luijks JACW, Hoevenaars B, Halilovic A, Nooijen P, Bladel EV, Jonge-Peeters S, Lensen C, Pruijt H, van der Spek E, Vermaat JSP, Hess C, Hebeda KM, Stevens WBC, van Krieken JHJM, van den Brand M, Groenen PJTA, Scheijen B. Detection of second primary lymphoma in late diffuse large B-cell lymphoma recurrences. Mod Pathol. 2023;36(5):100119. https://doi.org/10.1016/j.modpat.2023.100119. Epub 2023 Feb 1. PMID: 36805792.
24. Koizumi S, Togawa Y, Saeki Y, Shimizu R, Nakano M. A case of cutaneous variant of intravascular large B-cell lymphoma in which dermoscopy revealed telangiectasias associated with erythematous induration. Dermatol Reports. 2023;16(1):9731. https://doi.org/10.4081/dr.2023.9731. eCollection 2024 Mar 12. PMID: 38623370.
25. Miyabe C, Nomura J, Ikeda T, Takahashi K, Kawakami T. Skin biopsies using dermoscopy for earlier diagnosis of intravascular large B-cell lymphoma. J Dermatol. 2020;47(7):e276–8. https://doi.org/10.1111/1346-8138.15350. Epub 2020 Apr 10. PMID: 32275085.
26. Mascolo M, Piccolo V, Argenziano G, Costa C, Lo Presti M, De Rosa G, Scalvenzi M, Staibano S. Dermoscopy pattern, histopathology and immunophenotype of primary cutaneous B-cell lymphoma presenting as a solitary skin nodule. Dermatology. 2016;232(2):203–7. https://doi.org/10.1159/000442251. Epub 2015 Dec 23. PMID: 26694025.
27. Llamas-Velasco M, Held L, Gold R, Paredes B. Dermoscopy of primary cutaneous intravascular large B-cell lymphoma. Clin Exp Dermatol. 2020;45(2):269–72. https://doi.org/10.1111/ced.14073. Epub 2019 Sep 26. PMID: 31419326.
28. Behera B, Palit A, Nayak AK, Panigrahi A, Mishra P, Sethy M. Clinico-dermoscopic-pathological features of a rare case of locally invasive multifocal primary cutaneous diffuse large B cell lymphoma-leg type over the face and scalp. Indian J Dermatol. 2022;67(3):283–6. https://doi.org/10.4103/ijd.IJD_783_20. PMID: 36386119.
29. Mikami T, Ichikawa T, Kazama T, Aoyama Y, Mabuchi T, Ikoma H, Kajiwara H, Nagafuji Y, Sekiguchi Y, Kodama E, Fukuzawa T, Kuroki T, Nagao R, Hashimoto J. Cutaneous metastases from testicular diffuse large B-cell malignant lymphoma and Bowen disease: 18F-FDG PET-CT findings. Tokai J Exp Clin Med. 2020;45(2):58–62. PMID: 32602102.
30. Ribrag V, Bron D, Rymkiewicz G, Hoelzer D, Jørgensen J, de Armas-Castellano A, Trujillo-Martín M, Fenaux P, Malcovati L, Bolaños N, Ribera JM, Herbaux C, Sarkozy C, Zinzani PL, Walewski J, Chamuleau MED. Diagnosis and treatment of Burkitt lymphoma in adults: clinical practice guidelines from ERN-EuroBloodNet. Lancet Haematol. 2025;12(2):e138–50. https://doi.org/10.1016/S2352-3026(24)00351-X. PMID: 39909657.
31. Rogers A, Graves M, Toscano M, Davis L. A unique cutaneous presentation of Burkitt lymphoma. Am J Dermatopathol. 2014;36(12):997–1001. https://doi.org/10.1097/DAD.0000000000000004. PMID: 24562050.
32. Geller S, Myskowski PL, Pulitzer M. NK/T-cell lymphoma, nasal type, γδ T-cell lymphoma, and CD8-positive epidermotropic T-cell lymphoma-clinical and histopathologic features, differential diagnosis, and treatment. Semin Cutan Med Surg. 2018;37(1):30–8. https://doi.org/10.12788/j.sder.2018.020. PMID: 29719018.
33. Brüggen MC, Kerl K, Haralambieva E, Schanz U, Chang YT, Ignatova D, Dummer R, Cozzio A, Hoetzenecker W, French LE, Guenova E. Aggressive rare T-cell lymphomas with manifestation in the skin: a monocentric cross-sectional case study. Acta Derm Venereol. 2018;98(9):835–41. https://doi.org/10.2340/00015555-2950. PMID: 29693696.
34. Oluwole OO, Zic JA, Douds JJ, Ann Thompson M, Greer JP. Cutaneous manifestations and management of hematologic neoplasms. Semin Oncol. 2016;43(3):370–83. https://doi.org/10.1053/j.seminoncol.2016.02.021. Epub 2016 Feb 23. PMID: 27178691.
35. Natkunam Y, Smoller BR, Zehnder JL, Dorfman RF, Warnke RA. Aggressive cutaneous NK and NK-like T-cell lymphomas: clinicopathologic, immunohistochemical, and molecular analyses of 12 cases. Am J Surg Pathol. 1999;23(5):571–81. https://doi.org/10.1097/00000478-199905000-00012. PMID: 10328090.
36. Torres-Cabala CA. Diagnosis of T-cell lymphoid proliferations of the skin: putting all the pieces together. Mod Pathol. 2020;33(Suppl 1):83–95. https://doi.org/10.1038/s41379-019-0397-3. Epub 2019 Oct 29. PMID: 31664155.
37. Gerami P, Wickless SC, Querfeld C, Rosen ST, Kuzel TM, Guitart J. Cutaneous involvement with marginal zone lymphoma. J Am Acad Dermatol. 2010;63(1):142–5. https://doi.org/10.1016/j.jaad.2009.07.047. Epub 2010 May 11. PMID: 20462658.
38. Baldassano MF, Bailey EM, Ferry JA, Harris NL, Duncan LM. Cutaneous lymphoid hyperplasia and cutaneous marginal zone lymphoma: comparison of morphologic and immunophenotypic features. Am J Surg Pathol. 1999;23(1):88–96. https://doi.org/10.1097/00000478-199901000-00010. PMID: 9888708.
39. Matutes E, Montalban C. Clinical features and management of non-gastrointestinal non-ocular extranodal mucosa associated lymphoid tissue (ENMALT) marginal zone lymphomas. Best Pract Res Clin Haematol. 2017;30(1-2):99–108. https://doi.org/10.1016/j.beha.2016.07.005. Epub 2016 Nov 5. PMID: 28288723.
40. Cao Q, Li Y, Lin H, Ke Z, Liu Y, Ye Z. Mantle cell lymphoma of blastoid variant with skin lesion and rapid progression: a case report and literature review. Am J Dermatopathol. 2013;35(8):851–5. https://doi.org/10.1097/DAD.0b013e31828de73a. PMID: 23928453.

41. Wehkamp U, Pott C, Unterhalt M, Koch K, Weichenthal M, Klapper W, Oschlies I. Skin involvement of mantle cell lymphoma may mimic primary cutaneous diffuse large B-cell lymphoma, leg type. Am J Surg Pathol. 2015;39(8):1093–101. https://doi.org/10.1097/PAS.0000000000000445. PMID: 26034867.
42. Gru AA, Bacchi CE, Pulitzer M, Bhagat G, Kempf W, Robson A, Plaza JA, Pincus L, Raghavan S, Xu M, Vencato da Silva T, Salavaggione AL, Subtil A, Battistella M. Secondary skin involvement in classic Hodgkin lymphoma: results of an international collaborative cutaneous lymphoma working group study of 25 patients. J Cutan Pathol. 2021;48(11):1367–78. https://doi.org/10.1111/cup.14077. Epub 2021 Jul 5. PMID: 34089205.
43. Erkiliç S, Erbagci Z, Koçer NE, Bayazit YA, Camci C. Cutaneous involvement in Hodgkin's lymphoma: report of two cases. J Dermatol. 2004;31(4):330–4. https://doi.org/10.1111/j.1346-8138.2004.tb00680.x. PMID: 15187329.
44. Dhull AK, Soni A, Kaushal V. Hodgkin's lymphoma with cutaneous involvement. BMJ Case Rep. 2012;2012:bcr2012007599. https://doi.org/10.1136/bcr-2012-007599. PMID: 23195828.
45. Hsia CC, Howson-Jan K, Rizkalla KS. Hodgkin lymphoma with cutaneous involvement. Dermatol Online J. 2009;15(5):5. PMID: 19624983.
46. Introcaso CE, Kantor J, Porter DL, Junkins-Hopkins JM. Cutaneous Hodgkin's disease. J Am Acad Dermatol. 2008;58(2):295–8. https://doi.org/10.1016/j.jaad.2005.11.1055. PMID: 18222326.
47. de Leval L, Gaulard P, Dogan A. A practical approach to the modern diagnosis and classification of T- and NK-cell lymphomas. Blood. 2024;144(18):1855–72. https://doi.org/10.1182/blood.2023021786. PMID: 38728419.
48. Mraz-Gernhard S, Natkunam Y, Hoppe RT, LeBoit P, Kohler S, Kim YH. Natural killer/natural killer-like T-cell lymphoma, CD56+, presenting in the skin: an increasingly recognized entity with an aggressive course. J Clin Oncol. 2001;19(8):2179–88. https://doi.org/10.1200/JCO.2001.19.8.2179. PMID: 11304770.
49. Zhang X, Zhou J, Han X, Wang E, Zhang L. Update on the classification of and diagnostic approaches to mature T-cell lymphomas. Arch Pathol Lab Med. 2022;146(8):947–52. https://doi.org/10.5858/arpa.2021-0143-RA. PMID: 34524423.
50. Morón-Ocaña JM, Monsalve-Sosa P, Martínez-Barranca ML, Coronel-Pérez IM, Pérez-Gil A. Clinical characteristics and outcomes of pediatric systemic anaplastic large cell lymphoma. Pediatr Dermatol. 2025;42(3):487–91. https://doi.org/10.1111/pde.15850. Epub 2025 Jan 12. PMID: 39800860.
51. Lee WJ, Moon IJ, Lee SH, Won CH, Chang SE, Choi JH, Moon KC, Park CS, Huh J, Lee MW. Cutaneous anaplastic large-cell lymphoma (ALCL): a comparative clinical feature and survival outcome analysis of 52 cases according to primary tumor site. J Am Acad Dermatol. 2016;74(6):1135–43. https://doi.org/10.1016/j.jaad.2015.12.053. Epub 2016 Feb 17. PMID: 26897385.
52. Kadin ME, Carpenter C. Systemic and primary cutaneous anaplastic large cell lymphomas. Semin Hematol. 2003;40(3):244–56. https://doi.org/10.1016/s0037-1963(03)00138-0. PMID: 12876673.
53. Gable AD, Clark SH, Magro CM. Myxoid variant of anaplastic large cell lymphoma involving the skin: a case report. J Cutan Pathol. 2012;39(8):787–90. https://doi.org/10.1111/j.1600-0560.2012.01911.x. Epub 2012 May 22. PMID: 22612158.
54. Botros N, Cerroni L, Shawwa A, Green PJ, Greer W, Pasternak S, Walsh NM. Cutaneous manifestations of angioimmunoblastic T-cell lymphoma: clinical and pathological characteristics. Am J Dermatopathol. 2015;37(4):274–83. https://doi.org/10.1097/DAD.0000000000000144. PMID: 25794336.
55. Lee WJ, Won KH, Choi JW, Won CH, Chang SE, Choi JH, Lee MW. Cutaneous angioimmunoblastic T-cell lymphoma: Epstein-Barr virus positivity and its effects on clinicopathologic features. J Am Acad Dermatol. 2019;81(4):989–97. https://doi.org/10.1016/j.jaad.2018.08.053. Epub 2018 Sep 18. PMID: 30240776.
56. Oishi N, Sartori-Valinotti JC, Bennani NN, Wada DA, He R, Cappel MA, Feldman AL. Cutaneous lesions of angioimmunoblastic T-cell lymphoma: clinical, pathological, and immunophenotypic features. J Cutan Pathol. 2019;46(9):637–44. https://doi.org/10.1111/cup.13475. Epub 2019 May 3. PMID: 30980412.
57. Huang CT, Chuang SS. Angioimmunoblastic T-cell lymphoma with cutaneous involvement: a case report with subtle histologic changes and clonal T-cell proliferation. Arch Pathol Lab Med. 2004;128(10):e122–4. https://doi.org/10.5858/2004-128-e122-ATLWCI. PMID: 15387690.
58. Advani RH, Skrypets T, Civallero M, Spinner MA, Manni M, Kim WS, Shustov AR, Horwitz SM, Hitz F, Cabrera ME, Dlouhy I, Vassallo J, Pileri SA, Inghirami G, Montoto S, Vitolo U, Radford J, Vose JM, Federico M. Outcomes and prognostic factors in angioimmunoblastic T-cell lymphoma: final report from the international T-cell project. Blood. 2021;138(3):213–20. https://doi.org/10.1182/blood.2020010387. PMID: 34292324.
59. Pesqué D, Marcantonio O, Vázquez I, Papaleo N, Sánchez-González B, Gallardo F, Colomo L, Pujol RM. Cutaneous involvement of angioimmunoblastic T-cell lymphoma masquerading as B-cell reactive lymphoid hyperplasia. Am J Dermatopathol. 2022;44(4):e41–5. https://doi.org/10.1097/DAD.0000000000002110. PMID: 34966050.
60. Lachenal F, Berger F, Ghesquières H, Biron P, Hot A, Callet-Bauchu E, Chassagne C, Coiffier B, Durieu I, Rousset H, Salles G. Angioimmunoblastic T-cell lymphoma: clinical and laboratory features at diagnosis in 77 patients. Medicine (Baltimore). 2007;86(5):282–92. https://doi.org/10.1097/MD.0b013e3181573059. PMID: 17873758.

61. Lee WJ, Moon HR, Won CH, Chang SE, Choi JH, Moon KC, Lee MW. Precursor B- or T-lymphoblastic lymphoma presenting with cutaneous involvement: a series of 13 cases including 7 cases of cutaneous T-lymphoblastic lymphoma. J Am Acad Dermatol. 2014;70(2):318–25. https://doi.org/10.1016/j.jaad.2013.10.020. Epub 2013 Dec 4. PMID: 24314877.
62. Gru AA, McHargue C, Salavaggione AL. A systematic approach to the cutaneous lymphoid infiltrates: a clinical, morphologic, and immunophenotypic evaluation. Arch Pathol Lab Med. 2019;143(8):958–79. https://doi.org/10.5858/arpa.2018-0294-RA. PMID: 31339758.
63. Montes-Torres A, Llamas-Velasco M, Capusan TM, Aguado B, Adrados M. Cutaneous involvement as the first manifestation of T-lymphoblastic lymphoma and review of the literature. J Cutan Pathol. 2019;46(5):372–5. https://doi.org/10.1111/cup.13431. Epub 2019 Mar 7. PMID: 30680766.
64. Intermesoli T, Weber A, Leoncin M, Frison L, Skert C, Bassan R. Lymphoblastic lymphoma: a concise review. Curr Oncol Rep. 2022;24(1):1–12. https://doi.org/10.1007/s11912-021-01168-x. Epub 2022 Jan 20. PMID: 35059993.
65. Sander CA, Medeiros LJ, Abruzzo LV, Horak ID, Jaffe ES. Lymphoblastic lymphoma presenting in cutaneous sites. A clinicopathologic analysis of six cases. J Am Acad Dermatol. 1991;25(6 Pt 1):1023–31. https://doi.org/10.1016/0190-9622(91)70302-i. PMID: 1810981.
66. Shi Y, Wang E. Blastic plasmacytoid dendritic cell neoplasm: a clinicopathologic review. Arch Pathol Lab Med. 2014;138(4):564–9. https://doi.org/10.5858/arpa.2013-0101-RS. PMID: 24678689.
67. Shimony S, Luskin MR, Gangat N, LeBoeuf NR, Feraco AM, Lane AA. Blastic plasmacytoid dendritic cell neoplasm (BPDCN): 2025 update on diagnosis, pathophysiology, risk assessment, and management. Am J Hematol. 2025;100(8):1408–22. https://doi.org/10.1002/ajh.27737. Epub 2025 Jun 17. PMID: 40525728.
68. Gera S, Dekmezian MS, Duvic M, Tschen JA, Vega F, Cho-Vega JH. Blastic plasmacytoid dendritic cell neoplasm: evolving insights in an aggressive hematopoietic malignancy with a predilection of skin involvement. Am J Dermatopathol. 2014;36(3):244–51. https://doi.org/10.1097/DAD.0b013e318280de99. PMID: 24247574.
69. Brüggen MC, Valencak J, Stranzenbach R, Li N, Stadler R, Jonak C, Bauer W, Porkert S, Blaschke A, Meiss F, Nicolay JP, Wehkamp U, Schlaak M, Nguyen VA, Romani N, Cozzio A, Gayathri N, Dimitriou F, French LE, Dummer R, Guenova E. Clinical diversity and treatment approaches to blastic plasmacytoid dendritic cell neoplasm: a retrospective multicentre study. J Eur Acad Dermatol Venereol. 2020;34(7):1489–95. https://doi.org/10.1111/jdv.16215. Epub 2020 Mar 10. PMID: 31955469.
70. Cota C, Vale E, Viana I, Requena L, Ferrara G, Anemona L, Metze D, Fink-Puches R, Wiesner T, Cerroni L. Cutaneous manifestations of blastic plasmacytoid dendritic cell neoplasm-morphologic and phenotypic variability in a series of 33 patients. Am J Surg Pathol. 2010;34(1):75–87. https://doi.org/10.1097/PAS.0b013e3181c5e26b. PMID: 19956058.
71. Salva KA, Haemel AK, Pincus LB, Liu J, Sundram U, Guitart J, Longley BJ, Wood GS. Expression of CD31/PECAM-1 (platelet endothelial cell adhesion molecule 1) by blastic plasmacytoid dendritic cell neoplasms. JAMA Dermatol. 2014;150(1):73–6. https://doi.org/10.1001/jamadermatol.2013.7141. PMID: 24225899.
72. Nicklas C, Bellolio E, Lopez E, Goldberg I, Geller S, Navarrete-Dechent C. Dermoscopy of blastic plasmacytoid dendritic cell neoplasm in two patients. Clin Exp Dermatol. 2021;46(5):950–2. https://doi.org/10.1111/ced.14621. Epub 2021 Mar 17. PMID: 33639013.
73. Tokioka R, Saito-Sasaki N, Sawada Y. A case of cutaneous blastic plasmacytoid dendritic cell neoplasm on the chest. Cureus. 2024;16(9):e70288. https://doi.org/10.7759/cureus.70288. eCollection 2024 Sep. PMID: 39463539.
74. Pujol RM, Gallardo F, Servitje O, Martí RM, Bordes R, García-Muret MP, Estrach MT, Nomdedeu JF. Peripheral T-cell lymphoma with secondary epithelioid granulomatous cutaneous involvement: a clinicopathologic study of four cases. J Dermatol. 2005;32(7):541–8. https://doi.org/10.1111/j.1346-8138.2005.tb00796.x. PMID: 16335869.
75. Bekkenk MW, Vermeer MH, Jansen PM, van Marion AM, Canninga-van Dijk MR, Kluin PM, Geerts ML, Meijer CJ, Willemze R. Peripheral T-cell lymphomas unspecified presenting in the skin: analysis of prognostic factors in a group of 82 patients. Blood. 2003;102(6):2213–9. https://doi.org/10.1182/blood-2002-07-1960. Epub 2003 May 15. PMID: 12750155.
76. Kempf W, Petrella T, Willemze R, Jansen P, Berti E, Santucci M, Geissinger E, Cerroni L, Maubec E, Battistella M, Goodlad J, Guenova E, Lappalainen K, Ranki A, Craig P, Calonje E, Martin B, Whittaker S, Oschlies I, Wehkamp U, Nicolay JP, Wobser M, Scarisbruck J, Pimpinelli N, Stadler R, Kerl French K, Quaglino P, Lin J, Chen L, Beer M, Emanuel P, Dalle S, Robson A. Clinical, histopathological and prognostic features of primary cutaneous acral CD8+ T-cell lymphoma and other dermal CD8+ cutaneous lymphoproliferations: results of an EORTC cutaneous lymphoma group workshop. Br J Dermatol. 2022;186(5):887–97. https://doi.org/10.1111/bjd.20973. PMID: 34988968.
77. Kiyohara T, Makimura K, Nakamaru S, Miyamoto M, Shijimaya T, Nagano N, Tanimura H. B-cell lymphoblastic leukemia/lymphoma in infants: report of two cases on the face. J Dermatol. 2019;46(7):e255–6. https://doi.org/10.1111/1346-8138.14799. Epub 2019 Feb 5. PMID: 30719747.
78. Pemmaraju N, Lane AA, Sweet KL, Stein AS, Vasu S, Blum W, Rizzieri DA, Konopleva M. Tagraxofusp in blastic plasmacytoid dendritic-cell neoplasm. N Engl J Med. 2019;380(17):1628–37. https://doi.org/10.1056/NEJMoa1815105.

Part VIII

Skin Metastasis from Neuroendocrine Tumours

Cutaneous Metastasis from Neuroendocrine Tumors

20

Dimitra Koumaki

Abstract

Neuroendocrine tumors are a heterogeneous group of neoplasms derived from neuroendocrine cells, which are widely distributed throughout the body and predominantly arise in the gastrointestinal tract, bronchopulmonary system, and pancreas. Cutaneous metastases from neuroendocrine tumors are defined as secondary skin involvement by these tumors, distinct from primary cutaneous neuroendocrine carcinomas, and are rare clinical entities that may herald an occult internal malignancy or signify advanced disease. This chapter provides an overview of the classification, incidence, clinical presentation, diagnosis, management, and prognosis of cutaneous metastases from neuroendocrine tumors. We discuss the 2022 World Health Organization classification, which separates neuroendocrine neoplasms into well-differentiated tumors graded by mitotic rate and Ki-67 index, and poorly differentiated carcinomas, and highlights their differing molecular and prognostic profiles. Cutaneous metastases arise predominantly from bronchopulmonary and gastrointestinal primaries and present as erythematous to violaceous papules or nodules, with possible pain related to perineural invasion or vasoactive secretions. Diagnosis relies on histopathologic examination and immunohistochemical studies using markers such as chromogranin, synaptophysin, CD56, and cytokeratin panels, which help to differentiate these lesions from Merkel cell carcinoma and other mimics. Molecular profiling is increasingly informing prognosis and therapy, unveiling distinct mutational landscapes between neuroendocrine tumors (NETs) and neuroendocrine carcinomas (NECs), including a prognostic seven-gene signature and frequent TP53 and RB1 (retinoblastoma 1 gene) mutations in NECs. Management is multidisciplinary, encompassing surgical, systemic, and palliative strategies adapted to tumor grade and burden. The presence of cutaneous metastases generally portends poor prognosis despite the advancement in systemic therapy; however, well-differentiated tumors can demonstrate longer survival. Increasing recognition and precise characterization of these metastases are imperative for optimized patient outcomes.

Keywords

Neuroendocrine tumor · Cutaneous metastasis · Neuroendocrine carcinoma · Skin metastasis · Immunohistochemistry · Ki-67 · Bronchopulmonary neuroendocrine tumor · Gastrointestinal neuroendocrine tumor · Molecular profiling · Tumor classification

D. Koumaki (✉)
Dermatology Department, University Hospital of Heraklion, Heraklion, Greece

D. Koumaki et al. (eds.), *Cutaneous Metastases*, https://doi.org/10.1007/978-3-032-26764-1_20

20.1 Introduction

Neuroendocrine tumors (NETs) are a Cutaneous metastasis:neuroendocrine tumors (NETs) heterogeneous group of neoplasms arising from neuroendocrine cells distributed throughout the body, most commonly in the gastrointestinal tract, bronchopulmonary system, and pancreas [1–4]. Cutaneous metastasis from neuroendocrine tumors is defined as the spread of a visceral NET to the skin, distinct from primary cutaneous neuroendocrine carcinomas such as Merkel cell carcinoma [5–10]. These metastases may be the first manifestation of an otherwise occult internal malignancy or appear as a terminal feature of widespread disease.

20.2 Neuroendocrine Tumors: Classification

Neuroendocrine neoplasms are categorized by differentiation and grade, following the recommendation of the World Health Organization and the International Agency for Research on Cancer. The main categories are:

Well-differentiated NETs are graded by mitotic count and Ki-67 index into Grade 1 (low), Grade 2 (intermediate grade), and Grade 3 (high-grade well-differentiated, distinct from NECs) [11–20].

- Poorly differentiated NECs are always high-grade G3 and include the subtypes of small cell and large neuroendocrine cell.
- Mixed neuroendocrine-nonneuroendocrine neoplasms: lesions comprising both neuroendocrine and non-neuroendocrine components.

These neoplasms, NETs and NECs, may arise in any organ but most frequently arise in the following:

- Gastrointestinal tract: stomach, small intestine, appendix, rectum
- Pancreas

The lung/bronchopulmonary system includes a typical and atypical carcinoid, small-cell lung cancer, and large-cell neuroendocrine carcinoma.

20.2.1 Thymus

- Other sites: parathyroid, thyroid (medullary thyroid carcinoma), adrenal (pheochromocytoma), pituitary.

NETs are also classified according to functional status:

- Functional, that is, hormone-secreting, e.g., insulinoma and gastrinoma.
- Nonfunctional, that is, without symptoms related to hormones.

This classification informs prognosis and management, according to guidelines developed by the National Comprehensive Cancer Network (NCCN) and other expert societies.

20.3 Incidence

Skin metastases of neuroendocrine tumors (NETs) and neuroendocrine carcinomas (NECs) rarely occur. The present review focuses on 43 cases reported from 1980 to 2022 [21–30]. The cases show that there is a predominance of NETs/NECs with primary origins from the bronchopulmonary system (typical and atypical carcinoids, large-cell neuroendocrine carcinoma (LCNEC), and small-cell lung carcinoma (SCLC)) and from the gastrointestinal tract (ileal, rectal, gastric, and pancreatic cancers), larynx, breast/uterus cancers, and other rarer regions including prostate cancer, bladder cancer, mediastinal cancers, and sinus cancers. The distribution of cases among different regions was 44%, 21%, 21%, 21%, 21%, and 16%, respectively (Table 20.1). The patients were usually affected between 60 and 80 years of age (29–86 years old with an approxi-

Table 20.1a Patient demographics and primary tumor characteristics in skin metastases of neuroendocrine tumours

Case number	First author (Year)	Gender	Age (years)	Primary tumor type	Primary location	Time to skin metastasis
1	Keane J et al. (1980)	F	57	Bronchial carcinoid (type B, undifferentiated)	Bronchial	6.5 years
2	Archer CB et al. (1985)	M	68	Pulmonary carcinoid	Pulmonary	Unknown (diagnosed after skin metastasis)
3	Rodriguez G et al. (1992)	M	80	Unknown (probably gastric antrum)	Gastric?	Unknown (4-month history)
4	Fogaça MF et al. (1993)	F	33	Poorly differentiated cervical cancer	Cervix and lower uterine tumor	N/A
5	Schmidt U et al. (1994)	F	63	Oncocytoid laryngeal carcinoid	Larynx	15 months (post-recurrence)
6	Yoshimasu T et al. (2001)	M	46	Mediastinal NEC	Mediastinum	3 months
7	Ottinetti A et al. (2003)	M	61	Laryngeal NEC	Larynx	5 years
8	Bachmeyer C et al. (2004)	M	52	NEC, unknown primary	Unknown	N/A
9	Vidulich KA et al. (2007)	F	76	Breast NET	Breast	3 years
10	Santi R et al. (2008)	M	60	Lung typical carcinoid	Lung	N/A
11	Puri PK et al. (2008)	M	53	Metastatic carcinoid (post-liver transplant)	Liver/GEP?	N/A
12	Lee WJ et al. (2009)	F	49	Uterine small-cell NEC	Uterus	4 months
13	Blochin E et al. (2010)	F	55	Pulmonary atypical carcinoid (stage IV)	Lung	N/A (diagnosed 2007)
14	Jedrych J et al. (2011)—Case 1	F	50	Lung typical carcinoid (RUL, 1.1 cm, NB)	Lung	12 months
15	Jedrych J et al. (2011)—Case 2	M	74	Lung atypical carcinoid (RML)	Lung	N/A
16	Jedrych J et al. (2011)—Case 3	F	67	Pancreatic NET (1.3 cm, NB)	Pancreas	3 months
17	Jedrych J et al. (2011)—Case 4	M	67	Distal ileal WDNET (2.3 cm)	Ileum	12 months
18	Donati P et al. (2013)	F	43	Pulmonary atypical carcinoid (pT3N1)	Lung	N/A
19	Fluehler C et al. (2013)	M	65	Rectal poorly differentiated NEC	Rectum	2 years
20	Yuan C et al. (2014)	F	60	LCNEC (disseminated)	Lung?	N/A
21	Hong S et al. (2014)	M	62	Laryngeal poorly differentiated NEC	Larynx	6 years
22	Amorim GM et al. (2015)	N/A	N/A	NEC (inguinal LN)	Inguinal?	2 years
23	Wang KR et al. (2016)	F	54	Laryngeal atypical carcinoid	Larynx	N/A
24	Linhas R et al. (2018)	F	30	Lung atypical carcinoid (IA2)	Lung	7 years

(continued)

Table 20.1a (continued)

Case number	First author (Year)	Gender	Age (years)	Primary tumor type	Primary location	Time to skin metastasis
25	Dhingra R et al. (2018)	F	69	GEP-NETs	GEP	N/A
26	Munera-Campos M et al. (2019)	M	80	Prostate adenocarcinoma (NEC?)	Prostate	6 years
27	Pathoulas JT et al. (2021)	F	71	Pulmonary atypical carcinoid	Lung	11 years
28	Fiorio LM (2021)	M	64	Pulmonary carcinoid (unknown prior)	Lung (R bronchus)	N/A
29	Hobbs MM et al. (2022)—Pt 1	F	56	Ileal carcinoid	Ileum	Known cancer
30	Hobbs MM et al. (2022)—Pt 2	F	59	Breast NEC (presumed)	Breast	Unknown
31	Hobbs MM et al. (2022)—Pt 3	M	74	Ileal carcinoid	Ileum	Concurrent
32	Hobbs MM et al. (2022)—Pt 4	M	86	Ileum/esophagus poorly differentiated NEC	Ileum, esophagus	Known cancer
33	Hobbs MM et al. (2022)—Pt 5	F	68	Lung atypical carcinoid	Lung	Known cancer
34	Hobbs MM et al. (2022)—Pt 6	M	67	Lung small-cell carcinoma (presumed)	Lung	Concurrent
35	Hobbs MM et al. (2022)—Pt 7	M	56	Lung large-cell NEC	Lung	Concurrent
36	Hobbs MM et al. (2022)—Pt 8a	M	76	Lung small-cell carcinoma	Lung	Concurrent
37	Hobbs MM et al. (2022)—Pt 8b	M	76	Lung small-cell carcinoma	Lung	Concurrent
38	Hobbs MM et al. (2022)—Pt 9	F	29	Uterine small-cell carcinoma	Uterus	N/A
39	Hobbs MM et al. (2022)—Pt 10	F	75	Bladder poorly differentiated NEC (presumed)	Bladder	Unknown
40	Hobbs MM et al. (2022)—Pt 11	M	55	Lung atypical carcinoid	Lung	Concurrent
41	Hobbs MM et al. (2022)—Pt 12	M	55	Sinus small-cell carcinoma	Sinus	Known cancer
42	Hobbs MM et al. (2022)—Pt 13	M	61	Rectal poorly differentiated NEC	Rectum	N/A
43	Hobbs MM et al. (2022)—Pt 14	M	82	Prostate small-cell carcinoma	Prostate	Known cancer

Selected reported cases of cutaneous metastases from neuroendocrine tumors (NETs): patient demographics and primary tumor characteristics
Abbreviations: *F* female, *M* male, *NEC* neuroendocrine carcinoma, *NET* neuroendocrine tumor, *GEP* gastroenteropancreatic, *LCNEC* large-cell neuroendocrine carcinoma, *WDNET* well-differentiated neuroendocrine tumor, *RUL* right upper lobe, *RML* right middle lobe, *NB* not biopsied, *LN* lymph node, *N/A* not available

Table 20.1b Clinical features of skin metastases in neuroendocrine tumours

Case number	First author (Year)	No. of lesions	Duration of lesions	Color/morphology	Lesion type	Location	Dimensions	Symptoms
1	Keane J et al. (1980)	Solitary	N/A	Violaceous, firm	Nodule	Thigh	2.5 × 2.5 cm	N/A
2	Archer CB et al. (1985)	Numerous	N/A	N/A	Subcutaneous lumps with erosion	Neck, scalp, trunk, thighs	3 × 2 cm (main)	Tender, painful
3	Rodriguez G et al. (1992)	9	4 months	Red-brown	Cutaneous nodules	Forehead, neck, forearms, lateral chest, thighs	4–20 mm	Extremely painful
4	Fogaça MF et al. (1993)	Multiple	Rapidly growing; 2-week history post-surgery	Firm, non-ulcerated, moved with skin	Skin nodules	Scalp, neck, chest, axilla, abdomen	0.2–1.2 cm	Tender
5	Schmidt U et al. (1994)	Multiple	N/A	N/A	N/A	N/A	N/A	N/A
6	Yoshimasu T et al. (2001)	1	N/A	Nodular, erosive	Elevated nodule	Left palm	4.5 × 2.5 × 2 cm	N/A
7	Ottinetti A et al. (2003)	2	1 month, rapid	Red-violaceous, firm	Cutaneous nodules	Chest, back	2 cm and 1.2 cm	Asymptomatic
8	Bachmeyer C et al. (2004)	Numerous	N/A	Erythematous	Tender nodules	Eyelid, scalp, thorax	N/A	Tender
9	Vidulich KA et al. (2007)	Multiple	1 year	Erythematous, grouped	Nodules	Left inferior breast	N/A	N/A
10	Santi R et al. (2008)	1	Rapid	Violaceous-red, firm	Nodule	Back	2.5 × 1 cm	Painless
11	Puri PK et al. (2008)	1	N/A	Pearly with gray-blue speckles	Papule	Scalp	0.5 × 0.5 × 0.1 cm	N/A
12	Lee WJ et al. (2009)	Multiple	1 week	Skin-colored	Confluent nodules	Pubic area	N/A	N/A
13	Blochin E et al. (2010)	N/A	5 months	N/A	Alopecia (painful)	Scalp	N/A	Painful
14	Jedrych J et al. (2011)—Case 1	1	12 months	Flesh-colored, firm	Nodule	Scalp	0.5 cm	Painless
15	Jedrych J et al. (2011)—Case 2	1	N/A	N/A	Nodule	Scalp	1 cm	Painless

(continued)

Table 20.1b (continued)

Case number	First author (Year)	No. of lesions	Duration of lesions	Color/morphology	Lesion type	Location	Dimensions	Symptoms
16	Jedrych J et al. (2011)—Case 3	1	N/A	N/A	Nodule	Scalp	2.5 cm	Painless
17	Jedrych J et al. (2011)—Case 4	1	N/A	N/A	Subcutaneous nodule	Lower back	1 cm	Painless
18	Donati P et al. (2013)	1	Slow	Red-purplish	Nodule	Forehead	1.5 × 1 cm	Intensely painful
19	Fluehler C et al. (2013)	1	N/A	Pinkish-purple, exophytic	Nodule	Right rima oris	2 cm	Non-tender
20	Yuan C et al. (2014)	1	N/A	N/A	Nodule	Chest wall (L breast)	N/A	Back pain
21	Hong S et al. (2014)	Multiple	N/A	N/A	Subcutaneous/IM masses	Abdomen, back, thighs	N/A	Severe pain
22	Amorim GM et al. (2015)	Multiple	3 months	N/A	N/A	R thigh, buttock	N/A	N/A
23	Wang KR et al. (2016)	Multiple	N/A	N/A	Cutaneous/ subcutaneous nodules	Chest wall, abdomen	N/A	N/A
24	Linhas R et al. (2018)	1	N/A	N/A	Subcutaneous nodule	Back	0.5–1 cm	Painless
25	Dhingra R et al. (2018)	1	N/A	N/A	Nodule	Upper R flank	N/A	N/A
26	Munera-Campos M et al. (2019)	Numerous	1 month	Erythematous-violaceous	Plaques	Groin, scrotum	N/A	Painful, edema
27	Pathoulas JT et al. (2021)	2	10 months	Violaceous, firm	Nodules	R mid-flank	0.6 × 0.4 cm	Tender
28	Fiorio LM (2021)	1	7 months	Erythematous, exophytic, vascular	Nodule	Nasal tip	N/A	Painful
29	Hobbs MM et al. (2022)—Pt 1	1	N/A	N/A	N/A	Breast	1.8 cm	N/A
30	Hobbs MM et al. (2022)—Pt 2	1	N/A	N/A	N/A	Breast	2 cm	N/A
31	Hobbs MM et al. (2022)—Pt 3	1	N/A	N/A	N/A	Umbilicus	0.5 cm	N/A

(continued)

32	Hobbs MM et al. (2022)—Pt 4	1	N/A	N/A	N/A	Lip	2 cm	N/A
33	Hobbs MM et al. (2022)—Pt 5	1	N/A	N/A	N/A	Chest wall	1.5 cm	N/A
34	Hobbs MM et al. (2022)—Pt 6	1	N/A	N/A	N/A	Chest wall	1 cm	N/A
35	Hobbs MM et al. (2022)—Pt 7	1	N/A	N/A	N/A	Arm	0.7 cm	N/A
36	Hobbs MM et al. (2022)—Pt 8a	1	N/A	N/A	N/A	Temple	0.4 cm	N/A
37	Hobbs MM et al. (2022)—Pt 8b	1	N/A	N/A	N/A	Scalp	0.5 cm	N/A
38	Hobbs MM et al. (2022)—Pt 9	1	N/A	N/A	N/A	Scalp	1 cm	N/A
39	Hobbs MM et al. (2022)—Pt 10	1	N/A	N/A	N/A	Scalp	0.5 cm	N/A
40	Hobbs MM et al. (2022)—Pt 11	1	N/A	N/A	N/A	Axilla	0.9 cm	N/A
41	Hobbs MM et al. (2022)—Pt 12	1	N/A	N/A	N/A	Scalp	0.5 cm	N/A
42	Hobbs MM et al. (2022)—Pt 13	1	N/A	N/A	N/A	Inguinal	N/A	N/A
43	Hobbs MM et al. (2022)—Pt 14	1	N/A	N/A	N/A	Scalp	2 cm	N/A

Selected reported cases of cutaneous metastases from neuroendocrine tumors (NETs): clinical features of skin metastases including lesion number, morphology, location, size, and symptoms

Abbreviations: *F* female, *M* male, *R* right, *L* left, *IM* intramuscular, *N/A* not available

Table 20.1c Histopathological and immunohistochemical (IHC) findings in skin metastases of neuroendocrine tumours

Case number	First author (Year)	Biopsy performed	Positive IHC (skin metastasis)	Negative IHC (skin metastasis)	Positive IHC (primary tumor)
1	Keane J et al. (1980)	Yes	Ultrastructural neuroendocrine features	Negative special stains (PAS, mucicarmine, Sevier-Munger, Masson-Fontana)	N/A
2	Archer CB et al. (1985)	Yes; ↑5-HIAA	N/A	N/A	N/A
3	Rodriguez G et al. (1992)	Yes (H&E, PAS)	CgA, S-100, NSE; mild argyrophilia	N/A	N/A
4	Fogaça MF et al. (1993)	Yes (scalp nodule)	NSE, CAM5.2, CK AE1/AE3, SYN (focal)	LCA, S-100, vimentin, bombesin	NSE, CAM5.2, CK AE1/AE3, SYN (focal)
5	Schmidt U et al. (1994)	N/A	CK, CgA, NSE	N/A	CK, CgA, NSE
6	Yoshimasu T et al. (2001)	Yes	CgA, SYN, NSE, CK20 (partial)	S-100, CD57	Similar to skin
7	Ottinetti A et al. (2003)	Yes	CgA, NSE, SYN, low-MW CK, pan-CK	N/A	Similar (lower mitoses)
8	Bachmeyer C et al. (2004)	Yes	NSE, SYN, CgA	LCA, vimentin, S-100, CK7/20	N/A
9	Vidulich KA et al. (2007)	Yes	CgA, SYN	TTF-1, EGFR, HER2	N/A
10	Santi R et al. (2008)	Yes	CK AE1/3, CAM5.2, CgA, SYN; NSE/CK7 (weak)	CD56, CK20, TTF-1	Similar (low mitoses)
11	Puri PK et al. (2008)	Yes	CK MNF116, CgA, SYN	CK7, CK20, EMA, S-100	N/A
12	Lee WJ et al. (2009)	Yes	CD56, NSE; SYN/CgA (weak)	CK20, somatostatin	N/A
13	Blochin E et al. (2010)	Yes	CK AE1/3, CAM5.2, CK7, TTF-1, CgA, NSE, CD56	CK903, CK20, GCDFP-15	Similar
14	Jedrych J et al. (2011)—Case 1	Yes	CgA, TTF-1, CK AE1/3	CK20	N/A
15	Jedrych J et al. (2011)—Case 2	Yes	CgA, CAM5.2, CK7	SYN, TTF-1, CK20	N/A
16	Jedrych J et al. (2011)—Case 3	Yes	CgA, SYN, CAM5.2, CK AE1/3	TTF-1, CDX2, CK20	N/A
17	Jedrych J et al. (2011)—Case 4	Yes	CgA, SYN, CDX2, CAM5.2	TTF-1	N/A

(continued)

18	Donati P et al. (2013)	Yes	CgA, TTF-1, CK7, SYN, NSE, CD56 (focal)	S-100, CK20	CgA, SYN, CD57/56, TTF-1
19	Fluehler C et al. (2013)	Yes	SYN (strong)	CgA, CK7, CK20, NSE	SYN
20	Yuan C et al. (2014)	Yes	CK AE1/3, TTF-1, CD56, SYN, CgA	CK7, napsin, CK20, GATA-3, mammaglobin, CEA	N/A
21	Hong S et al. (2014)	Yes	Pan-CK, CgA, SYN; Ki67 slight	N/A	N/A
22	Amorim GM et al. (2015)	Yes	CgA, SYN; CK20 (focal dot); Ki67 60%	N/A	N/A
23	Wang KR et al. (2016)	Yes	CK, CgA, SYN, HIF-1α, p53, CD56; Ki-67 15%	GLUT-1, p-Akt, PI3K	N/A
24	Linhas R et al. (2018)	Yes	CAM5.2, CgA, SYN, CD56, TTF-1; Ki67 2%	N/A	CAM5.2, CD56, CgA, SYN
25	Dhingra R et al. (2018)	Yes	SYN, CDX2; Ki67 15%	N/A	N/A
26	Munera-Campos M et al. (2019)	Yes	SYN, CgA	PSA, ERG, CK20, AR, cyclin D1, TTF-1	N/A
27	Pathoulas JT et al. (2021)	Yes	CgA, SYN, TTF-1	N/A	N/A
28	Fiorio LM (2021)	Yes	CK (40/48/50/50.6 Golgi pattern), CgA, SYN	TTF-1, CK20	N/A
29	Hobbs MM et al. (2022)—Pt 1	Yes	SYN, INSM1	TTF-1, NF	N/A
30	Hobbs MM et al. (2022)—Pt 2	Yes	CK AE1/3, CK7, CgA, SYN, GATA3, ER	CK5/6, CK20, TTF-1, p63/p40, CDX2, PAX8, NF	N/A
31	Hobbs MM et al. (2022)—Pt 3	Yes	CK AE1/3, CK20 (focal), CgA, SYN, INSM1; Ki67 < 10%	CK7, NF	N/A
32	Hobbs MM et al. (2022)—Pt 4	Yes	CK7, CgA, SYN, p53	CK20, TTF-1, NF	N/A
33	Hobbs MM et al. (2022)—Pt 5	Yes	CK7, CgA, SYN, TTF-1, INSM1	CK20, CDX2, PSA, S-100, NF	N/A
34	Hobbs MM et al. (2022)—Pt 6	Yes	CK AE1/3, CK7, CgA, SYN, TTF-1, INSM1 (focal)	CK20, CDX2, NF	N/A

(continued)

Table 20.1c (continued)

Case number	First author (Year)	Biopsy performed	Positive IHC (skin metastasis)	Negative IHC (skin metastasis)	Positive IHC (primary tumor)
35	Hobbs MM et al. (2022)—Pt 7	Yes	CK AE1/3, CK7, CgA, SYN, INSM1	CK20, TTF-1, CDX2, NF	N/A
36	Hobbs MM et al. (2022)—Pt 8a	Yes	CK7, CgA, SYN, TTF-1, INSM1	CK20, S-100, NF	N/A
37	Hobbs MM et al. (2022)—Pt 8b	Yes	CK7, CgA, SYN, INSM1	CK20, NF	N/A
38	Hobbs MM et al. (2022)—Pt 9	Yes	CK AE1/3, CK20 (focal), CgA, SYN, CD56, CDX2, INSM1 (focal)	CK5/6, CK7, TTF-1, p63/p40, NF	N/A
39	Hobbs MM et al. (2022)—Pt 10	Yes	CK AE1/3, SYN	CK7, CK20, CD56, TTF-1, S-100, NF, INSM1	N/A
40	Hobbs MM et al. (2022)—Pt 11	Yes	CK AE1/3, CK7, CgA, SYN, TTF-1, INSM1	p63/p40, ER, PAX8, NF	N/A
41	Hobbs MM et al. (2022)—Pt 12	Yes	CK AE1/3, CK7, CgA, SYN, CD56, TTF-1, INSM1	CK20, p63/p40, NF	N/A
42	Hobbs MM et al. (2022)—Pt 13	Yes	SYN	CK7, CK20, CgA, p63/p40, NF, INSM1	N/A
43	Hobbs MM et al. (2022)—Pt 14	Yes	CK AE1/3, SYN, TTF-1, INSM1	CK7, CK20, PSA, NF	N/A

Selected reported cases of cutaneous metastases from neuroendocrine tumors (NETs): biopsy performance and immunohistochemical profile of skin metastases and primary tumors

Abbreviations: *IHC* immunohistochemistry, *CgA* chromogranin A, *SYN* synaptophysin, *NSE* neuron-specific enolase, *CK* cytokeratin, *TTF-1* thyroid transcription factor-1, *INSM1* insulinoma-associated protein 1, *NF* neurofilament, *LCA* leukocyte common antigen, *EMA* epithelial membrane antigen, *EGFR* epidermal growth factor receptor, *HER2* human epidermal growth factor receptor 2, *PSA* prostate-specific antigen, *AR* androgen receptor, *ERG* ETS-related gene, *H&E* hematoxylin and eosin, *PAS* periodic acid–Schiff, *5-HIAA* 5-hydroxyindoleacetic acid, *N/A* not available

Table 20.1d Management and clinical outcomes in skin metastases of neuroendocrine tumours

Case number	First author (Year)	Management	Clinical course	Outcome
1	Keane J et al. (1980)	N/A	Patient deteriorated	N/A
2	Archer CB et al. (1985)	Cyclophosphamide, MTX, lomustine (IV every 3 weeks)	New nodules at 3 months	Deceased (4 month post-skin metastasis)
3	Rodriguez G et al. (1992)	N/A	N/A	Deceased (2 years later)
4	Fogaça MF et al. (1993)	N/A	N/A	N/A
5	Schmidt U et al. (1994)	N/A	N/A	Deceased (33 month post-primary)
6	Yoshimasu T et al. (2001)	Cisplatin + etoposide (3 cycles)	Brain metastases, coma	Deceased (1 month post-op)
7	Ottinetti A et al. (2003)	N/A	Cachexia, heart failure	Deceased (6 months later)
8	Bachmeyer C et al. (2004)	None (died before chemotherapy)	Bone marrow hemorrhage	Deceased (2 weeks later)
9	Vidulich KA et al. (2007)	N/A	N/A	N/A
10	Santi R et al. (2008)	Octreotide	Liver/mediastinum/bone metastases	N/A
11	Puri PK et al. (2008)	N/A	N/A	N/A
12	Lee WJ et al. (2009)	Chemotherapy + radiotherapy	Disseminated metastases	Deceased (2 months later)
13	Blochin E et al. (2010)	N/A	N/A	N/A
14	Jedrych J et al. (2011)—Case 1	N/A	N/A	N/A
15	Jedrych J et al. (2011)—Case 2	N/A	N/A	Alive (60 months with progression)
16	Jedrych J et al. (2011)—Case 3	N/A	N/A	Deceased (36 months later)
17	Jedrych J et al. (2011)—Case 4	N/A	N/A	Alive (24 months with progression)
18	Donati P et al. (2013)	N/A	N/A	N/A
19	Fluehler C et al. (2013)	N/A	N/A	N/A
20	Yuan C et al. (2014)	Intrathecal pump, WBRT, chemotherapy	Poor prognosis	N/A
21	Hong S et al. (2014)	Surgery + chemotherapy (6 cycles)	N/A	N/A
22	Amorim GM et al. (2015)	Irinotecan salvage	Progression	Follow-up ongoing
23	Wang KR et al. (2016)	N/A	N/A	N/A

(continued)

Table 20.1d (continued)

Case number	First author (Year)	Management	Clinical course	Outcome
24	Linhas R et al. (2018)	Carboplatin + etoposide (4 cycles)	N/A	No relapse (12 month follow-up)
25	Dhingra R et al. (2018)	Octreotide → lanreotide	N/A	N/A
26	Munera-Campos M et al. (2019)	Docetaxel → palliative care	Progression	N/A
27	Pathoulas JT et al. (2021)	Palliative	N/A	N/A
28	Fiorio LM (2021)	Oncologist referral	Multi-organ metastases	Deceased (1 month later)
29	Hobbs MM et al. (2022)—Pt 1	N/A	N/A	Alive
30	Hobbs MM et al. (2022)—Pt 2	N/A	N/A	N/A
31	Hobbs MM et al. (2022)—Pt 3	N/A	Hepatic metastases	Deceased
32	Hobbs MM et al. (2022)—Pt 4	N/A	N/A	Deceased
33	Hobbs MM et al. (2022)—Pt 5	N/A	N/A	Deceased
34	Hobbs MM et al. (2022)—Pt 6	N/A	Liver and spine metastases	Deceased
35	Hobbs MM et al. (2022)—Pt 7	N/A	Liver metastases	Deceased
36	Hobbs MM et al. (2022)—Pt 8a	N/A	N/A	Deceased
37	Hobbs MM et al. (2022)—Pt 8b	N/A	N/A	Deceased
38	Hobbs MM et al. (2022)—Pt 9	N/A	N/A	Deceased
39	Hobbs MM et al. (2022)—Pt 10	N/A	Lung/liver/spine metastases + myeloma	Deceased
40	Hobbs MM et al. (2022)—Pt 11	N/A	N/A	Alive
41	Hobbs MM et al. (2022)—Pt 12	N/A	N/A	Deceased
42	Hobbs MM et al. (2022)—Pt 13	N/A	N/A	Deceased
43	Hobbs MM et al. (2022)—Pt 14	N/A	N/A	Deceased

Selected reported cases of cutaneous metastases from neuroendocrine tumors (NETs): therapeutic management, clinical course, and outcomes
Abbreviations: MTX methotrexate, *IV* intravenous, *WBRT* whole brain radiotherapy, *N/A* not available

mate mean of 60 years), with a slight predilection for males (24:16). However, there is no sex-specific predilection for the regions of NET/NEC. The time interval from malignant growth to the development of skin metastases is highly variable. These cases include synchronous (13 cases) ~30%, cases with 3–12 months (~8 cases), cases with more than 5–15 years (cases like: 11 years for atypical carcinoids of lungs and 6.5 years for carcinoids of bronchi), and approximately 40% where time is not estimated [31–40]. Diagnosis is often delayed on account of the heterogeneous clinical appearance of incidental cutaneous metastatic rashes. They present as vascular lesions with benign differentiation. Hence, one needs to have excellent suspicion for patients with NETs/NECs.

20.4 Clinical Characteristics of Skin Metastases Secondary to Neuroendocrine Tumors

Skin metastases of NETs are characterized by erythematous to violaceous papules, nodules, plaques, or subcutaneous masses ranging in size from 0.3 to 4.5 cm [41–50]. They come in either solitary (e.g., 0.5 cm nodule situated on the scalp of a patient having a pulmonary carcinoid) or multiple/numerous lesions (e.g., thighs, forehead, chest of a patient having a NET of an unspecified site). Skin lesions exhibit a wide range of morphologies, including shiny papules with pinkish-brown speckles, exophytic lesions of vascular nature, erosive yet elevated lesions, and lesions variably arranged in a linear pattern.

Lesions are painless, but they may vary from mild to severe pain. Pain occurs because of rapid growth, erosion, and vasoactive peptides such as serotonin, 5-hydroxyindoleacetic acid (5-HIAA), and kallikrein. For instance, they may present with extremely painful alopecia of the scalp, painful lesions in the thighs, or pain-free scalp lesions associated with areas of alopecia.

Cutaneous involvement may appear at any location and commonly follows lymphatic or vascular channels from their primary site:

- Pulmonary/large-cell neuroendocrine carcinoma (LCNEC)/SCLC
- Laryngeal NECs: chest
- Gastrointestinal (such as the ileum): breast
- Pelvic/utérine NECs
- Head/neck lesions (sinus primaries)

Examples include confluent lesions of the breast, umbilicus, and flank in small-cell uterine carcinoid, aggressive and erythematous scalp/axillary lesions of cervical NEC following surgery, and violaceous lesions of the flank in pulmonary carcinoid (Table 20.1). These skin manifestations may take anywhere from a week to a few months or more to become apparent or may be chronic for up to a year, sometimes ulcerating or showing erythema and edema. They may be mistaken for vascular neoplasms like angiosarcoma, inflammatory dermatoses like erythema nodosum, or adnexal lesions because of their clinical presentation.

20.5 Diagnosis

The diagnosis of cutaneous NET/NEC metastases is firmly made through a skin biopsy and immunohistopathological verification of dermal and/or subcutaneous infiltration with monomorphic NET/NEC tumor cells: small round/oval basaloid cells with low cytoplasmic volume, high nucleus-to-cytoplasm ratio, salt-and-pepper nuclei, and low or high mitotic indices (rare in carcinoids and high in NECs) [51–65]. The main histological patterns of metastases include nodular (usually most common; for instance, tough thigh/scalp lesions), infiltrative (confluent lesions of pubic regions), sheet-like, and intravascular patterns; moreover, aggressive morphological patterns of necrosis, crush effects, organoid nesting, and trabecular growth patterns of necrosis or argyrophilia may occur in aggressive lesions. Another decisive differentiation is against Merkel cell.

The diagnosis is definitively established by a skin biopsy with immunohistopathologic examination, which classically demonstrates dermal or subcutaneous infiltration by tumor cells of neuroendocrine morphology, small, round, or oval cells with scant cytoplasm and frequent mitoses. Four major histologic patterns are described: nodular, infiltrative, diffuse, and intravascular. Immunohistochemical confirmation of neuroendocrine differentiation and the distinction of metastatic neuroendocrine tumors from Merkel cell carcinoma, a primary cutaneous neuroendocrine carcinoma, are important. Useful markers include synaptophysin, chromogranin, CD56, CK7, CK20, and thyroid transcription factor-1 (TTF-1). Cytokeratin 20 (CK20) is usually negative in non-cutaneous neuroendocrine metastasis, whereas TTF-1 may be positive in both pulmonary and some extrapulmonary primaries. A panel approach is advocated since no single marker has specificity for the site of origin.

Clinical correlation and radiologic imaging studies (CT, PET, or MRI) are necessary for the detection of the primary tumor and other sites of metastatic disease. Molecular profiling and somatostatin receptor imaging, such as Gallium-DOTATATE PET-CT, may be performed in selected cases for further tumor characterization to inform management.

20.6 Histopathology

Histopathologically, cutaneous metastases of neuroendocrine tumors (NETs) usually show nodular, dermal, and occasionally subcutaneous infiltrates of rather monomorphic small- to medium-sized basaloid tumor cells. The overlying epidermis is typically uninvolved or atrophic, and epidermotropism is exceptional. Neoplastic cells can infiltrate the subcutaneous fat in the shape of a well defined, unencapsulated nodule or in a diffuse pattern along the septa of the connective tissue.

There can be various architectural patterns, such as the organoid, trabecular, nested, or sheet-like pattern, according to the growth pattern of the main tumor. Organoid nesting with palisading at the periphery or rossette formation can be observed in well-differentiated NETs, and the diffuse pattern or solid sheets can be observed in poorly differentiated and high-grade neuroendocrine carcinomas. There may be necrosis or apoptosis, predominantly in the highly aggressive tumors, due to the cytological fragility related to the small-cell morphology.

Tumor cells are characterized by a high N/C ratio, round to oval nuclei having finely stippled chromatin patterns described variably as "salt-and-pepper" chromatin, and inconspicuous nucleoli. The cytoplasm is small in amount and amphophilic, but more prominent and eosinophilic cytoplasm has also been observed in atypical carcinoid or large-cell variants of NEC. There may be variable numbers of mitoses/Ki-67 labeling index. Lymphatic infiltration/vascular invasion has also been observed, thus supporting hematogenous/lymphatic routes of spread, described above.

In some instances, the morphology may be very similar to Merkel cell carcinoma and/or metastatic small-cell carcinoma. Other possibilities in the histological differential diagnosis may include small round-cell metastatic sarcomas (for example, Ewing's sarcoma) and basaloid adnexal tumors. However, the presence of neuroendocrine cellular differentiation and immunoprofile helps to establish a diagnosis.

20.7 Immunohistochemistry

Immunohistochemistry studies provide an essential function in identifying neuroendocrine differentiation and also help determine the primary site of metastasis.

Neuroendocrine markers that are always expressed include:

- *Chromogranin A (CgA)*—a specific marker for dense-core neurosecretory granules
- *Synaptophysin (SYN)*—marker with high sensitivity for presynaptic terminals
- *CD56 (neural cell adhesion molecule) and neuron-specific enolase (NSE)*—supportive but not very specific markers of neuroendocrine differentiation.
- *Insulinoma-associated protein 1 (INSM1)*—a relatively newer nuclear marker that is quite

sensitive and specific for neuroendocrine tumors and shows diffuse positivity in both NETs and NECs.

The pattern of cytoplasmic keratin expression is also very helpful. The great majority of metastatic neuroendocrine tumors are CK7+/CK20–, while Merkel cell carcinomas are CK20+/CK7–, with a characteristic paranuclear dot-like staining.

Positivity for TTF-1 (thyroid transcription factor 1) may be suggestive of a lung or mediastinal primary malignancy; however, it may be rarely observed in extrapulmonary NECs. Positivity for CDX2 may help differentiate the intestinal origin. GATA3, ER, and PR positivity may be observed in neuroendocrine carcinomas of breast origin. Positivity for Prostate-Specific Antigen (PSA)/(NK3 Homeobox 1) NKX3.1 may be suggestive of a prostatic primary malignancy. Positivity for Paired Box Gene 8 (PAX8) may help indicate a renal, thyroid, or gynecologic primary cancer.

Ki-67 LI (Labeling Index) retains its importance to a great extent in the grading system. Values <20% may be observed in well-differentiated NETs, whereas poorly differentiated NECs may have values exceeding 50–90% in most cases with skin metastases, which correlate with a rapid clinical course (Table 20.1).

There were instances where insulinoma-associated protein 1(INSM1), TTF-1, and chromogranin A expression levels in the skin lesions reflected expression levels in the main tumor, thereby attesting to their metastatic source. Also, the absence of protein expression of Alpha-Thalassemia/Mental Retardation, X-linked (ATRX) or Death Domain Associated Protein (DAXX), when assessed, can be indicative of a pancreatic or well-differentiated NET, whereas p53 expression, along with the absence of RB1 expression, depicts a high-grade NEC.

As a result, integration of morphologic, immunophenotypic, and clinical data is required for accurate diagnoses and classification. A broad IHC profile, including both neuroendocrine and lineage-specific markers, is still considered the standard to use to differentiate metastatic NETs from morphologic mimics and to determine their site of origin, especially where skin metastasis is evident before or instead of the primary lesion.

20.8 Molecular Characteristics and Prognostic Biomarkers of Neuroendocrine Tumors

Molecular profiling of neuroendocrine neoplasms has revealed profound genetic and immunohistochemical heterogeneity that underpins their clinical behavior, therapeutic responsiveness, and metastatic potential, including spread to the skin. Well-differentiated neuroendocrine tumors and poorly differentiated neuroendocrine carcinomas represent distinct biological entities with separate molecular pathways of oncogenesis.

Poorly differentiated NECs often contain biallelic inactivation of tumor suppressor genes, including TP53 and RB1, combined with oncogenic alterations of MYC, KRAS, BRAF, and the PI3K–AKT–mTOR pathway. These molecular derangements promote uncontrolled proliferation, loss of cell-cycle regulation, and resistance to apoptosis, in keeping with the aggressive clinical course and short survival usually reported in patients with cutaneous metastases from small-cell or large-cell NECs reflected in Table 20.1. NECs generally exhibit high TMB and a high neoantigen load, but paradoxically often escape immune surveillance owing to LOH at loci encoding antigen presentation, leading to low responses to immune checkpoint blockade.

The malignant phenotype of poorly differentiated NETs contrasts with the more indolent molecular phenotype of well-differentiated NETs, which typically harbor mutations that affect MEN1, DAXX, ATRX, and TSC2 regulation of chromatin remodeling, telomere maintenance, and mTOR signaling. These alterations confer slower tumor kinetics and correlate with prolonged survival occasionally seen in patients with solitary or late-appearing skin metastases from typical or atypical carcinoids. SSTR2 expression and intact ATRX/DAXX protein expression support a well-differentiated phenotype and predict a favorable response to somatostatin analogs and PRRT.

Recent high-throughput analyses have identified a seven-gene expression prognostic signature (MLH3, NACA, NOTCH1, NPAP1, RANBP17, TSC2, and ZFHX4), the alterations of which are strongly predictive of poorer overall survival. Further dysregulation of the Notch and TSC2/mTOR pathways further delineates aggressive molecular subgroups and can also be considered targeted therapeutic options. Although uncommon, BRAF V600E mutations have recently been increasingly recognized in Grade 3 NETs and NECs and do represent a potentially actionable therapeutic target.

The Ki-67 proliferation index and mitotic count remain key histological surrogates of proliferative activity and are central to the 2022 WHO classification of NENs. However, for cases in which morphology or proliferation indices are indeterminate, molecular indices derived from NGS studies add an important layer of precision. Integration of immunohistochemical markers, namely TP53, RB1, SSTR2, INSM1, and Ki-67, with targeted NGS panels now allows not only for the accurate subclassification of high-grade lesions but also for the identification of putative therapeutic vulnerabilities.

In the context of cutaneous metastases, molecular testing provides critical diagnostic and prognostic information that allows confirmation of tumor origin, distinction from Merkel cell carcinoma or other small-cell malignancies, and determination of systemic therapy options. In many reported cases, skin metastases'immunohistochemical profiles mirrored that of the primary tumor, underlining clonal stability across metastatic sites.

The integration of genomic, transcriptomic, and epigenetic markers into clinical practice will increase diagnostic precision, further stratify prognosis, and allow for personalized therapies. Ultimately, the merging of molecular profiling and clinicopathological data has the prospect of improving patient outcomes for individuals affected by NETs and their infrequent yet important appearance as skin metastasis.

20.9 Mode of Spread

Metastasis of neuroendocrine tumors to the skin can occur by the hematogenous, lymphatic, or, less often, direct extension route. Of the various routes, hematogenous spread can be regarded as the most common, given the highly vascular nature of neuroendocrine tumors. The pattern of metastasis is in agreement with the presentation of many patients having skin metastases as a series of separate nodules, randomly distributed, often distant from the area of the primary lesion, on the scalp, chest, back, and legs.

By contrast, lymphatic spread would be implicated where the skin lesions are seen in a linear or grouped distribution, occasionally along dermal lymphatic channels. There have also been a few instances of a grouped or regional distribution, especially in the neck, axillary, or inguinal regions, presumably secondary involvement of skin lymph drainage routes, in addition to the possibility of being confined, as seen in a few instances of skin primaries, especially where the underlying organs have thoracic or pelvic involvement.

The skin distribution patterns may be related to the primary tumor site and the favored route of metastatic spread. For example, pulmonary/mediastinal NETs typically metastasize to the head, neck, or back of the upper body because of hematogenous or lymphatic spread to these areas via the superior vena cava or thoracic duct. On the other hand, gastrointestinal or pelvic NETs metastasize to the lower abdominal or perineal areas because of spread via the lymphatic system or the portal lymphatic system to the abdominal or perineal regions.

In several patients, skin metastasis appeared simultaneously with extensive visceral disease, thus confirming that skin metastasis can be a late phase of tumor spread. However, in a few patients, skin metastasis appeared to be the initial presentation of an occult NET, thus demonstrating a possible initial selective vascular spread to the skin.

The underlying biological processes for cutaneous metastasis of NETS are still poorly understood. Some of these processes may include adhesion of tumor cells to the cutaneous microvasculature, activation of particular integrins/chemokine receptors, and a favorable cutaneous vascular background for implantation of tumor cell dissemination.

In conclusion, it is evident that the lymphatic or hematogenous spread is also involved in the distribution of NETS in the skin. This can be inferred based on the distribution pattern of the skin involvement depending on the location of the malignancy. This is also very important in the diagnosis and staging in relation to the presentation of the malignancy in the skin.

20.10 Differential Diagnosis

Distinction from other cutaneous neuroendocrine neoplasms and mimickers is key:

- Merkel cell carcinoma (MCC) is positive for CK20, usually displaying a dot-like immunoreactivity pattern, negative for CK7, and does not have hormone receptors.
- Cutaneous lymphomas are negative for keratin and neuroendocrine markers but are positive for leukocyte common antigen.
- Variants of basal cell Ca may be BerEP4+ but negative for ER/PR and neuroendocrine markers.
- Metastatic small-cell carcinoma of the lung has similar neuroendocrine features but is predominantly TTF-1 positive.

20.11 Management

Management of skin metastases in NET is a combined approach based on the extent of systemic disease involvement and the grade of malignancy. Skin metastases indicate the dissemination of the disease and are generally palliative in nature.

1. Local Management
   - Surgical intervention can be considered in cases of isolated or symptomatic cutaneous metastatic disease. In diseases that are limited and accessible, complete resection can offer diagnostic confirmations and locoregional control.
   - Radiotherapy can be used to palliate painful or bleeding lesions. It can be given as an adjuvant following removal for patients presenting with limited metastases.
2. Systemic Therapy
   - Hormone analogs of somatostatin, such as octreotide and Lanreotide, are administered habitually in well-differentiated NETs. This may control the growth of the tumors and symptoms.

   Radioligand therapy in the form of PRRT with radiolabeled somatostatin analogs such as 177Lu-dotatate has achieved established efficacy in
   - For targeted therapies, everolimus (mTOR inhibitor) or sunitinib (tyrosine kinase inhibitor) could be considered in advanced pancreatic and gastrointestinal NETs.

   Chemotherapy, usually platinum-etoposide, is indicated only in cases of poorly differentiated and small-cell neuroendocrine carcinomas. These are aggressive, highly progressive tumors.
   - Immunotherapy: It is investigational but shows some hope in selected aggressive cases.
3. Supportive Care

Control of pain, treatment of the wound, and psychosocial support continue to be important aspects of care. Ulcerating or bleeding skin lesions may call for hemostatic agents or low-dose radiotherapy.

Given the tendency for cutaneous metastases to be associated with widespread systemic disease, it is most appropriate that the treatment plan be discussed in a multidisciplinary conference including dermatology, oncology, nuclear medicine, and palliative care. Intensive multimodality therapy can be effective in those with limited disease and good performance status.

20.12 Prognosis

Cutaneous metastasis from a neuroendocrine tumor (NET) generally signifies advanced disease and poor prognosis. Review of the published cases indicates that most patients succumbed within a few months after the appearance of skin lesions, although survival up to 2 to 3 years has been reported in some cases of well-differentiated or atypical carcinoids. The median survival after the diagnosis of cutaneous metastasis typically ranges from several weeks to less than 2 years, depending largely on tumor differentiation, extent of systemic disease, and response to therapy.

Patients with poorly differentiated or small-cell neuroendocrine carcinomas experienced rapid progression and early mortality, often within weeks to months. In contrast, those with typical or atypical carcinoids, particularly of pulmonary or ileal origin, occasionally demonstrated a more indolent course, with some patients remaining alive or stable beyond 1 year of follow-up. Overall, the occurrence of cutaneous metastasis is considered a late manifestation of disseminated NET, reflecting limited curative options and generally unfavorable outcomes.

20.13 Conclusion

In conclusion, cutaneous metastasis of neuroendocrine tumors, though rare, serves as a clinically significant indicator of disseminated disease. Awareness of this manifestation, combined with accurate histopathological and immunohistochemical evaluation, is essential for correct diagnosis and staging. As advances in systemic management continue to extend survival in patients with NETs, clinicians may encounter cutaneous involvement with increasing frequency, underscoring the importance of multidisciplinary evaluation and individualized treatment strategies.

References

1. Shah MH, Goldner WS, Benson AB, Bergsland E, Blaszkowsky LS, Brock P, Chan J, Das S, Dickson PV, Fanta P, Giordano T, Halfdanarson TR, Halperin D, He J, Heaney A, Heslin MJ, Kandeel F, Kardan A, Khan SA, Kuvshinoff BW, Lieu C, Miller K, Pillarisetty VG, Reidy D, Salgado SA, Shaheen S, Soares HP, Soulen MC, Strosberg JR, Sussman CR, Trikalinos NA, Uboha NA, Vijayvergia N, Wong T, Lynn B, Hochstetler C. Neuroendocrine and adrenal tumors, version 2.2021, NCCN Clinical Practice Guidelines in Oncology. J Natl Compr Canc Netw. 2021;19(7):839–68. https://doi.org/10.6004/jnccn.2021.0032. PMID: 34340212.
2. Klöppel G. Classification and pathology of gastroenteropancreatic neuroendocrine neoplasms. Endocr Relat Cancer. 2011;18(Suppl 1):S1–16. https://doi.org/10.1530/ERC-11-0013. Print 2011 Oct. PMID: 22005112.
3. Gheorghişan-Gălăţeanu AA, Ilieşiu A, Lambrescu IM, Ţăpoi DA. The complex histopathological and immunohistochemical spectrum of neuroendocrine tumors-an overview of the latest classifications. Int J Mol Sci. 2023;24(2):1418. https://doi.org/10.3390/ijms24021418. PMID: 36674939.
4. Loree JM, Chan D, Lim J, Stuart H, Fidelman N, Koea J, Posavad J, Cummins M, Doucette S, Myrehaug S, Naraev B, Bailey DL, Bellizzi A, Laidley D, Boyle V, Goodwin R, Del Rivero J, Michael M, Pasieka J, Singh S. Biomarkers to inform prognosis and treatment for unresectable or metastatic GEP-NENs. JAMA Oncol. 2024;10(12):1707–20. https://doi.org/10.1001/jamaoncol.2024.4330. PMID: 39361298.
5. Sun BL, Ding H, Sun X. Histopathologic and genetic distinction of well-differentiated grade 3 neuroendocrine tumor versus poorly-differentiated neuroendocrine carcinoma in high-grade neuroendocrine neoplasms. Am J Clin Pathol. 2025;163(6):804–14. https://doi.org/10.1093/ajcp/aqaf013. PMID: 40037757.
6. Rindi G, Inzani F. Differentiation versus grade for pancreatic neuroendocrine neoplasms. Arch Pathol Lab Med. 2025; https://doi.org/10.5858/arpa.2024-0410-RA. Online ahead of print. PMID: 40031961.
7. Tang H, Xia H, Sun N, Hernandez PV, Wang M, Adeniran AJ, Cai G. Selection of neuroendocrine markers in diagnostic workup of neuroendocrine neoplasms: the real-world data and machine learning model algorithms. Cancer Cytopathol. 2025;133(5):e70018. https://doi.org/10.1002/cncy.70018. PMID: 40289395.

8. Sultana Q, Kar J, Verma A, Sanghvi S, Kaka N, Patel N, Sethi Y, Chopra H, Kamal MA, Greig NH. A comprehensive review on neuroendocrine neoplasms: presentation, pathophysiology and management. J Clin Med. 2023;12(15):5138. https://doi.org/10.3390/jcm12155138. PMID: 37568540.
9. Hussein MR. Skin metastasis: a pathologist's perspective. J Cutan Pathol. 2010;37(9):e1–20. https://doi.org/10.1111/j.1600-0560.2009.01469.x. Epub 2009 Nov 17. PMID: 19922483.
10. Kamińska-Winciorek G, Pilśniak A, Piskorski W, Wydmański J. Skin metastases in the clinical and dermoscopic aspects. Semin Oncol. 2022;49(2):160–9. https://doi.org/10.1053/j.seminoncol.2022.04.005. Epub 2022 May 3. PMID: 35589424.
11. Keane J, Fretzin DF, Jao W, Shapiro CM. Bronchial carcinoid metastatic to skin. Light and electron microscopic findings. J Cutan Pathol. 1980;7(1):43–9. https://doi.org/10.1111/j.1600-0560.1980.tb00976.x. PMID: 7358881.
12. Archer CB, Wells RS, MacDonald DM. Metastatic cutaneous carcinoid. J Am Acad Dermatol. 1985;13(2 Pt 2):363–6. https://doi.org/10.1016/s0190-9622(85)70175-2. PMID: 2993380.
13. Sicsic JC, Moulin G, Vetter A, Lalo M, Bussone M. Cutaneous metastasis revealing carcinoid tumor in a 82-year-old patient. J Chir (Paris). 1989;126(12):699. PMID: 2621238.
14. Rodriguez G, Villamizar R. Carcinoid tumor with skin metastasis. Am J Dermatopathol. 1992;14(3):263–9. https://doi.org/10.1097/00000372-199206000-00014. PMID: 1510225.
15. Fogaça MF, Fedorciw BJ, Tahan SR, Johnson R, Federman M. Cutaneous metastasis of neuroendocrine carcinoma of uterine origin. J Cutan Pathol. 1993;20(5):455–8. https://doi.org/10.1111/j.1600-0560.1993.tb00671.x. PMID: 8300931.
16. Schmidt U, Metz KA, Schrader M, Leder LD. Well-differentiated (oncocytoid) neuroendocrine carcinoma of the larynx with multiple skin metastases: a brief report. J Laryngol Otol. 1994;108(3):272–4. https://doi.org/10.1017/s0022215100126519. PMID: 8169520.
17. Yoshimasu T, Yamamoto Y, Uede K, Furukawa F. Skin metastasis of neuroendocrine carcinoma derived from the mediastinum. J Dermatol. 2001;28(3):168–71. https://doi.org/10.1111/j.1346-8138.2001.tb00114.x. PMID: 11349471.
18. Ottinetti A, Colombo E, Dardano F, Migliora P, Picciotto F, Zaccagna A, Angeli G. Cutaneous metastasis of neuroendocrine carcinoma of the larynx: report of a case. J Cutan Pathol. 2003;30(8):512–5. https://doi.org/10.1034/j.1600-0560.2003.00062.x. PMID: 12950503.
19. Bachmeyer C, Henni AM, Cazier A, Putterman M, Morel X. Eyelid metastases indicating neuroendocrine carcinoma of unknown origin. Eye (Lond). 2004;18(1):94–5. https://doi.org/10.1038/sj.eye.6700545. PMID: 14707982.
20. Bell HK, Poston GJ, Vora J, Wilson NJ. Cutaneous manifestations of the malignant carcinoid syndrome. Br J Dermatol. 2005;152(1):71–5. https://doi.org/10.1111/j.1365-2133.2004.06273.x. PMID: 15656803.
21. Vidulich KA, Donley SE, Duvic M. Multinodular cutaneous spread in neuroendocrine tumor of the breast : an unusual presentation. Am J Clin Dermatol. 2007;8(6):379–83. https://doi.org/10.2165/00128071-200708060-00008. PMID: 18039021.
22. Santi R, Massi D, Mazzoni F, Antonuzzo L, Comin CE. Skin metastasis from typical carcinoid tumor of the lung. J Cutan Pathol. 2008;35(4):418–22. https://doi.org/10.1111/j.1600-0560.2007.00822.x. PMID: 18333904.
23. Puri PK, Galan A, Glusac EJ, Cowper SE. Metastatic cutaneous carcinoid tumor mimicking an adnexal poroid neoplasm. J Cutan Pathol. 2008;35(1):54–7. https://doi.org/10.1111/j.1600-0560.2007.00755.x. PMID: 18095995.
24. Lee WJ, Lee DW, Lee MW, Choi JH, Moon KC, Koh JK. Multiple cutaneous metastases of neuroendocrine carcinoma derived from the uterine cervix. J Eur Acad Dermatol Venereol. 2009;23(4):494–6. https://doi.org/10.1111/j.1468-3083.2008.02955.x. PMID: 19335736.
25. Blochin E, Stein JA, Wang NS. Atypical carcinoid metastasis to the skin. Am J Dermatopathol. 2010;32(7):735–9. https://doi.org/10.1097/DAD.0b013e3181d4d0fb. PMID: 20595888.
26. Donati P, Panetta C, Cota C, Paolino G, Muscardin L. Carcinoid metastasis of the skin appearing as painful tumor. J Dermatol. 2013;40(5):415–7. https://doi.org/10.1111/1346-8138.12084. Epub 2013 Feb 18. PMID: 23414140.
27. Fluehler C, Quaranta L, di Meo N, Ulessi B, Trevisan G. Cutaneous metastasis of neuroendocrine carcinoma. Indian J Dermatol. 2013;58(3):247. https://doi.org/10.4103/0019-5154.110890. PMID: 23723522.
28. Jedrych J, Busam K, Klimstra DS, Pulitzer M. Cutaneous metastases as an initial manifestation of visceral well-differentiated neuroendocrine tumor: a report of four cases and a review of literature. J Cutan Pathol. 2014;41(2):113–22. https://doi.org/10.1111/cup.12263. Epub 2013 Dec 3. PMID: 24218988.
29. Yuan C, Keating B, Farricielli LA, Zhang K. Large-cell neuroendocrine carcinoma (LCNEC) without pulmonary symptoms diagnosed in a cutaneous metastasis. Am J Case Rep. 2014;15:97–102. https://doi.org/10.12659/AJCR.890094. eCollection 2014. PMID: 24624250.
30. Hong S, Li L, Liu X, Tu C. Neuroendocrine carcinoma of the larynx with subcutaneous and intramus-

cular metastases: a case report. Int J Clin Exp Pathol. 2014;7(11):8217–22. eCollection 2014. PMID: 25550875.
31. Cohen JM, Nambudiri VE, Kulke MH, Todd DJ, Murphy GF, LeBoeuf NR. Cutaneous paraneoplastic granulomatous eruptions secondary to metastatic carcinoid tumour. Br J Dermatol. 2015;172(5):1451–4. https://doi.org/10.1111/bjd.13516. Epub 2015 Mar 27. PMID: 25388104.
32. Assi HA, Patel R, Mehdi S. Neuroendocrine carcinoma of the larynx with metastasis to the eyelid. J Community Support Oncol. 2015;13(10):378–80. https://doi.org/10.12788/jcso.0165. PMID: 26862914.
33. Amorim GM, Quintella D, Cuzzi T, Rodrigues R, Ramos-E-Silva M. Cutaneous metastasis of neuroendocrine carcinoma with unknown primary site: case report and review of the literature. Case Rep Dermatol. 2015;7(3):263–74. https://doi.org/10.1159/000440661. eCollection 2015 Sep-Dec. PMID: 26557073.
34. Wang KR, Jia YJ, Zhou SH, Wang QY, Bao YY, Feng ZY, Yao HT, Fan J. Cutaneous and subcutaneous metastases from atypical laryngeal carcinoids: case report and review of the literature. Medicine (Baltimore). 2016;95(7):e2796. https://doi.org/10.1097/MD.0000000000002796. PMID: 26886629.
35. Falto-Aizpurua L, Seyfer S, Krishnan B, Orengo I. Cutaneous metastasis of a pulmonary carcinoid tumor. Cutis. 2017;99(5):E13–5. PMID: 28632813.
36. Linhas R, Tente D, China N, Conde S, Barroso A. Subcutaneous metastasis of a pulmonary carcinoid tumor: a case report. Medicine (Baltimore). 2018;97(2):e9415. https://doi.org/10.1097/MD.0000000000009415. PMID: 29480829.
37. Dhingra R, Tse JY, Saif MW. Cutaneous metastasis of gastroenteropancreatic neuroendocrine tumors (GEP-Nets). JOP. 2018;19(5). http://pancreas.imedpub.com/cutaneous-metastasis-of-gastroenteropancreatic-neuroendocrine-tumors-gepnets.pdf. Epub 2018 Sep 18. PMID: 30405324.
38. Munera-Campos M, Bielsa I, Plana-Pla A, Posada R, Quer A, Ferrándiz C. Cutaneous metastases from prostate cancer revealing neuroendocrine differentiation. J Cutan Pathol. 2019;46(12):976–8. https://doi.org/10.1111/cup.13561. Epub 2019 Aug 27. PMID: 31393629.
39. Pathoulas JT, Flanagan KE, Walker CJ, Ly A, Krajewski KM, Pupo Wiss I, Senna MM. Subcutaneous metastasis from an atypical pulmonary carcinoid tumor. Dermatol Online J. 2021;27(5) https://doi.org/10.5070/D327553613. PMID: 34118814.
40. Fiorio LM, Diniz LM, Lucas EA. Cutaneous metastasis on the nasal tip: first clinical sign of pulmonary carcinoid tumor. An Bras Dermatol. 2021;96(5):578–80. https://doi.org/10.1016/j.abd.2021.03.002. Epub 2021 Jul 18. PMID: 34284938.
41. Hobbs MM, Snow JT, Shachner TR, Sokumbi O. Cutaneous metastases of non-cutaneous neuroendocrine neoplasms: a histopathologic review of 15 cases. J Cutan Pathol. 2022;49(11):960–70. https://doi.org/10.1111/cup.14294. Epub 2022 Aug 15. PMID: 36222210.
42. Filizoglu N, Ozguven S. Skin and subcutaneous tissue metastases of the pulmonary carcinoid tumor on 68 Ga-DOTATATE PET/CT. Clin Nucl Med. 2023;48(11):e554–5. https://doi.org/10.1097/RLU.0000000000004840. Epub 2023 Sep 18. PMID: 37796157.
43. Zuetenhorst JM, Taal BG. Metastatic carcinoid tumors: a clinical review. Oncologist. 2005;10(2):123–31. https://doi.org/10.1634/theoncologist.10-2-123. PMID: 15709214.
44. Cokonis CD, Green JJ, Manders SM. Primary carcinoid tumor of the skin. J Am Acad Dermatol. 2004;51(5 Suppl):S146–8. https://doi.org/10.1016/j.jaad.2004.03.043. PMID: 15577755.
45. Cuthbertson DJ, Shankland R, Srirajaskanthan R. Diagnosis and management of neuroendocrine tumours. Clin Med (Lond). 2023;23(2):119–24. https://doi.org/10.7861/clinmed.2023-0044. PMID: 36958842.
46. Raphael MJ, Chan DL, Law C, Singh S. Principles of diagnosis and management of neuroendocrine tumours. CMAJ. 2017;189(10):E398–404. https://doi.org/10.1503/cmaj.160771. PMID: 28385820.
47. Riihimäki M, Hemminki A, Sundquist K, Sundquist J, Hemminki K. The epidemiology of metastases in neuroendocrine tumors. Int J Cancer. 2016;139(12):2679–86. https://doi.org/10.1002/ijc.30400. Epub 2016 Sep 9. PMID: 27553864.
48. Leventhal JS, Braverman IM. Skin manifestations of endocrine and neuroendocrine tumors. Semin Oncol. 2016;43(3):335–40. https://doi.org/10.1053/j.seminoncol.2016.02.022. Epub 2016 Feb 23. PMID: 27178685.
49. Vernemmen AIP, Li X, Roemen GMJM, Speel EM, Kubat B, Hausen AZ, Winnepenninckx VJL, Samarska IV. Cutaneous metastases of internal malignancies: a single-institution experience. Histopathology. 2022;81(3):329–41. https://doi.org/10.1111/his.14705. Epub 2022 Jul 20. PMID: 35758186.
50. Alcaraz I, Cerroni L, Rütten A, Kutzner H, Requena L. Cutaneous metastases from internal malignancies: a clinicopathologic and immunohistochemical review. Am J Dermatopathol. 2012;34(4):347–93. https://doi.org/10.1097/DAD.0b013e31823069cf. PMID: 22617133.

51. Guanziroli E, Coggi A, Venegoni L, Fanoni D, Ercoli G, Boggio F, Veraldi S, Berti E, Gianotti R, Ferrero S, Del Gobbo A. Cutaneous metastases of internal malignancies: an experience from a single institution. Eur J Dermatol. 2017;27(6):609–14. https://doi.org/10.1684/ejd.2017.3142. PMID: 29160213.
52. Choate EA, Nobori A, Worswick S. Cutaneous metastasis of internal tumors. Dermatol Clin. 2019;37(4):545–54. https://doi.org/10.1016/j.det.2019.05.012. Epub 2019 Jul 10. PMID: 31466594.
53. Johnston MJ, Sachedina A, McDonald JE. A unique case of diffuse metastatic neuroendocrine cancer with subcutaneous nodules on (18)F-Fluorodeoxyglucose positron emission tomography/computer assisted tomography. World J Nucl Med. 2015;14(2):134–6. https://doi.org/10.4103/1450-1147.154232. PMID: 26097426.
54. Zhou N, Wang F, Yang L, Wang Q, Liu J, Chen Y. Primary high-grade neuroendocrine carcinoma with positive steroid hormone receptors arising in the inguinal skin: a case report of an exceedingly rare entity. Medicine (Baltimore). 2023;102(50):e36624. https://doi.org/10.1097/MD.0000000000036624. PMID: 38115331.
55. Chen TY, Morrison AO, Susa J, Cockerell CJ. Primary low-grade neuroendocrine carcinoma of the skin: an exceedingly rare entity. J Cutan Pathol. 2017;44(11):978–81. https://doi.org/10.1111/cup.13028. Epub 2017 Sep 4. PMID: 28815668.
56. Muntaner-Virgili C, Boronat-Cucarull J, Ferreres JR, Gamissans M, Marcoval J, Fernández-Calvo D, Penín RM, Bermejo J, Huesa-Barceló L, Manzano-Mora S, Ruzafa-Martínez E, Bajen-Lázaro MT, Benítez-Segura A, Notta PC, Jiménez-Colomo L, Martín-Liberal J, Araguas-Mora P, Juárez-Lozano M, Linares-Galiana I. Distant metastasis of Merkel cell carcinoma: a descriptive study. Dermatol Pract Concept. 2025;15(3):5134. https://doi.org/10.5826/dpc.1503a5134. PMID: 40790416.
57. Rekhi B, Saxena S, Chintamani. Gastric outlet obstruction and cutaneous metastasis in adenocarcinoid tumor of stomach - unusual presentations with cytologic and ultra structural findings. Indian J Cancer. 2005;42(2):99–101. https://doi.org/10.4103/0019-509x.16700. PMID: 16141510.
58. Wick MR, Millns JL, Sibley RK, Pittelkow MR, Winkelmann RK. Secondary neuroendocrine carcinomas of the skin. An immunohistochemical comparison with primary neuroendocrine carcinoma of the skin ("Merkel cell" carcinoma). J Am Acad Dermatol. 1985;13(1):134–42. https://doi.org/10.1016/s0190-9622(85)70155-7. PMID: 3161911.
59. Tasto O, Raitio A, Losty PD. Management and outcomes of pediatric neuroendocrine tumors - a systematic review of published studies. Eur J Surg Oncol. 2025;51(10):110388. https://doi.org/10.1016/j.ejso.2025.110388. Online ahead of print. PMID: 40819413.
60. McCrary MR, Garcia R, Jiang J, Morgan MB. Histopathologic and immunophenotypic properties of primary cutaneous large cell neuroendocrine carcinomas. J Cutan Pathol. 2025; https://doi.org/10.1111/cup.14853. Online ahead of print. PMID: 40887431.
61. Negris OR, Aqeel JA, Chan MP, Harms KL, Pedersen EA. A rare case of sweat gland carcinoma of the scalp with neuroendocrine differentiation: primary cutaneous malignancy versus breast cancer metastasis. JAAD Case Rep. 2025;65:183–6. https://doi.org/10.1016/j.jdcr.2025.07.014. eCollection 2025 Nov. PMID: 41143220.
62. Laschinger ME, Naga L, Gaspari AA. Cutaneous metastases of pancreatic neuroendocrine carcinoma. G Ital Dermatol Venereol. 2018;153(5):722–4. https://doi.org/10.23736/S0392-0488.17.05103-3. PMID: 30246953.
63. Liu M, Li N, Tang H, Chen L, Liu X, Wang Y, Lin Y, Luo Y, Wei S, Wen W, Chen M, Wang J, Zhang N, Chen J. The mutational, prognostic, and therapeutic landscape of neuroendocrine neoplasms. Oncologist. 2023;28(9):e723–36. https://doi.org/10.1093/oncolo/oyad093. PMID: 37086484.
64. Bodei L, Schöder H, Baum RP, Herrmann K, Strosberg J, Caplin M, Öberg K, Modlin IM. Molecular profiling of neuroendocrine tumours to predict response and toxicity to peptide receptor radionuclide therapy. Lancet Oncol. 2020;21(9):e431–43. https://doi.org/10.1016/S1470-2045(20)30323-5. PMID: 32888472.
65. Wee K, Yang KC, Schaeffer DF, Zhou C, Leung E, Feng X, Laskin J, Marra MA, Loree JM, Gorski SM. Genomic and transcriptomic landscapes of metastatic neuroendocrine neoplasms from distinct primary sites and their clinical implications. Sci Rep. 2025;15(1):15770. https://doi.org/10.1038/s41598-025-00549-7. PMID: 40328872.

Part IX

Skin Metastasis from Unknown Primary Tumours

21 Skin Metastases of Unknown Primary Tumors

Eirini Kyrmanidou and Elizabeth Lazaridou

Abstract

Management of a cutaneous metastasis exhibits great difficulty, let alone cutaneous metastases from an unknown primary tumor. The identification of a cutaneous metastasis is of high importance since it is an indication of increased oncogenic burden. Internal malignancies that often metastasise to the skin include breast, lung, and colon cancer. Skin metastases show morphological variation and can present as rapidly growing solitary or multiple papules, nodules, indurated plaques, or ulcers. Through histopathological examination and carefully selected immunohistochemical stains, the site of the primary tumor can be suspected.

Keywords

Skin metastasis · Unknown primary tumor · Cutaneous metastasis

E. Kyrmanidou (✉) · E. Lazaridou
Second Dermatology Department, School of Health Sciences, Aristotle University of Thessaloniki, Thessaloniki, Greece
e-mail: bethlaz@auth.gr

21.1 Introduction

Management of a cutaneous metastasis exhibits great difficulty, let alone cutaneous metastases from an unknown primary tumor. Often, the first question to be answered is whether the tumor is a primary cutaneous neoplasm or a metastasis from a visceral malignancy. The identification of a cutaneous metastasis is of high importance since it is an indication of increased oncogenic burden. Cutaneous metastasis has been identified in between 0.7% and 10% of cancer patients according to various case series [1, 2]. Skin metastases often present unique challenges and opportunities in the clinical setting, as they can be detected earlier than metastatic lesions in other organs. This early detection emphasizes the importance for clinicians to be alert in recognizing the diverse appearances of skin metastases. Through careful pathology examination, valuable insights into the probable origin of the primary tumor can be gleaned. Histological analysis serves as a cornerstone in this process, offering a deeper understanding of the tumor's characteristics and behavior, which can be further enhanced through advanced histological stainings and imaging modalities.

D. Koumaki et al. (eds.), *Cutaneous Metastases*, https://doi.org/10.1007/978-3-032-26764-1_21

21.2 Epidemiology

21.2.1 Incidence

Cutaneous manifestations of internal malignancies encompass a diverse range of skin-related symptoms and conditions. Research indicates that between 0.2% and 9% of patients with cancer develop skin metastases, which frequently correlate with already known primary cancers [3]. Skin metastases from unknown primary tumors are estimated to account for 4.4% of all cases of cutaneous metastases.

The incidence of cutaneous metastases significantly varies among different neoplasms, with metastatic melanoma exhibiting particularly high rates, since up to 45% of melanoma patients develop skin metastases. Excluding melanoma, internal malignancies that often metastasise to the skin include breast, lung, and colon cancer. Metastases from malignant tumors are a common occurrence, particularly near the original site of the primary cancer. Research indicates that the chest is the most frequent location for these secondary tumors, with approximately 32% of metastases found there. The abdomen follows closely behind, accounting for 20% of cases, while the scalp is affected in about 15% of instances. These patterns of spread not only highlight the aggressive nature of certain cancers but also provide valuable clues for identifying the source of the malignancy. One specific area of concern is the umbilical region, which can serve as a key indicator of underlying malignancies, particularly ovarian and genitourinary cancers. The presence of Sister Mary Joseph nodules in this region is particularly orienting, as these tumors arise from cancer that has infiltrated the peritoneum. This phenomenon underscores the importance of thorough clinical evaluation when such nodules are observed, as they may signify advanced metastatic disease. Understanding these patterns is critical for early detection and appropriate management of malignancies, ultimately improving patient outcomes.

In summary, skin metastases can serve as significant indicators of underlying malignancies, highlighting the intricate relationship between internal diseases and their external manifestations. Understanding these interactions is crucial for early detection and management of cancer.

21.2.2 Demographics

Excluding melanoma, lung cancer in men and breast carcinoma in women stand out as the most prevalent origins of skin metastases. These cancers frequently spread to the skin, highlighting the importance of vigilant monitoring for skin changes in patients with these primary malignancies. Lookingbill et al. reported that after reviewing 4020 patients' files, the primary tumor in women with skin metastases had the following distribution: breast (70%), ovary (3.3%), oral cavity (2.3%), lung (2%), and colon (1.3%). Additionally, in men, the distribution was recorded as follows: lung (11.8%), large intestine (11%), oral cavity (8.7%), kidney (4.7%), breast (2.4%), esophagus (2.4%), and pancreas, stomach, and liver with 0.8% each [2, 4]. Incidence rates reported by Marcoval et al. showed similar results for women: breast (66.5%), melanoma (13.4%), colon (3.6%), and head and neck (3.2%). Respectively, for men, the distribution was melanoma (19.1%), head and neck (19.1%), lung (18.3%), and colon (9.5%) [5]. Generally, there is a correlation between the frequency of cutaneous metastases and that of primary cancer in each sex. Hu et al. report the incidence of skin metastases, without referral to sex differences, as follows: breast (36.2%), lung (16.3%), colorectal (11.3%), oral mucosa (7.8%), and gastric (7.1%) [1] (Table 21.1).

Table 21.1 Rates of skin metastases of unknown primary origin from various studies

	No. of patients with metastatic disease	No. of patients with skin metastases	Percentage (%)
Lookingbill [2]	271	20	7.4%
Marcoval [5]	381	20	5.2%
Hu [1]	141	9	6.4%

21.3 Clinical Presentation-Dermoscopical Features

Skin metastases show morphological variation and can present as rapidly growing solitary or multiple papules, nodules, indurated plaques, or ulcers. It is usually not possible to determine the primary tumor from the clinical presentation of a skin metastasis, and in some cases, this is the first sign of internal malignancy. Nonetheless, well-differentiated metastases often show typical morphological characteristics of the primary tumor. Vernemmen et al. recently reported that in male patients with lung or gastrointestinal malignancy, the head and scalp regions were the most common sites of skin metastasis. Whereas, in female breast cancer patients, the anterior chest wall was the most common anatomical site of skin metastasis. Most often, the metastatic skin lesions present within the anatomical region of the primary malignancy. This regional preference of cutaneous metastases is of great significance in evaluating cutaneous metastases of unknown primary origin.

Hu et al. analyzed the characteristics of cutaneous metastases from internal malignancies over 20 years. They report that cutaneous metastasis appeared as a first indicator of malignancy in 13.5% of cases, and the time interval between diagnosis of primary tumor and cutaneous metastasis ranged from less than 1 month to 10 years (mean time 27.9 months). Although in most cases the primary clinical diagnosis was correctly recognized as metastasis, in some lesions the morphological characteristics directed toward benign lesions such as epidermal cyst, pyogenic granuloma, hemangioma, or herpes zoster [1].

Dermoscopy can provide valuable information for the diagnosis of skin metastasis. Tiodorovic et al. examined 632 cutaneous metastases from 583 patients using dermoscopy. In general, prominent vessels were recognized as the most common dermoscopic feature. Non-pigmented lesions with linear serpentine vessels were detected in over half of all lesions (56.3%). Structureless brown and structureless white areas were noted in 57.2% and 68.6%, respectively [6]. Chernoff et al. also reported the vascular pattern of the lesions to be the most frequent dermoscopic feature in skin metastasis, appearing in 88% of cases. The most frequent vascular pattern was serpentine (77%) and arborizing vessels (53%). Dotted and comma vessels were also observed in 24% and 18% of cases. In lesions showing hyperpigmentation, brown streaks and blue-gray globules were present [7]. In a standard dermoscopic examination, the visualization of vascular structures within a nodule that reveals distinctive patterns and features can aid in the assessment and diagnosis of potential cutaneous metastases in cancer patients.

Histopathologic examination remains the gold standard for the diagnosis. When examining a skin biopsy histologically, some features indicate cutaneous metastasis, e.g., the absence of epidermal involvement, necrosis, ulceration, vascular infiltration, and the extent of inflammatory infiltrate.

We present a partial biopsy of a sizable lesion on the left arm of a 93-year-old female patient. Figure 21.1a, b shows the hematoxylin and eosin (H&E)-stained neoplastic cells forming solid structures and branching cords. Oval, dark or clear nuclei, visible nucleoli, basophilic cytoplasm, and numerous mitoses can be detected. Angiolymphatic invasion and luminal formation can also be seen. The epidermis is intact. In Figs. 21.2 and 21.3 shows immunohistochemical staining using CK18 and CEA, respectively. The immunomorphological findings are compatible with a metastatic focus of a poorly differentiated adenocarcinoma.

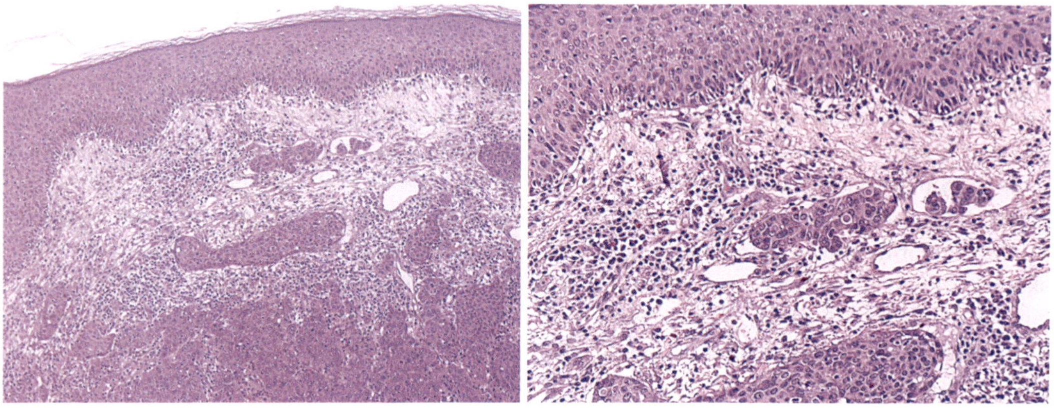

Fig. 21.1 A partial biopsy was obtained from a sizable lesion of the patient's left arm. Neoplastic cells form solid structures and branching cords. The cells exhibit oval nuclei with dark or clear chromatin, visible nucleoli, basophilic cytoplasm, and numerous mitoses. Angiolymphatic invasion and luminal formation are observed. Dermal invasion by a poorly differentiated adenocarcinoma is observed. (**a**) H&E, ×100 and (**b**) H&E, ×200

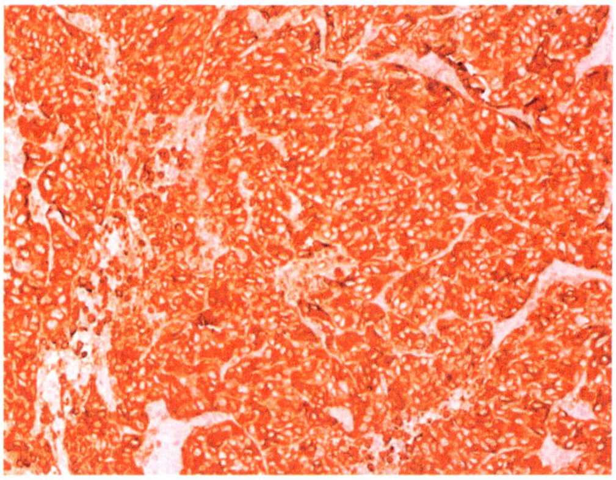

Fig. 21.2 Immunohistochemical staining for CK18. The neoplastic cells are positive for CK18 (×200)

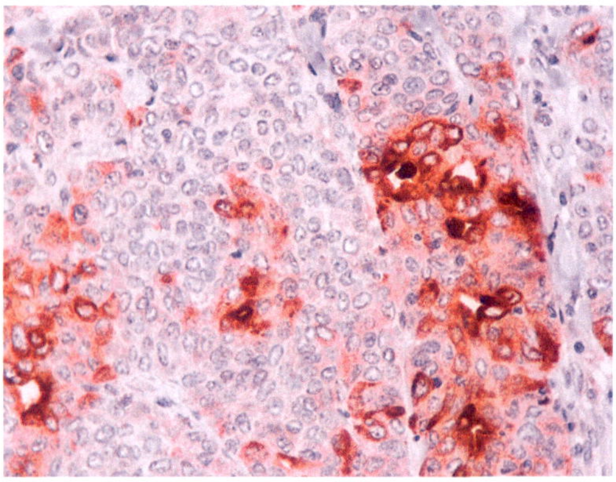

Fig. 21.3 Immunohistochemical staining of CEA. The neoplastic cells are partially positive for CEA. The immunomorphological findings are compatible with a metastatic focus of a poorly differentiated adenocarcinoma

21.4 Immunohistochemistry

Immunohistochemistry (IHC) is a laboratory technique used to detect specific antigens in skin lesion biopsies, aiding in the diagnosis and classification of dermatologic conditions, particularly skin cancers. The process begins with the collection of a skin biopsy, which is fixed in formalin, embedded in paraffin, and sectioned onto slides. These sections are deparaffinized, rehydrated, and subjected to antigen retrieval to expose target epitopes. Endogenous enzymatic activity is blocked to prevent background staining, followed by the application of a primary antibody specific to the antigen of interest. A secondary antibody conjugated to an enzyme such as horseradish peroxidase is then applied. Upon adding a chromogenic substrate like diaminobenzidine (DAB), , a colored precipitate forms at the antigen site. The slides are counterstained with hematoxylin, dehydrated, and mounted for microscopic evaluation. The staining pattern helps pathologists identify cell types and characterize lesions, distinguishing between entities such as melanoma, basal cell carcinoma, and inflammatory dermatoses.

Primary cutaneous adnexal malignancies often present with clinical and histological features similar to those of cutaneous metastases, making accurate diagnosis challenging. To differentiate between these entities, pathologists utilize immunohistochemical panels that include markers such as cytokeratins (CKs). Cytokeratin expression patterns, especially CK7 and CK20, serve as important diagnostic tools in pathology. These intermediate filament proteins are expressed in various epithelial tissues, and their distinct patterns help identify epithelial differentiation within tumors. Keratins' tissue-specific expression persists during various stages of development, maintaining structural integrity and specialized functions across tissues even after malignant transformation. By analyzing the presence or absence of CK7 and CK20, tumor cells can be accurately subclassified, gaining insights into their origin. This information is particularly valuable when determining the primary site of metastatic carcinomas, especially in cases where the primary tumor remains unknown. .).

CK20 is a highly tissue-specific marker predominantly found in gastrointestinal mucosa. Its expression is characteristic of cells within this tissue. Tumors originating from the gastrointestinal tract tend to show the highest levels of CK20 positivity, aiding in the accurate identification and differentiation of these neoplasms in pathological studies. CK7 is less tissue-specific and is expressed across a broader range of epithelial tissues and tumors. Studies indicate that CK7 is positive in approximately 69% of epithelial tumors. Its primary utility lies in its ability to help distinguish among various carcinomas, especially because it is rarely expressed in prostate and colorectal adenocarcinomas, thereby aiding in ruling out these origins. Conversely, CK7 shows higher positivity in tumors arising from the gastrointestinal tract, pancreas, and other glandular tissues [8].

In the context of diagnostic pathology, CK-7 and CK-20 immunohistochemical staining serve as valuable tools. They effectively distinguish pulmonary adenocarcinomas, which typically show CK-7 positivity and CK-20 negativity, from colorectal adenocarcinomas, often exhibiting a reverse staining profile, thereby assisting in accurate tumor origin identification. Lung carcinomas are a significant source of metastatic tumors to the skin, with adenocarcinomas and small cell carcinomas being the most commonly identified subtypes. These metastases often present concurrently with or even before the primary lung tumor is diagnosed, making clinical detection particularly important. When skin metastases occur, they can mimic primary cutaneous neoplasms, posing diagnostic challenges for clinicians and pathologists. To differentiate between metastatic lung carcinomas and primary skin tumors, immunohistochemical markers are invaluable. Notably, lung adenocarcinomas tend to show positive staining for CK7, which is a useful marker in this context. Additionally, thyroid transcription factor-1 (TTF-1) is frequently expressed in lung-origin tumors, assisting in confirming their pulmonary origin. However, squamous cell carcinomas of the lung can be more difficult to distinguish because they often share similar staining patterns, including CK7 positivity and variable TTF-1 expression. Accurate identification of these metastatic lesions is crucial for proper staging, underscoring the importance of immunohistochemical analysis in such cases.

Similar cytokeratin staining to lung cancer displays breast cancer cells. Both CK-7 and CK-20 negative staining can be seen in most cases of prostatic carcinomas.

Breast adenocarcinoma is a common and often aggressive form of breast cancer that frequently exhibits a propensity to metastasize beyond the primary site. Among the sites involved in metastatic spread, the skin represents a notable and sometimes early location, especially in advanced stages of the disease. The occurrence of cutaneous metastases from breast adenocarcinoma presents considerable diagnostic challenges for clinicians and pathologists alike. This is primarily due to the morphological and immunohistochemical similarities that metastatic breast cancer shares with primary skin neoplasms, making it difficult to distinguish between a metastasis and a primary cutaneous tumor solely based on routine histopathology. Morphologically, metastatic breast adenocarcinoma to the skin can mimic various primary skin tumors, including sweat gland carcinomas, adnexal tumors, and other adenocarcinomas originating from skin structures. These similarities can lead to diagnostic ambiguity, which is critical to resolve because treatment strategies and prognostic considerations differ significantly between primary skin cancers and metastatic disease. Accurate diagnosis hinges upon integrating histological findings with immunohistochemical profiles. Traditional IHC markers such as estrogen receptor (ER), progesterone receptor (PR), and human epidermal growth factor receptor 2 (HER2) are often positive in breast adenocarcinoma and can support the diagnosis of metastasis when the clinical history is suggestive. However, these markers are not entirely specific, as some primary skin tumors can express similar hormonal receptors or related markers, complicating the differentiation process. To improve diagnostic accuracy, additional markers such as p63 and p40 are utilized. Both are nuclear transcription factors involved in the development and differentiation of basal and myoepithelial cells. p63 is expressed in various epithelial tissues and is commonly positive in primary cutaneous adnexal tumors, including certain sweat gland carcinomas [9]. p40, a more specific isoform of p63, has gained prominence owing to its higher specificity for squamous and basal cell differentiation. When used in combination with other markers, p63 and p40 can help distinguish primary skin neoplasms from metastatic carcinomas. Moreover, the incorporation of podoplanin, a glycoprotein expressed in lymphatic endothelial cells and some tumor cells, further refines diagnostic accuracy [10]. The combined use of p40 and podoplanin can enhance the ability to differentiate primary cutaneous tumors, which typically express these markers, from metastatic breast adenocarcinoma, which usually lacks expression of p40 and podoplanin. Notably, p40 has demonstrated higher specificity and positive predictive value compared to p63, making it a more reliable marker in this diagnostic setting. In summary, the challenge of distinguishing metastatic breast adenocarcinoma to the skin from primary cutaneous neoplasms can be addressed with a strategic panel of immunohistochemical markers [11]. The combined use of p40 and podoplanin provides a powerful approach, with p40 offering superior specificity and positive predictive value. This nuanced immunoprofile is essential for guiding appropriate clinical management and ensuring accurate diagnosis, ultimately improving patient outcomes in cases of cutaneous metastatic disease.

Ovarian carcinomas infrequently metastasize to the skin; however, when such metastases do occur, they are most commonly found on the abdominal skin, surgical scars, or the umbilical region. These cutaneous metastases often present as nodular or ulcerative lesions, sometimes mimicking other skin conditions. Histologically, these metastases typically display glandular or papillary structures characteristic of ovarian origin. Immunohistochemistry usually reveals positivity for CK7 and negativity for CK20 [12]. Additionally, patients often have elevated serum CA125 levels, which serve as a tumor marker for ovarian carcinoma [13]. Recognizing these features is crucial for accurate diagnosis and appropriate management of such rare metastatic presentations.

Squamous cell carcinoma of the oral cavity is a common malignancy in males that tends to invade locally and has the potential to metastasize to distant sites. One notable pattern of metastasis involves the skin, particularly on the neck and face regions. These cutaneous metastases often appear near previous surgical sites, reflecting the tumor's aggressive nature and its ability to spread via lymphatic or hematogenous routes. Accurate diagnosis of such metastases is crucial. Immunohistochemical markers play a vital role in confirming the origin of these skin lesions. Markers such as p63, MNF116, and p40 are frequently employed due to their high specificity for squamous cell carcinoma cells [14]. However, their use is not without limitations; issues like false-positive results for MNF116 and nonspecific cytoplasmic staining for p63 in cases of leiomyosarcomas can pose diagnostic challenges [15]. Despite these limitations, immunohistochemistry remains an essential tool in distinguishing SCC metastases from other cutaneous malignancies, aiding clinicians in devising appropriate treatment plans.

Immunohistochemistry should be used carefully within the appropriate morphological context, as improper application or interpretation may lead to misleading results. Although IHC is used almost as a routine staining method, there are no antibodies that are pathognomonic for a specific tumor, and the specific antibody for every case should be chosen upon clinical and morphological suspicion.).

21.5 Conclusion

Although uncommon, cutaneous metastases may appear in dermatology clinics, underscoring the importance of vigilant assessment. Clinicians should perform comprehensive examinations, both clinically and dermoscopically, paying particular attention to the head and neck areas, where such lesions often manifest. Recognizing subtle histologic features is crucial for accurate diagnosis, since the morphologic pattern of the metastatic tissue can guide towards the identification of the primary malignancy. The use of appropriate diagnostic tools, including biopsies and immunohistochemical staining, plays a vital role in differentiating metastatic lesions from primary skin conditions. Early identification of cutaneous metastases allows for timely management and may provide valuable insights into an underlying internal malignancy, emphasizing the need for thorough clinical and histopathological evaluation in atypical dermatologic presentations.

Acknowledgement The pictures for this chapter were kindly provided by Eleni Lappa, melina-d@hotmail.com
Pathology Department, University Hospital of Heraklion, 71 500, Heraklion, Greece.

References

1. Hu SS, Chen GS, Lu YW, Wu CS, Lan CC. Cutaneous metastases from different internal malignancies: a clinical and prognostic appraisal. J Eur Acad Dermatol Venereol. 2008;22(6):735–40.
2. Lookingbill DP, Spangler N, Helm KF. Cutaneous metastases in patients with metastatic carcinoma: a retrospective study of 4020 patients. J Am Acad Dermatol. 1993;29(2):228–36.
3. Freedberg IM, Eisen AZ, Wolff K, Austen KF, Goldsmith LA, Katz SI, et al. Fitzpatrick's dermatology in general medicine. 5th ed. New York: McGraw-Hill; 1999.
4. Brownstein MH, Helwig EB. Metastatic tumors of the skin. Cancer. 1972;29(5):1298–307.
5. Marcoval J, Moreno A, Peyrí J. Cutaneous infiltration by cancer. J Am Acad Dermatol. 2007;57(4):577–80.
6. Tiodorovic D, Stojkovic-Filipovic J, Marghoob A, Argenziano G, Puig S, Malvehy J, et al. Dermatoscopic patterns of cutaneous metastases: a multicentre cross-sectional study of the International Dermoscopy Society. J Eur Acad Dermatol Venereol. 2024;38(7):1432–8.
7. Chernoff KA, Marghoob AA, Lacouture ME, Deng L, Busam KJ, Myskowski PL. Dermoscopic findings in cutaneous metastases. JAMA Dermatol. 2014;150(4):429.
8. Dum D, Menz A, Völkel C, De Wispelaere N, Hinsch A, Gorbokon N, et al. Cytokeratin 7 and cytokeratin 20 expression in cancer: a tissue microarray study on 15,424 cancers. Exp Mol Pathol. 2022;126:104762.
9. Ivan D, Nash JW, Prieto VG, Calonje E, Lyle S, Diwan AH, et al. Use of p63 expression in distinguishing primary and metastatic cutaneous adnexal neoplasms from metastatic adenocarcinoma to skin. J Cutan Pathol. 2007;34(6):474–80.
10. Plaza JA, Ortega PF, Stockman DL, Suster S. Value of p63 and podoplanin (D2-40) immunoreactivity in the distinction between primary cutaneous tumors and adenocarcinomas metastatic to the skin: a clinicopathologic and immunohistochemical study of 79 cases. J Cutan Pathol. 2010;37(4):403–10.
11. Lee JJ, Mochel MC, Piris A, Boussahmain C, Mahalingam M, Hoang MP. p40 exhibits better specificity than p63 in distinguishing primary skin adnexal carcinomas from cutaneous metastases. Hum Pathol. 2014;45(5):1078–83.
12. Chu PG, Weiss LM. Keratin expression in human tissues and neoplasms. Histopathology. 2002;40(5):403–39.
13. Tornos C, Soslow R, Chen S, Akram M, Hummer AJ, Abu-Rustum N, et al. Expression of WT1, CA 125, and GCDFP-15 as useful markers in the differential diagnosis of primary ovarian carcinomas versus metastatic breast cancer to the ovary. Am J Surg Pathol. 2005;29(11):1482–9.
14. Alomari AK, Glusac EJ, McNiff JM. p40 is a more specific marker than p63 for cutaneous poorly differentiated squamous cell carcinoma. J Cutan Pathol. 2014;41(11):839–45.
15. Dotto JE, Glusac EJ. p63 is a useful marker for cutaneous spindle cell squamous cell carcinoma. J Cutan Pathol. 2006;33(6):413–7.

Part X

Skin Metastases from Head and Neck Cancer

22 Head and Neck Cancer Metastases

Xekardakis Dimitrios

Abstract

Although rare, cutaneous metastases from head and neck carcinomas are highly aggressive and often signal a poor prognosis. These metastases are typically categorized based on the primary tumor site: oral/oropharyngeal, nasopharyngeal, or laryngeal carcinomas. The skin lesions most often appear on the head, neck, and upper chest regions closest to the original tumor but they can affect other areas as well. Clinically, their presentation is diverse. These metastases may appear as nodules, plaques, patches, or even blisters (bullae), sometimes resembling infections or benign skin tumors, which can make diagnosis challenging. Patients are most commonly older men with a history of heavy tobacco use, alcohol consumption, or both highlighting the importance of lifestyle factors in disease risk and progression.

Keywords

Head and Neck cancer · Oral · Nasopharyngeal · Laryngeal carcinoma · Cutaneous metastases

X. Dimitrios (✉)
Venizeleio General Hospital, Dermatology Clinic, Heraklion, Greece

22.1 Introduction

Head and neck cancer ranks as the sixth most common type of cancer worldwide [1], with squamous cell carcinoma (SCC) being the most frequently diagnosed histological type. Among the various complications associated with these cancers, cutaneous metastasis, the spread of cancer cells from the primary tumor to the skin, is both uncommon and clinically significant. Notably, when it occurs, it is usually more aggressive than the original tumor itself [2]. Skin involvement from head and neck cancers is rare but tends to indicate advanced disease and a poor prognosis. According to a study by Calhoun et al., the average survival for patients with cutaneous metastases from head and neck cancers is only around 4 months [3]. While cutaneous metastases occur in just 1–2% of patients with head and neck SCC [4, 5], they account for more than 10% of all distant metastases in these patients [6]. Overall, head and neck cancer contributes to about 15% of all skin metastases identified across cancers [7]. These lesions may appear as single or multiple nodules [8]. Cutaneous metastases are not unique to head and neck cancers. They can also be seen in other malignancies, most notably kidney, colon, bronchus, and breast cancers [4]. In fact, nearly 0.7–9% of all cancer patients may develop skin metastases during the course of their illness. Among women, breast cancer is the most com-

D. Koumaki et al. (eds.), *Cutaneous Metastases*, https://doi.org/10.1007/978-3-032-26764-1_22

mon source of cutaneous metastases, while in men, it's typically lung cancer [9]. Within head and neck cancers, oral cavity cancers are the most likely to spread to the skin, followed by laryngeal carcinomas. Although the mechanisms behind cutaneous metastases in head and neck cancers are not fully understood, several pathways have been proposed. These include direct extension from the primary tumor, local dissemination through intradermal lymphatics, and hematogenous spread [10]. Head and neck carcinomas are generally classified into three main categories: oral cavity/oropharyngeal, nasopharyngeal, and laryngeal carcinomas. While cutaneous metastases from these cancers most commonly appear on the head, neck, and upper chest, they can, in rare cases, spread to more distant areas, including the extremities. In the following sections, we will explore the patterns and clinical presentations of cutaneous metastases associated with each of these cancer types. This discussion will be guided by a review of sporadic case reports published in the medical literature, highlighting the variability and rarity of these metastatic pathways.

22.1.1 Oral Cavity and Oropharyngeal Cancer

Cancers of the oral cavity and oropharynx account for approximately 30% of all head and neck malignancies. These cancers are particularly prevalent in Southeast Asia, especially in India, where the habitual use of betel nut is a major contributing risk factor [11]. The most common histological subtype is squamous cell carcinoma (SCC), with the basaloid variant known for its aggressive behavior and widespread metastatic potential [12]. Distant metastases typically involve the liver, bones, and lungs [13]. Although cutaneous metastases from oral cavity and oropharyngeal cancers are extremely rare, accounting for less than 10% of all distant metastases [2], several case reports have documented such occurrences. These skin metastases usually appear close to the primary tumor site, most often on the neck and scalp. The majority of reported cases involve male patients, often with a history of tobacco use, reinforcing the well-established link between smoking and the development and progression of head and neck cancers.

Among the various subtypes of head and neck cancers, oral cavity tumors appear to have a higher incidence of cutaneous (dermal) metastases, although this observation is based on limited data from small sample sizes [2]. In a single-institution cohort study by Chaitanya et al., involving 2430 patients with oral cancer, 68 cases of skin metastases were identified. Most of these metastases occurred on the neck (accounting for approximately 50%), followed by the face (17.6%), and less frequently on the chest wall and abdomen [2]. This pattern aligns with earlier findings by Brownstein and Helwig, who noted the face and neck as the most common sites for skin metastases originating from oral cavity carcinomas [14, 15]. Although extremely rare, there are also case reports documenting upper limb and digital (acrocutaneous) metastases, particularly from squamous cell carcinoma of the tongue [13, 16, 17], highlighting the potential for unusual metastatic spread.

In patients who have undergone surgery for oral cancer, the incidence of dermal metastases is reported to be around 2.83%. Furthermore, among all advanced-stage (T-stage) head and neck tumors, those arising from the oral cavity, oropharynx, and hypopharynx show the highest likelihood of developing skin metastases [12].

Primary tumors of the oral cavity and oropharynx most commonly arise in areas such as the tongue (particularly the base), tonsils, and buccal mucosa. Among these, cancers of the floor of the mouth and tongue are more frequently associated with the early development of cutaneous metastases [2]. Another significant risk factor for early skin involvement is the presence of extracapsular extension, indicating more aggressive disease behavior [2].

The clinical presentation of skin metastases from oral cavity and oropharyngeal carcinomas is variable and often polymorphic. Lesions may appear as patches, papules, plaques, or nodules, and in many cases, these different lesion types coexist in the same patient. As the disease progresses, ulceration of the skin lesions is also commonly observed, further complicating diagnosis and management.

Cancers of the tongue, including both the anterior tongue and base of tongue, represent one of the most common sites of distant metastases in head and neck cancers, second only to laryngeal carcinoma [11]. These tumors are associated with a particularly poor prognosis, especially in advanced stages. Nearly 80% of patients with advanced tongue cancer already present with lymph node metastases at the time of diagnosis [13].

In most cases, cancer of the base of the tongue remains localized above the clavicles, consistent with the typical pattern of spread seen in head and neck malignancies [18]. Reported cases of cutaneous metastases from tongue cancer most frequently involve the head and neck, where lesions often present as plaques, papules, or nodules with variable coloration.

Other affected areas include:

- The face (e.g., lips, zygomatic region, chin, etc.) [8, 11]
- The scalp [18]
- The neck and upper chest [11]

These skin lesions are often ulcerated, with features such as yellowish slough, hemorrhagic crusting, and surface erosions [11], making them both clinically alarming and diagnostically challenging.

In extremely rare cases, metastases may appear on the abdomen or upper limbs. Among the most uncommon presentations are acrometastases, metastases to the distal extremities. Although these account for just 0.1% of all metastatic cases, there are rare reports of such lesions originating from base of tongue squamous cell carcinoma.

Examples include:

- A case described by Rastogi et al. (2005) involving multiple subcutaneous nodules on the forearm [13]
- A nonhealing lesion on the fifth finger reported by Mandadi and Kudva [16]
- A painful, erythematous plaque on a finger with spontaneous bleeding, extending to the nail fold and subungual tissue, described by Aiempanakit [17]

These acral metastases are highly aggressive and often misdiagnosed, as they tend to mimic inflammatory or infectious conditions such as:

- Osteomyelitis
- Pyogenic granuloma
- Paronychia
- Rheumatoid arthritis [16, 17]

The thumb's distal phalanx is the most commonly affected site in such cases [17].

Diagnosis of acral metastases is frequently delayed due to their nonspecific presentation. Additionally, nail changes from chemotherapeutic agents such as taxanes or epidermal growth factor inhibitors (EGFRIs) can obscure clinical suspicion, further complicating early recognition [17].

Tonsillar carcinoma is an uncommon subset of head and neck cancers, and cutaneous metastases from this tumor are exceptionally rare. To date, only five cases have been documented in the medical literature [19]. All reported patients were male, with a median age of 55 years at diagnosis, and three of them had a history of smoking. The interval between the initial cancer diagnosis and the development of skin metastases ranged from 6 to 54 months [19].

While the exact pathogenesis of tonsillar carcinoma remains unclear, there is a strong association with high-risk human papillomavirus (HPV) subtypes, particularly HPV-16 and HPV-18. Both have been implicated in the development of oropharyngeal cancers, including tonsillar carcinoma, as supported by meta-analyses of epidemiological data [12, 19].

Histologically, the most common type of tonsillar carcinoma associated with cutaneous spread is squamous cell carcinoma, which accounts for approximately 75% of cases, followed by lymphoma [19].

Tonsillar squamous cell carcinoma represents around 10% of all head and neck malignancies. Though rare, cutaneous metastases may sometimes be the initial presenting feature of recurrence, or even the first sign of the disease, prompting patients to seek medical attention.

Skin metastases typically involve regions close to the primary tumor, such as the head and chest, but can also appear at distant sites, including the extremities.

The morphology of these lesions is highly variable. Reported clinical presentations include:

- Confluent erythematous papules, nodules, and plaques on the left periorbital, temporal, and malar regions [19]
- Swelling and nodular plaques on the right fronto-parietal scalp [19, 20]
- Ulcerated proliferative nodules on the scalp and left thigh [19, 21]
- Erythematous papules and plaques on the chest, and ulcerated/crusted nodules on the neck, within previous radiation fields, mimicking varicella zoster virus (VZV) infection [19]
- A blanchable erythematous patch across the right chest and abdomen, with reddish-yellow papules over the clavicle, chest, and shoulder [12, 19]

These diverse and sometimes deceptive skin manifestations highlight the importance of including cutaneous metastasis in the differential diagnosis, particularly in patients with a history of tonsillar or other oropharyngeal cancers.

In Table 22.1, we represent case reports describing patients with Oral Cavity and Oropharyngeal Cancer Cutaneous Metastases.

Cutaneous metastases from oral cavity and oropharyngeal cancers are rare but clinically significant. When they do occur, they are typically aggressive and strongly associated with advanced disease, serving as a poor prognostic indicator. These metastases show a predominant male distribution, often related to established risk factors such as smoking and alcohol use.

Clinically, the skin lesions can mimic benign or infectious conditions, such as epidermoid cysts, pyogenic granulomas, cellulitis, osteomyelitis, or even varicella zoster virus infection. This wide spectrum of appearances increases the risk of misdiagnosis, especially when the lesion is painless or deceptively simple in presentation.

Importantly, cutaneous metastases may be the first sign of disease recurrence in patients previously treated for oral or oropharyngeal cancers. Therefore, clinicians, particularly dermatologists, oncologists, and head and neck specialists, must maintain a high index of suspicion when evaluating new or unusual skin lesions in this patient population. Early recognition can lead to more timely staging, intervention, and appropriate palliative care.

22.1.2 Nasopharyngeal Cancer

Nasopharyngeal carcinoma (NPC) is a relatively rare malignancy in Western countries, with an age-standardized incidence rate of fewer than one case per 100,000 population per year [22, 23]. In contrast, NPC is much more prevalent in certain regions, particularly Southern China, Southeast Asia, and Northern Africa, where it is considered a common cancer of the upper aerodigestive tract [23–25].

Although NPC accounts for less than 1% of all malignancies globally [26], it is one of the most frequent tumors to arise in the nasopharyngeal region. Clinically, it is known for its aggressive behavior and propensity for distant metastasis, most commonly affecting the lungs, liver, and bones [27].

Skin metastasis from nasopharyngeal carcinoma is extremely rare, with only a few cases reported in the literature [22, 27]. When cutaneous involvement does occur, it typically signifies advanced, systemic disease and is associated with a very poor prognosis [24]. In fact, these patients often experience a rapidly fatal disease course once skin metastases appear.

Historically, Markson and Pack were the first to report cases of cutaneous metastases from NPC in 1949 [28]. Later, Meltzer described a case of a metastatic skin lesion occurring within the radiation treatment field [29], and Robey was among the first to highlight the poor prognosis associated with this pattern of metastasis [30].

Table 22.1 Cases describing patients with Oral Cavity and Oropharyngeal Cancer Cutaneous Metastases

Clinical Information	Oral Cancer Histopathology	Cutaneous Metastases Clinical Presentation	Cutaneous Metastases Histology
46-year-old male, invasive tumor of the lateral border of the tongue	Moderately differentiated Squamous Cell Carcinoma	Erosions, hemorrhagic crusting and yellowish slough, single well to ill-defined ulcer of the lower lip (4 × 2 cm), well to ill-defined erythematous to violaceous non-tender nodulo-plaques, asymptomatic to mildly itchy, over the chest region	Punch biopsy of the chest. Normal epidermis, pleomorphic tumor epithelial cells, hyperchromatic plump spindle-shaped nuclei infiltrating the dermis (poorly differentiated Squamous Cell Carcinoma)
55-year-old male, chronic tobacco chewing, hoarseness, sore throat, base of the tongue mass	Stage IV Squamous Cell Carcinoma with bilateral secondary neck nodes	Nodule of the left side of the thigh (5 × 5 cm), hard, tender, fixed, and ulcerated and nodule of the left zygomatic (4 × 4 cm) region, mobile, firm, tender, and inflamed	Fine needle aspiration of both the two nodules. Metastatic Squamous Cell Carcinoma, clusters of neoplastic cells, irregular hyperchromatic nuclei, variable amount of cytoplasm
58-year-old male, chronic smoker, alcoholic, beetle chewer, sore throat and bilateral neck swelling, ulcerated tumor of the right side of the tongue with extension to the right pharyngeal wall and vallecula	Stage IVA Well-differentiated Squamous Cell Carcinoma	Multiple cutaneous nodules of the left forearm (below the elbow region)	Fine needle aspiration. Metastatic Squamous Cell Carcinoma consistent with primary Squamous Cell Carcinoma of base tongue, group of atypical squamous epithelial cells with big, hyperchromatic nuclei
30-year-old male, irregular mass of the base of the tongue extending to epiglottis, pre-epiglottic space, and left vallecula	Poorly differentiated Squamous Cell Carcinoma	Multiple cutaneous nodules of the neck, scalp, abdomen, and right hand	Fine needle aspiration. Metastatic Squamous Cell Carcinoma consistent with primary Squamous Cell Carcinoma of the base tongue
61-year-old male, mass of the base of the tongue	Stage III Squamous Cell Carcinoma	Erythematous patch, tender, ill-defined of the left index finger, firm consistency on the radial side of the lateral nail fold and 1/3 of the adjacent subungual tissue, painful with spontaneous bleeding	Skin biopsy. Digital Squamous Cell Carcinoma metastasis, multiple fragments of squamous epithelial cells with some prominent nucleoli, mitosis, and foci of keratinization
66-year-old male, base of the tongue ulcer with bleeding	Moderately differentiated Squamous Cell Carcinoma	Nonhealing ulcerated lesion in the distal phalanx of right fifth finger, 2.5 × 2.5 cm, tenderness around the ulcer, minimal discharge	Confluent clusters and nest of malignant cells scattered among dyskeratotic cells, atypical mitoses, keratin pearls, areas of hyalinization, areas of necrosis surrounded by fibrocollagenous stroma with myxoid change (moderately differentiated Squamous Cell Carcinoma)

(continued)

Table 22.1 (continued)

Clinical Information	Oral Cancer Histopathology	Cutaneous Metastases Clinical Presentation	Cutaneous Metastases Histology
59-year-old male, invasive tumor of the right tonsil, no history of smoking or alcohol	Stage IV Squamous Cell Carcinoma	Ulcerated, crusted nodules on the neck (within radiation port, beneath tracheostomy collar) initially painful, multiple erythematous plaques (> 6 × 4 cm), consisting of individual, confluent papules on the neck and proximal chest	Two chest punch biopsies. Atypical keratinocytes in the superficial dermis that do not extend from the overlying epidermis, central necrosis, and multiple dyskeratotic cells. Immunohistochemistry (+) cytokeratin 5/6, p40 (Squamous Cell Carcinoma markers). Metastatic Squamous Cell Carcinoma
40-year-old male, bilateral neck swelling and dysphagia, history of smoking, tumor of the tonsils	Well-differentiated Squamous Cell Carcinoma	Individual, confluent papules, nodules on the left periocular, temple, malar cheek with erythematous plaques, papules	Fine needle aspiration. Metastatic Squamous Cell Carcinoma
70-year-old male, weight loss and dysphagia, left tonsil tumor, smoker	Moderately differentiated Squamous Cell Carcinoma	Plaques, nodules, swelling of the right frontoparietal region	Fine needle aspiration. Cutaneous metastasis of Squamous Cell Carcinoma
55-year-old male, sore throat, weight loss, dysphagia, right tonsil tumor, history of smoking	Moderately differentiated Squamous Cell Carcinoma	Three ulcerated nodules of the scalp, one ulcerated nodule of the left thigh	Squamous Cell Carcinoma
70-year-old male, history of prostate cancer, tumor of the right tonsil	Stage IV Squamous Cell Carcinoma, (+) p16	Asymptomatic Cutaneous rash, reddish-yellow papules overlying right lateral, chest, shoulder, clavicle, and a large erythematous patch, blanchable of the right chest and upper abdomen, extended across the midline	Patch punch biopsy. Squamous Cell Carcinoma with (+) p16, p40, high expression of PD-L1, only in angiolymphatic spaces. Papule punch biopsy. Squamous Cell Carcinoma, basaloid morphology, (+) p16, p40, high expression PD-L1.
46-year-old male, progressive, painless, insidious ulcer over the left side buccal mucosa, chronic tobacco chewer	Well-differentiated Squamous Cell Carcinoma with no extra-nodular extension or perineural/ lymphovascular invasion	Multiple nodular, non-tender, painless, progressive deposits over chest wall, abdomen, thigh, shoulders and upper back	Metastatic Squamous Cell Carcinoma

22.1.2.1 Histological Subtypes of Nasopharyngeal Carcinoma

Nasopharyngeal carcinoma (NPC) is classified into three main histological types:

1. Squamous Cell Carcinoma (SCC), a non-lymphomatous type that arises from the epithelial lining of the nasopharynx [31]
2. Mucin-secreting Adenocarcinoma
3. Undifferentiated Carcinoma [22]

The distribution of histological subtypes varies significantly across populations. In non-Hispanic white populations, the keratinizing squamous cell carcinoma is the most common form. In contrast, among Chinese populations, particularly in endemic regions, the predominant types are undifferentiated carcinoma and non-keratinizing squamous cell carcinoma [23].

Most nasopharyngeal tumors are of the undifferentiated carcinoma type, which is strongly associated with Epstein-Barr virus (EBV) infection [24, 25, 32]. In fact, undifferentiated carcinoma is the only NPC subtype consistently linked to EBV. The other histological types, including keratinizing SCC and adenocarcinoma, are not associated with EBV, but rather with environmental and lifestyle-related risk factors such as:

- Smoking
- Tobacco chewing
- Genetic predisposition
- Racial and ethnic background [33]

22.1.2.2 Clinical Presentation of Cutaneous Metastases in Nasopharyngeal Carcinoma

Cutaneous metastases from nasopharyngeal carcinoma (NPC) are rare, and their presentation can be clinically diverse. In most reported cases, lesions appear as single or multiple nodules, which are typically painless, although painful and ulcerated lesions have also been described. Some case reports have noted other morphologies, including:

- Solitary masses
- Papules
- Papulonodules
- Plaques

In 2001, Swan et al. described three Chinese patients who presented with atypical facial swelling, which was later confirmed by biopsy as metastatic undifferentiated NPC [23]. These cases emphasize the subtle and sometimes misleading appearance of skin metastases, particularly in endemic regions.

Interestingly, in the majority of published cases, patients with cutaneous NPC metastases have been male, with only one female patient reported in the literature, highlighting a potential gender predominance in these presentations.

The most frequently reported morphology remains that of nodular lesions, either solitary or multiple. These nodules are often asymptomatic, making early detection challenging. Metastatic lesions can occur both near the primary tumor (e.g., face, neck) and at distant sites (e.g., trunk, limbs).

A notable case by Jacyk et al. (1998) described a patient who developed multiple small nodules simultaneously on the trunk, thighs, right forearm, and flexor surfaces, reflecting a widespread and aggressive dissemination pattern [34].

Though rare, cutaneous metastases from nasopharyngeal carcinoma (NPC) exhibit a wide spectrum of clinical presentations and anatomical distributions, often mimicking benign or inflammatory conditions.

In 1999, Ycel et al. reported two cases:

- One patient presented with multiple asymptomatic nodules on the scalp and right forearm.
- The other had a solitary metastatic nodule located at the periumbilical area, an uncommon site for NPC skin metastasis [27].

Two decades later, in 2019, Bohli et al. described two patients with extensive disseminated cutaneous and subcutaneous nodules affecting the trunk and lower limbs, highlighting a more widespread disease pattern [24].

In 2003, Luk et al. presented a series of four Chinese patients with metastatic NPC who developed a variety of cutaneous metastases, including:

- Hard, painful nodules located in multiple regions simultaneously, such as the right axilla, chest wall, epigastrium, and periareolar region
- Solitary subcutaneous masses on less typical sites such as the buttock and left upper back [25]

Caloglu et al. (2005) reported a patient with a complex combination of lesions, including erythematous plaques, ulcerated skin lesions, and multiple nodules involving the upper body, neck, scapula, and upper arm, further emphasizing the morphologic variability of NPC skin metastases [22].

One particularly rare and unique case was documented by Garcia et al. in 2015, involving a patient with lymphoepithelioma-like NPC who developed zosteriform erythematous papular metastases. These followed a metameric distribution on the chest and posterior neck, clinically resembling herpes zoster, and representing an unusual dermatologic mimic [32].

While cutaneous metastases from nasopharyngeal carcinoma (NPC) most often present as nodules, atypical morphologies have also been described. In some cases, metastasis may mimic benign conditions, delaying diagnosis.

One striking example involves diffuse facial swelling. As reported by Swan et al., three Chinese patients with a history of undifferentiated NPC presented with nonspecific swelling of the face, which could easily be misinterpreted as an allergic reaction, facial cellulitis, or other inflammatory condition. In all three cases, the correct diagnosis of cutaneous metastasis was only confirmed after a skin biopsy [23].

Cutaneous metastases from NPC can also involve unusual anatomical locations. Pack and Booher [35], as well as Robey and Schellhamer [36], reported extremely rare cases of nasopharyngeal squamous cell carcinoma metastasizing to the skin of the penis. Although extraordinarily uncommon, such cases underscore the unpredictable nature of metastatic spread in NPC.

In addition to true skin metastases, nasopharyngeal carcinoma may also be associated with paraneoplastic syndromes that manifest with cutaneous findings. These skin lesions are not caused by direct tumor infiltration but instead represent indirect effects of tumor-derived metabolites, immune responses, or cytokine activity [33]. The most notable dermatologic paraneoplastic syndrome associated with NPC is dermatomyositis. Though rare, it occurs in approximately 1 in 1000 patients with nasopharyngeal carcinoma [26]. Because dermatomyositis can serve as a clinical clue to an underlying malignancy, NPC should be specifically excluded during cancer screening in any patient who presents with dermatomyositis of unknown origin.

In Table 22.2, we present case reports describing patients with Nasopharyngeal Cancer Cutaneous Metastases.

In conclusion Cutaneous metastases of nasopharyngeal carcinoma (NPC) are extremely rare but carry a grave prognosis when they occur. They show a clear male predominance and are typically associated with the undifferentiated carcinoma subtype, which is strongly linked to Epstein-Barr virus (EBV) infection.

The skin lesions most commonly present as nodules, either solitary or multiple, and can appear at a wide range of anatomical sites, both regional and distant. However, as with metastases from oral cavity tumors, these lesions may mimic common dermatologic conditions, including inflammatory or infectious processes such as erysipelas, herpes zoster, or even allergic reactions. This resemblance can lead to delayed recognition of metastatic disease.

Given the aggressive nature of NPC and its poor survival outcomes once cutaneous metastases develop, early and accurate diagnosis is critical. Clinicians should maintain a high index of suspicion when evaluating new or unusual skin findings in patients with a history of NPC, even years after initial treatment.

22.1.3 Laryngeal Cancer

Carcinoma of the larynx is the most common malignancy of the head and neck region, accounting for approximately 45% of all head and neck cancers. Within the larynx, tumors most commonly arise in the glottis (65%), followed by the supraglottic region (30%)—particularly the epiglottis and hypopharynx, and much less frequently in the subglottic area (5%) [37].

Table 22.2 Cases describing patients with Nasopharyngeal Cancer Cutaneous Metastases

Clinical Information	Nasopharyngeal Cancer Histopathology	Cutaneous Metastases Clinical Presentation	Cutaneous Metastases Histology
46-year-old male, nasopharyngeal tumor, heavy smoker	Nasopharyngeal adenocarcinoma	Small, asymptomatic nodules on the trunk, right forearm, thighs, flexor surface (0.5–1 cm)	Periodic acid-Schiff staining: abundant intraluminal, focal intracytoplasmic mucus. Histology: metastatic adenocarcinoma, well-formed adenoid structures, molding of the cells
34-year-old male, masses in the nasopharynx and neck with paralysis	Non-keratinized undifferentiated carcinoma, clear cells with high mitotic activity	Multiple subcutaneous, erythematous painless nodules in the scalp, right forearm (1–2 cm)	Non-keratinized undifferentiated carcinoma, clear cells with high mitotic activity
40-year-old male, history of moderately differentiated supraglottic laryngeal Squamous Cell Carcinoma, mass in the nasopharynx	Non-keratinized differentiated carcinoma	Erythematous cutaneous nodule at the periumbilical region	Non-keratinized differentiated carcinoma
63-year-old male, right nasopharyngeal mass	Stage IV undifferentiated Nasopharyngeal Carcinoma (identifiable EBV RNA), ciliated columnar epithelium, cohesive sheets of polygonal to spindle tumor cells, prominent nucleoli in six lymphoplasmacytic stroma, (+) nuclear staining for EBV RNA	Multiple skin nodules, painful over the right axilla, epigastrium, right upper chest wall, and near the right nipple (0.5–2 cm)	Fine needle aspirate. Metastatic undifferentiated Nasopharyngeal Carcinoma, sheets of polygonal to spindle tumor cells, prominent nucleoli (similar to nasopharyngeal biopsy)
47-year-old female, nasopharyngeal mass	Stage II undifferentiated Nasopharyngeal Carcinoma	Single subcutaneous nodule over left chest wall, slowly increased in size, hard, painful	Fine needle aspiration cytology. Metastatic undifferentiated Nasopharyngeal Carcinoma
32-year-old male, nodular mass over left nasopharyngeal wall, left upper cervical lymphadenopathy, blood-stained nasal discharge	Stage IV undifferentiated Nasopharyngeal Carcinoma	Subcutaneous mass of left buttock slowly enlarged to 10 cm	Fine needle aspiration. Metastatic undifferentiated Nasopharyngeal Carcinoma
30-year-old male, nasopharyngeal mass	Undifferentiated Nasopharyngeal Carcinoma	Asymptomatic cutaneous mass over the left upper back	Fine needle aspiration. Metastatic undifferentiated Nasopharyngeal Carcinoma

(continued)

Table 22.2 (continued)

Clinical Information	Nasopharyngeal Cancer Histopathology	Cutaneous Metastases Clinical Presentation	Cutaneous Metastases Histology
63-year-old male, enlargement neck masses	Lymphoepithelioma-like carcinoma (distinctive subtype of Nasopharyngeal Carcinoma). Polymorphic lymphoid cell population, poorly differentiated syncytial groups of atypical cells of epithelial lineage, large vesicular nuclei, prominent nucleoli surrounded/ infiltrated by dense lymphoplasmocytic infiltrates (mainly T lymphocytes)	Painful erythematous papulo-nodular lesions following a metameric distribution in the left side of the chest, several lesions in the posterior neck area	Metastatic non-keratinizing Lymphoepithelioma-like carcinoma. Infiltration of deep dermis syncytial groups of large cells, vesicular nuclei, and vacuolated clear cytoplasm
54-year-old male, nasopharyngeal mass	Stage III undifferentiated Nasopharyngeal Carcinoma	Disseminated cutaneous nodules on the trunk (1–2 cm)	Metastatic undifferentiated Nasopharyngeal Carcinoma
53-year-old male, nasopharyngeal mass	Stage IV undifferentiated Nasopharyngeal Carcinoma	Painless subcutaneous nodules on the trunk, lower limbs, large erythematous plaque on the abdomen	Excision-biopsy. Metastatic undifferentiated Nasopharyngeal Carcinoma
40-year-old male, fatigue, weight loss, bilateral swelling of the neck, multiple enlarged lymph nodes in both upper cervical chains, nasopharyngeal mass on the right side of the nasopharyngeal roof infiltrating the bony structures into the sphenoid sinus, heavy smoker	Stage III undifferentiated Nasopharyngeal Carcinoma. Well-defined aggregates of epithelial cells surrounded by fibrous tissue and lymphoid cells, rich vascular network, vesicular nuclei with smooth outline, single, large, sharply etched eosinophilic nucleolus	Hard, erythematous, nonmobile skin nodules of the chest, followed by multiple nodules over the skin of the upper body, the right upper arm, right side of the neck and right scapula, forming widespread erythematous plaques with ulcers and purulent discharge	Skin biopsy of the chest. Metastatic undifferentiated Nasopharyngeal Carcinoma. Solid cords, thin strands of anaplastic cells infiltrating the lymphatic vessel, reticular dermis and interfascicular spaces of the dermis. (+) for cytokeratin, (−) HMB45, LC
35-year-old male, right ear tinnitus, cervical lymphadenopathy, serous median otitis, postnasal mass	Undifferentiated Nasopharyngeal Carcinoma	Diffuse facial swelling involving the face, periorbital, and perioral area, including the lips, the tongue, was spared	Biopsy of the skin. Metastatic Undifferentiated Nasopharyngeal Carcinoma, malignant cells within the dermal lymphatics, infiltrative strands of tumor cells between collagen bundles in the subcutaneous layer
50-year-old male, mass of paranasopharynx, pterygoid plate, base of skull, level II cervical lymph nodes bilaterally	Undifferentiated Nasopharyngeal Carcinoma	Diffuse facial swelling involving the face, mild erythema over the neck, and the tongue was spared.	Biopsy of the skin. Metastatic Undifferentiated Nasopharyngeal Carcinoma within the dermis, few reactive lymphocytes, dermal lymphatic tumor emboli

(continued)

Table 22.2 (continued)

Clinical Information	Nasopharyngeal Cancer Histopathology	Cutaneous Metastases Clinical Presentation	Cutaneous Metastases Histology
47-year-old male, postnasal mass, left cervical lymph nodes	Undifferentiated Nasopharyngeal Carcinoma	Swelling, erythema, and induration of the lower part of the face, the submental region and the neck	Metastatic Undifferentiated Nasopharyngeal Carcinoma

Supraglottic tumors are often referred to as "silent tumors" due to their atypical early symptoms. Early clinical signs may be subtle, including:

- Odynophagia (painful swallowing)
- Otalgia (ear pain)
- Persistent sore throat

Symptoms such as voice changes or airway obstruction typically appear only at advanced stages, contributing to delays in diagnosis and treatment.

22.1.3.1 Histological Subtypes

While a range of non-epidermoid carcinomas have been described in the larynx, including:

- Small cell carcinoma
- Adenocarcinoma
- Atypical carcinoid
- Mucoepidermoid and adenosquamous carcinoma
- Acinic cell carcinoma
- Salivary duct carcinoma
- Anaplastic and lobular variants [38]

More than 90% of all laryngeal cancers are squamous cell carcinomas (SCC), making it the most common malignancy of the upper respiratory tract [39].

Among all histological variants, SCC, adenocarcinoma, and atypical carcinoid tumors have been most commonly reported to metastasize to distant sites [37]. Squamous cell carcinoma of the larynx most frequently spreads to the:

- Bones
- Liver
- Lungs

with reported rates of distant metastasis ranging between 6.5% and 7.2% [37, 39].

22.1.3.2 Cutaneous Metastases fromLaryngealCarcinoma

Cutaneous metastases from laryngeal carcinoma are exceedingly rare, but when they do occur, they often signal advanced disease, cancer recurrence, or, in some cases, serve as the first clinical sign of a previously undiagnosed "silent" laryngeal cancer. Because of this, their presence is considered a poor prognostic indicator.

Among laryngeal cancers, squamous cell carcinoma (SCC), particularly the basaloid variant, is the histological type most commonly associated with cutaneous metastases. Basaloid squamous cell carcinoma is a rare, high-grade, and aggressive subtype of SCC, with a strong predilection for metastasis, especially in tumors arising from the vocal cords [40, 41].

These cases predominantly affect older male patients, typically with a history of tobacco and/or alcohol use [41], aligning with well-known risk profiles for head and neck cancers.

Another histological type that may give rise to cutaneous metastases is the atypical carcinoid, part of the broader category of neuroendocrine carcinomas (NECs) of the larynx. These tumors are extremely rare, accounting for less than 1% of all laryngeal cancers [42].

NECs are classified into four subtypes, based on cellular differentiation and size:

1. Typical carcinoid (well-differentiated)
2. Atypical carcinoid (moderately differentiated)
3. Small cell NEC (poorly differentiated)
4. Large cell NEC (poorly differentiated)

Among these, the atypical carcinoid is the most frequent and also the most aggressive, often originating in the supraglottic region and exhibiting a high rate of distant metastasis [42, 43].

In fact, after lymph nodes, the skin is the second most common site of metastasis for atypical carcinoid tumors [42]. This pattern makes dermatologic findings a potentially important clue in detecting or staging these rare neoplasms.

22.1.3.3 Clinical Presentation and Distribution of Cutaneous Metastases in Laryngeal Carcinoma

As with other head and neck cancers, cutaneous metastases from laryngeal carcinoma can present with variable morphologies, making clinical recognition challenging. The most common presentation involves single or multiple nodules, which are typically:

- Firm
- Rubbery
- Fixed to underlying tissue [44]

These nodules are often non-tender and painless, although painful lesions have also been described in the literature [40]. In more advanced or aggressive cases, nodules may become ulcerated [45].

Other less common morphologies include:

- Papules and plaques, particularly around the tracheostoma, which are referred to as stromal recurrences [37]
- Sclerodermoid plaques, which may mimic fibrosing skin conditions [46]
- Zosteriform patterns, where bullae and vesicles appear in a dermatomal distribution, mimicking herpes zoster [37, 39]

A particularly rare and unusual presentation was described by Ellis et al. (2014), who reported a patient with multiple cutaneous metastases within the prior radiation field, clinically resembling eruptive keratoacanthomas [47]. This case emphasizes how these lesions can imitate benign or inflammatory skin conditions, potentially delaying diagnosis.

22.1.3.4 Common and Uncommon Sites of Involvement

Cutaneous metastases from laryngeal carcinoma are most frequently found on the:

- Scalp
- Face
- Neck
- Upper chest [37, 44]

However, other anatomical sites have also been reported, including:

- Abdomen
- Extremities
- Penis

In some patients, multiple cutaneous metastases may present simultaneously at different body sites, reflecting widespread hematogenous or lymphatic dissemination.

Although cutaneous metastases from laryngeal cancer most commonly occur on the head, neck, and upper chest, a number of case reports describe unusual or acral sites of involvement. These atypical presentations often complicate diagnosis and may mimic benign or inflammatory conditions.

22.1.3.5 Acral Metastases

Acral cutaneous metastases, involving the fingers, toes, or distal extremities, are exceedingly rare but clinically significant. Documented cases include:

- Bhandarkar et al. (1997): Reported metastatic nodules on the right hand and little toe [46].
- Das et al. (2014): Described multiple painful eruptions on the left thigh and little finger [40].
- Nayak et al. (2011): Noted hard, erythematous, tender swellings involving several finger pulps, particularly the third finger of both hands [48].
- Kumar et al. (2011): Described a supraglottic squamous cell carcinoma that metastasized to

all five distal phalanges of the left hand [45].

- Lewin et al. (1997): Reported a rare case of thumb metastasis originating from a true vocal fold squamous cell carcinoma [49].

These acral lesions may be misdiagnosed as infections (e.g., paronychia, cellulitis) or inflammatory conditions such as rheumatoid nodules or osteomyelitis, especially in the absence of known widespread disease.

Other rare sites of cutaneous spread have also been reported:

- Nasal tip metastases have been described in three separate cases of laryngeal SCC by Shvili et al. (1990), Koutis et al. (2008), and Shindo et al. (2013) [38, 41, 44]. The nasal tip is an uncommon site and may initially be mistaken for basal cell carcinoma or rhinophyma.
- Abdominal skin metastases were documented by Krunic et al. (2005) and Wang et al. (2016) [37, 42], further demonstrating the capacity of laryngeal tumors to spread to distant cutaneous locations.
- In an especially unusual case, Perez et al. (1992) reported penile skin metastasis from a supraglottic carcinoma, underscoring the importance of considering metastatic disease in atypical presentations [50].

In Table 22.3, we present case reports describing patients with Laryngeal Cancer Cutaneous Metastases.

In conclusion, Laryngeal carcinoma is a relatively rare but highly aggressive malignancy, often associated with a poor prognosis, particularly in its advanced stages. The predominant his-

Table 22.3 Cases describing patients with Laryngeal Cancer Cutaneous Metastases

Clinical Information	Laryngeal Cancer Histopathology	Cutaneous Metastases Clinical Presentation	Cutaneous Metastases Histology
55-year-old male, supraglottic larynx mass	Stage IV laryngeal squamous cell carcinoma	Swelling on the tip of all fingers, nail bed of the left hand, multiple cutaneous nodules in the upper/lower limb	Tip of fingers/subcutaneous swelling, fine needle aspiration Metastatic squamous cell carcinoma, a cluster of malignant cells, extensive necrosis, and apoptosis in background
50-year-old male, laryngeal mass	Stage IV laryngeal squamous cell carcinoma	Hard, fixed cutaneous nodules non-tender over left clavicle, left parietal scalp region, on the dorsum of the right hand (overlying the base of the first metacarpal), ulcerated, inflamed nodule of the left little toe	Biopsies from all the lesions showed metastatic squamous cell carcinoma
60-year-old male, tumor of the vocal cords	Stage IV moderately differentiated laryngeal squamous cell carcinoma	Multiple painful, inflamed, tender nodules on the trunk, neck, thigh, chin, left little finger (1–1.5 cm)	Fine needle aspiration from multiple lesions Metastatic squamous cell Carcinoma, cellular clusters of neoplastic cells, hyperchromatic nuclei, variable amount of cytoplasm

(continued)

Table 22.3 (continued)

Clinical Information	Laryngeal Cancer Histopathology	Cutaneous Metastases Clinical Presentation	Cutaneous Metastases Histology
54-year-old female, sore throat, radiating pain in the right ear, denied hoarseness, dysphagia, fever, respiratory distress, reddish mass on the laryngeal surface of the epiglottis	Stage II laryngeal atypical carcinoid, tumor cells uniform in size with heteromorphy, arranged into nests/cords with eosinophilic cytoplasm (+), chromogranin A, cytokeratin, synaptophysin, HIF-1a, p53, CD56 (−) PI3K, p-Akt, GLUT-1	Multiple cutaneous/ subcutaneous nodules of the chest/abdomen with additional pain	Biopsy of an abdominal nodule Atypical metastatic carcinoid (both cutaneous/ subcutaneous areas of the abdomen)
49-year-old male, supraglottic larynx mass	Stage IV moderately differentiated laryngeal squamous cell carcinoma	Multiple reddish/purple, hard, non-tender nodules on the forehead, left side of the nose, posterior neck, scalp, right lower abdomen	Biopsy of two nodules (scalp, lower abdomen) Metastatic squamous cell carcinoma, poorly differentiated epithelial neoplasm, reticular dermis, no connection to the overlying epidermis, cells with squamous differentiation, eosinophilic cytoplasm, intercellular bridges, and keratin pearls
68-year-old male, laryngeal mass	Laryngeal squamous cell carcinoma	Painful enlarging flesh colored/red nodules (several ulcerated, some crater form with keratin-filled central areas clinically suggestive of keratoacanthomas) within the radiotherapy area (right side of the face, neck, mid-chest), erythema that outlined the distribution of radiation port	Keratin-filled right chest nodule biopsy Metastatic keratinizing laryngeal squamous cell carcinoma, orthokeratosis, mild acanthosis of epidermis, flattening of rete ridges, perivascular lymphocytic inflammation of papillary dermis, and metastatic keratinizing squamous cells with large/ atypical nuclei in the dermis without attachment to the overlying epidermis
69-year-old male, proliferative growth in right arytenoepiglottic folds, fixed right vocal cord	Laryngeal squamous cell carcinoma	Multiple shiny, hyperpigmented/skin colored grouped papules, nodules, plaques over left side of the neck (upper margin into the left submandibular, mandibular region, lower margin into clavicular supraclavicular, presternal area	Metastatic squamous cell carcinoma, extensive invasion of dermis by groups of atypical tumor cells with large, hyperchromatic, pleomorphic nuclei with a halo, intact epidermis

(continued)

Table 22.3 (continued)

Clinical Information	Laryngeal Cancer Histopathology	Cutaneous Metastases Clinical Presentation	Cutaneous Metastases Histology
69-year-old male, laryngeal mass	Locoregionally advanced laryngeal squamous cell carcinoma	Erythematous, hard, tender swelling of several finger pulps in both hands, most pronounced in the third finger of both hands, erythematous mass in the left thigh	Fine needle aspiration Metastatic squamous cell carcinoma
51-year-old male, sore throat, neck swelling, weight loss, anorexia, tumor of the epiglottis	Poorly differentiated laryngeal squamous cell carcinoma	Nodules dome-shaped (3 cm) on the right flank, left posterior thigh, left anterior rib cage	Right flank skin biopsy Poorly differentiated squamous cell carcinoma, thin nests of tumor cells in the dermis, rare intercellular bridges, nuclear pleomorphism, and uptake of keratin stain
77-year-old male, smoker, dysphagia, hoarseness, exophytic mass of right false vocal fold, right vocal fold, right ventricle	Basaloid squamous cell carcinoma, invasive tumor islands, small, closely packed basaloid cells, peripheral palisading, comedonecrosis, thick basement membrane, lack of epidermal connection, immunoreactivity for high molecular weight keratin	Exophytic tumor (3 cm) at the midline of the nasal tip	Metastatic basaloid squamous cell carcinoma, palisade arrangement of peripheral cells
72-year-old male, hoarseness, exophytic tumor (3 cm) of the epiglottis, extension to right aryepiglottic fold, right ventricular band, and right pyriform sinus	Basaloid squamous cell carcinoma, hyperchromatic nuclei, scant cytoplasm, anaplasia, many mitoses, small areas of focal squamous differentiation, single-cell keratinization, pearl formation, (+) cytokeratin, cells of squamous differentiation (+) for epithelial membrane antigen, palisade arrangement,	Exophytic tumor (2 cm) at the midline of the nasal tip	Metastatic basaloid squamous cell carcinoma

(continued)

Table 22.3 (continued)

Clinical Information	Laryngeal Cancer Histopathology	Cutaneous Metastases Clinical Presentation	Cutaneous Metastases Histology
74-year-old male, hypopharyngeal mass, esophageal mass	Poorly differentiated squamous cell carcinoma of the larynx, moderately to well-differentiated squamous cell carcinoma of the esophagus	Red nodule on the nasal tip (clown nose), dermoscopy with dilated follicular openings, yellow-white area, vasodilation	Metastasis of poorly differentiated squamous cell carcinoma of the Atypical squamous cell nests from the dermis to the subcutaneous tissue, vasodilation in the upper dermis
72-year-old female, tumor in the supraglottic region affecting the submucosa	Atypical carcinoid of the larynx (moderately differentiated neuroendocrine neoplasm), trabecular, organoid, and pseudoglandular pattern, proliferating cells arranged in nests/ribbons, regular polygonal shape, deeply eosinophilic cytoplasm, hyperchromatic nuclei, frequent mitoses, focal hyaline sclerosis/mild chronic inflammatory infiltrate of the stroma, argyrophilic neoplastic cells, (+) keratins, calcitonin, CEA, and EMA immunostaining	Several nodules in the scalp (1–2 cm) within the dermis and subdermis	Metastatic atypical carcinoid of the larynx
70-year-old male, hoarseness, tumor of the right true vocal fold	Poorly differentiated laryngeal squamous cell carcinoma	Fever, weight loss, painful, nonhealing ulcer on the volar surface of the left thumb	Metastatic poorly differentiated laryngeal squamous cell carcinoma
64-year-old male, alcohol and tobacco abuse, left arytenoid edema, decreased left vocal cord mobility	Biopsy of the left laryngeal surface of the epiglottis, poorly differentiated non-keratinizing squamous cell carcinoma	Indurated dorsal penile lesion (3 cm), darkened band along parts of the induration	Punch biopsy, metastatic squamous cell carcinoma, ulceration, lymphatic involvement

tological type is squamous cell carcinoma (SCC), with the basaloid variant representing a notably aggressive subtype that carries a higher metastatic potential.

Although cutaneous metastases from laryngeal cancer are rare, they can occasionally serve as the first clinical sign of disease, prompting the patient to seek medical evaluation. These skin lesions may occur in atypical and distant anatomical sites, including the abdomen, extremities, and even the penis, and are frequently misdiagnosed as benign conditions or infections due to their nonspecific appearance.

Because of this, clinicians, especially dermatologists, oncologists, and ENT specialists, must maintain a high index of suspicion when evaluating persistent or unusual skin lesions in patients with a history of laryngeal cancer. If a lesion is unresponsive to standard treatments such as antibiotics, a biopsy should be strongly considered to rule out metastatic disease.

Early identification of cutaneous metastases, though rare, is crucial for timely management and may help guide palliative or systemic treatment decisions in advanced laryngeal cancer.

References

1. Gil Z, Fliss DM. Contemporary management of head and neck cancers. Isr Med Assoc J. 2009;11(5):296–300.
2. Chaitanya SA, Kumar AA, Dalakoti P, Basude M, Kumar S, Jonathan GT, Rao TS, Rao LMCS, Nemade H. Dermal metastases in oral cancer after curative treatment: a single institution cohort study. Br J Oral Maxillofac Surg. 2021;59(6):677–80.
3. Calhoun KH, Fulmer P, Weiss R, et al. Distant metastases from head and neck squamous cell carcinoma. Laryngoscope. 1994;104:1199–205.
4. Yoskovitch A, et al. Skin metastases in squamous cell carcinoma of the head and neck. Otolaryngol Head Neck Surg. 2001;124(3):248–52.
5. Ferlito A, Shaha AR, Silver CE, Rinaldo A, Mondin V. Incidence and sites of distant metastases from head and neck cancer. ORL—J Oto-Rhino-Laryngol Relat Spec. 2001;63(4):202–7.
6. Pitman JT, Johnson JT. Skin metastases from head and neck squamous cell carcinoma: incidence and impact. Head Neck. 1999;21:560–5.
7. Emanuel H, Emanuel P. Cutaneous metastasis of head and neck malignancy. Int J Head Neck Surg. 2015;6(2):57–63.
8. Rahman T, Krishnatreya M, Sarma A, Kumar M, Kataki A. Cutaneous metastasis from squamous carcinoma of the base of tongue. N Am J Med Sci. 2015;7(1):24–6.
9. Ritusha M, Sovan SD, Himanshu M, Anupam KA. Carcinoma buccal mucosa with multiple cutaneous metastases. Ann Int Med Dental Res. 2017;3(2)
10. Dragan AD, Nixon IJ, Orabi AA, Manganaris A, Jeannon J-P, Guerrero-Urbano MT, Simo R. Direct skin involvement of cervical lymph node metastasis from mucosal squamous cell carcinoma of the head and neck. J Laryngol Otol. 2013;127(2):181–6.
11. Verma K, Gupta M, Gulati A, Sharma RK. Cutaneous metastasis of carcinoma tongue: a rare case report. J Dermatol Dermatol Surg. 2019;23(2):99–101.
12. Ramser AE, Craig EM, Delost GR, Baron E. Cutaneous metastasis of tonsillar carcinoma: report of a rare case. J Am Acad Dermatol Case Rep. 2018;4(6):551–4.
13. Rastogi M, Srivastava K, Srivastava M, Chufal KS, Bhatt MLB, Srivastava AN. Multiple skin metastases in forearm from base tongue carcinoma. Oral Oncol Extra. 2005;41(8):188–90.
14. Brownstein MH, Helwig EB. Patterns of cutaneous metastasis. Arch Dermatol. 1972;105:862–8.
15. Schwartz RA. Cutaneous metastatic disease. J Am Acad Dermatol. 1995;33:161–86.
16. Mandadi SR, Kudva A. Acrocutaneous metastasis—a rare presentation. Int J Surg Case Rep. 2018;51:178–80.
17. Aiempanakit K. Digital metastasis of tongue squamous cell carcinoma. J Am Acad Dermatol Case Rep. 2018;4(2):200–2.
18. Bedi N, Garg P, Gupta Y. Multiple cutaneous metastases from squamous cell carcinoma of the base of the tongue: a very rare case report. Int J Case Rep Images. 2016;7(1):20–3.
19. Bari O, Cohen PR. Cutaneous metastasis from tonsillar squamous cell carcinoma: report and review of the literature. Cureus. 2017;9(3):e1122.
20. Chikkannaiah P, Boovalli MM, Kumar RP, Murthy VS. Unusual cases of carcinoma of palatine tonsil. J Oral Maxillofac Pathol. 2015;19(2):242–6. https://doi.org/10.4103/0973-029X.164539. PMID: 26604503
21. Singh GK, Yadav V, Singh P, Bhowmik KT. Multiple cutaneous metastases in a patient of carcinoma tonsil – Report of a rare case. J Egypt Natl Canc Inst. 2016;28(3):191–3. https://doi.org/10.1016/j.jnci.2016.04.004. Epub 2016 May 10. PMID: 27177839
22. Caloglu M, Uygun K, Altaner S, Uzal C, Kocak Z, Piskin S. Nasopharyngeal carcinoma with extensive nodular skin metastases: a case report. Tumori. 2006;92(2):181–4.
23. Leong SS, Tan EH, Khoo-Tan HS, Yang TL, Wee J, Tan SH, Poh WT, Tan NG. Recurrent nasopharyngeal carcinoma presenting as diffuse dermal lymphatic infiltration in the neck: three case reports. Head Neck. 2001;23(2):160–5.
24. Bohli M, Tebra S, Bouaouina N. Nasopharyngeal carcinoma with cutaneous metastases. Eur Ann Otorhinolaryngol Head Neck Dis. 2019;136(5):409–11.
25. Luk NM, Yu KH, Choi CL, Yeung WK. Skin metastasis from nasopharyngeal carcinoma in four Chinese patients. Clin Exp Dermatol. 2004;29(1):28–31.
26. Chakroun A, Guigay J, Lusinchi A, Marandas P, Janot F, Hartl DM. Paraneoplastic dermatomyositis accompanying nasopharyngeal carcinoma: diagnosis, treatment and prognosis. Eur Ann Otorhinolaryngol Head Neck Dis. 2011;128(3):127–31.
27. Yücel ÖT, Hoşal AŞ, Önerci M, Sökmensüer C. Skin: an unusual site of metastases in nasopharyngeal carcinoma. Otolaryngol–Head Neck Surg. 1999;121(6):833–4.
28. Markson LS, Stoops CW, Kanter J. Metastatic transitional carcinoma of penis simulating chancre. Arch Dermatol Syphilis. 1949;59:50–4.
29. Meltzer J, Ahmed SA, Archambeau JO. The development of metastases within a field of previous irradiation: a case report. Cancer. 1981;48:717–20.

30. Robey EL, Schellhammer PF. Four cases of metastases to the penis and a review of the literature. J Urol. 1984;132:992–4.
31. Tomao F, Miele E, Spinelli GP, Caprio G, Ranieri E, Mingazzini P, Zullo A, Tomao S. Axillary and subcutaneous breast metastases from rhinopharyngeal carcinoma: a case report and literature review. Anticancer Res. 2008;28(1B):419–23.
32. González García A, Grillo Fernández E, Barbolla Díaz I, Ballester A, Pian H, Fraile G. A rare case of zosteriform cutaneous metastases from a nasopharyngeal carcinoma. Case Rep Dermatol Med. 2015;2015(415393):1–3.
33. Toro C, Rinaldo A, Silver CE, Politi M, Ferlito A. Paraneoplastic syndromes in patients with nasopharyngeal cancer. Auris Nasus Larynx. 2009;36(5):513–20.
34. Jacyk WK, Dinkel DE, Becker GJ. Cutaneous metastases from carcinoma of the nasopharynx. Br J Dermatol. 1998;139(2):344–5.
35. Pack GT, Booher RJ. Localization of metastatic cancer by trauma. NY State J Med. 1949;49:1839–41.
36. Robey EL, Schellhamer PF. Four cases of metastases to the penis and review of the literature. J Urol. 1984;132:982–4.
37. Krunic AL, Cockerell CJ, Truelson J, Taylor RS. Laryngeal squamous cell carcinoma with infradiaphragmatic presentation of skin metastases. Clin Exp Dermatol. 2006;31(2):242–4.
38. Shvili Y, Talmi YP, Gal R, Kessler E, Kolkov Z, Zohar Y. Basaloid-squamous carcinoma of the larynx metastatic to the skin of the nasal tip. J Craniofac Surg. 1990;18(7):322–4.
39. Aravamuthan R, Gurusamy R, Rajendrabose A, Barburam Krishna A, Palanisamy AP. Cutaneous metastases from primary carcinoma larynx: a rare presentation. Otolaryngol Online J. 2013;3(2)
40. Das K, Krishnatreya M, Baishya N, Sarma A, Kataki A. Multiple cutaneous metastases in laryngeal carcinoma: a rare occurrence. Clin Cancer Investig J. 2014;3(6):533–5.
41. Koutis EV, Assimakopoulos DA, Doukas MG, Zinovieva I. A rare nasal tip skin metastasis of a basaloid squamous cell carcinoma of the larynx. Am J Med. 2008;121(9):e3–4.
42. Wang K-R, Jia Y-J, Zhou S-H, Wang Q-Y, Bao Y-Y, Feng Z-Y, Yao H-T, Fan J. Cutaneous and subcutaneous metastases from atypical laryngeal carcinoids: case report and review of the literature. Medicine. 2016;95(7):e2796.
43. Ereño C, López JI, Sánchez JM. Atypical carcinoid of the larynx: presentation with scalp metastases. J Laryngol Otol. 1997;111(1):89–91.
44. Shindo M, Yoshida Y, Tominaga K, Yamamoto O. Skin metastasis of hypopharyngeal carcinoma to the nasal tip. Yonago Acta Med. 2013;56(2):57–8.
45. Kumar N, Bera A, Kumar R, Ghoshal S, Angurana SL, Srinivasan R. Squamous cell carcinoma of supraglottic larynx with metastasis to all five distal phalanges of left hand. Indian J Dermatol. 2011;56(5):578–80.
46. Bhandarkar P, Green KMJ, de Carpentier JP. Multiple cutaneous metastases from laryngeal carcinoma. J Laryngol Otol. 1997;111(7):654–5.
47. Ellis DL, Riahi RR, Murina AT, Cohen PR. Metastatic laryngeal carcinoma mimicking eruptive keratoacanthomas: report of keratoacanthoma-like cutaneous metastases in a radiation port. Dermatol Online J. 2014;20(9)
48. Nayak J, Zhong Y, Haigentz M Jr. Acral metastases from laryngeal carcinoma. J Clin Oncol. 2011;29(9):e220–1.
49. Lewin JS, Cleary KR, Eicher SA. An unusual metastasis to the thumb in a laryngectomized tracheoesophageal speaker. Arch Otolaryngol–Head Neck Surg. 1997;123(9):1007–9.
50. Perez LM, Shumway RA, Carson CC, Fisher SR, Hudson WR. Penile metastasis secondary to supraglottic squamous cell carcinoma: review of the literature. J Urol. 1992;147(1):157–60.

Part XI

Cutaneous Metastases from Sarcoma

Skin Metastases from Soft Tissue Sarcomas

23

Eirini Kyrmanidou and Elizabeth Lazaridou

Abstract

Soft tissue sarcomas (STS) are a heterogeneous group of malignant tumors arising from mesenchymal tissues and thus may originate from the fascia, elastic tissue, fat, smooth muscle, fibrous capsule, blood vessels, and nerves. While pulmonary, hepatic, and osseous metastases are well-documented, cutaneous and subcutaneous metastases from STS are rare and typically occur in the context of disseminated disease, indicating a poor prognosis. They present in diverse forms, including painless, firm nodules that can be skin-colored or pigmented, ulcerations that may be tender or bleeding, and cellulitis-like lesions that appear red, edematous, and inflamed.

Keywords

Soft tissue sarcomas · Metastasis · Skin · Cutaneous

E. Kyrmanidou (✉) · E. Lazaridou
Second Dermatology Department, School of Health Sciences, Aristotle University of Thessaloniki, Thessaloniki, Greece
e-mail: bethlaz@auth.gr

23.1 Introduction

Soft tissue sarcomas (STS) are a heterogeneous group of malignant tumors arising from mesenchymal tissues, representing less than 1% of adult cancers [1]. Many of the STS emerge from normal soft tissue structures, so that the lesions may originate from the fascia, elastic tissue, fat, smooth muscle, fibrous capsule, blood vessels, and nerves.

While pulmonary, hepatic, and osseous metastases are well-documented, cutaneous and subcutaneous metastases from STS are rare and often overlooked [2, 3]. These metastases typically occur in the context of disseminated disease and may indicate a poor prognosis. Clinically, cutaneous metastases from STS can present in various forms, including firm dermal or subcutaneous nodules, plaques, or ulcerated lesions. Due to their variable morphology and nonspecific appearance, they are frequently misdiagnosed as benign skin conditions or primary cutaneous malignancies. Histopathological analysis, supported by immunohistochemistry, is crucial for definitive diagnosis, particularly given the diversity of STS subtypes.

Although uncommon, skin metastases can be the first sign of recurrence or systemic spread in patients with a prior history of sarcoma. In rare cases, they may even precede the identification of the primary tumor. Prompt recognition of this presentation is vital for staging, prognosis, and

D. Koumaki et al. (eds.), *Cutaneous Metastases*, https://doi.org/10.1007/978-3-032-26764-1_23

treatment planning. This chapter will review the epidemiology, pathogenesis, clinical manifestations, diagnostic approach, and management of cutaneous metastases from soft tissue sarcomas.

23.2 Epidemiology of STS

STSs are uncommon malignant tumors that originate in the connective tissues of the body. These tumors have an estimated incidence of approximately five cases per 100,000 people each year, making them relatively rare in the adult population [4, 5]. They most frequently develop in the extremities—such as the arms and legs—as well as in the trunk and head and neck regions. In adults, soft tissue sarcomas account for about 90% of all sarcoma cases, underscoring their significance within this category of malignancies. Conversely, in children, these tumors are much more common, comprising almost 7% of pediatric cancers. When they do occur in the pediatric age group, they are most often represented by rhabdomyosarcoma, a highly aggressive form that arises from skeletal muscle tissue [6]. Despite their rarity, soft tissue sarcomas require prompt diagnosis and treatment, as they can be aggressive and have the potential to metastasize if not managed effectively.

Disease staging for soft tissue sarcomas is a crucial process that guides treatment planning and prognostic assessment. A primary focus of staging involves evaluating the presence of distant metastases, which significantly influence management decisions. To detect metastasis, a chest computed tomography (CT) scan is typically performed, as the lungs are the most common site for sarcoma spread. In cases where the lesion is classified as low risk, a chest X-ray may suffice, reducing patient exposure to radiation and cost. However, for tumors with a higher likelihood of metastasizing, additional imaging studies are often needed. An abdomen CT scan is used to evaluate potential spread to intra-abdominal organs (e.g., round cell/myxoid liposarcoma, angiosarcoma, epithelioid sarcoma, and leiomyosarcoma) , while brain magnetic resonance imaging (MRI) and spine MRI are reserved for tumors known to metastasize to the central nervous system or spine, respectively (e.g., angiosarcoma, alveolar soft part sarcoma, and clear cell sarcoma). Assessment of regional lymph nodes is also an important consideration, especially for certain high-risk subtypes (e.g., clear cell sarcoma, epithelioid sarcoma, synovial sarcoma, and rhabdomyosarcoma). Techniques such as ultrasound-guided lymph node evaluation or sentinel lymph node biopsy can help determine nodal involvement, which impacts staging and treatment strategies. The role of positron emission tomography (PET) and combined PET/CT imaging remains investigational, with ongoing research exploring their utility in detecting occult metastases and guiding therapy [7]. Cutaneous metastasis of STS is rare and, in some cases, the first indication of internal malignancy.

Follow-up imaging is tailored to the individual's disease stage and tumor aggressiveness. Typically, patients undergo periodic scans every 4–8 months to monitor for recurrence or progression, ensuring early detection and intervention if the disease recurs. This comprehensive approach to staging and follow-up helps optimize outcomes for patients with soft tissue sarcomas [8].

23.3 Clinical presentation

Soft tissue tumors present a wide range of clinical manifestations, reflecting their remarkable ability to originate from almost any part of the body. Their presentation often depends significantly on the tumor's location, size, and growth rate. For instance, tumors situated near vital structures such as nerves or blood vessels may cause pain, numbness, or swelling, while those located superficially might be noticed as a palpable mass. As these neoplasms grow, they can exert pressure on surrounding tissues, leading to functional impairments or discomfort. Because of this variability, accurate diagnosis typically necessitates a combination of radiological imaging—such as MRI or CT scans—to assess the extent and nature of the lesion, along with histological examination of biopsy samples to determine the tumor's structural characteristics. This comprehensive approach helps distinguish benign from malignant tumors and guides appropriate treatment strategies.

Accordingly, cutaneous metastases from soft tissue tumors can appear at any anatomical region, although there is a predilection for the scalp skin, probably due to the increased blood inflow of this area. Cutaneous metastases typically occur following the diagnosis of a primary malignancy, serving as an indication that cancer has spread to the skin. However, in some cases, these metastases can be detected simultaneously with the primary tumor or even before its identification [9]. They present in diverse forms, including painless, firm nodules that can be skin-colored or pigmented, ulcerations that may be tender or bleeding, and cellulitis-like lesions that appear red, edematous, and inflamed. Wang et al. analyzed 65 patients with skin metastases from soft tissue sarcomas and reported that leiomyosarcoma was the most common primary tumor to give skin metastases, and the majority of patients already had metastases elsewhere [10].

23.4 Histopathology

Histopathological examination remains the gold standard diagnostic method to define the tumor type, since, according to the diagnosis, the prognosis and therapeutic management can differ vastly. In Table 23.1, all malignant soft tissue sarcomas with metastatic potency are listed according to the WHO classification published in 2020 [11].

The diagnosis of sarcoma relies upon the evaluation as well as the integration of four main features:

1. Predominant shape of the neoplastic cells: spindle, epithelioid, round, and pleomorphic cells.
2. Pattern of growth: fascicular, herringbone, storiform, alveolar, solid, and biphasic growth pattern.
3. Quality of the background: fibrous, sclerotic, myxoid, myxochondroid, and osteogenic extracellular stroma.
4. Architecture of the vascular network: plexiform, archiform, and hemangiopericytoma-like architecture.

Integrating the abovementioned specified morphological features often narrows down the diagnostic options and may reduce the necessity for additional diagnostic techniques [12]. However, achieving an accurate and definitive diagnosis typically still requires a comprehensive evaluation, including supplementary methods, such as immunohistochemical staining, to ensure precise identification and appropriate treatment planning.

Table 23.1 WHO classification of malignant soft tissue tumors, NOS: Not Otherwise Specified

Adipocytic tumors	Liposarcoma, well differentiated, not otherwise specified (NOS) Dedifferentiated liposarcoma Myxoid liposarcoma Pleomorphic liposarcoma
Fibroblastic/myofibroblastic tumors	Adult fibrosarcoma Myxofibrosarcoma Low-grade fibromyxoid sarcoma Sclerosing epithelioid fibrosarcoma
So-called fibrohistiocytic tumors	Malignant tenosynovial giant cell tumor
Smooth muscle tumors	Leiomyosarcoma (excluding skin)
Pericytic (perivascular) tumors	Malignant glomus tumor
Skeletal muscle tumors	Embryonal rhabdomyosarcoma Alveolar rhabdomyosarcoma Pleomorphic rhabdomyosarcoma Spindle cell/sclerosing rhabdomyosarcoma
Vascular tumors of soft tissue	Epithelioid hemangioendothelioma Angiosarcoma of soft tissue
Nerve sheath tumors	Malignant peripheral nerve sheath tumor Epithelioid malignant peripheral nerve sheath tumor Malignant perineurioma Malignant Triton tumor Malignant granular cell tumor Ectomesenchymoma (currently classified among skeletal muscle tumors)
Tumors of uncertain differentiation	Synovial sarcoma NOS Synovial sarcoma, spindle cell Synovial sarcoma, biphasic Epithelioid sarcoma Alveolar soft part sarcoma Clear cell sarcoma of soft tissue Extraskeletal myxoid chondrosarcoma Extraskeletal Ewing sarcoma Desmoplastic small round cell tumor Extrarenal rhabdoid tumor Neoplasms with perivascular epithelioid cell differentiation (PEComa) PEComa NOS, benign PEComa NOS, malignant Intimal sarcoma
Undifferentiated/unclassified sarcomas	Undifferentiated spindle cell sarcoma Undifferentiated pleomorphic sarcoma Undifferentiated round cell sarcoma Undifferentiated epithelioid sarcoma Undifferentiated sarcoma NOS

23.5 Immunohistochemistry

Immunohistochemical (IHC) characterization plays a crucial role in the accurate diagnosis of soft tissue sarcomas, providing vital information about tumor differentiation and aiding in classification. This technique involves using specific antibodies to detect various antigens within tumor cells, aiding in the identification of the tissue of origin and the tumor's lineage. However, reliance solely on broad, morphology-unsupervised markers can be problematic, as such markers may lack specificity and lead to diagnostic misinterpretations. Therefore, it is essential to evaluate IHC results within the broader clinical and morphological context, considering the morphological features, clinical presentation, and other diagnostic data. Although

Table 23.2 IHC Differentiation Markers commonly used in the diagnosis of soft tissue sarcomas

Myogenic Differentiation Markers	Smooth muscle actin, muscle specific actin (HHF-35), desmin, h-caldesmon, myogenin (MYF4), and MyoD1 (MYF3)
Neural Differentiation Markers	Glial fibrillary acidic protein (GFAP), SOX10, and H3K27me3 (histone 3K27 trimethylation)
Epithelial Differentiation Markers	Cytokeratin and epithelial membrane antigen (EMA)
Endothelial Differentiation Markers	CD34, CD31, FLI1, ERG, and HHV-8 (Kaposi sarcoma)

Table 23.3 Cases describing patients with cutaneous metastases from liposarcomas

Reference	Age/ Gender	Diagnosis	Location of primary	Location of metastasis	Time to metastasis
[20]	50/M	PLPS	Retroperitoneal	Scalp	N/A
[21]	73/F	PLPS	Retroperitoneal	Multifocal	At time of diagnosis
[22]	63/M	DDL	Retroperitoneal	Multifocal	3 years
[23]	63/M	PLPS	Retroperitoneal	Scalp	3 years
[24]	58/M	DDL	Anterior abdomen/ Groin	Groin/Abdomen skin	15 days postoperatively of the primary tumor

PLPS pleomorphic liposarcoma, *DDL* Dedifferentiated liposarcoma

many classic markers demonstrate high sensitivity, their specificity can be limited, especially as newer markers and molecular tools continue to evolve. Differentiation IHC markers used in the evaluation of soft tissue sarcomas are listed in Table 23.2.

23.6 Cutaneous Metastases from Liposarcomas in the Medical Literature

Liposarcomas represent the most prevalent type of soft tissue sarcomas. Among them, the atypical lipomatous tumor, also known as well-differentiated liposarcoma (WDL) and dedifferentiated liposarcoma (DDL), constitutes the largest subgroup. WDL typically appears as a mass that closely resembles mature fat tissue, making it somewhat challenging to distinguish from benign lipomas on imaging and histological examination. Despite its seemingly indolent behavior, WDL has a propensity for local recurrence after surgical removal, although it rarely metastasizes. A notable aspect of WDL is its potential to undergo dedifferentiation; approximately 10% of cases may transform into DDL over time. DDL is markedly more aggressive, exhibiting a higher likelihood of invasion and metastasis. Histologically, DDL can display a wide range of high-grade features, often resembling other types of high-grade sarcomas, which complicates accurate diagnosis. This diversity in appearance underscores the importance of thorough pathological evaluation, especially when prior evidence of WDL is lacking. The most frequent site of DDL is the retroperitoneum [13–16].

WDL tends to recur locally with a rate of approximately 30–50% of tumors, depending on site, but has no metastatic potential. WDL at any site can dedifferentiate, with an incidence of up to 10%, with those arising at the retroperitoneum showing a higher risk of dedifferentiation [17]. Metastases of DDL can be within the retroperitoneum or to distant sites (liver, lungs, brain, and bone) and soft tissue sites (including the paratesticular region, the back, and thigh) [14, 18, 19]. Cutaneous metastases are reported in five cases in the medical literature, listed in Table 23.3.

23.7 Cutaneous Metastases from Leimyosarcomas in the Medical Literature

Cutaneous leiomyosarcoma is an uncommon malignant neoplasm that arises from smooth muscle cells within the skin. This tumor can present in various forms, typically classified based on its origin within the skin layers. The dermal form of cutaneous leiomyosarcoma tends to be less aggressive compared to its subcutaneous counterpart. Patients with dermal lesions often experience a slower disease progression, and while these tumors tend to recur locally after excision, they rarely metastasize to distant sites. Conversely, subcutaneous leiomyosarcomas are more invasive and exhibit a higher propensity for recurrence and metastasis, which significantly impacts patient outcomes. When the tumor spreads beyond the primary site, the prognosis worsens considerably. Metastatic cases of cutaneous leiomyosarcoma usually derive from a primary tumor located in the retroperitoneum, the uterus, or the subfascial muscle fibers of the extremities and are associated with a particularly poor prognosis [25–28]. Winchester et al. in a retrospective review of 21 cases of skin metastases of leiomyosarcoma, reported that the majority of primary tumor locations were superficial leiomyosarcoma of the skin, followed by the uterus and vena cava. As expected for this kind of tumor that metastasizes hematogenously, the most common location for the first cutaneous metastasis was the scalp, followed by the trunk. [29] In a case series of 130 patients with uterine leiomyosarcoma, Bartosch et al reported that lung metastases were the most common (55%), followed by skin and soft tissue metastases (13%) distributed on the trunk [30].

23.8 Cutaneous Metastases from Rhabdomyosarcoma in the Medical Literature

Rhabdomyosarcomas (RMS) represent the most prevalent type of soft tissue sarcoma found in children, making up approximately 5–8% of all pediatric cancers. RMS holds the distinction of being the third most common extracranial solid tumor in children, following neuroblastoma and Wilms tumor. Notably, it accounts for about half of all pediatric soft tissue sarcomas and approximately 7% of all childhood cancers, underscoring its clinical importance [31]. Skin metastases are rare and mainly affect children. Adult cases of rhabdomyosarcoma metastases to the skin are presented in Table 23.4.

Table 23.4 Cases describing adult patients with cutaneous metastases from rhabdomyosarcomas.

Reference	Age/ gender	Primary site tumor	Site of skin metastasis	Immunohistochemistry
[32]	51/M	Nasal cavity	Face	N/A
[33]	28/M	Unknown	Scalp, upper lip	Positive: vimentin, MyoD1, and myogenin Negative: leukocyte common antigen, desmin, and HHF35 (muscle actin)
[34]	20/M	Orbit	Lumbar area	Positive: desmin, myogenin Negative: cytokeratin, leukocyte common antigen(LCA)
[35]	34/F	Right dorsal region	Right ring finger, right index finger	Positive: vimentin, desmin, myoglobin, and actin Negative: S100 protein, CD68

Table 23.5 Case describing patient with cutaneous metastasis from MPNST

Reference	Age/Gender	Primary site tumor	Site of skin metastasis	Immunohistochemistry
[37]	60/F	Pancreas	Right thigh	Positive: S100, Microphthalmia transcription factor (MITF), and SOX10 Negative: TTF1, CK7, CK20, HMB45, melan-A, and CK903

23.9 Cutaneous Metastases from Nerve Sheath Tumors in the Medical Literature

Malignant peripheral nerve sheath tumors (MPNSTs) are uncommon, highly aggressive types of sarcomas that develop from the cells surrounding peripheral nerves. This tumor is highly associated with neurofibromatosis type I [36]. These tumors are characterized by their rapid growth and potential to invade surrounding tissues, making them particularly challenging to treat [37]. MPNSTs account for approximately 4–10% of all soft tissue sarcomas, highlighting their rarity. Due to their aggressive nature, they tend to metastasize frequently, often spreading to distant organs such as the lungs and liver. Cutaneous metastases are uncommon, and one published case is presented in Table 23.5.

References

1. Clark MA, Fisher C, Judson I, Thomas JM. Soft-tissue sarcomas in adults. N Engl J Med. 2005;353(7):701–11.
2. Plaza JA, Perez-Montiel D, Mayerson J, Morrison C, Suster S. Metastases to soft tissue. Cancer. 2007;112(1):193–203.
3. Staser K, Mount CE, Solus J, Musiek A. Pleomorphic soft tissue sarcoma metastatic to the skin of the scalp and groin. JAAD Case Rep. 2015;1(2):96–8.
4. Hui JYC. Epidemiology and etiology of sarcomas. Surg Clin N Am. 2016;96(5):901–14.
5. Gatta G, van der Zwan JM, Casali PG, Siesling S, Dei Tos AP, Kunkler I, et al. Rare cancers are not so rare: The rare cancer burden in Europe. Eur J Cancer. 2011;47(17):2493–511.
6. Gatta G, Trama A. RARECAREnet: Information network on rare cancers in Europe. Eur J Public Health. 2018;28(suppl_4).
7. Lim HJ, Johnny Ong C-A, Tan JW-S, Ching Teo MC. Utility of positron emission tomography/computed tomography (PET/CT) imaging in the evaluation of sarcomas: a systematic review. Critic Rev Oncol/Hematol. 2019;143:1–13.
8. Simone M. Soft tissue tumors a practical and comprehensive guide to sarcomas and benign neoplasms. Cham: Springer; 2021. p. 823.
9. Prieto Muñoz I, Pardo MJ. Scalp metastasis from leiomyosarcoma of the inferior vena cava sign as the first clinical sign: a case report. Case Rep Oncol Med. 2012;2012:1–3.
10. Wang WL, Bones-Valentin RA, Prieto VG, Pollock RE, Lev DC, Lazar AJ. Sarcoma metastases to the skin. Cancer. 2011;118(11):2900–4.
11. Choi JH, Ro JY. The 2020 WHO classification of tumors of soft tissue: selected changes and new entities. Adv in Anatomic Pathol. 2020;28(1):44–58.
12. Tos APD. Soft tissue sarcomas a pattern-based approach to diagnosis. Cambridge, United Kingdom: Cambridge University Press; 2019.
13. Dei TA. Liposarcoma: new entities and evolving concepts. Ann Diagn Pathol. 2000;4(4):252–66.
14. Iwasa Y, Nakashima Y. Dedifferentiated liposarcoma with lipoma-like well-differentiated liposarcoma. Int J Surg Pathol. 2012;21(1):15–21.
15. Lucas DR, Nascimento AG, Sanjay BKS, Rock MG. Well-differentiated liposarcoma: the Mayo Clinic experience with 58 cases. Am J Clin Pathol. 1994;102(5):677–83.
16. Thway K. Well-differentiated liposarcoma and dedifferentiated liposarcoma: an updated review. Semin Diagn Pathol. 2019;36(2):112–21.
17. Weiss SW, Rao VK. Well-differentiated liposarcoma (atypical lipoma) of deep soft tissue of the extremities, retroperitoneum, and miscellaneous sites. Am J Surg Pathol. 1992;16(11):1051–8.
18. Montgomery E, Fisher C. Paratesticular liposarcoma. Am J Surg Pathol. 2003;27(1):40–7.
19. Huang H-Y, Brennan MF, Singer S, Antonescu CR. Distant metastasis in retroperitoneal dedifferentiated liposarcoma is rare and rapidly fatal: a clinicopathological study with emphasis on the low-grade myxofibrosarcoma-like pattern as an early sign of dedifferentiation. Modern Pathol. 2005;18(7):976–84.
20. Peison B. Retroperitoneal liposarcoma metastatic to scalp. Arch Dermatol. 1978;114(9):1358.
21. Alcalá Pedrajas JN, Jiménez Murillo L, Clemente Millan MJ. Liposarcoma retroperitoneal con metástasis pulmonares, cutáneas y pancreáticas. Archivos de Bronconeumología. 1996;32(6):313–5.
22. Ben Salha I, Zaidi S, Noujaim J, Miah AB, Fisher C, Jones RL, et al. Rare aggressive behavior of MDM2-

amplified retroperitoneal dedifferentiated liposarcoma, with brain, lung and subcutaneous metastases. Rare Tumors. 2016;8(3):105–8.
23. Yu J, Sokumbi O. Cutaneous metastasis of pleomorphic liposarcoma to the scalp: an elusive diagnosis. J Cutaneous Pathol. 2016;43(6):526–30.
24. Chambers M, Badin DJ, Sriharan AA, Linos KD. Expanding the differential of cutaneous epithelioid tumors: a case of dedifferentiated liposarcoma with epithelioid features involving the skin, with review of the literature. J Cutaneous Pathol. 2020;47(6):554–60.
25. Helbig D, Dippel E, Erdmann M, Frisman A, Kage P, Leiter U, et al. S1-guideline cutaneous and subcutaneous leiomyosarcoma. JDDG. Journal der Deutschen Dermatologischen Gesellschaft. 2023;21(5):555–63.
26. Llombart B, Serra-Guillén C, Requena C, Alsina M, Morgado-Carrasco D, Machado I, et al. Leiomyosarcoma and pleomorphic dermal sarcoma: guidelines for diagnosis and treatment. Actas Dermo-Sifiliográficas (English Edition). 2019;110(1):4–11.
27. Rodríguez-Lomba E, Molina-López I, Parra-Blanco V, Suárez-Fernández R, Pulido-Pérez A. Clinical and histopathologic findings of cutaneous leiomyosarcoma: correlation with prognosis in 12 patients. Actas Dermo-Sifiliográficas (English Edition). 2018;109(2):140–7.
28. Soares Queirós C, Filipe P, Soares de Almeida L. Cutaneous leiomyosarcoma: a 20-year retrospective study and review of the literature. Anais Brasileiros de Dermatologia. 2021;96(3):278–83.
29. Winchester DS, Hocker TL, Roenigk RK. Skin metastases of leiomyosarcoma (LMS): a retrospective review of 21 cases. J Am Acad Dermatol. 2015;72(5):910–2.
30. Bartosch C, Afonso M, Pires-Luís AS, Galaghar A, Guimarães M, Antunes L, et al. Distant metastases in uterine leiomyosarcomas: the wide variety of body sites and time intervals to metastatic relapse. Int J Gynecol Pathol. 2017;36(1):31–41.
31. Leiner J, Le Loarer F. The current landscape of rhabdomyosarcomas: an update. Virchows Archiv. 2019;476(1):97–108.
32. Simsir A, Ioffe OB, Henry M. Adult rhabdomyosarcoma with skin metastases: diagnosis by fine needle aspiration biopsy. Acta Cytol. 2001;45(1):106–8.
33. Shimizu S, Yasui C, Minauchi K, Tsuchiya K. Metastatic rhabdomyosarcoma of the skin. J Am Acad Dermatol. 2008;58(5):S118–S20.
34. Elomrani F, Touri S, Ouziane I, Berrada N, Boutayeb S, Mrabti H, et al. Orbital rhabdomyosarcoma with skin metastasis: a case report BMC Res Notes. 2014;7(1).
35. Meneses M, Copparoni C, Samper A. Cutaneous metastasis of rhabdomyosarcoma. J Eur Acad Dermatol Venereol. 2017;31(1):e20–e1.
36. Evans DG, Baser ME, McGaughran J, Sharif S, Howard E, Moran A. Malignant peripheral nerve sheath tumours in neurofibromatosis 1. J Med Genet. 2002;39(5):311–4.
37. Yanofsky VR, Ng E, Ratner D. Cutaneous metastasis of malignant peripheral nerve sheath tumor arising from the pancreas: a rarity. Dermatol Surg. 2019;45(8):1107–9.

24 Cutaneous Metastases from Bone Sarcomas

Nikolaos Sideris

Abstract

Bone sarcoma (BS) is an umbrella term comprising a variety of heterogeneous and rare malignant mesenchymal tumors that arise primarily from osseous tissue. They are characterized by the production of osteoid, cartilaginous, or fibrous matrix and exhibit a wide spectrum of histological subtypes, molecular profiles, and clinical behavior. Despite their rarity, they represent the majority of primary malignant tumors of bone, especially in younger populations. Cutaneous metastases from primary bone sarcomas are exceedingly uncommon and may mimic a broad spectrum of benign and malignant skin lesions, posing therapeutic and diagnostic challenges for both clinicians and pathologists.

Keywords

Bone sarcoma · Osteosarcoma · Chondrosarcoma · Ewing sarcoma · Cutaneous metastases · Immunohistochemistry · Histopathology

N. Sideris (✉)
First Department of Dermatology and Venereology, School of Medicine, Aristotle University, Thessaloniki, Greece

24.1 Introduction to Bone Sarcomas

Primary BSs account for less than 0.2% of all malignant neoplasms across age groups [1, 2], with an overall incidence ranging between 0.8 and 0.9 cases per 100,000/year. Among these, no single subtype exceeds 0.3/100,000/year in incidence [3]. Osteosarcoma is the most common histological subtype, followed by chondrosarcoma and Ewing sarcoma (ES) . These tumors display distinct age distributions and site predilections, which have implications for diagnosis and management. These three types are also, by far, the most common types of BS. The remaining types, known as rare primary malignant bone sarcomas (RPMBS), have a wide variety of clinical and radiographical presentations and are actually so rare that they pose serious diagnostic and treatment challenges.

Osteosarcoma typically affects adolescents and young adults, with a peak incidence of 0.8–1.1 per 100,000/year in the 15–19 age group, where it accounts for more than 10% of all solid tumors [2]. A second, smaller peak is observed in older adults, often in the context of predisposing conditions such as Paget's disease or previous radiotherapy. The male-to-female ratio is approximately 1.4:1. Most tumors arise in the metaphyseal regions of long bones in the young, while axial involvement becomes more common with advancing age. Established risk factors include:

D. Koumaki et al. (eds.), *Cutaneous Metastases*, https://doi.org/10.1007/978-3-032-26764-1_24

Paget's disease of the bone, hereditary cancer syndromes (Li–Fraumeni, Rothmund–Thomson, Werner, Bloom), hereditary retinoblastoma, and prior exposure to ionizing radiation [4].

Chondrosarcoma is the most common bone sarcoma of adulthood, with an incidence of approximately 0.2/100,000/year and peak presentation between 30 and 60 years of age. In contrast to osteosarcoma and ES, there is no significant gender predilection. While conventional chondrosarcomas dominate the spectrum, rarer subtypes such as dedifferentiated, mesenchymal, and clear cell chondrosarcomas each occur with an incidence of <0.1/100,000/year [2]. These variants often demonstrate more aggressive clinical behavior and can mimic other sarcoma types.

ES, a round cell sarcoma driven by EWSR1 gene fusions, is the third most common bone sarcoma, with an annual incidence of approximately 0.1–0.3 per 100,000/year. It primarily affects children and adolescents (median age at diagnosis: 15 years) and exhibits a male predominance (1.5:1). While 50% of cases involve the long bones of the extremities, pelvic bones, ribs, and vertebral column are also frequent sites of origin. Although classically considered a bone tumor, soft-tissue involvement is present in up to 30% of adult cases. ES has been increasingly distinguished from other round cell sarcomas with overlapping morphology but distinct molecular alterations, such as CIC-rearranged sarcomas and BCOR-altered tumors [5].

Other rare BSs include chordomas (arising from notochordal remnants, typically at the skull base or sacrum), undifferentiated high-grade pleomorphic sarcomas, fibrosarcomas, etc., which together constitute a small fraction of malignant bone tumors. Chordomas, for example, are extremely rare, with an incidence of ~0.8/1,000,000/year, and tend to present in older adults (median age ~ 60 years), with a slight male predominance.

Taken together, BSs pose unique diagnostic and therapeutic challenges due to their rarity, histological variability, and tendency for aggressive local and/or distant spread. The most common metastatic sites are the lungs; however, cutaneous metastases, although extremely rare, represent a clinically significant phenomenon with important diagnostic and prognostic implications.

24.2 Metastatic Behavior of Bone Sarcomas

BSs, despite their rarity, demonstrate distinct patterns of metastatic behavior that are critical for prognosis and treatment planning. Metastatic spread typically occurs via hematogenous routes, with the lungs being by far the most common site of dissemination across all major histological subtypes [6–8]. Lymphatic spread is extremely rare, and bone-to-bone metastasis, although possible, is generally a late manifestation of disseminated disease.

Osteosarcoma, the most frequent primary malignant bone tumor, metastasizes in approximately 15–20% of patients at initial diagnosis, with over 85% of these cases involving pulmonary metastases [9]. Metastatic disease may also affect other organs, such as bones or, very rarely, the skin and brain. The presence of metastasis at diagnosis is a strong negative prognostic factor, with 5-year survival rates falling below 30% in such cases, compared to 60–70% in localized disease [10–12].

ES is also highly aggressive and prone to early dissemination. Around 25% of patients present with metastatic disease at diagnosis, [13, 14] most commonly affecting the lungs, bones, and bone marrow [8, 15]. Unlike osteosarcoma, bone and marrow involvement are more common in ES, reflecting its predilection for systemic spread through microscopic foci. Prognosis in metastatic ES is generally poor, particularly in cases with extrapulmonary metastases [8].

Chondrosarcoma exhibits a more indolent behavior overall, especially in its conventional form, but dedifferentiated and mesenchymal variants are associated with a higher risk of metastasis. Pulmonary metastases are again the most common, though the risk and timeline of dissemination are more variable, often occurring late in the disease course [16].

Cutaneous metastases from bone sarcomas are exceedingly rare, with only sporadic case reports available in the literature. These metastases usually occur in the setting of widespread systemic disease and indicate a poor prognosis. Their rarity may reflect both true biological behavior and potential underdiagnosis, especially when not biopsied or mistaken for primary skin lesions.

24.3 General Aspects of Cutaneous Metastases

Cutaneous metastases are an uncommon manifestation of internal malignancies, occurring in approximately 0.7–10% of all cancer patients, depending on tumor type and stage [17, 18]. They may present as the first sign of occult malignancy or, more frequently, arise during the progression of advanced disease. Breast, lung, colon, melanoma, and renal cell carcinomas are among the most frequent primary tumors associated with skin metastases [19].

The mechanisms by which cancer cells reach the skin include hematogenous or lymphatic spread, direct invasion from underlying structures, and iatrogenic seeding along surgical or procedural tracts. Hematogenous dissemination is particularly relevant in sarcomas, given their typical route of metastasis.

The development of skin metastases is generally associated with a poor prognosis, often reflecting disseminated systemic disease [17, 20, 21]. However, their recognition can provide important diagnostic and therapeutic information, particularly when they serve to diagnose a previously unidentified primary malignant tumor, an early indicator of recurrence, or disease progression [18].

24.4 Clinical Presentation

The lesions typically present as rapidly growing, firm, painless nodules in the dermis or subcutaneous tissue. Less commonly, they may present as plaques, papules, ulcers, or inflammatory eruptions [22]. They may be skin-colored, erythematous, violaceous, or ulcerated and range in size from a few millimeters to several centimeters [17].

Most patients present with one or a few lesions, although multiple metastases may occur. The scalp, trunk, and extremities are the most common sites, but lesions have also been reported in less typical areas such as the face and genitalia. Areas previously subjected to surgery or radiotherapy are also sites of predilection for metastasis.

In some cases, the metastatic nodules may mimic benign skin conditions, such as epidermal cysts, dermatofibromas, or pyogenic granulomas, leading to diagnostic delays [23]. Pain is not a consistent feature, but some lesions can be tender or associated with local inflammation.

The time interval between primary tumor diagnosis and the appearance of cutaneous metastases is variable. In osteosarcoma, cutaneous lesions may appear months to years after the initial diagnosis, often in the context of pulmonary or other systemic metastases. Most appear within 2 years of treatment initiation [24]. In general, the median time for pulmonary metastases is 5–6 months, and for extrapulmonary metastases, including cutaneous lesions, 9–10 months [25] .

For ES, precise estimates regarding the timing of cutaneous metastases are not really feasible due to the rarity of the cases. Reports [26, 27] suggest that, similar to osteosarcoma, skin lesions generally develop after a few months, although both shorter and longer intervals have been observed. For other, rarer primary BSs, the available data are extremely limited.

24.5 Diagnosis and Histopathology

The diagnostic approach to suspected cutaneous metastasis from bone sarcomas relies on a combination of clinical suspicion, histopathological confirmation, and systemic staging. Given their rarity and often non-specific clinical appearance, these lesions can easily be misdiagnosed.

Clinical evaluation begins with a thorough history and physical examination. The presence of firm, non-tender nodules, especially in a patient with a known history of sarcoma, should raise suspicion. Particular attention should be paid to areas of prior surgical intervention or radiotherapy, which may serve as sites of tumor seeding or recurrence.

Histopathological diagnosis relies on biopsy and immunohistochemical analysis. The metastatic lesions generally reflect the histology of the primary tumor, although they may be more poorly differentiated:

In *osteosarcoma*, metastatic lesions show malignant osteoid deposition with pleomorphic osteoblastic cells, occasionally forming lace-like trabeculae. *ES* metastases typically consist of sheets of uniform small round blue cells with scant cytoplasm and PAS-positive glycogen. *Chondrosarcoma* metastases reveal lobulated hyaline cartilage with atypical chondrocytes in lacunae, sometimes with myxoid change. As for some other important but exceedingly rare subtypes: *Undifferentiated pleomorphic sarcoma* presents as highly pleomorphic spindle and giant cells in a storiform or fascicular pattern, often with brisk mitoses and necrosis. *Fibrosarcoma of bone* shows intersecting fascicles of monomorphic spindle cells with a herringbone pattern. *Angiosarcoma of bone* demonstrates anastomosing vascular channels lined by atypical endothelial cells, with possible epithelioid morphology. Malignant *giant cell tumor of bone* shows mononuclear stromal cells with numerous scattered multinucleated giant cells. *Chordoma* metastases are characterized by physaliphorous cells with vacuolated cytoplasm in a myxoid stroma, often arranged in cords and lobules.

Summary information on the histopathologic and immunohistochemical features of cutaneous metastases from primary bone sarcomas is presented in Tables 24.1, 24.2, and 24.3 [24, 27–40]. For three of the exceedingly rare histologic subtypes (fibrosarcoma of bone, angiosarcoma of bone, and malignant giant cell tumor of bone), no documented cases of cutaneous metastases have been reported in the literature; therefore, the histopathologic and immunohistochemical features presented are extrapolated from the description of the primary tumors. We also excluded some extremely rare and distinct entities, such as osteoblastoma (usually benign, with rare and even controversial malignant transformation) and hemangiopericytoma (exceptionally rare in bone). Naturally, cutaneous metastases of these tumor types have never been reported.

Table 24.1 Histopathologic features of cutaneous metastases from primary bone sarcomas

Primary bone sarcoma	Histopathologic features in cutaneous metastases
Osteosarcoma	Malignant spindle/pleomorphic cells with osteoid production; lace-like eosinophilic osteoid; frequent atypical mitoses; necrosis is common.
Ewing sarcoma	Sheets of small, round blue cells; scant cytoplasm; fine nuclear chromatin; possible Homer-Wright rosettes.
Chondrosarcoma	Lobulated pattern; malignant chondrocytes in lacunae; cartilaginous matrix (blue/purple, basophilic); nuclear atypia; binucleation; possible myxoid change.
Undifferentiated pleomorphic sarcoma of bone	Storiform/pleomorphic arrangement; spindle and bizarre multinucleated giant cells; marked atypia; high mitotic index; necrosis.
Fibrosarcoma of bone	Intersecting fascicles of spindle cells (herringbone pattern); eosinophilic cytoplasm; elongated nuclei with variable atypia.
Angiosarcoma of bone	Anastomosing vascular channels; atypical endothelial cells lining irregular spaces; erythrocyte extravasation; possible solid epithelioid areas.
Giant cell tumor of bone	Mononuclear stromal cells with numerous scattered multinucleated osteoclast-like giant cells.
Chordoma	Lobules of physaliphorous cells with vacuolated cytoplasm; myxoid stroma; cords/nests separated by fibrous septa.

The differential diagnosis includes other cutaneous neoplasms, metastatic carcinomas, lymphomas, other sarcomas, and, of course, the benign conditions mentioned above (cysts, dermatofibromas, pyogenic granulomas, etc.). Given

Table 24.2 Immunohistochemical features of cutaneous metastases from primary bone sarcomas

Primary bone sarcoma	Immunohistochemical features in cutaneous metastases
Osteosarcoma	SATB2+, osteocalcin+, osteonectin+, alkaline phosphatase+, vimentin+; negative for cytokeratins, EMA, S100.
Ewing sarcoma	CD99+, FLI-1+, NKX2.2+; PAS+ glycogen; negative for keratins and LCA.
Chondrosarcoma	S100+, SOX9+, type II collagen+; negative for cytokeratins, EMA.
Undifferentiated pleomorphic sarcoma of bone	Vimentin+; variably CD68+, α1-antichymotrypsin+; negative for lineage-specific markers (keratins, S100, desmin).
Fibrosarcoma of bone	Vimentin+; occasionally SMA+; negative for S100, keratins, desmin.
Angiosarcoma of bone	CD31+, ERG+, FLI-1+, factor VIII-related antigen+; CD34 often+; keratins may be focally positive.
Giant cell tumor of bone	RANKL+, CD68+, H3F3A G34W+
Chordoma	Brachyury (nuclear)+, cytokeratins (AE1/AE3)+, EMA+, S100+ (often focal), vimentin+.

Table 24.3 Histopathology and immunohistochemistry notes for cutaneous metastases from primary bone sarcomas

Primary bone sarcoma	Histology notes/differential/pitfalls	IHC notes/differential/pitfalls
Osteosarcoma	May mimic reactive bone formation, ossifying dermatofibroma, or metastatic carcinoma with osteoid production.	SATB2 is relatively specific for osteoblastic differentiation, though not entirely exclusive.
Ewing sarcoma	Can resemble lymphoma, rhabdomyosarcoma, neuroblastoma, Merkel cell carcinoma, or small cell melanoma.	CD99 is sensitive but not specific; FLI-1 and NKX2.2 improve diagnostic accuracy.
Chondrosarcoma	May be confused with chondroid syringoma, myxoid soft-tissue sarcoma, or extraskeletal myxoid chondrosarcoma.	Must be distinguished from melanoma (also S100+); melanocytic markers (HMB45, Melan-A) aid in differential diagnosis.
Undifferentiated pleomorphic sarcoma of bone	Overlaps with cutaneous pleomorphic sarcoma, atypical fibroxanthoma, leiomyosarcoma, or melanoma (spindle cell type).	Diagnosis of exclusion; broad panel required to rule out other sarcomas.
Fibrosarcoma of bone	Mimics dermatofibrosarcoma protuberans, fibrosarcomatous transformation of DFSP, or low-grade myofibroblastic sarcoma.	No pathognomonic marker; relies on morphology and exclusion.
Angiosarcoma of bone	May resemble primary cutaneous angiosarcoma, Kaposi sarcoma, or epithelioid hemangioendothelioma.	CD31 is the most specific vascular marker; differentiation from epithelioid hemangioendothelioma is essential.
Giant cell tumor of bone	May mimic aneurysmal bone cyst or osteoclast-rich sarcomas; malignant transformation is rare and usually shows conventional sarcoma morphology.	RANKL expression in stromal cells drives recruitment of osteoclast-like giant cells.
Chordoma	Can be mistaken for metastatic mucinous adenocarcinoma, myoepithelial carcinoma, or clear cell neoplasms.	Brachyury is highly specific, helping distinguish between metastatic adenocarcinoma and chondrosarcoma.

the rarity of skin metastases from BSs, a high index of suspicion and careful clinical-pathological correlation are necessary for accurate diagnosis.

Radiologic imaging is crucial to assess both the extent of cutaneous involvement and systemic disease burden. In known cancer patients, a new skin lesion warrants a whole-body imaging workup — typically with contrast-enhanced CT, PET/CT, or MRI as indicated. These studies help determine whether the cutaneous lesion is an isolated recurrence or part of a broader metastatic spread. PET/CT is particularly useful in BSs due to their high metabolic activity.

In some cases, fine-needle aspiration (FNA) may be performed initially, but its diagnostic yield is often lower than that of excisional biopsy, particularly in lesions with dense matrix components such as chondroid or osteoid tissue.

24.6 Therapeutic Considerations for Cutaneous Metastases of Bone Sarcomas

Management of cutaneous metastases from bone sarcomas requires a multidisciplinary approach, ideally within a sarcoma board including dermatology, medical oncology, radiation oncology, pathology, and surgery. Once the diagnosis is confirmed, staging and treatment should follow established sarcoma guidelines and be tailored according to disease extent, symptoms, performance status, and patient preferences.

In most cases, the presence of skin metastases indicates disseminated disease, and systemic therapy remains the cornerstone of treatment. Multi-agent chemotherapy addresses both the primary tumor and metastatic deposits, including skin. Responses in cutaneous sites are generally limited, but systemic therapy is essential since local measures alone are insufficient. Typical examples include MAP-based approaches as front-line therapy for osteosarcoma (Methotrexate-Adriamycin-Cisplatin), interval-compressed (every 2 weeks) VDC/IE for ES (Vincristine-Doxorubicin-Cyclophosphamide/Ifosfamide—Etoposide), irinotecan-temozolomide or high-dose busulfan-melphalan for relapsed ES, etc. Tyrosine kinase inhibitors, like cabozantinib, have demonstrated some activity and improved progression-free survival in studies. Many other targeted agents (pazopanib, anlotinib, regorafenib, etc.) are under investigation for various types and stages of BSs [2, 41–43].

Skin-directed treatments are mainly considered adjunctive, aiming to alleviate symptoms such as bleeding, pain, malodor, or functional impairment. Electrochemotherapy, most commonly with bleomycin, represents an effective modality in cases of painful, bleeding, or ulcerated skin lesions not amenable to excision and has consistently provided meaningful symptom relief and local control across cutaneous metastases of different origins [44–46]. Radiotherapy also holds a palliative role, with short hypofractionated courses reducing pain, bleeding, or mass effect; dose and fractionation are individualized depending on lesion size, location, and expected benefit [47, 48]. Surgical excision or debulking may be considered in selected patients, particularly when lesions are isolated, accessible, and symptomatic, or when systemic disease is indolent or controlled [49]. Although rare cases of isolated cutaneous metastasectomy with curative intent have been reported, surgery primarily serves palliative and hygienic purposes.

Finally, supportive measures are integral to comprehensive care. Meticulous wound management, hemostatic dressings, infection and odor control, and adequate analgesia often provide disproportionate improvements in quality of life and should be initiated early [50–52].

References

1. Gatta G, Capocaccia R, Botta L, Mallone S, De Angelis R, Ardanaz E, et al. RARECAREnet working group. Burden and centralised treatment in Europe of rare tumours: results of RARECAREnet-a population-based study. Lancet Oncol. 2017;18(8):1022–39. https://doi.org/10.1016/S1470-2045(17)30445-X.
2. ESMO/European Sarcoma Network Working Group. Bone sarcomas: ESMO clinical prac-

tice Guidelines for diagnosis, treatment and follow-up. Ann Oncol. 2014;25(Suppl 3):iii113–23. https://doi.org/10.1093/annonc/mdu256.
3. Strauss SJ, Frezza AM, Abecassis N, Bajpai J, Bauer S, Biagini R, et al.; ESMO Guidelines Committee, EURACAN, GENTURIS and ERN PaedCan. Bone sarcomas: ESMO-EURACAN-GENTURIS-ERN PaedCan clinical practice guideline for diagnosis, treatment and follow-up. Ann Oncol 2021;32(12):1520–1536. https://doi.org/10.1016/j.annonc.2021.08.1995.
4. Fuchs B, Pritchard DJ. Etiology of osteosarcoma. Clin Orthop Relat Res. 2002;397:40–52. https://doi.org/10.1097/00003086-200204000-00007.
5. WHO Classification of Tumours Editorial Board. WHO Classification of Tumours, 5th ed, Volume 3: Soft Tissue and Bone Tumours. WHO Classification of Tumours series. Lyon: International Agency for Research on Cancer; 2020. ISBN-13: 978-92-832-4502-5.
6. Crombé A, Simonetti M, Longhi A, Hauger O, Fadli D, Spinnato P. Imaging of osteosarcoma: presenting findings, metastatic patterns, and features related to prognosis. J Clin Med. 2024;13(19):5710. https://doi.org/10.3390/jcm13195710.
7. Odri GA, Tchicaya-Bouanga J, Yoon DJY, Modrowski D. Metastatic progression of osteosarcomas: a review of current knowledge of environmental versus oncogenic drivers. Cancers (Basel). 2022;14(2):360. https://doi.org/10.3390/cancers14020360.
8. Zhang L, Xiong L, Wu LM, Shen WH, Zhou P, Lian CL, et al. The patterns of distant metastasis and prognostic factors in patients with primary metastatic Ewing sarcoma of the bone. J Bone Oncol. 2021;30:100385. https://doi.org/10.1016/j.jbo.2021.100385.
9. Isakoff MS, Bielack SS, Meltzer P, Gorlick R. Osteosarcoma: current treatment and a collaborative pathway to success. J Clin Oncol. 2015;33(27):3029–35. https://doi.org/10.1200/JCO.2014.59.4895.
10. Smeland S, Bielack SS, Whelan J, Bernstein M, Hogendoorn P, Krailo MD, et al. Survival and prognosis with osteosarcoma: 2023 outcomes in more than 2000 patients in the EURAMOS-1 (European and American Osteosarcoma Study) cohort. Eur J Cancer. 2019;109:36–50. https://doi.org/10.1016/j.ejca.2018.11.027.
11. Kager L, Zoubek A, Pötschger U, Kastner U, Flege S, Kempf-Bielack B, et al.; Cooperative German-Austrian-Swiss Osteosarcoma Study Group. Primary metastatic osteosarcoma: presentation and outcome of patients treated on neoadjuvant Cooperative Osteosarcoma Study Group protocols. J Clin Oncol 2003;21(10):2011–2018. https://doi.org/10.1200/JCO.2003.08.132.
12. American Cancer Society. Survival rates for osteosarcoma. Available from: https://www.cancer.org/cancer/types/osteosarcoma/detection-diagnosis-staging/survival-rates.html. Accessed 24 Aug 2025.
13. Ozaki T. Diagnosis and treatment of Ewing sarcoma of the bone: a review article. J Orthop Sci. 2015;20(2):250–63. https://doi.org/10.1007/s00776-014-0687-z.
14. Grier HE, Krailo MD, Tarbell NJ, Link MP, Fryer CJ, Pritchard DJ, et al. Addition of ifosfamide and etoposide to standard chemotherapy for Ewing's sarcoma and primitive neuroectodermal tumor of bone. N Engl J Med. 2003;348(8):694–701. https://doi.org/10.1056/NEJMoa020890.
15. Oberlin O, Rey A, Desfachelles AS, Philip T, Plantaz D, Schmitt C, et al.; Société Française des Cancers de l'Enfant. Impact of high-dose busulfan plus melphalan as consolidation in metastatic Ewing tumors: a study by the Société Française des Cancers de l'Enfant. J Clin Oncol 2006;24(24):3997–4002. https://doi.org/10.1200/JCO.2006.05.7059.
16. de Camargo OP, Baptista AM, Atanásio MJ, Waisberg DR. Chondrosarcoma of bone: lessons from 46 operated cases in a single institution. Clin Orthop Relat Res. 2010;468(11):2969–75. https://doi.org/10.1007/s11999-010-1368-7.
17. Lookingbill DP, Spangler N, Helm KF. Cutaneous metastases in patients with metastatic carcinoma: a retrospective study of 4020 patients. J Am Acad Dermatol. 1993;29(2 Pt 1):228–36. https://doi.org/10.1016/0190-9622(93)70173-q.
18. Fernández-Antón Martínez MC, Parra-Blanco V, Avilés Izquierdo JA, Suárez Fernández RM. Cutaneous metastases of internal tumors. Actas Dermosifiliogr. 2013;104(10):841–53. English, Spanish. https://doi.org/10.1016/j.ad.2012.06.005.
19. Brownstein MH, Helwig EB. Patterns of cutaneous metastasis. Arch Dermatol. 1972;105(6):862–8.
20. Teyateeti P, Ungtrakul T. Retrospective review of cutaneous metastasis among 11,418 patients with solid malignancy: a tertiary cancer center experience. Medicine (Baltimore). 2021;100(29):e26737. https://doi.org/10.1097/MD.0000000000026737.
21. Schoenlaub P, Sarraux A, Grosshans E, Heid E, Cribier B. Survie après métastases cutanées: étude de 200 cas [Survival after cutaneous metastasis: a study of 200 cases]. Ann Dermatol Venereol. 2001;128(12):1310–5.
22. Alcaraz I, Cerroni L, Rütten A, Kutzner H, Requena L. Cutaneous metastases from internal malignancies: a clinicopathologic and immunohistochemical review. Am J Dermatopathol. 2012;34(4):347–93. https://doi.org/10.1097/DAD.0b013e31823069cf.
23. Schwartz RA. Cutaneous metastatic disease. J Am Acad Dermatol. 1995;33(2 Pt 1):161–82.; quiz 183–6. https://doi.org/10.1016/0190-9622(95)90231-7.
24. Larsen S, Davis DM, Comfere NI, Folpe AL, Sciallis GF. Osteosarcoma of the skin. Int J Dermatol. 2010;49(5):532–40. https://doi.org/10.1111/j.1365-4632.2010.04315.x.
25. Jeffree GM, Price CH, Sissons HA. The metastatic patterns of osteosarcoma. Br J Cancer. 1975;32(1):87–107. https://doi.org/10.1038/bjc.1975.136.

26. Biswas G, Khadwal A, Kulkarni P, Bakshi A, Nair C, Kurkure P, et al. Ewing's sarcoma with cutaneous metastasis—a rare entity: report of three cases. Indian J Dermatol Venereol Leprol. 2005;71(6):423–5. https://doi.org/10.4103/0378-6323.18950.
27. Izquierdo MJ, Pastor MA, Carrasco L, Requena C, Fariña MC, Martín L, et al. Cutaneous metastases from Ewing's sarcoma: report of two cases. Clin Exp Dermatol. 2002;27(2):123–8. https://doi.org/10.1046/j.1365-2230.2002.00973.x.
28. Patterson JW, Maygarden SJ. Extraskeletal Ewing's sarcoma with cutaneous involvement. J Cutan Pathol. 1986;13(1):46–58. https://doi.org/10.1111/j.1600-0560.1986.tb00460.x.
29. Covello SP, Humphreys TR, Lee JB. A case of extraskeletal osteosarcoma with metastasis to the skin. J Am Acad Dermatol. 2003;49(1):124–7. https://doi.org/10.1067/mjd.2003.297.
30. Ouseph MM, Sharan GK, Sharma P, Rathi AK, Shyama J, Singh K, et al. Osteosarcoma with cutaneous metastases. A case report. Acta Cytol. 2007;51(1):102–6. https://doi.org/10.1159/000325695.
31. Collier DA, Busam K, Salob S. Cutaneous metastasis of osteosarcoma. J Am Acad Dermatol. 2003;49(4):757–60. https://doi.org/10.1067/s0190-9622(03)00460-2.
32. Ragsdale MI, Lehmer LM, Ragsdale BD, Chow WA, Carson RT. Cutaneous metastasis of osteosarcoma in the scalp. Am J Dermatopathol. 2011;33(6):e70–3. https://doi.org/10.1097/DAD.0b013e318214a7ea.
33. Correia C, Fernandes S, Filipe P, Kutzner H, Soares-de-Almeida L. A rare case of cutaneous metastasis of distal phalanx chondrosarcoma. Dermatol Online J. 2022;28(2). https://doi.org/10.5070/D328257397.
34. Karabela-Bouropoulou V, Patra-Malli F, Agnantis N. Chondrosarcoma of the thumb: an unusual case with lung and cutaneous metastases and death of the patient 6 years after treatment. J Cancer Res Clin Oncol. 1986;112(1):71–4. https://doi.org/10.1007/BF00394943.
35. Arce FP, Pinto J, Portero I, Echevarría S, Val-Bernal JF. Cutaneous metastases as initial manifestation of dedifferentiated chondrosarcoma of bone. An autopsy case with review of the literature. J Cutan Pathol. 2000;27(5):262–7. https://doi.org/10.1034/j.1600-0560.2000.027005262.x.
36. Suarez Conde MF, Vallone MG, González VM, Vigovich FA, Casas JG, Cermignan L, et al. Metastatic chordoma. JAAD Case Rep. 2019;5(10):852–4. https://doi.org/10.1016/j.jdcr.2019.07.029. PMID: 31649971; PMCID: PMC6804473.
37. Dimopoulos YP, Ivan D, Prieto VG, Aung PP. Chordoma metastatic to skin: a report of two cases and a brief review of the literature. J Cutan Pathol. 2023;50(6):500–4. https://doi.org/10.1111/cup.14348.
38. D'Amuri A, Brunelli M, Floccari F, De Caro F, Crisman G, Sanguedolce F, et al. On a rare cutaneous metastasis from a sacrococcygeal chordoma. Case Rep Pathol. 2017;2017:5281239. https://doi.org/10.1155/2017/5281239.
39. Harish M, Yadala A, Joshi RP, Parameswari R. A rare presentation of a cutaneous metastasis from an undifferentiated pleomorphic sarcoma. J Cancer Res Ther. 2025;21(3):743–5. https://doi.org/10.4103/jcrt.jcrt_1771_24.
40. Yamamoto H, Ishihara S, Toda Y, Oda Y. Histone H3.3 mutation in giant cell tumor of bone: an update in pathology. Med Mol Morphol. 2020;53(1):1–6. https://doi.org/10.1007/s00795-019-00238-1.
41. Gerrand C, Amary F, Anwar HA, Brennan B, Dileo P, Kalkat MS, et al. UK guidelines for the management of bone sarcomas. Br J Cancer. 2025;132(1):32–48. https://doi.org/10.1038/s41416-024-02868-4.
42. Womer RB, West DC, Krailo MD, Dickman PS, Pawel BR, Grier HE, et al. Randomized controlled trial of interval-compressed chemotherapy for the treatment of localized Ewing sarcoma: a report from the Children's Oncology Group. J Clin Oncol. 2012;30(33):4148–54. https://doi.org/10.1200/JCO.2011.41.5703.
43. Italiano A, Mir O, Mathoulin-Pelissier S, Penel N, Piperno-Neumann S, Bompas E, et al. Cabozantinib in patients with advanced Ewing sarcoma or osteosarcoma (CABONE): a multicentre, single-arm, phase 2 trial. Lancet Oncol. 2020;21(3):446–55. https://doi.org/10.1016/S1470-2045(19)30825-3.
44. Gehl J, Sersa G, Matthiessen LW, Muir T, Soden D, Occhini A, et al. Updated standard operating procedures for electrochemotherapy of cutaneous tumours and skin metastases. Acta Oncol. 2018;57(7):874–82. https://doi.org/10.1080/0284186X.2018.1454602.
45. Ferioli M, Lancellotta V, Perrone AM, Arcelli A, Galuppi A, Strigari L, et al. Electrochemotherapy of skin metastases from malignant melanoma: a PRISMA-compliant systematic review. Clin Exp Metastasis. 2022;39(5):743–55. https://doi.org/10.1007/s10585-022-10180-9.
46. Cabula C, Campana LG, Grilz G, Galuppo S, Bussone R, De Meo L, et al. Electrochemotherapy in the treatment of cutaneous metastases from breast cancer: a multicenter cohort analysis. Ann Surg Oncol. 2015;22(Suppl 3):S442–50. https://doi.org/10.1245/s10434-015-4779-6.
47. Johnstone C, Lutz ST. The role of hypofractionated radiation in the management of non-osseous metastatic or uncontrolled local cancer. Ann Palliat Med. 2014;3(4):291–303. https://doi.org/10.3978/j.issn.2224-5820.2014.10.01.
48. Keatts SA, Salem AF, Swanson DM, Farooqi AS, Bishop AJ, Amaria RN, et al. Durable local control with hypofractionated radiation therapy for unresectable or metastatic melanoma. Clin Transl Radiat Oncol. 2024;49:100856. https://doi.org/10.1016/j.ctro.2024.100856.
49. Huang S, Parekh V, Waisman J, Jones V, Yuan Y, Vora N, et al. Cutaneous metastasectomy: is there a role in breast cancer? A systematic review and overview of current treatment

modalities. J Surg Oncol. 2022;126(2):217–38. https://doi.org/10.1002/jso.26870.
50. da Costa Santos CM, de Mattos Pimenta CA, Nobre MR. A systematic review of topical treatments to control the odor of malignant fungating wounds. J Pain Symptom Manag. 2010;39(6):1065–76. https://doi.org/10.1016/j.jpainsymman.2009.11.319.
51. Furka A, Simkó C, Kostyál L, Szabó I, Valikovics A, Fekete G, et al. Treatment algorithm for cancerous wounds: a systematic review. Cancers (Basel). 2022;14(5):1203. https://doi.org/10.3390/cancers14051203.
52. Firmino F, Villela-Castro DL, Santos JD, de Gouveia C, Santos VL. Topical management of bleeding from malignant wounds caused by breast cancer: a systematic review. J Pain Symptom Manag. 2021;61(6):1278–86. https://doi.org/10.1016/j.jpainsymman.2020.10.020.

Part XII

Cutaneous Metastases from Primary Cutaneous Malignancies

Cutaneous Metastases from Primary Cutaneous Malignancies

25

Daniel Micallef, David Pisani, and Michael J. Boffa

Abstract

Cutaneous malignancies, particularly melanoma, rank among the most frequent cancers to metastasize to the skin. Up to one-fifth of patients with primary melanoma develop cutaneous metastases, which may manifest as microsatellites, satellite lesions, in-transit metastases, or distant deposits. The clinical appearance of metastatic cutaneous melanoma is highly variable, ranging from dark brown or black lesions to skin-colored papules and nodules, sometimes accompanied by pruritus, ulceration, bleeding, pain, or paresthesia. Dermoscopy can aid in diagnosis, especially when features such as a homogeneous blue pattern, globules, uniform brown pigmentation, red or purple lacunae, and irregular vessels are present. Histologically, lesions typically consist of a well-circumscribed dermal proliferation of malignant melanocytes, although cases may also rarely exhibit an epidermal component. Conversely, primary dermal melanomas have been documented, underscoring the need to integrate clinical context and imaging findings to confirm the diagnosis.

Beyond melanoma, cutaneous metastases can also occur with Merkel cell carcinoma and, less frequently, squamous cell carcinoma (SCC). SCC metastases often present as in-transit lesions from head and neck primaries, while Merkel cell carcinoma—though rare—not uncommonly gives rise to in-transit or distant cutaneous deposits.

Management of cutaneous metastatic disease extends beyond surgery, with modalities such as targeted therapy and immunotherapy offering the potential for durable responses and improved survival outcomes.

Keywords

Cutaneous metastases · melanoma · squamous cell carcinoma · Merkel cell carcinoma · targeted therapy · immunotherapy

D. Micallef (✉)
Department of Dermatology, Mater Dei Hospital, Msida, Malta
e-mail: daniel.b.micallef@gov.mt

D. Pisani
Department of Pathology, Mater Dei Hospital, Msida, Malta
e-mail: david.c.pisani@gov.mt

M. J. Boffa
Department of Dermatology, Mater Dei Hospital, Msida, Malta

University of South Wales, Wales, UK
e-mail: michael.boffa@gov.mt

D. Koumaki et al. (eds.), *Cutaneous Metastases*, https://doi.org/10.1007/978-3-032-26764-1_25

25.1 Introduction

Cutaneous metastatic deposits are often presumed to originate from an internal malignancy, however, metastatic deposits, however, metastatic deposits from primary cutaneous melanomas are, in fact, depending on the series analysed, either the commonest or amongst the commoner malignancies that metastasise to skin [1–3]. Additionally, the skin may also harbor metastases from other cutaneous primaries, including squamous cell carcinomas, Merkel cell carcinomas, and adnexal malignancies.

25.2 Cutaneous Metastasis from Melanoma

25.2.1 Epidemiology

The incidence of cutaneous melanoma metastases (CMM) shows significant gender and geographic variance. In a cohort of 420 patients with cutaneous metastases in the United States, CMM represented 18.3% of all cases. CMM was preceded only by breast cancer in females but was the commonest primary disease site in males [4]. CMM frequencies as low as 7% were documented in a cohort of 115 Filipino patients [5], rising to 27.1% in a cohort of 96 Chilean patients [6].

In patients with a known primary melanoma, the incidence of CMM ranges widely from 2% to 20% depending on the cohorts studied [7], with one of the largest long-term cohort studies of 4030 melanoma patients in Italy documenting cutaneous metastases in 18.2% of cases [8]. A mean interval of 1.3 and 2.9 years from primary diagnosis has been documented for regional and distant metastasis, respectively [9]. Importantly, CMM may represent the first manifestation of melanoma in up to 5% of cases [10].

25.2.2 Classification of Cutaneous Metastatic Disease

Classification of CMM bears critical importance in patient prognostication and is outlined in the ninth edition of the American Joint Committee on Cancer (AJCC). Locoregional CMM occurs anywhere between the primary melanoma and the draining lymph node basin, while distant CMM occurs beyond the nodal basin [11]. The presence of locoregional CMM upstages a melanoma to a pN1c, stage IIIB category in the absence of locoregional nodal spread [12], implying a significantly increased risk of locoregional recurrence, lymph node metastasis, and decreased disease-free survival (DFS) and overall survival (OS) [13–17].

25.2.3 Melanoma Microsatellites

The AJCC defines microsatellites as any histologically identified foci of metastatic melanoma in microscopic proximity to the primary tumor but irrespective of size or distance, present in the skin or subcutaneous adipose tissue, and separated from the primary tumor by normal stroma (i.e., in the absence of inflammation or fibrosis) (Figs. 25.1 and 25.2) [11]. Microsatellites are an independent risk factor of 5- and 10-year DFS (36% / 27%, respectively, with microsatellites vs. 90% / 60% without) [18, 19] and correlate with locoregional recurrence, in-transit metastasis, and sentinel lymph node positivity, although, curiously, not distant metastasis [18, 20, 21].

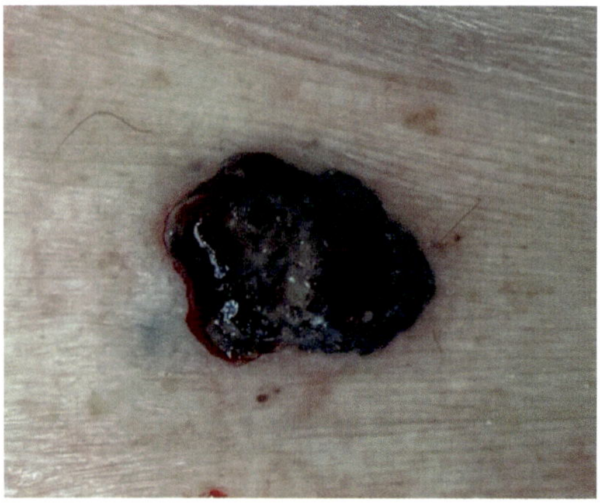

Fig. 25.1 Clinical photograph of an ulcerated nodular melanoma on the upper back with a separate bluish nodule to the 8 o'clock region, representing a satellite lesion

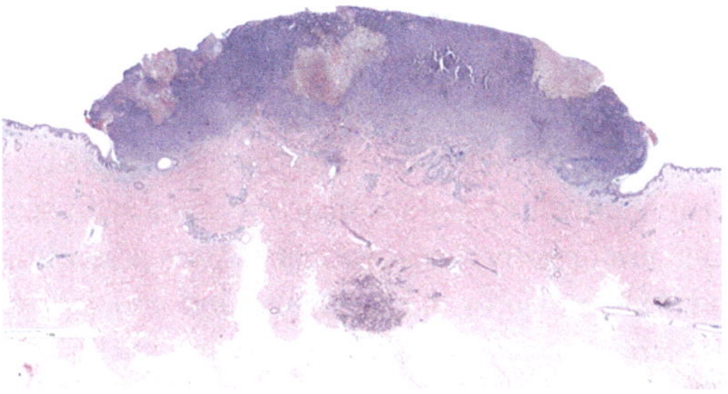

Fig. 25.2 An ulcerated nodular melanoma together with a microsatellite, separated from the main tumor by normal skin, centered on the deep dermis and abutting the subcutaneous adipose tissue (hematoxylin and eosin [H&E], ×15)

Microsatellites have been documented with increased frequencies in superficial spreading and nodular melanomas, with a higher prevalence suggested in head and neck regions [18], with their incidence being extremely low in thin melanomas (Breslow <1.0 mm) [22]. While neither microsatellite number nor size has a clear prognostic impact, the distance between the microsatellite and the main tumor is significant, with worse prognoses at intervals of 1 and 3.75 mm from the primary tumor [21].

25.2.4 Satellite Deposits and In-transit Metastases

The AJCC defines any cutaneous or subcutaneous metastatic deposit of melanoma occurring within the confines of the regional nodal basin as a *satellite deposit* if lying within a 2 cm radius from the primary tumor or its scar and as an *in-transit metastasis* if beyond this radius [11]. Satellite deposits and in-transit metastases (ITM-S) will be considered together in this review given that there appear to be no clear prognostic differences to date. ITM-S develop in approximately 2–13% of melanoma patients [23] and occur, in decreasing frequency, on the extremities, trunk, and head and neck [24]. Risk factors associated with locoregional cutaneous dissemination include a Breslow thickness >2 mm and primary tumor locations on acral sites, the lower extremities, and the head and neck [25].

ITM-S represent a pattern of melanoma cell dissemination and subsequent cutaneous seeding, presumably through cutaneous angiolymphatic channels [23]. ITM-S are clonally related to, and thus share similar mutational burdens as the parent primary melanoma [24], with loss of heterozygosity in 9p23–22 and 9p21 (likely involving the *NFIB*, *CDKN2A*, and *CDKN2B* tumor suppressor genes) being common in primary melanomas and found in around 50% of ITM-S [26, 27]. Additional loss in regions 1p, 10q, and 11q is found in around 35% of ITM-S [24, 28], with these regions encoding genes involved in cell cycle regulation (*NPAT*), cell cycle progression (*PPP2R1B*), and matrix degradation (*MMP23B*), among others. Furthermore, *NRAS* Q61 driver mutations are harbored at higher frequencies than primary melanomas and distant metastases, and, conversely, *NF1* function appears to be retained in ITM-S [29].

ITM-S are particularly strong predictors of locoregional lymph node involvement [23, 24], in the absence of which, ITM-S carry a 5-year survival of around 60%, this dropping to 36% in the presence of nodal disease. In the presence of ITM-S, the worst outcome is borne by patients with four or more involved nodes and primary tumors with Breslow thickness more than 3 mm [30].

25.2.5 Distant Cutaneous Melanoma Metastases

Present beyond the draining lymph node basin of the primary melanoma, distant cutaneous melanoma metastases (DCMM) represent AJCC pM1a stage IV disease [11]. While still overall poor, prognosis is marginally better than in the presence of pulmonary (pM1b), non-central nervous system visceral (pM1c), and central nervous system (pM1d) metastatic disease [31].

In the Caucasian population, melanomas are often non-acral (typically superficial spreading) in type, associated with ultraviolet radiation and consequently carrying a high mutational burden, and are frequently *BRAF/NRAS*-driven. Conversely, a higher incidence of acral melanomas with unclear pathogenesis and lower mutational burdens and *KIT* mutations is described in the Asian and Hispanic populations [32, 33]. DCMMs are more common in the non-acral melanoma subgroup, with metastatic disease occurring more often on the trunk and regularly more extensive in nature. Conversely, acral melanomas harbor ITM-S more frequently than distant metastases, with these often presenting slightly earlier than in non-acral melanomas (16 vs. 20 months). The number of DCMM, together with the frequencies of concomitant nodal and visceral metastatic disease, appears similar between the two categories. Furthermore, patients presenting with cutaneous involvement within 12 months of diagnosis appear to have a higher tendency for multiple cutaneous metastases and have a significantly poorer median overall survival (36 vs. 76 months) [34].

The pathogenesis of DCMM is unclear, with very few comparative studies available between the parent melanoma, ITM-S, regional lymph node metastasis, and DCMM. While the frequencies of *BRAF* and *KIT* appear similar across these groups, DCMM are often enriched in *NF1* (especially when compared to ITM-S), with this subgroup often carrying particular poor DFS and OS rates [29, 35].

25.2.6 Clinical and Dermoscopic Features

The clinical diagnosis of CMM requires a high index of suspicion and may be diagnostically challenging. While the morphological spectrum is similar for ITM-S and DCMM, anatomical distributions differ significantly. A United States-based cohort of 195 patients with CMM showed, with decreasing prevalence, involvement of the lower extremities (37.2%), the head and neck (31.4%), the upper extremities (18.6%), and the trunk (12.8%), although the pattern of spread was not stratified by melanoma subtype [10]. In a Korean-based cohort of 61 patients, acral melanomas (38% of the cohort) showed a much higher frequency of lower limb ITM-S, while non-acral melanomas showed more frequent truncal metastatic deposits (60.5%), followed by involvement of the limbs (31.6%) and head and neck regions (28.9%) [34].

The morphological spectrum of CMM is astounding, and lesions may vary greatly in size and multiplicity across patients. Cases presenting as dark brown or black papules and nodules are generally easier to diagnose than amelanotic, flesh-colored lesions, which may mimic dermatofibromas or benign nevi. While often asymptomatic, lesions may be complicated with pruritus, ulceration, bleeding, pain, and paresthesia [36, 37]. Rarer presentations include erysipeloid, well-demarcated, apigmented patches or plaques [38], a pattern of diffuse sclerodermoid infiltration (a pattern more often associated with breast carcinoma) termed melanoma en cuirasse [39], dermatomally distributed vesiculobullous zosteriform lesions [40], alopecia neoplastica [41] and livedo reticularis-like patterns (occurring secondary to widespread vascular emboli) [42].

While dermoscopic features lack a universally diagnostic pattern, certain features may assist in differentiating metastatic lesions from benign mimickers. Five global dermoscopic patterns have been proposed [43, 44], as summarized in Table 25.1. The presence of a homogeneous blue pattern, globules, homogeneous brown pigmentation, red and/or purple lacunae and irregular vessels has been reported to have an overall sensitivity (68%) and specificity (76%) for the diagnosis of CMM [45].

25.2.7 Pathological Features and Histologic Mimics

While CMMs do not typically pose a significant histological diagnostic challenge, an appreciation of the broad morphological spectrum that underpins the pseudonym often given to melanoma as "the grand mimicker" is warranted. The typical CMM deposit is represented by a well-circumscribed proliferation of neoplastic melanocytes, with epithelioid cytology predominating over spindled cytology (Figs. 25.3 and 25.4). Epidermal collarettes may be present in superfi-

Table 25.1 Dermoscopic patterns observed in cutaneous metastatic melanoma

Pattern	Features	Mimics
Homogenous	Structureless, uniform, diffuse pigmentation (red, brown, gray or gray-black)	Clark nevus Blue nevus Primary melanoma Pigmented basal cell carcinoma Hemangioma
Saccular	Comprising small, rounded, sac-like structures in blue, red-brown, or gray tones. Marked chromatic variability was noted due to the disorganized proliferation of nests, not respecting anatomic boundaries.	
Vascular	Punctate vessels are noted in superficial metastases and corkscrew vessels in deeper lesions.	Blue nevus Hemangioma Primary melanoma
Amelanotic	Lack discernible global dermoscopic structures, with variable vascular patterns including serpentine, corkscrew, arborizing, dotted, or milky-red patterns.	Regressing primary melanoma Regressing blue nevus
Polymorphic	Chaotic mix of dermoscopic structures and pigmentation	Several mimics, depending on structure, adopted

cial lesions; however, dense inflammatory reactions, dermal fibrosis, and myxoid stromal degeneration are uncommon [10]. Unusual histological patterns include balloon cell change [46], nevoid deposits akin to intradermal nevi but exhibiting atypia [10], lesions mimicking blue nevi, except for often subtle cytological atypia, [47] and florid regressive features reminiscent of halo nevi [10]. The notorious plasticity of melanoma may yield unusual morphologies, ranging from signet ring carcinoma-like features to neuroendocrine transdifferentiation [48] to lesions mimicking spindle cell neoplasms like dermatofibromas, leiomyosarcomas, angiosarcomas, atypical fibroxanthomas, and giant cell-rich

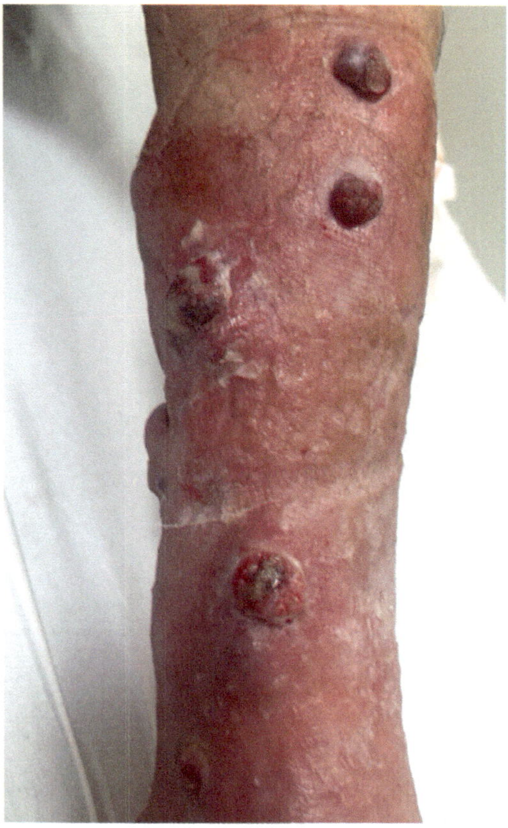

Fig. 25.3 Multiple cutaneous metastatic deposits of melanoma along the leg. The original melanoma was on the calf, and over months this patient developed multiple nodules with variable pigmentation, some of which ulcerated

tumors [10, 49]. While expression of S100 protein, Melan-A, HMB-45, and PRAME facilitates diagnosis in most cases, lineage infidelity is well recognized, with aberrant expression of epithelial, mesenchymal, histiocytic, and even hematopoietic markers described [50].

Epidermotropic metastatic melanomas (EMM) were described in 1978 by Korberg and colleagues [51], challenging the dogma that CMM invariably lack an epidermal component by demonstrating cases with both neoplastic epidermal and dermal melanocytic components, proven to be genetically clonally related to the parent melanoma in subsequent studies [52]. The absence of extension of the atypical epidermal component beyond the lateral confines of the malignant dermal component, the presence of

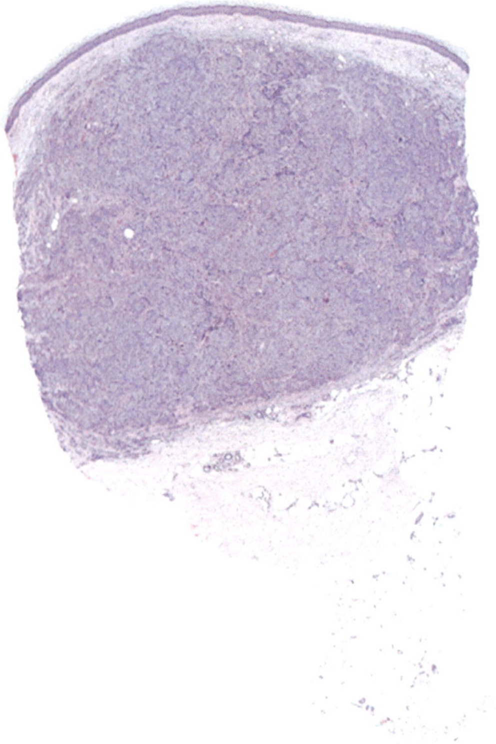

Fig. 25.4 A punch biopsy of skin showing a dermal-based satellite tumoral nodule, completely disparate from the overlying epidermis, comprised of nests of neoplastic melanocytes (hematoxylin and eosin [H&E], ×30)

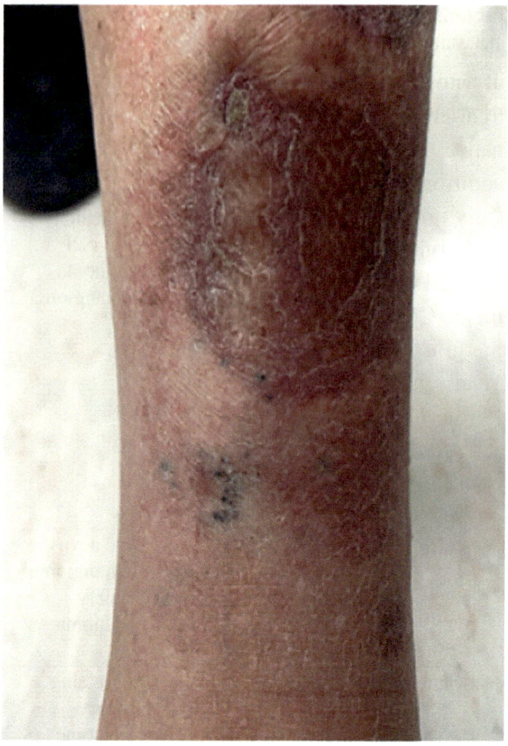

Fig. 25.5 Multiple bluish papules and nodules surrounding the graft site of previous excision of a primary melanoma on the leg

epidermal collarettes flanking the intradermal component, and lymphovascular space invasion should favor a diagnosis of EMM over a new primary melanoma in the appropriate clinical setting (Figs. 25.5 and 25.6) [51].

Conversely, rare scenarios exist describing cases of exclusively intradermal neoplastic melanocytic proliferations, histologically labeled as metastatic melanomas, in which no primary tumor or additional metastatic foci (cutaneous or otherwise) are identified despite thorough assessment. Such cases have been termed *primary dermal melanomas* (PDM). Despite often fulfilling histological criteria suggesting aggressive behavior, including high Breslow thicknesses, they appear to carry excellent prognostic outcomes with survival rates in the region of 80–100% even with surgery alone, far exceeding that expected of a pM1a melanoma [52, 53].

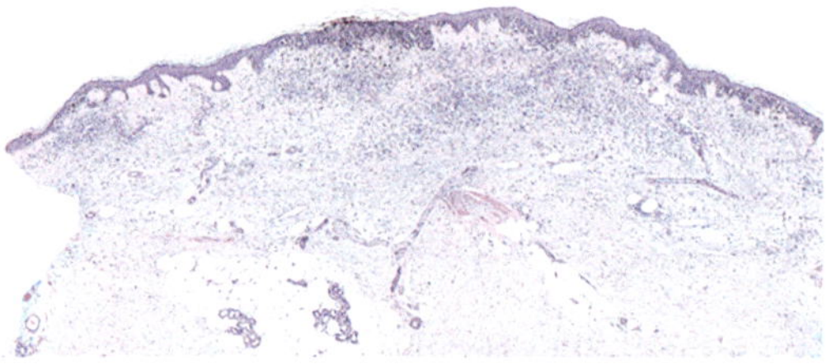

Fig. 25.6 Histological representation of an epidermotropic melanoma metastasis in the patient. Dermal infiltration by metastatic melanoma is apparent with multifocal infiltration of the epidermis and no evidence of regression, a pattern inconsistent with primary melanoma. (H&E, ×15)

25.2.8 Treatment of Cutaneous Metastatic Melanoma

Treatment of CMM remains complex given disease heterogeneity, high recurrence rates, and variable treatment response. Choice of treatment should be guided by patient performance status, patient preference, access to treatment, and disease extent; the latter underpins the importance of positron emission tomography–computed tomography (PET-CT) and brain magnetic resonance imaging (MRI) in the identification of additional foci of metastasis, which may radically impact the treatment approach.

Surgical excision is indicated in patients with isolated CMM in the absence of visceral involvement. Complete surgical resection with narrow margins has been associated with prolonged survival in up to 40% of selected patients. Furthermore, palliative excision may be performed for symptom alleviation in ulcerated, painful, or hemorrhagic lesions [54].

Despite historically being described as radioresistant, melanoma may exhibit favorable responses to radiotherapy, with reported response rates ranging from 52% to 90% [55]. Radiotherapy is often employed in the palliative setting, alleviating symptoms in irresectable lesions. Higher doses (> 30 Gy) have been associated with improved local disease control but may be associated with typically well-tolerated erythema and dermal fibrosis [54]. Furthermore, favorable abscopal responses (shrinkage of tumors at unirradiated sites) to radiotherapy have been documented in patients on immunotherapy [56].

Isolated limb perfusion (ILP) enables the administration of chemotherapy to a single limb at concentrations up to 25-fold higher than that achieved with systemic administration [56], providing a treatment option in patients with confined locoregional CMM. ILP involves open surgical cannulation of the limb artery and vein and isolation of the limb circulation by a tourniquet, followed by infusion with either melphalan monotherapy or a combination with tumor necrosis factor-α (TNF-α), dactinomycin, or dacarbazine, often at mildly hyperthermic temperatures (39 °C–40 °C) [54, 56]. Complete response rates of up to 65% have been documented, with rates similar between monotherapy and combination treatment [56]. Acute complications include erythema and blistering, epidermolysis, and compartment syndrome, while chronic complications include lymphedema, muscle atrophy, neuropathy, and recurrent infections [54]. A less invasive variation of ILP, termed isolated limb infusion (ILI), involves radiologically guided percutaneous catheterization of limb vessels with infusion of high-dose melphalan with or without actinomycin-D in a hypoxic, acidotic, and hyperthermic environment [54, 56]. While overall response rates are slightly lower for ILI, it is associated with reduced morbidity and systemic toxicity and is particularly effective in cases with lower tumor burden [54].

Electrochemotherapy combines the administration of chemotherapeutic agents like bleomycin or cisplatin with the application of local electrical pulses to increase cell membrane permeability (electroporation), with an increased cytotoxic effect of bleomycin up to 1000-fold and of cisplatin 80-fold [57]. An overall response rate of 78% has been reported, with complete remission in up to 58% of cases. Patients with ≤10 lesions <3 cm in diameter, or ≤20 lesions <1 cm in diameter, localized to a single limb segment within a 10 cm area, are ideal candidates [54].

Topical and intralesional therapies may be effective in melanoma. Talimogene laherparepvec (T-VEC) is an oncolytic herpes simplex virus modified to replicate selectively within melanoma cells, causing cell lysis and eliciting T-cell–mediated immunity, and which may induce an abscopal effect when combined with immunotherapy. This well-tolerated drug is approved for advanced cutaneous melanoma with reported response rates between 57% and 89% [58]. Topical imiquimod applied once daily, five times a week, often used in conjunction with other topical or systemic agents, may achieve partial or complete response in around 85% of patients and may represent a palliative or adjunctive treatment option [59]. Topical diphencyprone (DPCP) has demonstrated response rates ranging from 63% to 85%, with enhanced efficacy when used in conjunction with PD-1 inhibitors [54].

Systemic therapy forms the cornerstone of advanced melanoma treatment. Targeted therapies directed against the *MAPK* pathway, including *BRAF* inhibitors like dabrafenib and *MEK* inhibitors like trametinib, have significantly improved patient outcomes in stage III/IV BRAF-mutant melanoma [54]. Specific data for CMM are limited, but clinical trials in patients with ITM-S support the use of dabrafenib-trametinib in this cohort [60]. Immune checkpoint blockade has revolutionized melanoma treatment, with regimens incorporating anti-PD-1 agents (nivolumab and pembrolizumab) with or without anti-CTLA-4 inhibitors (ipilimumab) yielding response rates of 56% in patients with ITM-S. Despite their efficacy, immune-related adverse effects necessitate careful patient selection and monitoring [61].

25.3 Cutaneous Metastasis from Cutaneous Squamous Cell Carcinoma

Cutaneous squamous cell carcinoma (cSCC) represents the second most common form of non-melanoma skin cancer and is primarily associated with ultraviolet radiation [62]. Cutaneous metastases of cSCC are vanishingly rare, and staging is not outlined in the AJCC 8th Edition, which, coupled with limited data, makes management challenging.

Patients with in-transit metastases (ITM) carry a cumulative 2-year risk of cSCC recurrence of 55% and a 5-year disease-specific survival of 30%, with survival curves comparable to those of patients with node-positive disease [63]. Of four case series of ITM, totaling 125 patients, 1-year survival was between 45.5 and 69% [64]. This poor prognostic outcome has also been corroborated by other smaller cohort studies [65–67], with limited data also suggesting higher ITM frequencies in patients with head and neck primary tumors, underlying immunoparesis, [65, 68] and organ transplantation [66]. Indeed, of 125 patients with ITMs secondary to cutaneous SCC, at least a third were organ transplant recipients, and over 90% were head and neck cSCCs [64]. A risk of progression to new ITMs and nodal metastasis has also been reported, with disease-specific death associated with ITM diameters exceeding 2 cm and the presence of more than five ITMs [68].

Distant cutaneous metastatic disease from cSCC is exceptional and the subject of single case reports, exemplified by a case of poorly differentiated cSCC of the lip presenting with extensive nodal disease and multiple distant metastatic subcutaneous deposits [69].

Histologically, cutaneous metastases show deposits of squamous cell carcinoma, often morphologically similar to the parent tumor, centered on the dermis or subcutis, lacking epidermal connection (Fig. 25.7). A limited case series of 11 aggressive scalp cSCC, a subset of which were complicated with tumor satellites [70], together with a case of upper limb acral cSCC complicated with cutaneous metastases [71] suggest, counterintuitively, that the degree of tumour differentiation correlates poorly with ITM risk, with all tumors in this limited cohort exhibiting well to moderate degrees of differentiation.

Limited data suggest that a combined approach with surgery and radiotherapy may achieve better outcomes than monotherapy [63, 65, 66, 68]. European consensus-based guidelines recommend surgical removal of ITMs if number, size, and location permit complete excision. Amputation, which used to be a common option, is no longer recommended as it does not afford a positive impact on prognosis. Radiotherapy, intralesional chemotherapy (5-fluorouracil, bleomycin, or methotrexate), intralesional recombi-

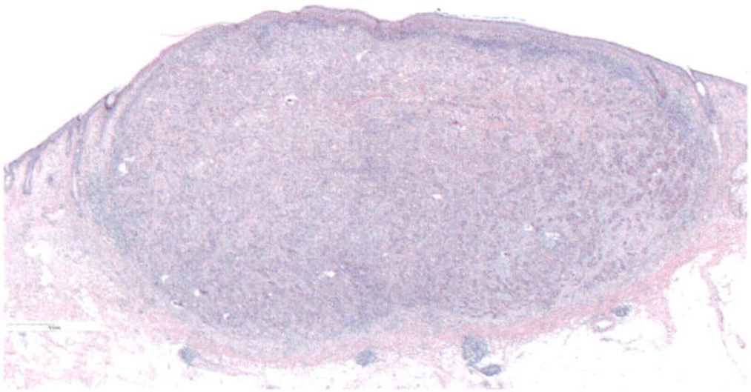

Fig. 25.7 A well-circumscribed dermal metastatic deposit of moderately differentiated squamous cell carcinoma, completely discontinuous from the overlying epidermis (H&E × 30)

nant interferon-alpha, electrochemotherapy, or isolated limb perfusion are all local options. The only licensed systemic agent is the anti-PD-1 agent cemiplimab [72]. In a pivotal randomized controlled trial [73], which included patients with metastatic or locally advanced, unresectable cutaneous SCC, cemiplimab was associated with an overall response rate of 47.2%, 17.1% representing complete responses and the remainder partial responses. In addition, a further 22.8% had stable disease [73].

25.4 Cutaneous Metastasis from Merkel Cell Carcinoma

Merkel cell carcinoma (MCC) represents a rare, aggressive cutaneous neuroendocrine carcinoma of the elderly, mediated by ultraviolet exposure and Merkel cell polyomavirus infection [74]. MCC ITMs are cutaneous metastases within the confines of the draining nodal basin and represent pN2 or pN3 disease depending on locoregional nodal involvement, with both scenarios comprising stage IIIB disease. DCM represents pM1a, stage IV disease [75]. While locoregional nodal metastasis occurs in approximately 70% of patients, ITMs are seen in around 10% [76], with nodal, visceral, and DCM seen in approximately 33% of patients [77].

Histologically, both primary and metastatic MCC lack an epidermal connection, with diagnosis of cutaneous metastasis depending on a prior disease history. Deposits show a neuroendocrine morphology and variably express synaptophysin, chromogranin, CD56 and/or INSM1. MCC often shows paranuclear dot positivity with cytokeratin 20 and is negative for thyroid transcription factor-1 (TTF-1), facilitating differentiation from metastatic extracutaneous neuroendocrine carcinomas (Figs. 25.8 and 25.9) [78].

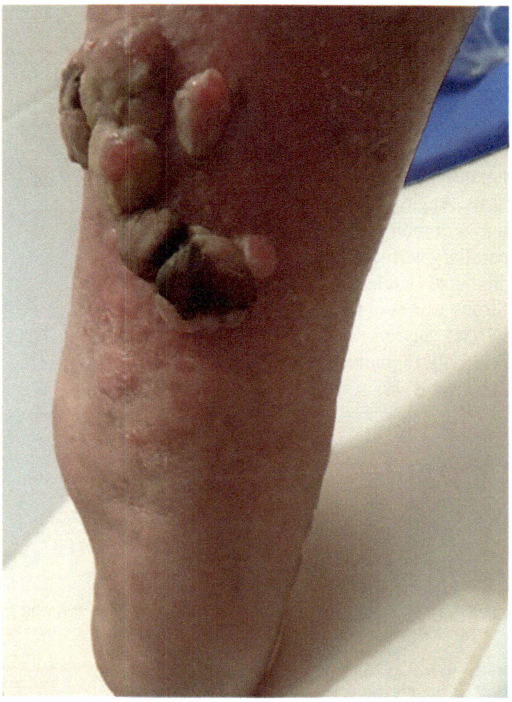

Fig. 25.8 Multiple ulcerated nodules on the leg in a patient who 6 months previously had excision of Merkel cell carcinoma

Recommended treatment for isolated MCC ITMs includes surgery and/or radiotherapy, with MCC being highly radiosensitive [79, 80]. Before the advent of immunotherapy, management relied on supportive care or chemotherapy regimens, usually employing a combination of cisplatin, carboplatin, and etoposide. Response rates varied between 23% and 61% without durable response and with an overall survival of approximately 9 months [80]. Immunotherapy, especially with avelumab (anti-PD-L1) or pembrolizumab (anti-PD1) shows more promising results with overall response rates of 56% for avelumab and 40% for pembrolizumab in the first-line setting. Response rates may be durable; for example, the median progression-free survival is 16.8 months [80].

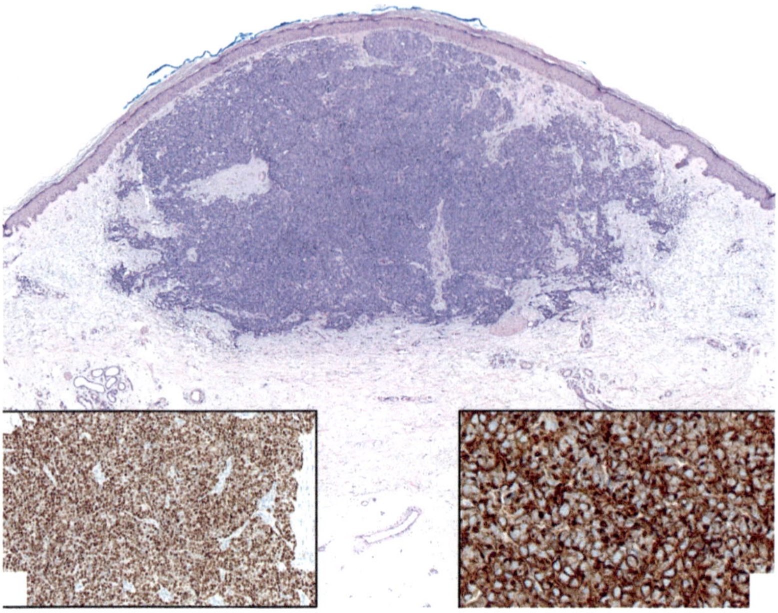

Fig. 25.9 Metastatic cutaneous deposit of Merkel cell carcinoma, comprising hyperchromatic, basaloid neoplastic cells organized in angulated nests. Angiolymphatic tumor emboli within papillary dermal vessels are noted (H&E, ×15). Strong expression of INSM1 (inset A) and dot positivity for cytokeratin 20 (inset B) are seen

25.5 Cutaneous Metastasis from Other Cutaneous Neoplasms

The presence of cutaneous satellites and metastases in the setting of sebaceous carcinoma [81], porocarcinoma [82], syringocystadenocarcinoma [83] and sweat gland adenocarcinoma [84] exemplifies exceptional cases of cutaneous metastases from other rare primary cutaneous adnexal carcinomas. Management is on a case-by-case basis and is often multimodal, including surgery, radiotherapy, and chemotherapy. The prognosis is, overall, poor, with high rates of local recurrence and distant metastases.

References

1. Queirós CS, Filipe PL, Soares de Almeida L. Cutaneous metastases from solid neoplasms in the 21st century: a retrospective study from a Portuguese tertiary care center. J Eur Acad Dermatol Venereol. 2020;34(6):1218–24.
2. Fernandez-Flores A. Cutaneous metastases: a study of 78 biopsies from 69 patients. Am J Dermatopathol. 2010;32(3):222–39.
3. Saeed S, Keehn CA, Morgan MB. Cutaneous metastasis: a clinical, pathological, and immunohistochemical appraisal. J Cutan Pathol. 2004;31(6):419–30.
4. Lookingbill DP, Spangler N, Helm KF. Cutaneous metastases in patients with metastatic carcinoma: a retrospective study of 4020 patients. J Am Acad Dermatol. 1993;29(2 Pt1):228–36.
5. Dumlao JKG, Cubillan ELA, Villena JPDS. Clinical and histopathologic profile of patients with cutaneous metastasis in a tertiary Hospital in The Philippines. Dermatopathology (Basel). 2022;9(4):392–407.
6. Kaplan V, Morales C, Bobadilla F, Fernández J, Segovia L, Vera V, Sanhueza I. Epidemiologic and histopathologic characterization of cutaneous metastases in patients who visited 2 hospitals in Santiago de Chile between 2005 and 2017. Actas Dermosifiliogr (Engl Ed). 2019;110(3):220–6.
7. Strickley JD, Jenson AB, Jung JY. Cutaneous Metastasis. Hematol Oncol Clin North Am. 2019;33(1):173–97.
8. Savoia P, Fava P, Nardò T, Osella-Abate S, Quaglino P, Bernengo MG. Skin metastases of malignant melanoma: a clinical and prognostic survey. Melanoma Res. 2009;19(5):321–6.
9. Jaros J, Hunt S, Mose E, Lai O, Tsoukas M. Cutaneous metastases: A great imitator. Clin Dermatol. 2020;38(2):216–22.
10. Plaza JA, Torres-Cabala C, Evans H, Diwan HA, Suster S, Prieto VG. Cutaneous metastases of malignant melanoma: a clinicopathologic study of 192 cases with emphasis on the morphologic spectrum. Am J Dermatopathol. 2010;32(2):129–36.

11. TNM Classification of Malignant Tumours (UICC). 9th ed. Oxford: Wiley-Blackwell; 2025.
12. Keung EZ, Gershenwald JE. The eighth edition American joint committee on cancer (AJCC) melanoma staging system: implications for melanoma treatment and care. Expert Rev Anticancer Ther. 2018;18(8):775–84.
13. Kimsey TF, Cohen T, Patel A, Busam KJ, Brady MS. Microscopic satellitosis in patients with primary cutaneous melanoma: implications for nodal basin staging. Ann Surg Oncol. 2009;16:1176–83.
14. Kelly JW, Sagebiel RW, Calderon W, Murillo L, Dakin RL, Blois MS. The frequency of local recurrence and microsatellites as a guide to reexcision margins for cutaneous malignant melanoma. Ann Surg. 1984;200:759–63.
15. Mraz-Gernhard S, Sagebiel RW, Kashani-Sabet M, Miller JR 3rd, Leong SP. Prediction of sentinel lymph node micrometastasis by histological features in primary cutaneous malignant melanoma. Arch Dermatol. 1998;134:983–7.
16. Nagore E, Oliver V, Botella-Estrada R, Moreno-Picot S, Insa A, Fortea JM. Prognostic factors in localized invasive cutaneous melanoma: high value of mitotic rate, vascular invasion and microscopic satellitosis. Melanoma Res. 2005;15:169–77.
17. Rao UN, Ibrahim J, Flaherty LE, Richards J, Kirkwood JM. Implications of microscopic satellites of the primary and extracapsular lymph node spread in patients with high-risk melanoma: pathologic corollary of Eastern Cooperative Oncology Group Trial E1690. J Clin Oncol. 2002;20:2053–7.
18. Shaikh L, Sagebiel RW, Ferreira CMM, Nosrati M, Miller JR, Kashani-Sabet M. The role of microsatellites as a prognostic factor in primary malignant melanoma. Arch Dermatol. 2005;141(6):739–42.
19. Leon P, Daly JM, Synnestvedt M, Schultz DJ, Elder DE, Clark WH Jr. The prognostic implications of microscopic satellites in patients with clinical stage I melanoma. Arch Surg. 1991;126:1461–8.
20. Day CL Jr, Harrist TJ, Gorstein F, Sober AJ, Lew RA, Friedman RJ, et al. Malignant melanoma. Prognostic significance of "microscopic satellites" in the reticular dermis and subcutaneous fat. Ann Surg. 1981;194:108–12.
21. Niebling MG, Haydu LE, Lo SN, Rawson RV, Lamboo LGE, Stollman JT, Karim RZ, Thompson JF, Scolyer RA. The prognostic significance of microsatellites in cutaneous melanoma. Mod Pathol. 2020;33(7):1369–79.
22. Wennberg E, Bittar R, Svensson H, Paoli J. The frequency of microsatellite metastases, satellite metastases, and residual tumor in thin melanomas: a retrospective cohort study. Dermatol Pract Concept. 2025;15(2):5157.
23. Russano F, Rastrelli M, Dall'Olmo L, Del Fiore P, Gianesini C, Vecchiato A, Mazza M, Tropea S, Mocellin S. Therapeutic treatment options for in-transit metastases from melanoma. Cancers (Basel). 2024;16(17):3065.
24. Bann DV, Chaikhoutdinov I, Zhu J, Andrews G. Satellite and in-transit metastatic disease in melanoma skin cancer: A retrospective review of disease presentation, treatment, and outcomes. Dermatologic Surg. 2019;45(3):371–80.
25. Messeguer F, Agustí-Mejías A, Traves V, Alegre V, Oliver V, Nagore E. Risk factors for the development of locoregional cutaneous metastases as the sole form of recurrence in patients with melanoma. Actas Dermosifiliogr. 2013;104(1):53–60.
26. Fountain JW, Karayiorgou M, Ernstoff MS, Kirkwood JM, Vlock DR, Titus-Ernstoff L, Bouchard B, Vijayasaradhi S, Houghton AN, Lahti J, et al. Homozygous deletions within human chromosome band 9p21 in melanoma. Proc Natl Acad Sci USA 1992;89(21):10557–10561.
27. Herbst RA, Larson A, Weiss J, Cavenee WK, Hampton GM, Arden KC. A defined region of loss of heterozygosity at 11q23 in cutaneous malignant melanoma. Cancer Res. 1995;55(12):2494–6.
28. Nakayama T, Taback B, Turner R, Morton DL, Hoon DS. Molecular clonality of in-transit melanoma metastasis. Am J Pathol. 2001;158(4):1371–8.
29. El Moheb M, Kim S, Cao C, Zhang Y, Shafiei MS, Shen C, Haden K, Dengel LT, Fallahi-Sichani M, Tsung A, Slingluff C, Witt R. Characterization of driver oncogenic mutations of in-transit melanoma metastases. JCO. 2024;42:9586.
30. Weide B, Faller C, Büttner P, Pflugfelder A, Leiter U, Eigentler TK, Bauer J, Forschner A, Meier F, Garbe C. Prognostic factors of melanoma patients with satellite or in-transit metastasis at the time of stage III diagnosis. PLoS One. 2013;8(4):e63137.
31. Tas F. Metastatic behavior in melanoma: timing, pattern, survival, and influencing factors. J Oncol. 2012;2012:647684.
32. Kwon MR, Choi SH, Jang KT, Kim JH, Mun GH, Lee J, Lee DY. Acral malignant melanoma; emphasis on the primary metastasis and the usefulness of preoperative ultrasound for sentinel lymph node metastasis. Sci Rep. 2019;9(1):15894.
33. Vicente ALSA, Novoloaca A, Cahais V, Awada Z, Cuenin C, Spitz N, Carvalho AL, Evangelista AF, Crovador CS, Reis RM, Herceg Z, de Lima Vazquez V, Ghantous A. Cutaneous and acral melanoma cross-OMICs reveals prognostic cancer drivers associated with pathobiology and ultraviolet exposure. Nat Commun. 2022;13(1):4115.
34. Kang HJ, Choi ME, Won CH, Chang SE, Lee MW, Choi JH, Lee WJ. Clinicoprognostic characteristics of cutaneous metastatic melanoma: a retrospective comparative study between acral and nonacral melanoma. Int J Dermatol. 2020;59(10):1249–57.
35. Cirenajwis H, Lauss M, Ekedahl H, Törngren T, Kvist A, Saal LH, Olsson H, Staaf J, Carneiro A, Ingvar C, Harbst K, Hayward NK, Jönsson G. NF1-mutated melanoma tumors harbor distinct clinical and biological characteristics. Mol Oncol. 2017;11(4):438–51.

36. Reed KB, Cook-Norris RH, Brewer JD. The cutaneous manifestations of metastatic malignant melanoma. Int J Dermatol. 2012;51(3):243–9.
37. Savoia P, Fava P, Grazia M. Cutaneous metastases from malignant melanoma: clinical features and new therapeutic perspectives [Internet]. Treatment of metastatic melanoma. INTECH; 2011. Available from: https://doi.org/10.5772/19228.
38. Rekik M, Kouki C, Kammoun N, Sellami K, Triki M, Boudaya S, Bahloul E, Amouri M, Boudawara T, Turki H. A rare case of melanoma erysipeloides. Clin Case Reports. 2022;10(9):e6315.
39. Dimitrowa J, Kirjakowa N, Michailow I, Balabanowa M. Melanoma malignum en cuirasse. Z Hautkr. 1988;63(10):828–30.
40. Itin PH, Lautenschlager S, Buechner SA. Zosteriform metastases in melanoma. J Am Acad Dermatol. 1995;32(5 Pt2):854–7.
41. Chansky P, Micheletti RG. Alopecia neoplastica. BMJ Case Rep. 2017;2017:bcr2017220215.
42. Primka EJ, King C, O'Keefe EJ. Malignant melanoma of Unkown origin presenting as a systemic vasculitis. Arch Dermatol. 1993;129(9):1205–7.
43. Rubegni P, Lamberti A, Mandato F, Perotti R, Fimiani M. Dermoscopic patterns of cutaneous melanoma metastases. Int J Dermatol. 2014;53(4):404–12.
44. Bono R, Giampetruzzi AR, Concolino F, Puddu P, Scoppola A, Sera F, Marchetti P. Dermoscopic patterns of cutaneous melanoma metastases. Melanoma Res. 2004;14(5):367–73.
45. Costa J, Ortiz-Ibañez K, Salerni G, Borges V, Carrera C, Puig S, Malvehy J. Dermoscopic patterns of melanoma metastases: interobserver consistency and accuracy for metastasis recognition. Br J Dermatol. 2013;169(1):91–9.
46. Bertlich I, Bidier M, Brandt R, Enk A, Hassel JC. Nevoid cutaneous melanoma with balloon cell metastasis. Ann Case Report. 2024;9:1847.
47. Helm MF, Bax MJ, Bogner PN, Chung CG. Metastatic melanoma with features of blue nevus and tumoral melanosis identified during pembrolizumab therapy. JAAD Case Rep. 2017;3(2):135–7.
48. Pisani D, Micallef D, Scerri J, Betts A, Degaetano J, Baldacchino S. Neuroendocrine transdifferentiation in cutaneous melanoma: a case report and review of the literature. Am J Dermatopathol. 2023;45(4):264–8.
49. Lowe L. Metastatic melanoma and rare melanoma variants: a review. Pathology. 2023;55(2):236–44.
50. Saliba E, Bhawan J. Aberrant expression of Immunohistochemical markers in malignant melanoma: a review. Dermatopathology (Basel). 2021;8(3):359–70.
51. Kornberg R, Harris M, Ackerman AB. Epidermotropically metastatic malignant melanoma: differentiating malignant melanoma metastatic to the epidermis from malignant melanoma primary in the epidermis. Arch Dermatol. 1978;114(1):67–9.
52. Swetter SM, Ecker PM, Johnson DL, Harvell JD. Primary dermal melanoma: A distinct subtype of melanoma. Arch Dermatol. 2004;140(1):99–103.
53. Sidiropoulos M, Obregon R, Cooper C, Sholl LM, Guitart J, Gerami P. Primary dermal melanoma: a unique subtype of melanoma to be distinguished from cutaneous metastatic melanoma: a clinical, histologic, and gene expression-profiling study. J Am Acad Dermatol. 2014;71(6):1083–92.
54. Di Raimondo C, Lozzi F, Di Domenico PP, Campione E, Bianchi L. The diagnosis and Management of Cutaneous Metastases from melanoma. Int J Mol Sci. 2023;24(19):14535.
55. Shi W. Radiation therapy for melanoma. In: Ward WH, Farma JM, editors. Cutaneous melanoma: etiology and therapy [internet]. Brisbane: Codon Publications; 2017. Chapter 8. Available: https://www.ncbi.nlm.nih.gov/books/NBK481863/. https://doi.org/10.15586/codon.cutaneousmelanoma.2017.ch8.
56. Testori A, Ribero S, Bataille V. Diagnosis and treatment of in-transit melanoma metastases. Eur J Surg Oncol. 2017;43(3):544–60.
57. Wichtowski M, Murawa D. Electrochemotherapy in the treatment of melanoma. Contemp Oncol (Pozn). 2018;22(1):8–13.
58. Ferrucci PF, Pala L, Conforti F, Cocorocchio E. Talimogene Laherparepvec (T-VEC): an Intralesional cancer immunotherapy for advanced melanoma. Cancers (Basel). 2021;13(6):1383.
59. Scarfì F, Patrizi A, Veronesi G, Lambertini M, Tartari F, Mussi M, Melotti B, Dika E. The role of topical imiquimod in melanoma cutaneous metastases: a critical review of the literature. Dermatol Ther. 2020;33(6):e14165.
60. Long GV, Hauschild A, Santinami M, Atkinson V, Mandalà M, Chiarion-Sileni V, Larkin J, Nyakas M, Dutriaux C, Haydon A, Robert C, Mortier L, Schachter J, Schadendorf D, Lesimple T, Plummer R, Ji R, Zhang P, Mookerjee B, Legos J, Kefford R, Dummer R, Kirkwood JM. Adjuvant Dabrafenib plus Trametinib in stage III BRAF-mutated melanoma. N Engl J Med. 2017;377(19):1813–23.
61. Holmberg CJ, Ny L, Hieken TJ, Block MS, Carr MJ, Sondak VK, Örtenwall C, Katsarelias D, Dimitriou F, Menzies AM, Saw RP, Rogiers A, Straker RJ 3rd, Karakousis G, Applewaite R, Pallan L, Han D, Vetto JT, Gyorki DE, Tie EN, Vitale MG, Ascierto PA, Dummer R, Cohen J, Hui JY, Schachter J, Asher N, Helgadottir H, Chai H, Kroon H, Coventry B, Rothermel LD, Sun J, Carlino MS, Duncan Z, Broman K, Weber J, Lee AY, Berman RS, Teras J, Ollila DW, Long GV, Zager JS, van Akkooi A, Olofsson Bagge R. The efficacy of immune checkpoint blockade for melanoma in-transit with or without nodal metastases – a multicenter cohort study. Eur J Cancer. 2022;169:210–22.
62. Jiang R, Fritz M, Que SKT. Cutaneous squamous cell carcinoma: an updated review. Cancers (Basel). 2024;16(10):1800.
63. Smile TD, Ruiz ES, Kus KJB, Murad F, Wei W, Xiong DD, Vidimos AT, Schmults CD, Koyfman SA. Implications of Satellitosis or in-transit metastasis in cutaneous squamous cell carcinoma: a prog-

nostic omission in cancer staging systems. JAMA Dermatol. 2022;158(4):390–4.
64. Klein JC, McKesey J, Srivastava D, Nijhawan RI. In transit metastases of cutaneous squamous cell carcinoma: a single institution case series. J Am Acad Derm. 2022;88(4):943–5.
65. Ma JH, Wu A, Veness M, et al. In-transit metastasis from squamous cell carcinoma. Dermatologic Surg. 2016;42(11):1285–92.
66. Carucci JA, Martinez JC, Zeitouni NC, et al. In-transit metastasis from primary cutaneous squamous cell carcinoma in organ transplant recipients and nonimmunosuppressed patients: clinical characteristics, management, and outcome in a series of 21 patients. Dermatologic Surg. 2004;30(4 Pt 2):651–5.
67. Xu MJ, Lazar AA, Garsa AA, et al. Major prognostic factors for recurrence and survival independent of the American Joint Committee on Cancer eighth edition staging system in patients with cutaneous squamous cell carcinoma treated with multimodality therapy. Head Neck. 2018;40(7):1406–14.
68. Marti-Marti I, Podlipnik S, Cañueto J, Ferrándiz-Pulido C, Deza G, Sanmartín O, Jaka A, Beà-Ardèbol S, Botella-Estrada R, Redondo P, Turrión-Merino L, Ruiz-Salas V, Masferrer E, Yébenes M, Sánchez-Schmidt JM, Gracia-Darder I, Altemir-Vidal A, Aguayo-Ortiz RS, Becerril S, Bodet-Castillo D, Leal L, Fuente MJ, Moreno-Arrones OM, Abril-Pérez C, Tomás-Velázquez A, Sandoval-Clavijo A, Toll A. Prognostic factors for satellitosis or in-transit metastasis in cutaneous squamous cell carcinoma: a multicentric cohort study. J Am Acad Dermatol. 2023;89(1):119–27.
69. Trivedi V, Abdul khalam M, Ghosh M, Chauhan R, Naseera S. An exceptional case of cutaneous metastasis of squamous cell carcinoma of the lip. J Cancer Res Pract. 2017;4(4):156–8.
70. Lang PG Jr, Braun MA, Kwatra R. Aggressive squamous carcinomas of the scalp. Dermatologic Surg. 2006;32(9):1163–70.
71. Lowe E, Brown T, Geary WA. A rare case of acral cutaneous squamous cell carcinoma with multiple late cutaneous metastases and extensive neurotropic spread. JAAD Case Rep. 2016;2(1):34–6.
72. Stratigos AJ, Garbe C, Dessinioti C, Lebbe C, van Akkooi A, Bataille V, et al. European consensus-based interdisciplinary guideline for invasive cutaneous squamous cell carcinoma: part 2. Treatment-update 2023. Eur J Cancer. 2023;193:113252.
73. Hughes BGM, Guminski A, Bowyer S, Migden MR, Schmults CD, Khushalani NI, et al. A phase 2 open-label study of cemiplimab in patients with advanced cutaneous squamous cell carcinoma (EMPOWER-CSCC-1): final long-term analysis of groups 1, 2, and 3, and primary analysis of fixed-dose treatment group 6. J Am Acad Dermatol. 2024;92(1):68–77.
74. Becker JC, Stang A, DeCaprio JA, Cerroni L, Lebbé C, Veness M, Nghiem P. Merkel cell carcinoma. Nat Rev Dis Primers. 2017;3:17077.
75. Trinidad CM, Torres-Cabala CA, Prieto VG, Aung PP. Update on eighth edition American Joint Committee on Cancer classification for Merkel cell carcinoma and histopathological parameters that determine prognosis. J Clin Pathol. 2019;72(5):337–40.
76. Song Y, Azari FS, Tang R, Shannon AB, Miura JT, Fraker DL, Karakousis GC. Patterns of metastasis in Merkel cell carcinoma. Ann Surg Oncol. 2021;28(1):519–29.
77. Lewis CW, Qazi J, Hippe DS, Lachance K, Thomas H, Cook MM, Juhlin I, Singh N, Thuesmunn Z, Takagishi SR, McEvoy A, Doolittle-Amieva C, Bhatia S, Paulson KG, O'Malley RB, Wang CL, Nghiem P. Patterns of distant metastases in 215 Merkel cell carcinoma patients: implications for prognosis and surveillance. Cancer Med. 2020;9(4):1374–82.
78. Jaeger T, Ring J, Andres C. Histological, immunohistological, and clinical features of merkel cell carcinoma in correlation to Merkel cell polyomavirus status. J Skin Cancer. 2012;2012:983421.
79. Lugowska I, Becker JC, Ascierto PA, Veness M, Blom A, Lebbe C, Migliano E, Hamming-Vrieze O, Goebeler M, Kneitz H, Nathan P, Rutkowski P, Slowinska M, Schadendorf D, Piulats JM, Petrelli F, van Akkooi ACJ, Berruti A, ESMO Guidelines Committee. Merkel-cell carcinoma: ESMO-EURACAN Clinical Practice Guideline for diagnosis, treatment and follow-up. ESMO Open. 2024;9(5):102977.
80. Gauci ML, Aristei C, Becker JC, Blom A, Bataille V, Dreno B, et al. Diagnosis and treatment of Merkel cell carcinoma: European consensus-based interdisciplinary guideline—update 2022. Eur J Cancer. 2022;171:203–31.
81. Campos LM, Dias JAF, Lima PB, Marques SA. Extraocular sebaceous carcinoma: tumor presentation of rapid evolution. An Bras Dermatol. 2022;97(2):268–71.
82. Snow SN, Reizner GT. Eccrine porocarcinoma of the face. J Am Acad Dermatol. 1992;27(2 Pt2):306–11.
83. Satter E, Grady D, Schlocker CT. Syringocystadenocarcinoma papilliferum with locoregional metastases. Dermatol Online J. 2014;20(4):22335.
84. Chintamani, Sharma R, Badran R, Singhal V, Saxena S, Bansal A. Metastatic sweat gland adenocarcinoma: a clinico-pathological dilemma. World J Surg Oncol. 2003;1(1):13.

Part XIII

Paediatric Cutaneous Metastases

Pediatric Cutaneous Metastases 26

Chrysi Karelaki and Marios Papadakis

Abstract

Cutaneous metastases in pediatric cancers are rare but often indicate advanced disease. While most commonly associated with leukemias and lymphomas, they may also arise from non-hematopoietic tumors, including neuroblastoma and rhabdomyosarcoma, which are the most frequent causes in children. These metastases typically present as bluish-red subcutaneous nodules, or "blueberry muffin" lesions, most often on the trunk and face. Accurate diagnosis requires careful clinical evaluation, deep biopsy, and cytogenetic or molecular studies. Neuroblastoma, arising from neural crest cells, primarily affects infants and toddlers, presenting with abdominal, mediastinal, or paraspinal masses and frequent metastases to liver, bone marrow, and skin; diagnosis is supported by urinary catecholamines, imaging, and immunocytochemical markers such as PHOX2B, neuron-specific enolase (NSE), synaptophysin, and chromogranin, with MYCN amplification common. Rhabdomyosarcoma, the most common pediatric soft tissue sarcoma, arises from mesenchymal precursors of skeletal muscle, with embryonal and alveolar subtypes predominating; cutaneous metastases are rare and associated with poor prognosis, and diagnosis relies on histology and immunohistochemical markers including vimentin, desmin, myogenin, and MyoD1. Management of both tumors involves surgery, chemotherapy, and, in selected cases, radiotherapy. This chapter reviews the epidemiology, clinical features, cytology, molecular characteristics, and management of neuroblastoma and rhabdomyosarcoma with cutaneous metastases, emphasizing their diagnostic challenges and prognostic significance.

Keywords

Cutaneous metastases · Pediatric tumors · Neuroblastoma · Skin cancer · Rhabdomyosarcoma · Immunocytochemistry · Nodules · "Blueberry muffin" rash

Cutaneous metastases in pediatric cancers are most frequently associated with hematologic malignancies, such as leukemias and lymphomas. However, rare cases have also been reported in non-hematopoietic tumors, including neuroblastoma, rhabdomyosarcoma, rhabdoid tumor,

C. Karelaki
National and Kapodistrian University of Athens, School of Medicine, First Department of Dermatology-Venereology, Andreas Sygros Hospital, Athens, Greece

M. Papadakis (✉)
University of Ioannina, Department of Plastic Surgery, Ioannina, Greece

D. Koumaki et al. (eds.), *Cutaneous Metastases*, https://doi.org/10.1007/978-3-032-26764-1_26

choriocarcinoma, Ewing sarcoma, osteosarcoma, adrenocortical carcinoma, and primitive neuroectodermal tumor (PNET) [1, 2]. The primary skin manifestation is typically a "blueberry muffin" rash, appearing as bluish-red nodules most commonly located on the trunk and face, with possible involvement of the extremities, neck, and head [3].

These nodules are not pathognomonic, as similar lesions may occur in various other conditions; therefore, establishing a differential diagnosis is essential. There is a clear association between the location of cutaneous metastases and the site of the primary tumor. Accurate diagnosis generally requires a large, deep skin biopsy, often supplemented by cytogenetic or molecular analyses [3, 4].

It is important to recognize that malignant conditions can occur even in neonates, sometimes presenting with cutaneous metastases as the first clinical sign. The presence of such skin lesions is often associated with a poor prognosis [1]. Compared to older children, neonates are more likely to present with skin nodules as an early manifestation of malignancy [2]. When multiple or suspicious skin lesions are identified, clinicians should promptly investigate to rule out serious underlying conditions, including cancer.

The distinguishing features of pediatric tumors with cutaneous metastases can be summarized by age of onset, clinical presentation, cytology, molecular genetics, and immunocytochemistry [4].

Neuroblastoma typically affects children aged 0–2 years and presents with an abdominal, mediastinal, or paraspinal mass. Metastatic disease may involve hepatomegaly, lymphadenopathy, subcutaneous nodules, bone pain, or neurological manifestations. Cytologically, neuroblastoma shows loose clusters of pleomorphic small round cells with stippled chromatin, many karyorrhectic nuclei, and occasional Homer–Wright rosettes with neuropil in the background. Molecular abnormalities include MYCN amplification, 1p deletion, and trisomy 17q. Immunocytochemically, tumor cells are positive for PHOX2B, neuron-specific enolase (NSE), synaptophysin, and chromogranin, and negative for WT1, CD45, desmin, and FLI1.

Alveolar rhabdomyosarcoma (ARMS) usually occurs in adolescents and young adults, presenting as painless, rapidly enlarging soft tissue masses, most often in the extremities. Cytology reveals small round cells with hyperchromatic nuclei and scant cytoplasm, sometimes with identifiable rhabdomyoblasts. Molecularly, ARMS is associated with PAX3–FOXO1 or PAX7–FOXO1 fusion genes. Immunocytochemical markers include vimentin, desmin, myogenin, and MyoD1.

Langerhans cell histiocytosis (LCH) occurs predominantly in children and can involve multiple organs, presenting with generalized lymphadenopathy, skin lesions, bone involvement, and cytopenias. Cytologically, LCH is characterized by scattered large atypical histiocytes with longitudinal nuclear grooves ("coffee-bean nuclei") in a background of eosinophils, lymphocytes, and multinucleated histiocytic giant cells. Molecular alterations often involve BRAF V600E mutations or other MAPK pathway mutations. Tumor cells are immunoreactive for CD68, CD1a, Langerin (CD207), and S100.

Acute lymphoblastic leukemia/lymphoma (ALL) commonly affects children aged 2–6 years. Clinical features include cytopenias, generalized lymphadenopathy, mediastinal mass, CNS involvement, and occasionally skin, liver, or testicular involvement. Cytologically, ALL is characterized by small atypical lymphoid cells with a high nuclear-to-cytoplasmic ratio, opened-up chromatin, prominent nucleoli, and scant basophilic granular cytoplasm. Molecular alterations include t(12;21), t(9;22), t(1;19), t(5;14), hyperdiploidy, or hypodiploidy. Tumor cells are immunopositive for CD45, TdT, and lineage-specific markers such as CD3 in T-ALL and CD20 in B-ALL.

Ewing sarcoma primarily affects children and young adults (5–25 years), presenting with bone pain, fever, leukocytosis, and soft tissue masses. Cytologically, it shows small, round, monomorphic cells with scant or vacuolated cytoplasm. Molecularly, it is associated with characteristic translocations including t(11;22)(EWSR1–

FLI1), t(21;22), t(7;22), and t(22;12). Tumor cells express CD99, FLI1, and NKX2.2.

Acute myeloid leukemia (AML) can occur at any age. Clinical involvement includes blood and bone marrow infiltration, subcutaneous nodules, and gingival hyperplasia. Cytology reveals myeloblasts with opened-up chromatin, prominent nucleoli, granular cytoplasm, and sometimes Auer rods. Molecular abnormalities include t(8;21), inv(16), t(15;17), t(9;11), t(6;9), t(3;3), and t(1;22). Immunophenotypically, AML cells are positive for myeloperoxidase, lysozyme, and CD45.

This chapter focuses on neuroblastoma and rhabdomyosarcoma, as they are the most frequent causes of cutaneous metastases in the pediatric population [5]. Detailed analyses of these tumors, including their epidemiology, clinical presentation, prognostic factors, and diagnostic approaches, are presented in the following sections.

26.1 Neuroblastoma

Neuroblastoma is a subtype of the group of tumors known as neuroblastic tumors, which also includes ganglioneuroblastoma and ganglioneuroma. It is the most common extracranial solid tumor of childhood, ranking after leukemia and brain tumors in overall incidence [6]. Neuroblastoma accounts for approximately 8–10% of all childhood cancers [7]. It arises from neural crest cells during embryonic development, most commonly in the adrenal medulla (40% of cases), but it may occur anywhere along the sympathetic chain of the peripheral sympathetic nervous system. Other frequent sites include the abdominal ganglia (25%), thoracic ganglia (15%), pelvic ganglia (5%), and cervical sympathetic ganglia (3–5%) [6]. Rare cases have been reported in the paratesticular region and urinary bladder, and about 1% present without an identifiable primary site. Approximately 90% of cases occur in children younger than 6 years, with an estimated 80% diagnosed by the age of four; the median age at diagnosis is 22 months [8]. Notably, onset after the age of five is associated with a poorer prognosis. The precise mechanisms underlying tumorigenesis remain unclear.

Clinical presentation varies depending on the site of the primary tumor and the presence of metastases, which may involve the lymph nodes, skin, liver, bone marrow, cortical bone, intracranial structures, orbits, lungs, and central nervous system [7, 9]. Notably, approximately 75% of neuroblastoma cases are metastatic at the time of diagnosis [7]. As a result, patients may present with diverse symptoms, including abdominal distension, ptosis, miosis, facial or upper body swelling, headache, dizziness, altered consciousness, bone pain, fever, anemia, hypertension, tachycardia, opsoclonus, myoclonus, flushing, sweating, or watery diarrhea, some of which are associated with paraneoplastic syndromes [8, 9].

Cutaneous metastases, though rare (about 1% of cases in infants), may serve as an important diagnostic clue [10]. They most commonly appear as painless, purple, firm, mobile subcutaneous nodules, usually on the trunk and extremities, though reports also describe involvement of the palms, soles, and scrotum [7, 8]. A distinctive phenomenon is central blanching with an erythematous halo after 2–3 minutes of palpation, attributed to catecholamine-induced vasoconstriction [9–11]. Another recognized feature is "raccoon eyes," or periorbital ecchymoses caused by orbital metastases. Rarely, heterochromia iridis may occur due to invasion of the ophthalmic sympathetic nerve. Interestingly, cutaneous metastases of neuroblastoma have occasionally been misdiagnosed as subcutaneous hemangiomas because of their similar morphology [11, 12].

Cutaneous metastases are most often observed within the first 6 months of life, particularly in Stage IV-S disease, which characteristically involves the liver, bone marrow, and skin. Despite its widespread dissemination, Stage IV-S paradoxically carries a high likelihood of spontaneous remission [9].

Diagnostic evaluation of neuroblastoma typically begins with biochemical testing, including urinary catecholamines and their metabolites, vanillylmandelic acid (VMA) and homovanillic acid (HVA), as well as serum neuron-specific enolase (NSE). While VMA and HVA are primarily used to monitor treatment response, elevated NSE levels are associated with a poorer prognosis but are not recommended for follow-up. Imaging studies, such as contrast-enhanced MRI of the abdomen and subcutaneous lesions, provide essential information on tumor location and extent.

Definitive diagnosis relies on tissue analysis through biopsy or fine-needle aspiration cytology (FNAC) of cutaneous or primary tumors. These specimens are evaluated using immunohistochemistry and immunocytochemistry [13]. Microscopically, Homer–Wright rosettes—neuroblasts arranged around a central core of neuropil (eosinophilic fibrillary material)—may be observed, supporting suspicion for neuroblastoma. Immunocytochemical analysis further aids diagnosis: PHOX2B is highly specific but not a maturational marker; Chromogranin-A is a maturational marker strongly expressed in adrenal chromaffin-derived and peripheral sympathetic neurons; Synaptophysin is a common neuronal marker present in synaptic vesicles and during axoplasmic transport; Somatostatin marks sympathetic neuron maturation; and SOX2, currently under investigation, indicates cellular immaturity. Tumors frequently exhibit N-myc oncogene amplification, which is strongly associated with disease biology [8, 13].

Cutaneous metastases in neuroblastoma are treated with chemotherapy and, in some cases, with radiation therapy and surgery when necessary.

26.2 Rhabdomyosarcoma

Rhabdomyosarcoma (RMS) is the most prevalent soft tissue sarcoma in children, arising from mesenchymal precursor cells of skeletal muscle. It accounts for approximately 4.4 cases per one million individuals younger than 20 years and represents about 3% of all pediatric malignancies [14–16]. There are four histological subtypes: embryonal, botryoid, alveolar, and pleomorphic [15, 16]. Neonatal RMS is extremely rare, comprising 1–2% of pediatric cases, and usually presents as the embryonal subtype [14, 17].

RMS can develop anywhere soft tissue is present, although it most commonly arises in the head and neck, genitourinary tract (including paratesticular tissues, urinary bladder, prostate, vagina, and vulva), extremities, trunk, and retroperitoneum [15]. A study by Kim et al. showed that the most frequent primary tumor sites in children are the trunk, head and neck, and extremities [18]. RMS is aggressive, with 37.7% of patients developing distant metastases; 27.5% present with metastases at diagnosis. The bone is the most common metastatic site, followed by the lung and lymph nodes. RMS of the extremities appears more aggressive and is associated with lymph node metastases, whereas metastases to the skin, perineum, testis, and epidural space are uncommon [15, 18]. Cutaneous and brain metastases have been reported, particularly in alveolar RMS [18, 19]. Cutaneous metastases are extremely rare, with seven cases described in the literature presenting as a "blueberry muffin" rash—diffuse multiple subcutaneous nodules with a purple-bluish color—and are associated with poor prognosis [14, 16]. Other poor prognostic factors include older age at presentation or age younger than 1 year, unfavorable primary tumor sites, larger tumor size, alveolar subtype, regional lymph node metastasis, and FOXO1 fusion-positive tumors, which indicate alveolar RMS [14, 17, 19].

Diagnosis is made via biopsy of the primary or cutaneous lesions, combined with immunohistochemical analysis. Histology typically reveals small round to spindle-shaped cells with hyperchromatic nuclei and scant eosinophilic cytoplasm, along with cytoplasmic filamentous structures and Z-bands, characteristic of rhabdomyoblasts. In the alveolar subtype, alveolar nest structures are present, and rhabdomyoblasts are observed in only about 30% of cases [15].

Key immunohistochemical markers in RMS include vimentin, an intermediate filament protein indicating mesenchymal origin and present in undifferentiated cells; desmin, an intermediate filament protein found in skeletal and smooth muscle cells and expressed in differentiated cells;

myoglobin, expressed in differentiated skeletal muscle cells; and myogenic muscle-specific actin, a marker of muscle differentiation [15].

Most patients with rhabdomyosarcoma are treated surgically. Radiotherapy may also be applied for local control, palliative therapy, or both. Other treatments, i.e., chemotherapy agents and blood stem cell transplantation, have also been described.

References

1. Wesche WA, Khare VK, Chesney TM, Jenkins JJ. Non-hematopoietic cutaneous metastases in children and adolescents: thirty years experience at St. Jude Children's Research Hospital. J Cutan Pathol. 2000;27(10):485–92.
2. Isaacs H Jr. Cutaneous metastases in neonates: a review. Pediatr Dermatol. 2011;28(2):85–93.
3. Fraitag S, Boccara O. What to look out for in a newborn with multiple Papulonodular skin lesions at birth. Dermatopathology (Basel). 2021;8(3):390–417.
4. Saharan N, Gupta P, Roy PS, Jain R. Subcutaneous swellings as the initial presentation of malignancy in an infant: highlighting the cytological mimics at the metastatic site. Cytopathology. 2021;32(5):695–9.
5. Souza BCE, Miyashiro D, Pincelli MS, Sanches JA. Cutaneous metastases from solid neoplasms - literature review. An Bras Dermatol. 2023;98(5):571–9.
6. Suleiman DE, Adamu ZA, Mohammed A. Multiple subcutaneous nodules leading to a diagnosis of metastatic neuroblastoma in an infant: a case report. Int J Med Health Dev. 2023;28(1):77–80.
7. Metin MS, Akdeniz N, Elmas ÖF, Gündoğdu B, Kızılyel O, Taş F, Bilici Ş, Efe H, Büyükavcı M. A case report of Neuroblastoma with cutaneous metastasis in a two-month-old infant. J Turk Acad Dermatol. 2015;9(1)
8. Singh M, Khan L, Sachan S, Mishra V, Sachan A. Cutaneous presentation of neuroblastoma in 8 months old boy: a rare case report. SSR Inst Int J Life Sci. 2019;5(4):2365–8.
9. Maher-Wiese VL, Wenner NP, Grant-Kels JM. Metastatic cutaneous lesions in children and adolescents with a case report of metastatic neuroblastoma. J Am Acad Dermatol. 1992;26(4):620–8.
10. Nowak E, Ostojska M, Osial N, Psiuk D, Nurzyńska-Flak J. Skin lesions as the first manifestation of metastatic neuroblastoma in an infant-case report. J Pre-Clin Clin Res. 2024;18(3)
11. Hassanein AH, Fishman SJ, Mulliken JB, Alomari AI, Kurek KC, Padua HM, Greene AK. Metastatic neuroblastoma mimicking infantile hemangioma. J Pediatr Surg. 2010;45(10):2045–9.
12. Ozawa MG, Cooney T, Rangaswami A, Hazard FK. Synchronous hepatoblastoma, neuroblastoma, and cutaneous capillary hemangiomas: a case report. Pediatr Dev Pathol. 2016;19(1):74–9.
13. Sarnat HB, Chan ES, Ng D, Yu W. Maturation of metastases in peripheral neuroblastic tumors (neuroblastoma) of children. J Neuropathol Exp Neurol. 2023;82(10):853–64.
14. Strah D, Stanley K, Oatmen K, Kylat RI, Dishop M, de la Maza M. An unusual presentation of neonatal rhabdomyosarcoma: a case report. Front Pediatr. 2023;11:1233334.
15. Wiss K, Solomon AR, Raimer SS, Lobe TE, Gourley W, Headington JT. Rhabdomyosarcoma presenting as a cutaneous nodule. Arch Dermatol. 1988;124(11):1687–90.
16. Ansari S, Yousefian S, Miri-Aliabad G, Ramim T. Rhabdomyosarcoma with skin metastasis: report of a case. Acta Med Iran. 2014;52(2):170–2.
17. Rodriguez-Galindo C, Hill DA, Onyekwere O, Pin N, Rao BN, Hoffer FA, Kun LE, Pappo AS, Santana VM. Neonatal alveolar rhabdomyosarcoma with skin and brain metastases. Cancer. 2001;92(6):1613–20.
18. Kim JR, Yoon HM, Koh KN, Jung AY, Cho YA, Lee JS. Rhabdomyosarcoma in children and adolescents: patterns and risk factors of distant metastasis. AJR Am J Roentgenol. 2017;209(2):409–16.
19. Hayashi K, Ohtsuki Y, Takahashi K, Sonobe H, Nakamura S, Kitagawa N, Arata J, Shimanouchi Y, Kurashige T. Congenital alveolar rhabdomyosarcoma with multiple skin metastases. Report of a case. Acta Pathol Jpn. 1988;38(2):241–8.

Part XIV

Cutaneous Metastasis from Central Nervous System Tumours

27 Cutaneous Metastases from Central Nervous System Tumors

Marios Papadakis

Abstract

Cutaneous metastases from central nervous system (CNS) tumors are rare clinical entities that can present diagnostic and therapeutic challenges. This chapter provides a comprehensive review of the main CNS tumors associated with cutaneous metastases, including meningiomas, embryonal tumors (medulloblastomas), and gliomal tumors (glioblastomas and ependymomas). True cutaneous metastases from meningiomas are exceedingly uncommon (<0.1%), often arising at prior surgical sites or as slow-growing nodules overlying cranial bones, and can occur even in WHO grade I tumors. Histologically, cutaneous meningiomas exhibit whorled arrangements of spindled-to-epithelioid cells, with characteristic immunohistochemical profiles including positivity for epithelial membrane antigen (EMA), vimentin, S100, and progesterone receptors. Management typically involves surgical resection and radiotherapy, with limited evidence for systemic chemotherapy. Medulloblastomas rarely metastasize extraneurally, with common sites including bone, lymph nodes, and, less frequently, skin, often via surgical seeding or shunt-assisted dissemination. Glioblastomas and ependymomas also demonstrate rare extracranial metastases, predominantly at surgical sites, with poor prognosis for glioblastoma metastases and variable outcomes for ependymoma scalp lesions. The pathophysiology, histopathology, clinical presentation, and management strategies for these tumors are reviewed to aid in early recognition and appropriate treatment of cutaneous metastases from CNS tumors.

Keywords

Cutaneous metastases · Central nervous system tumors · Meningioma · Medulloblastoma · Glioblastoma · Ependymoma · WHO grading · Scalp lesions · Surgical seeding

27.1 Meningioma

27.1.1 General

Meningiomas are localized, slow-growing tumors that account for approximately 37% of all primary CNS tumors [8]. They arise from arachnoid cap cells and typically grow along the outer surface of the brain or within the ventricular system [2].

Histologically, they are classified as:

M. Papadakis (✉)
University of Ioannina, Ioannina, Greece
e-mail: marios_papadakis@uoi.gr

D. Koumaki et al. (eds.), *Cutaneous Metastases*, https://doi.org/10.1007/978-3-032-26764-1_27

- WHO Grade I (benign, ~89%).
- WHO Grade II (atypical, ~6%).
- WHO Grade III (malignant, ~5%).

Grade I tumors can be subdivided into nine histological subtypes (e.g., meningothelial, transitional). Grade II tumors include chordoid and clear cell variants, while Grade III tumors comprise papillary, rhabdoid, and anaplastic subtypes. The diagnostic criteria for anaplastic meningioma include ≥20 mitotic figures per 10 high-power fields (HPF), or focal/diffuse loss of meningothelial differentiation, resulting in a carcinoma-, sarcoma-, or melanoma-like appearance [9].

All grades of meningioma have metastatic potential; therefore, the presence of metastasis is not a criterion for WHO grading [8].

27.1.2 Definitions

Cutaneous meningiomas have been described for more than 50 years. Based on their clinical and histological features, they have been classified into three types. Type 1 consists of congenital lesions located in the scalp, forehead, or paravertebral region with no connection to the CNS. This type can be further subclassified into two subtypes: true meningiomas with infiltrative characteristics and rudimentary/sequestered meningoceles [4].

Cutaneous meningiomas were first described more than 50 years ago. Based on their clinical and histological features, they have been classified into three types:

- *Type I* consists of congenital lesions located in the scalp, forehead, or paravertebral region, with no connection to the CNS. This type can be further subclassified into two subtypes: (1) true meningiomas with infiltrative characteristics, and (2) rudimentary or sequestrated meningoceles [4].
- *Type II* consists of acquired tumors that arise from arachnoid cells located along the course of cranial or spinal nerves. These tumors originate from nests of arachnoid cells that remain after the nerves penetrate the dura [6].
- *Type III* includes all cutaneous extensions or metastases of intracranial meningiomas [4].

Meningioma-related cutaneous lesions are not uncommon, and multiple entities have been described. Unfortunately, the term metastasis has often been used inconsistently and interchangeably. The differential diagnosis includes: (a) Recurrence of intracranial meningiomas with extracranial extension following resection, (b) Primary extracranial tumors (e.g., primary cutaneous meningiomas and heterotopic meningeal nodules), (c) Benign metastasizing meningiomas, (d) Angioblastic meningiomas, and (e) True cutaneous metastases (secondary cutaneous meningiomas).

Extracranial meningiomas are generally considered extensions of primary intracranial tumors, in contrast to heterotopic cutaneous meningeal nodules, which do not represent direct extensions of intracranial meningiomas [10]. While intracranial meningiomas may predispose to the development of subsequent extracranial tumors, there is insufficient evidence to suggest an increased risk of heterotopic recurrence. The scalp is the most common site of extracranial meningeal nodules; however, these tumors are unlikely to represent true metastases, given their differences in morphology and histologic grade [5].

"Benign metastasizing meningiomas" refer to synchronous intracranial and extracranial tumors that share identical benign histologic features in both the primary lesion and the so-called "metastatic" site, most commonly the lungs. Retrospective analyses have shown that a number of such cases were in fact hemangiopericytomas (angioblastic meningiomas) [5].

27.1.3 True Metastases

True cutaneous metastases from meningiomas (secondary cutaneous meningiomas) are extremely rare (<0.1%) [8]. When they do occur, they often present as nodules at previous surgical sites or as slow-growing masses overlying cranial bones [2]. Indeed, many previously reported cases represent other clinical entities, as noted above. Meningioma metastases are typically disseminated through the systemic circulation (i.e., cerebrospinal fluid, blood, or lymph), although iatrogenic spread has also been documented [3]. The location of the primary tumor appears to have limited significance in the occurrence of distant metastasis, although proximity to a major venous sinus may be a contributing factor. Simultaneous local recurrence and distant skin metastasis have been described in an atypical meningioma, with the metastasis located just beneath the scar of the previous incision and showing no continuity with the original mass [1]. Interestingly, 43% of all reported scalp metastases are observed in patients with WHO grade I primary tumors, challenging the notion that meningioma metastasis occurs only in high-grade lesions [8].

The median interval from diagnosis to metastasis reported in the literature is 3.5 years. As expected, this interval is shorter in patients with high-grade meningiomas (WHO II, WHO III) [8].

27.1.4 Histology

Histologically, cutaneous meningioma metastases present as discrete nodules of spindled-to-epithelioid cells arranged in whorls or short fascicles, often exhibiting an infiltrative pattern in the dermis. Primary cutaneous type II meningiomas may be histologically and immunophenotypically identical to type III intracranial meningiomas, making it crucial to exclude intracranial lesions in patients presenting with cutaneous meningiomas [6]. Intranuclear pseudoinclusions and nuclear vacuolization may be observed, along with psammoma bodies.

Immunohistochemical staining typically shows positivity for vimentin, epithelial membrane antigen (EMA), S100 protein, progesterone receptors, cytokeratins, and carcinoembryonic antigen (CEA) [2]. Decreased EMA expression may indicate recurrence or malignant progression to grade III anaplastic meningioma. The Ki-67/MIB-1 proliferative index has been shown to increase from grade I to grade III meningiomas [9].

Type II and type III cutaneous meningiomas may express p63, which is important to recognize to avoid misinterpreting p63 positivity as squamous cell carcinoma or adnexal tumors. As a general rule, the absence of keratin reactivity in cutaneous meningiomas effectively excludes an epithelial neoplasm; however, p63 expression does not distinguish primary extracranial tumors from those associated with intracranial meningiomas [6].

In general, when the diagnosis of cutaneous meningioma is not readily apparent histologically, it is rarely suspected clinically [4]. Excisional biopsy is therefore essential to establish the diagnosis.

27.1.5 Management

In all reported cases, patients underwent surgical resection followed by radiotherapy, resulting in a 100% survival rate at a mean follow-up of 18 months [7]. Chemotherapeutic agents, including hydroxyurea and sunitinib, have also been used to treat metastatic meningiomas; however, there is limited evidence supporting their efficacy [8].

27.2 Embryonal Tumors—Medulloblastoma

Medulloblastoma is a primitive neuroectodermal tumor of the central nervous system, typically arising in the cerebellum. It is the most common pediatric CNS malignancy [14]. Although the peak incidence occurs between 6 and 8 years of age, approximately 30% of cases are diagnosed in adults [13].

Extraneural metastasis is extremely rare. This rarity may be attributed to the absence of intraparenchymal lymphatic vessels, the collapse of tumor-adjacent intracerebral veins, the inability of the intracerebral environment to support metastatic malignant clones, the protective role of the blood–brain barrier, and the generally short survival time of affected patients [11]. Direct tumor seeding remains the most common mechanism of spread [12, 14]. The potential role of permanent shunting in facilitating metastasis and influencing the time to dissemination remains unclear [13].

Systemic metastasis occurs in 5–10% of patients. The most common sites are bone (77%) and lymph nodes (33%), though skin metastases have also been reported. In one case, a 22-year-old patient with a history of ventriculoperitoneal shunting, surgery, radiotherapy, and chemotherapy for a posterior fossa medulloblastoma developed a 4 × 2 cm firm, irregular, erythematous, nodular lesion with intratumoral hemorrhage, without associated lymphadenopathy [11, 14]. Another case described a lesion involving the skin and soft tissues of the posterior cervical region in a 48-year-old man previously treated for a WHO grade 4 medulloblastoma. The lesion was surgically excised, followed by cervical radiotherapy (36 Gy), and no relapse was observed at 3-year follow-up [14]. Metastases may also involve the soft tissues of the occipital bone [11].

The interval between initial diagnosis and systemic metastasis typically ranges from 2 to 4 years [13, 14]. Prognosis is generally poor, with reported 2- and 5-year overall survival rates following the diagnosis of extraneural metastasis of 31% and 26%, respectively [11].

27.3 Gliomal Tumors

Gliomal tumors are a group of primary neoplasms that arise from glial cells in the brain or spinal cord. Common types of gliomas include astrocytomas, oligodendrogliomas, and ependymomas. Glioblastoma is an aggressive subtype of astrocytoma, while gliosarcoma is now considered a variant of glioblastoma rather than a distinct tumor entity.

27.3.1 Glioblastoma

Glioblastoma multiforme (GBM) is the most common malignant CNS tumor, accounting for up to 25% of all primary CNS tumors [17]. The median overall survival is approximately 20 months, regardless of the treatment modality used [19].

Extracranial metastases of glioblastoma are observed in up to 3% of cases [18]. These metastases typically occur at a median of 9 months following the initial diagnosis [20] and are most commonly located in the lungs and pleura (60%). More than 70% of affected patients are male. The most probable pathogenic mechanisms for extracranial spread include surgical seeding, dural invasion, hematogenous dissemination, and subependymal spread of tumor cells through the cerebrospinal fluid [15].

Cutaneous metastases are extremely rare, comprising only about 7% of all extracranial metastases [20], and are almost always located at previous surgical sites. Their scarcity is thought to be due to the high mortality of GBM, which limits the time for metastases to develop, and to the inherent barriers to spread outside the CNS, including the blood–brain barrier, strong basement membrane, and robust dura [19]. The extent of primary tumor resection (gross total, subtotal, partial, or biopsy) does not appear to correlate with the time to metastasis [16].

Extracranial lesions can be diagnosed either through subtotal or total resection of the lesion or by fine-needle aspiration biopsy followed by surgical excision. Glioblastoma shares immunohistochemical markers such as S100 with melanoma [17]. Compared with primary tumors, extracranial lesions exhibit significantly lower expression of hypoxia-inducible factor-1α (HIF-1α), VEGFA, and EGFR, but significantly higher Ki-67 positivity. These findings may indicate alterations in the tumor microenvironment and enhanced tumor cell proliferation under the scalp, possibly due to its rich vascular supply [21].

The most commonly employed treatment strategies are surgery combined with radiotherapy or chemoradiation alone. Median survival after the diagnosis of extracranial metastasis is approximately 6 months [20].

27.3.2 Ependymal Tumors—Ependymoma

Ependymoma is a glial neoplasm that accounts for approximately 10% of all intracranial tumors in adults and 10% in children. More than 90% of cases arise intracranially and generally exhibit benign characteristics [22, 24].

Traditionally, ependymomas have been histologically classified into four groups: subependymoma, myxopapillary ependymoma, ependymoma with cellular, papillary, or clear cell variants, and anaplastic ependymoma. Since 2016, however, the classification has undergone significant restructuring. Tumors are now categorized based on a combination of histological, molecular, and anatomical features (supratentorial, posterior fossa, spinal) [25]. The current subtypes are [25]:

- Supratentorial ependymoma, ZFTA fusion–positive.
- Supratentorial ependymoma, YAP1 fusion–positive.
- Posterior fossa group A (PFA) ependymoma.
- Posterior fossa group B (PFB) ependymoma.
- Spinal ependymoma, MYCN-amplified.

Most ependymomas are classified as CNS WHO grade 2 or 3, although assigning a WHO grade is no longer required in the pediatric population due to the limitations of histological grading. Approximately two-thirds of intracranial ependymomas arise in the posterior fossa, with the remainder typically located in the supratentorial space [27]. Rarely, tumors may originate from soft tissue sites such as the sacrococcygeal or mediastinal regions, and these should be distinguished from extraneural metastases (see Table 27.1).

Table 27.1 Main differences between primary extracranial ependymomas and extracranial metastases from primary intracranial ependymomas

Parameter	Primary extracranial ependymomas [28]	Extracranial metastases from primary intracranial ependymomas [26]
Median age (y)	32	13
Gender	Female predominance	Male predominance
Most common site	Subcutaneous sacrococcygeal or pre-sacral region	Hilar/mediastinal lymph nodes (67%), lungs and pleura (48%), scalp (29%)
Histology type	Grade I (myxopapillary variant, 47%)	Grade III (formerly anaplastic, 79%)
Treatment	No standard of care *Surgery*: Solitary lesions *Radiotherapy*: Recurrent local disease. *Chemotherapy agents*: Carboplatin, etoposide, lapatinib, temozolomide, cyclophosphamide, adriamycin, cisplatin, procarbazine, paclitaxel, bevacizumab	*Primary tumor*: Surgery (98%), locoregional radiotherapy (30%), chemotherapy (8%) *Metastasis*: No treatment (58%), surgery (31%), chemotherapy (31%), locoregional radiotherapy (19%)
Median overall survival	27 years	3 months

Two thirds of intracranial ependymomas occur in the posterior fossa and some in the supratentorial space [27]. Rarely, tumors can primarily originate from soft tissue sites, e.g. sacrococcygeal, and mediastinal region and should be distinguished from extraneural metastases (see Table 27.1).

Although the lungs and lymph nodes are the most common sites of extracranial metastasis in ependymomas, scalp lesions are observed in up to 29% of cases. Proposed mechanisms for extracranial dissemination include hematogenous spread through abnormal vessels of the primary tumor, infiltration of major dural sinuses, and lymphatic or hematogenous dissemination following skull invasion [27]. The relatively high incidence of scalp metastases suggests a possible favorable skin microenvironment for the implantation of ependymoma cells [22, 23, 26].

Most patients with scalp metastases are managed with serial surgical resections and external beam radiotherapy. Chemotherapy is generally ineffective for CNS tumors due to the limited penetration across the blood–brain barrier [26]. However, total regression of scalp and cervical lymph node metastases in response to etoposide has been reported [23], suggesting a more favorable response in selected cases [27]. Since surgery is considered the most important risk factor for extracranial dissemination, prophylactic irradiation of surgical incision sites—similar to strategies used in mesothelioma—has also been proposed [26].

References

1. Akai T, Shiraga S, Iizuka H, Kishibe M, Kawakami S, Ueda Y. Recurrent meningioma with metastasis to the skin incision—case report. Neurol Med Chir (Tokyo). 2004;44(11):600–2.
2. Alcaraz I, Cerroni L, Rütten A, Kutzner H, Requena L. Cutaneous metastases from internal malignancies: a clinicopathologic and immunohistochemical review. Am J Dermatopathol. 2012;34(4):347–93.
3. Avecillas-Chasin JM, Saceda-Gutierrez J, Alonso-Lera P, Garcia-Pumarino R, Issa S, López E, Barcia JA. Scalp metastases of recurrent meningiomas: aggressive behavior or surgical seeding? World Neurosurg. 2015;84(1):121–31.
4. Courville P, Cappèle O, Bachy B, Hemet J, Métayer J. Type 1-primary cutaneous meningioma of the scalp. Eur J Pediatr Surg. 2000;10(6):387–9.
5. Enwereuzo C, Moral L, Henneberry JM. Heterotopic cutaneous meningioma: an unusual presentation occurring in a patient with a remote history of intracranial meningioma. Am J Dermatopathol. 2018;40(4):e57–9.
6. Fox MD, Billings SD, Gleason BC, Thomas AB, Cibull TL. Cutaneous meningioma: a potential diagnostic pitfall in p63 positive cutaneous neoplasms. J Cutan Pathol. 2013;40(10):891–5.
7. Javed S, Khan A, Khalid A, Scalia G, Umana GE, Mahmood A, Yaqoob E, Pahwa B, Chaurasia B. Scalp metastasis from atypical meningioma: a case report and literature review. Clin Case Reports. 2024;12(5):e8789.
8. Liu Y, Li J, Duan Y, Ye Y, Xiao L, Mao R. Subcutaneous metastasis of atypical meningioma: case report and literature review. World Neurosurg. 2020;138:182–6.
9. Thomas RZ, Dalal I. Extracranial metastases of anaplastic meningioma. BJR Case Rep. 2017;3(2):20150092.
10. Theaker JM, Fletcher CD, Tudway AJ. Cutaneous heterotopic meningeal nodules. Histopathology. 1990;16(5):475–9.
11. Geng D, Song X, Liu J, Yu Z, Ning F. Medulloblastoma with soft-tissue and skeletal metastases in an adult: a case report. Oncol Lett. 2015;10(4):2295–8.
12. Ranjani S, Mehdi I, Sreenath C, Palassery R. Subcutaneous metastasis secondary to surgical tract seeding in a child with medulloblastoma-a case report. Pediatr Hematol Oncol J. 2016;1(4):96–8.
13. Topham EJ, Francis N, Bunker CB. Medulloblastoma metastasizing to the skin. Br J Dermatol. 2006;154(3):554–5.
14. Vega-Moreno DA, Fernández JON, Reyes-Soto G, et al. Extracranial metastatic medulloblastoma: two case reports and systematic literature review. SN Compr Clin Med. 2025;7:101. https://doi.org/10.1007/s42399-025-01853-z.
15. Chang H, Ding Y, Wang P, Wang Q, Lin Y, Li B. Cutaneous metastases of the glioma. J Craniofac Surg. 2018;29(1):e94–6.
16. Ciscar-Fabuel M, De Vilalta-Bufurull A, Blanch-Pujol G, Romero-Quintela M, Plans-Ahicart G, Gabarros-Canals A. Metastatic glioblastoma multiforme on skin and subcutaneous tissue. Explor Neurosci. 2024;3(6):539–50.
17. Lewis GD, Rivera AL, Tremont-Lukats IW, Ballester-Fuentes LY, Zhang YJ, Teh BS. GBM skin metastasis: a case report and review of the literature. CNS Oncol. 2017;6(3):203–9.
18. Magdaleno-Tapial J, Valenzuela-Oñate C, Pérez-Pastor G, Alegre de Miquel V. Skin metastasis of glioblastoma multiforme: a case report and literature review. Actas Dermosifiliogr (Engl Ed). 2019;110(9):780–3.
19. Nakib CE, Hajjar R, Zerdan MB, Darwish H, Zeidan Y, Alame S, Kassouf HK, Chamseddine N, Assi HI. Glioblastoma multiforme metastasizing to the skin, a case report and literature review. Radiol Case Rep. 2021;17(1):171–5.
20. Pietschmann S, von Bueren AO, Kerber MJ, Baumert BG, Kortmann RD, Müller K. An individual patient

data meta-analysis on characteristics, treatments and outcomes of glioblastoma/ gliosarcoma patients with metastases outside of the central nervous system. PLoS One. 2015;10(4):e0121592.
21. Wang F, Dong J, Zhang J, Zhao H, Wang N, Jin J, Yan X, Gao X, Liu H, Hu S. Rapid progression of subcutaneous glioblastoma: a case report and literature review. Front Oncol. 2023;13:935944.
22. Chao MM, Packer RJ, Myseros JS, Rood BR. Isolated extracranial recurrence of anaplastic ependymoma. Pediatr Blood Cancer. 2011;56(2):317–8.
23. Kumar P, Rastogi N, Jain M, Chhabra P. Extraneural metastases in anaplastic ependymoma. J Cancer Res Ther. 2007;3(2):102–4.
24. Marsecano C, Bruno F, Michelini G, Perri M, Calvisi G, Di Cesare E, Splendiani A. Systemic metastases from central nervous system ependymoma: case report and review of the literature. Neuroradiol J. 2017;30(3):274–80.
25. McNamara C, Mankad K, Thust S, Dixon L, Limback-Stanic C, D'Arco F, Jacques TS, Löbel U. 2021 WHO classification of tumours of the central nervous system: a review for the neuroradiologist. Neuroradiology. 2022;64(10):1919–50.
26. Palmisciano P, Ferini G, Barone F, Chavda V, Romano F, Amico P, Emmanuele D, Nicoletti GF, Pompili G, Giammalva GR, Maugeri R, Iacopino DG, Strigari L, Yeo TT, Cicero S, Scalia G, Umana GE. Extra-neural metastases from primary intracranial Ependymomas: a systematic review. Front Oncol. 2022;12:831016.
27. Scalia G, Ferini G, Chaurasia B, Graziano F, Priola S, Amico P, Umana GE. Recurrent intracranial anaplastic ependymoma with late-onset giant scalp metastasis. Clin Case Reports. 2023;11(12):e8324.
28. Yust Katz S, Cachia D, Kamiya-Matsuoka C, Olar A, Theeler B, Penas Prado M, Gilbert MR, Armstrong T. Ependymomas arising outside of the central nervous system: a case series and literature review. J Clin Neurosci. 2018;47:202–7.

Part XV

Tissue-Based Diagnostic Techniques in Cutaneous Metastases: Immunohistochemistry, Molecular Pathology, and Cytogenetics

Tissue-Based Diagnostic Techniques in Cutaneous Metastases: Immunohistochemistry, Molecular Pathology, and Cytogenetics

28

Vaia Tsangari, Dimitra Koumaki, Galateia Datseri, and Mattheos Bobos

Abstract

Cutaneous metastases refer to secondary involvement of the skin by internal malignant neoplasms. Their presence usually indicates advanced disease, and less frequently, they represent the initial manifestation of malignancy. Evaluation of histopathological and immunohistochemical findings in combination with molecular and cytogenetic testing is required for an accurate diagnosis. In this chapter, we provide an overview of the diagnostic techniques used by pathologists to evaluate such specimens, aligned with the World Health Organization (WHO) Classification of Tumors, fifth edition, and present detailed descriptions of skin metastases from a variety of malignancies, supported by case-based illustrations. Pathologists are trained to recognize different histopathologic growth patterns and subsequently perform immunophenotypic profiling and molecular testing, which are essential for identifying the primary tumor and guiding therapeutic decisions. Discussion of cutaneous metastases from breast, lung, stomach, colon, prostate, kidney, bladder, ovary, thyroid, and uterine carcinomas, as well as melanoma, together with illustrative cases, highlights the practical diagnostic process followed in routine dermatopathology and surgical pathology practice.

Keywords

Cutaneous metastases · Immunohistochemistry · Molecular pathology · Cytogenetics · WHO classification · Metastatic tumors

V. Tsangari (✉)
Department of Pathology, General Hospital of Veria, Veria, Greece

D. Koumaki
Dermatology Department, University Hospital of Heraklion, Heraklion, Greece

G. Datseri
Pathology Department, University Hospital of Heraklion, Heraklion, Greece

M. Bobos (✉)
Department of Biomedical Sciences, School of Health Sciences, International Hellenic University, Alexandrian Campus, Thessaloniki, Greece

28.1 Introduction

Cutaneous metastases refer to secondary malignant deposits in the skin that originate from internal malignancies. Their reported incidence ranges from approximately 0.7% to 10% among patients with cancer, depending on tumor type and disease stage, and accounts for 1.2–10% of

D. Koumaki et al. (eds.), *Cutaneous Metastases*, https://doi.org/10.1007/978-3-032-26764-1_28

all surgical and biopsy specimens [1–6]. In most cases, cutaneous metastases signify disseminated disease and are associated with an adverse prognosis; however, in up to one-third of patients, they may be the first clinical manifestation of an underlying malignancy [1, 2]. Regarding pathogenesis, most cases are attributed to hematogenous spread, but lymphatic and angiotropic extravascular spread, as well as, rarely, iatrogenic implantation, have also been described [5]. The fifth edition of the WHO Classification of Tumors emphasizes the combination of morphology, immunohistochemistry, and molecular pathology as a valid diagnostic approach [7–9].

28.2 Histopathologic Evaluation

The first step in evaluating a skin biopsy is examining slides stained with hematoxylin–eosin (H&E), a method widely used in daily routine diagnosis. Skin metastases most commonly present as relatively well-circumscribed lesions that usually involve the dermis and/or subcutis without affecting the epidermis and lacking an in situ component [3–6]. Architectural patterns that are commonly observed include nodular growth, infiltrative single-cell or cord-like growth, diffuse sheet-like replacement, intravascular tumor emboli, and rarely epidermotropic growth [1, 3]. Cytologic features usually mimic those of the primary tumor and may include gland formation, mucin production, clear-cell change, keratinization, or spindle-cell morphology [4, 7].

28.3 Immunohistochemistry

Immunohistochemical examination is crucial for confirming lineage and narrowing the differential diagnosis of cutaneous metastases. The diagnostic strategy recommended begins with broad-spectrum epithelial markers followed by lineage-specific antibodies (Tables 28.1 and 28.2; Diagram 28.1) [5, 8]. The use of cytokeratins CK7 and CK20 provides a useful framework for initial categorization of the tumor. A CK7-positive/CK20-negative immunohistochemical pattern is seen in breast, lung, ovarian, thyroid, and most renal carcinomas, whereas CK7-negative/CK20-positive tumors may indicate colorectal origin. CK7-positive/CK20-positive

Table 28.1 Immunohistochemical lineage classification in cutaneous metastases

Lineage	Immunohistochemical markers
Carcinoma	CKAE1/AE3, EMA, CAM5.2, EpCAM, Claudin-4
Lymphoid	CD45
Melanoma	SOX10
Sarcoma	No specific markers
Germ cell	OCT3/4, SALL4
Mesothelioma	Calretinin

Adapted from Krämer et al. [10]

Table 28.2 Cytokeratin profile for tumor categorization in cutaneous metastases

CK7+/CK20+	CK7+/CK20−	CK7−/CK20+	CK7−/CK20-
Upper gastrointestinal/ pancreatobiliary	Colorectal cancer with MMR deficiency	Colorectal, upper astrointestinal	Adrenocortical carcinoma
Bladder	Breast	Merkel cell carcinoma	Renal cell carcinoma
Rectum	Thyroid		Hepatocellular carcinoma
	Upper gastrointestinal/ pancreatobiliary		Germ cell tumors
	Salivary gland		Prostate
	Renal (papillary, chromophobe)		Gastric
	Bladder		Small-cell lung carcinoma
	Endometrial, endocervical, ovaryerous)		Squamous cell carcinoma
	Lung		Neuroendocrine neoplasms

Adapted from Krämer et al. [10]

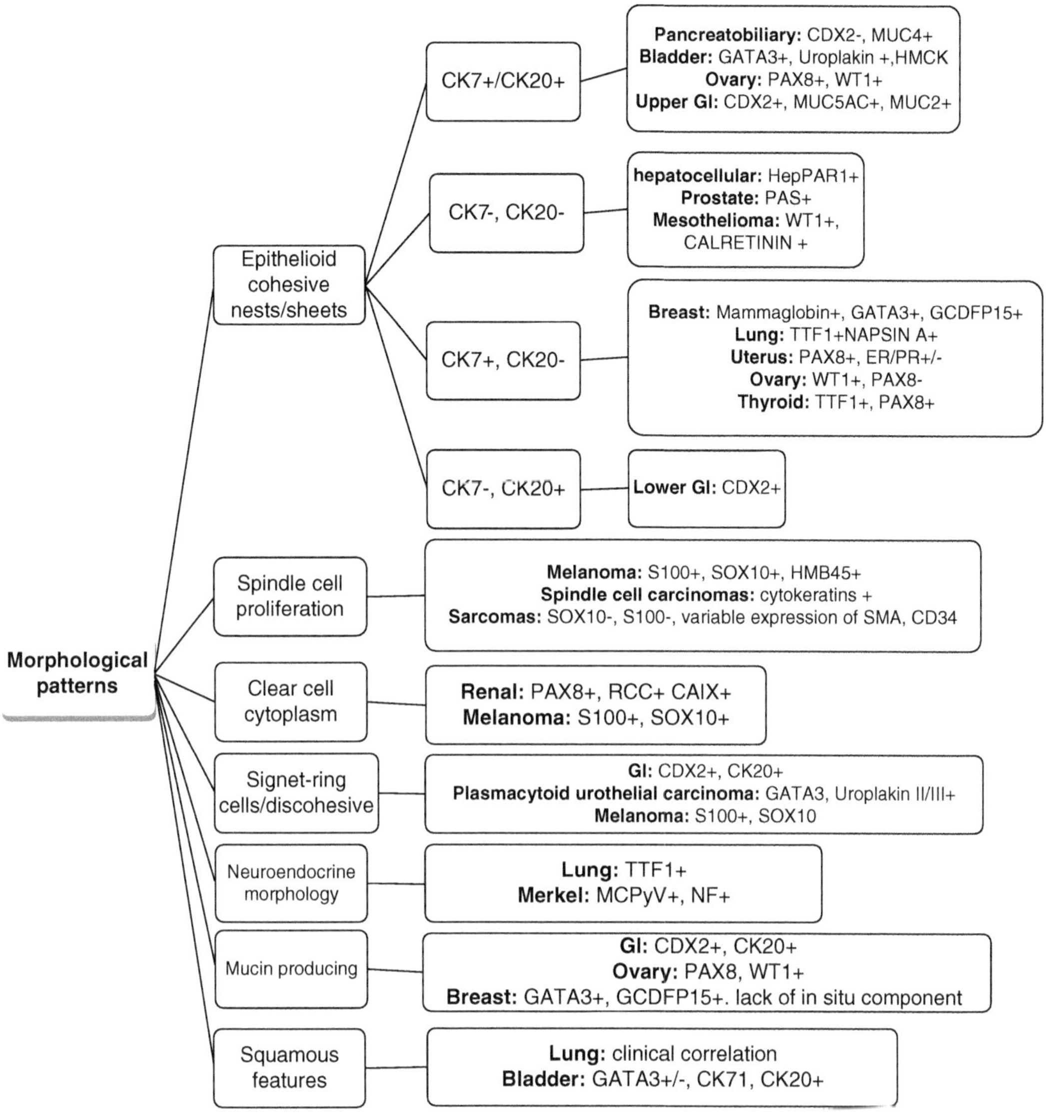

Diagram 28.1 Diagnostic algorithm of cutaneous metastases based on tumor cell morphology and immunohistochemistry. (Adapted from: Prieto et al. [5])

profiles are typical of upper gastrointestinal and urothelial carcinomas, while CK7-negative/CK20-negative tumors include prostate carcinoma and selected renal cell carcinomas [8, 9]. Expression of GATA3 and hormone receptors supports a breast origin; positivity for TTF-1 and Napsin A suggests pulmonary adenocarcinoma; CDX2 expression supports gastrointestinal origin; PAX8 is expressed in renal, thyroid, and Müllerian tumors; NKX3.1 is a highly sensitive marker for prostate carcinoma; and thyroglobulin confirms thyroid origin. In poorly differentiated carcinomas, there is loss of marker expression that impedes final diagnosis [5, 8, 11–13]. Positivity for cytokeratin 5/6 and p63 or p40 in tumor cells is suggestive of a primary cutaneous adnexal tumor over adenocarcinoma metastatic to the skin.

28.4 Molecular Pathology in Cutaneous Metastases

Pathology has incorporated molecular techniques into the diagnostic evaluation of cutaneous metastases, in line with WHO classification principles [4–7]. Next-generation sequencing (NGS) is a method applied to skin biopsy specimens that enables the detection of mutations, copy-number alterations, and gene rearrangements.

Molecular alterations provide valuable diagnostic information, and their detection can guide targeted therapy. Some examples of molecular alterations include PIK3CA mutations in breast carcinoma, EGFR mutations and ALK or ROS1 rearrangements in lung adenocarcinoma, CDH1 mutations in diffuse gastric carcinoma, TMPRSS2–ERG fusion and PTEN loss in prostate carcinoma, VHL gene inactivation in clear cell renal cell carcinoma, TP53 mutations in ovarian high-grade serous carcinoma, and BRAF V600E mutation in papillary thyroid carcinoma [11, 12, 15–17].

28.5 Cytogenetics

Cytogenetic techniques, such as fluorescence in situ hybridization (FISH), are used to detect gene rearrangements (e.g., ALK, ROS1), gene amplifications (e.g., ERBB2/HER2), and chromosomal alterations, including chromosome 3p loss in renal cell carcinoma [15]. These techniques are supplementary to immunohistochemistry and molecular findings providing a complete diagnostic approach.

28.6 Cutaneous Metastases of a Variety of Primary Origins and Case-Based Illustrations

28.6.1 Cutaneous Metastases from Breast Carcinoma

Cutaneous metastases from breast carcinoma represent the most common form of skin metastasis in women and account for a significant proportion of secondary cutaneous malignancies in dermatopathology practice [1, 2]. They usually occur in the setting of advanced disease but may occasionally represent the first clinical manifestation of an underlying breast carcinoma. Common anatomic sites include the chest wall, surgical scars, abdomen, scalp, and upper extremities. Cutaneous metastases occur predominantly by lymphatic dissemination and less commonly by hematogenous spread. Clinically, lesions may present as firm dermal or subcutaneous nodules, indurated plaques, erythematous inflammatory changes, or, less commonly, as telangiectatic or ulcerated lesions [1–3].

28.6.1.1 Histopathological Findings

Histopathologic examination reveals infiltration of the dermis and/or subcutis with relative sparing of the epidermis and absence of an in situ component, a feature that helps differentiate metastatic disease from primary cutaneous adnexal carcinomas [4, 6]. A variety of architectural patterns may be observed, reflecting the histological subtype of the primary breast carcinoma. The two most common subtypes are ductal and lobular carcinoma (Figs. 28.1 and 28.2).

Invasive ductal carcinoma consists of atypical epithelial cells arranged in cohesive nests, cords, or tubular structures within desmoplastic stroma. In contrast, invasive lobular carcinoma, as defined in the WHO Classification of Breast Tumours, is characterized by infiltrative growth of discohesive, small to medium-sized tumor cells, arranged in single-file linear cords that invade the stroma. Nuclei are round to oval with inconspicuous nucleoli.

Mucinous carcinoma consists of nests or sheets of malignant cells in abundant extracellular mucin, separated by delicate fibrous septa. In invasive papillary carcinomas, the histologic pattern consists of dilated ducts and microcysts containing papillary protrusions. Micropapillary carcinoma consists of morula-like aggregates of cuboidal to columnar neoplastic cells without true fibrovascular cores. Cytologic atypia, mitotic activity, and necrosis vary according to tumor grade and prior therapy [7].

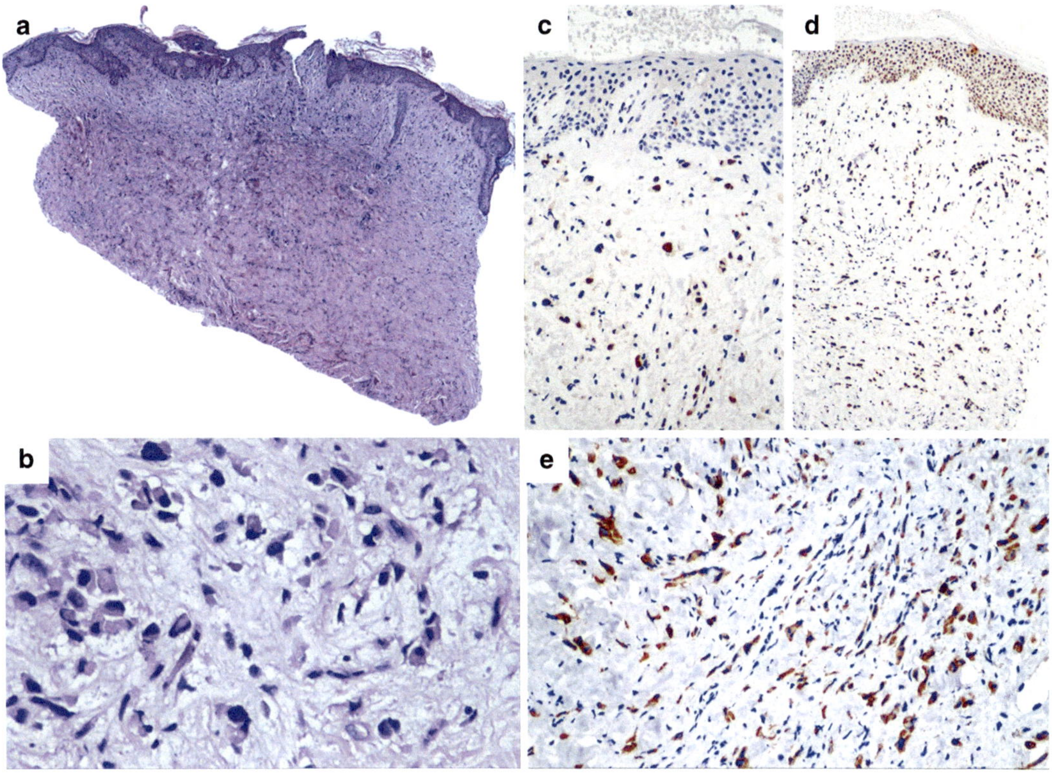

Fig. 28.1 Cutaneous metastasis from lobular breast carcinoma, pleomorphic type (pleomorphic lobular carcinoma). (**a**) Diffuse dermal invasion from the tumor. (**b**) The tumor cells show loss of cohesion, nuclear hyperchromasia, and intracytoplasmic mucin and display a signet ring cell appearance. (**c**) The neoplastic cells exhibit strong nuclear positivity for estrogen receptors (ER). (**d**) GATA3 strong nuclear expressions. (**e**) Cytokeratin 19 intense cytoplasmic expression. **a**, **b**: Hematoxylin and eosin stain. **c**–**e**: Immunohistochemistry. DAB chromogen

28.6.1.2 Immunohistochemical Profile

Immunohistochemical examination is essential for confirming mammary origin. Tumor cells typically express cytokeratin 7 (membrane/cytoplasmic staining) and cytokeratin 19, while cytokeratin 20 is negative in most cases [9].

One of the most sensitive and widely used markers for breast carcinoma is GATA3, with strong nuclear expression [9, 18]. Estrogen receptor (ER) and progesterone receptor (PR) expression are frequently retained in cutaneous metastases, although loss of hormone receptor expression may occur in high-grade or therapy-resistant tumors [7]. Mammaglobin and GCDFP-15 may support mammary differentiation but are less sensitive than GATA3, while the expression of both GATA3 and SOX10 is useful for the diagnosis of metastatic triple-negative breast cancer [19].

In metastatic invasive lobular carcinoma, loss of E-cadherin expression is a characteristic immunohistochemical feature and correlates with the discohesive growth pattern [20]. Assessment of HER2 (ERBB2) expression by immunohistochemistry, with confirmatory in situ hybridization when indicated, remains important for therapeutic stratification.

Chemotherapeutic and hormonal treatment may result in reduced or heterogeneous expression of hormone receptors and GATA3; there-

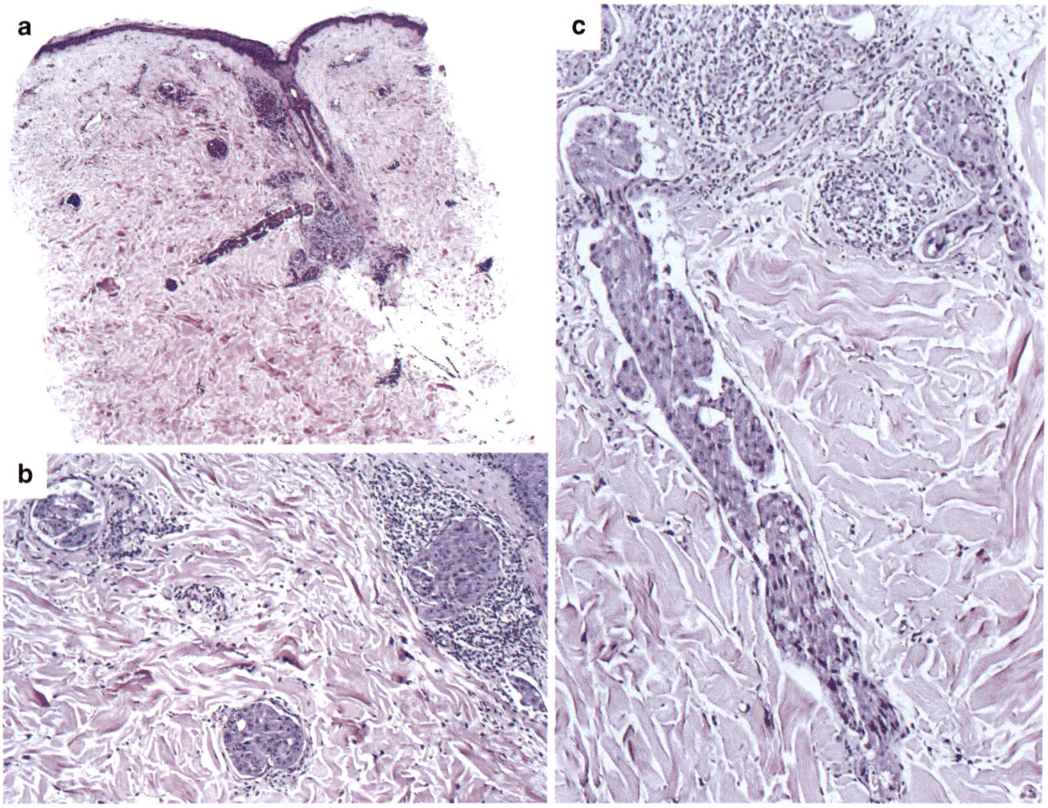

Fig. 28.2 Dermal metastasis from breast carcinoma of no special type (NST) with numerous lymphovascular emboli. (**a**) The tumor cells are mainly observed within the lumina of small vessels and invade as single cells or small units into the dermis. (**b**, **c**) Tumor cells filling vascular spaces. **a**–**c**: Hematoxylin and Eosin stain

fore, clinical correlation and molecular techniques are necessary in these cases [7].

28.6.1.3 Molecular Pathology

Molecular alterations detected in cutaneous metastases from breast carcinoma reflect intrinsic molecular subtypes and are useful for diagnostic, prognostic, and therapeutic purposes [7].

There are two divergent molecular pathways in breast cancer related to hormone receptors. One of them is the ER-positive pathway, and the molecular findings detected in this pathway include gains of 1q, loss of 16q, infrequent amplification of 17q12, and a gene expression signature enriched in genes associated with the ER-positive phenotype. These lesions express hormone receptors, lack HER2 overexpression and basal marker expression, and have relatively simple diploid or near-diploid karyotypes. The second, the ER-negative pathway, is characterized by loss of 13q, gain of chromosomal region 11q13, amplification of 17q12, and a gene expression signature enriched in genes associated with cellular proliferation. PIK3CA mutations can be present in both pathways, while TP53 mutations are detected more frequently in the ER-negative pathway. The ER-negative breast cancers include both HER2-positive and HER2-negative groups [7, 21].

28.6.2 Cutaneous Metastases from Lung Carcinoma

Lung carcinoma in men is the most frequent primary tumor to metastasize to the skin. The metastases may occur on any cutaneous surface, but mainly present on the trunk as a single nodule or a cluster of papules. Small cell carcinoma shows a predilection for the skin of the back [22]. Cutaneous involvement may occur at any stage of disease, and usually indicates a poor outcome [22, 23].

28.6.2.1 Histopathological Findings

The histological appearance is similar to that of the subtype of the primary lung carcinoma. Lung adenocarcinoma typically shows glandular, acinar, papillary, or solid growth patterns. Tumor cells are polygonal to columnar with moderate nuclear pleomorphism and prominent nucleoli. Intracytoplasmic mucin may be present and can be highlighted using special histochemical stains. Necrosis may be present, especially in poorly differentiated tumors [4, 8].

In squamous cell carcinoma, the tumor consists of nests and sheets of atypical squamous cells with varying degrees of keratinization and the presence or absence of intercellular bridges, depending on the tumor grade. Keratin pearl formation may be present but is often less prominent than in the primary tumor [8, 23]. Small cell lung carcinoma shows diffuse sheets of small-sized blue cells with scant cytoplasm, finely granular chromatin, nuclear molding, high mitotic rate, extensive necrosis, and crush artifact. There are rare subtypes, like hepatoid lung adenocarcinoma, which exhibit similar histopathological features to hepatocellular carcinoma and usually elevated alpha-fetoprotein in serum (Fig. 28.3). In cases of pleomorphic carcinoma in which none of the above morphological patterns are present, large cell carcinoma should be excluded by immunohistochemistry (Fig. 28.4) [8].

28.6.2.2 Immunohistochemical Profile

Most lung carcinomas show a CK7-positive/CK20-negative immunophenotype, which provides an initial diagnostic framework [7].

Thyroid transcription factor-1 (TTF-1) is a key marker for pulmonary adenocarcinoma and small cell lung carcinoma, showing strong nuclear expression. Napsin A is highly specific for lung adenocarcinoma and is frequently co-expressed with TTF-1, providing strong evidence of pulmonary origin when both markers are positive [5, 8]. In contrast, squamous cell carcinoma of the lung is typically negative for TTF-1 and Napsin A and positive for CK5/6, p40, and p63, with p40 considered a highly specific marker for squamous differentiation.

Markers of squamous differentiation, including p40 and p63, are useful in identifying metastatic squamous cell carcinoma and distinguishing it from adenocarcinoma. p40 is preferred due to its higher specificity for squamous differentiation. Cytokeratin 5/6 may also be expressed in squamous cell carcinoma [8].

In poorly differentiated cancers where standard H&E or IHC markers are inconclusive, PAS-diastase (Periodic Acid-Schiff with diastase) stain can reveal subtle mucin, confirming adenocarcinoma.

Small cell lung carcinoma (SCC) is positive for neuroendocrine markers, such as synaptophysin, chromogranin A, and INSM1, in conjunction with TTF-1 expression in most cases [8]. TTF-1 positivity CK20 and neurofilament negativity can also be used as a useful adjunct in distinguishing SCC from Merkel cell carcinoma of the skin [24].

28.6.2.3 Molecular Pathology

Lung adenocarcinoma frequently harbors activating EGFR mutations, which predict response to EGFR tyrosine kinase inhibitors [8]. Rearrangements of ALK and ROS1 can be detected by fluorescence in situ hybridization and next-generation sequencing (NGS), but also by immunochemistry [8, 14, 25]. KRAS mutations represent the most common oncogenic drivers in lung adenocarcinoma and have recently become therapeutically actionable [15].

Less frequent alterations include BRAF V600E mutations, RET rearrangements, ERBB2 (HER2) mutations, and NTRK gene fusions, all of which may guide targeted therapy in selected patients [8, 14]. TP53 alterations are frequent in squamous cell carcinoma and small cell lung carcinoma [8]. Furthermore, patients with PDL1 expression and tumor proportional scores above 50% are considered suitable for anti-PDL1 therapy [8].

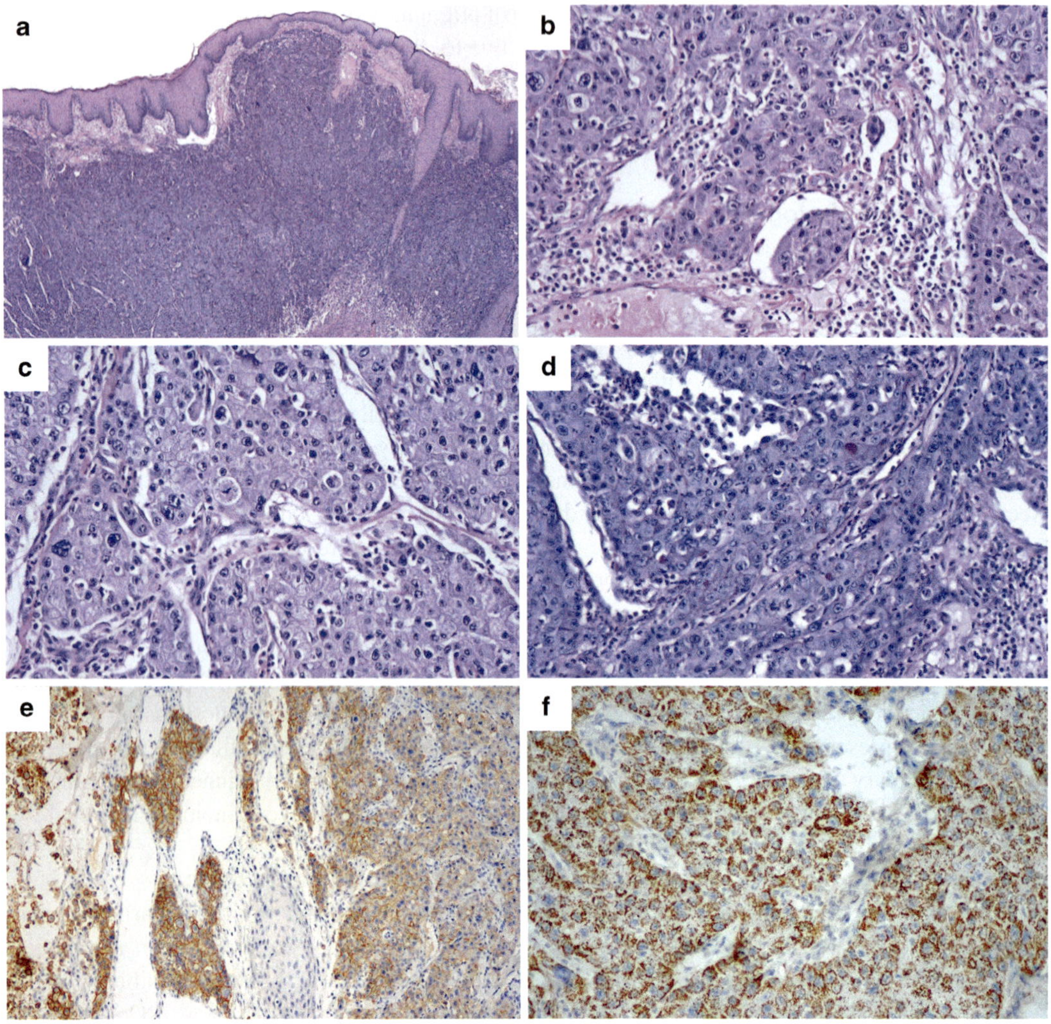

Fig. 28.3 Cutaneous metastasis from hepatoid lung adenocarcinoma. (**a**) A bulky tumor invades the dermis and elevates the overlying epidermis. (**b**) High magnification of a poorly differentiated carcinoma with solid sheets and nests of polygonal cells with pleomorphic vesicular nuclei and abundant cytoplasm. Note the tumor emboli within the lumina of small vessels. (**c**) The tumor cells show distinct cytoplasmic membranes, atypical nuclei, high mitotic activity, and prominent nucleoli. (**d**) Intra and extracellular periodic acid-Schiff (PAS)-positive diastase-resistant hyaline globules were noted in a few of the tumor cells. (**e**) Anti-BerEP4 antibody reactivity against adenocarcinoma cells. F. Hepatocyte paraffin 1 (HepPar1) antibody shows intense cytoplasmic granular positivity in the neoplastic cells. **a–c**: Hematoxylin and eosin stain. **d**: PAS diastase. **e–f**: Immunohistochemistry. DAB chromogen

28.6.3 Cutaneous Metastases from Gastric Carcinoma

Cutaneous metastases from gastric carcinoma are generally uncommon and usually involve the abdominal wall, including the umbilical region (Sister Mary Joseph nodule), but may also affect the trunk, scalp, and extremities. The majority of them are poorly differentiated carcinomas [1, 2, 4, 26].

28.6.3.1 Histopathological Findings

The morphological findings may include invasion of the dermis by cuboidal to columnar neoplastic cells with intracytoplasmic mucin, arranged in tubular and sometimes acinar structures, suggesting tubular gastric adenocarcinoma as the primary tumor, or arrangement in solid sheets with no clear tubular formation, as seen in poorly differentiated

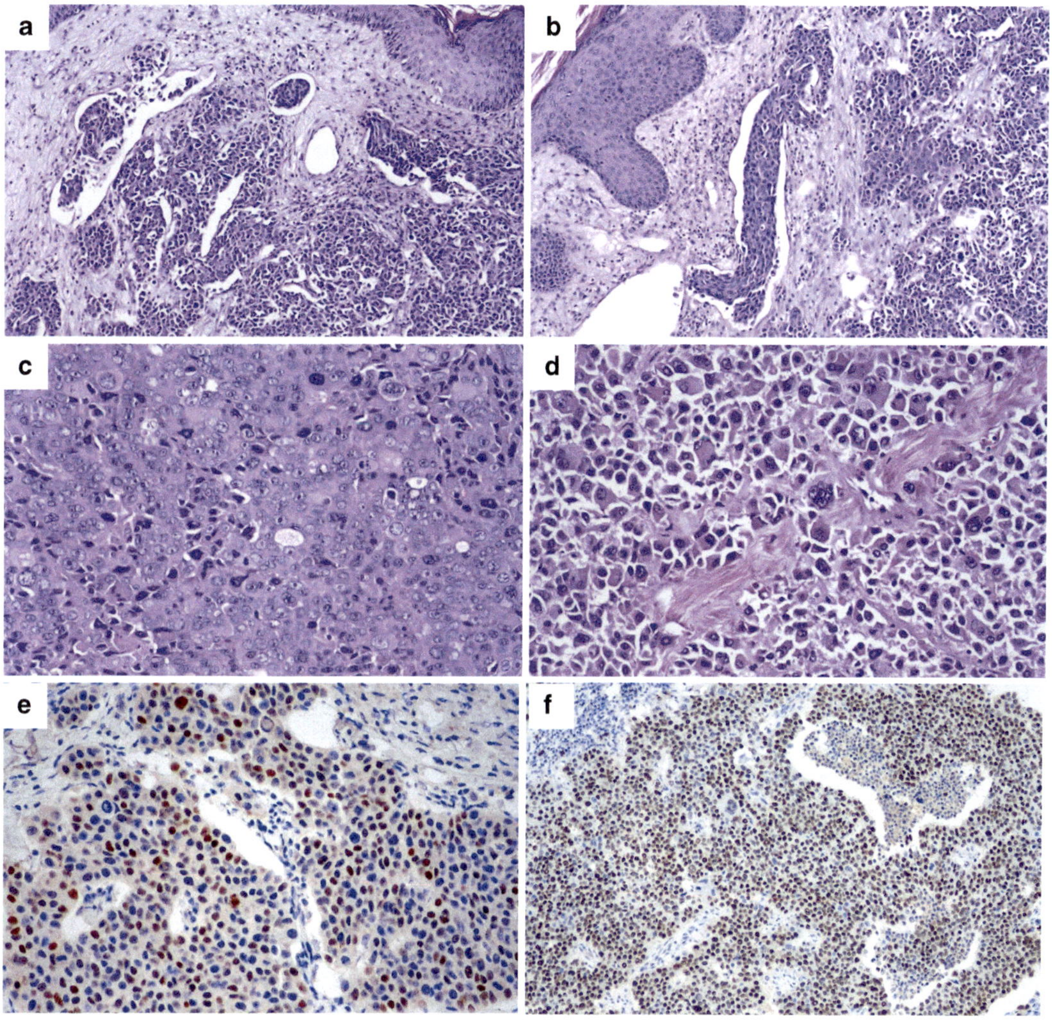

Fig. 28.4 Pleomorphic carcinoma of the lung metastatic to the skin. (**a**, **b**) The tumor cells invade the dermis as solid sheets and nests and are also located within dilated lymphatic vessels. (**c**) Large, pleomorphic, multinuclear, and giant tumor cells with eosinophilic cytoplasm and high mitotic activity. (**d**) Area of tumor with rhabdoid phenotype. (**e**) Insulinoma-associated protein 1 (INSM1) expression in a fraction of tumor cells. (**f**) Immunoperoxidase stain for thyroid transcription factor 1 (TTF1) shows the typical nuclear positivity. **a**–**d**: Hematoxylin and eosin stain. **e**–**f**: Immunohistochemistry. DAB chromogen

solid carcinoma. Another pattern is diffuse infiltration by solitary malignant cells or small aggregates, frequently with signet ring morphology, due to displacement of the nucleus from intracytoplasmic mucin (Fig. 28.5). Desmoplastic stromal response is variable, and lymphovascular invasion is commonly observed. In some cases, extensive dermal infiltration may produce indurated plaques or nodules clinically [12, 26, 27].

28.6.3.2 Immunohistochemical Profile

Gastric carcinoma metastases usually express cytokeratin 7 and cytokeratin 20, with variable expression patterns depending on tumor subtype [6]. CDX2 is a marker that supports gastrointestinal origin. In poorly cohesive carcinomas, reduction or loss of E-cadherin expression is usually noted [12]. Claudin 18, and especially the isoform Claudin 18.2, is highly expressed in most gastric cancers and, in conjunction with other

IHC markers, can be used in the histologic distinction of gastric carcinoma from other cancers.

Immunohistochemical assessment of HER2 (ERBB2) is recommended in metastatic gastric carcinoma, as HER2 overexpression or amplification may be retained in cutaneous metastases and has therapeutic implications [17].

28.6.3.3 Molecular Pathology

The Cancer Genome Atlas suggests a molecular classification of gastric adenocarcinomas that includes four categories: microsatellite-unstable, genomically stable, EBV-positive, and chromosomally unstable.

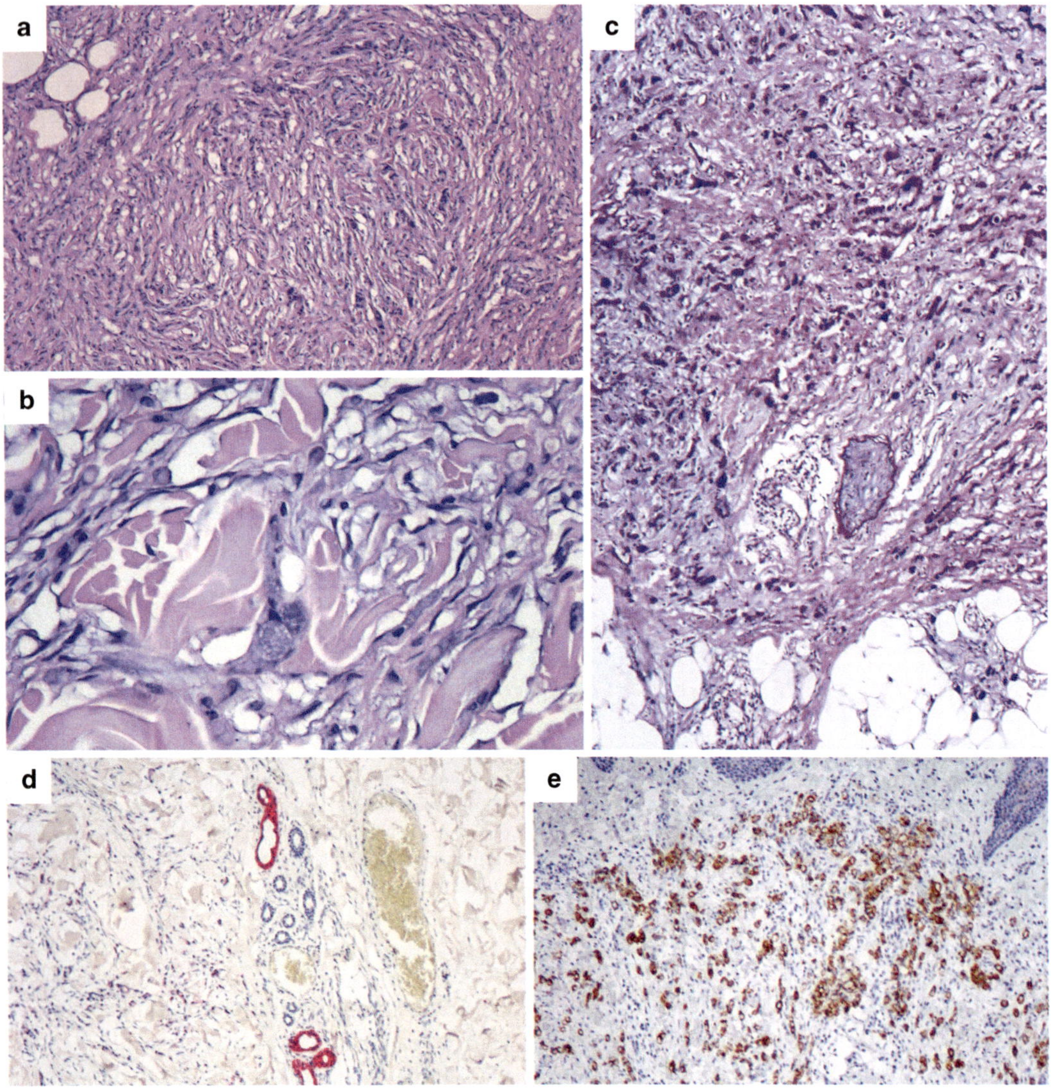

Fig. 28.5 Cutaneous metastasis from a poorly cohesive gastric carcinoma, signet-ring cell type. (**a**) The tumor invades the dermis widely with marked desmoplasia. (**b**) The tumor is composed predominantly of "signet-ring cells," cells with a central, globoid droplet of cytoplasmic mucin and an eccentrically placed nucleus. (**c**) Periodic acid-Schiff (PAS)-positive diastase-resistant mucin was noted in tumor cells. (**d**) Diffuse labeling of the tumor cells for cytokeratin 7. (**e**) Anti-Claudin-18 antibody has intense reactivity against carcinoma cells. **a**, **b**: Hematoxylin and eosin stain. **c**: PAS diastase. **d**: Immunohistochemistry. Fast red chromogen. E: Immunohistochemistry. DAB chromogen

The EBV-positive subtype displays genome-wide hypermethylation, PIK3CA and ARID1A mutations, and amplification of the CD274 gene. Genomically stable carcinomas show a lower frequency of genetic aberrations. The fourth subtype, chromosomally unstable, shows DNA copy-number abnormalities. These include amplification of receptor tyrosine kinase genes, such as EGFR, ERBB2, FGFR2, and MET [12].

28.6.4 Cutaneous Metastases from Colorectal Adenocarcinoma

Cutaneous metastases from colorectal carcinoma are rare and usually involve the abdominal wall, particularly surgical scars and the periumbilical region [1, 2, 4].

28.6.4.1 Histopathological Findings

Tumor growth is most often nodular or infiltrative, arranged in irregular glands, cribriform structures, or solid nests within a desmoplastic stroma (Figs. 28.6 and 28.7) [4, 6]. Tumor cells are columnar to cuboidal with elongated, hyperchromatic nuclei and variable cytoplasmic mucin. Extracellular mucin pools and signet-ring cells may be present, mimicking primary mucinous carcinoma of the skin.

28.6.4.2 Immunohistochemical Profile

Most cases of gastric carcinomas express CK20 but are CK7-negative, although exceptions occur, particularly in high-grade tumors [9]. Rectal carcinoma may stain positive for both or with CK7 only.

CDX2 shows strong nuclear expression in most colorectal adenocarcinomas and is a key marker of intestinal differentiation [28]. SATB2 is highly sensitive and specific for colorectal origin and is especially valuable in metastatic settings, including cutaneous lesions. Co-expression of CK20, CDX2, and SATB2 strongly supports a colorectal primary. Mismatch repair (MMR) can be detected by immunohistochemistry (MLH1,

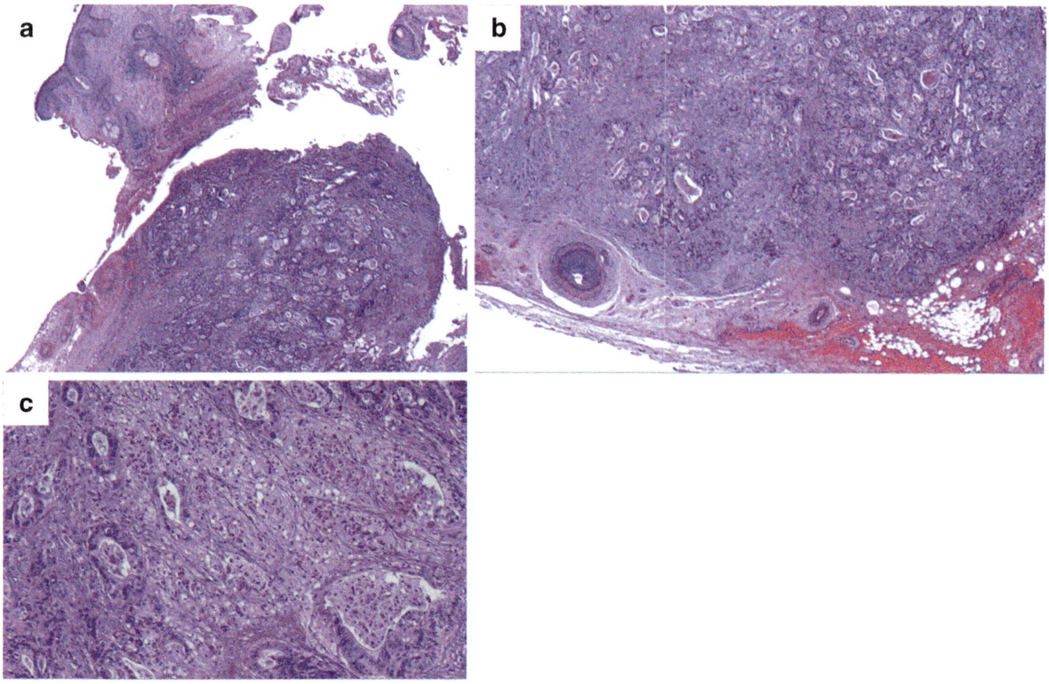

Fig. 28.6 Cutaneous metastasis from moderately differentiated colon adenocarcinoma. (**a**, **b**) The tumor cells invade the deep dermis and subcutis. (**c**) High magnification of a tumor area with extensive necrosis. **a**–**c**: Hematoxylin and eosin stain

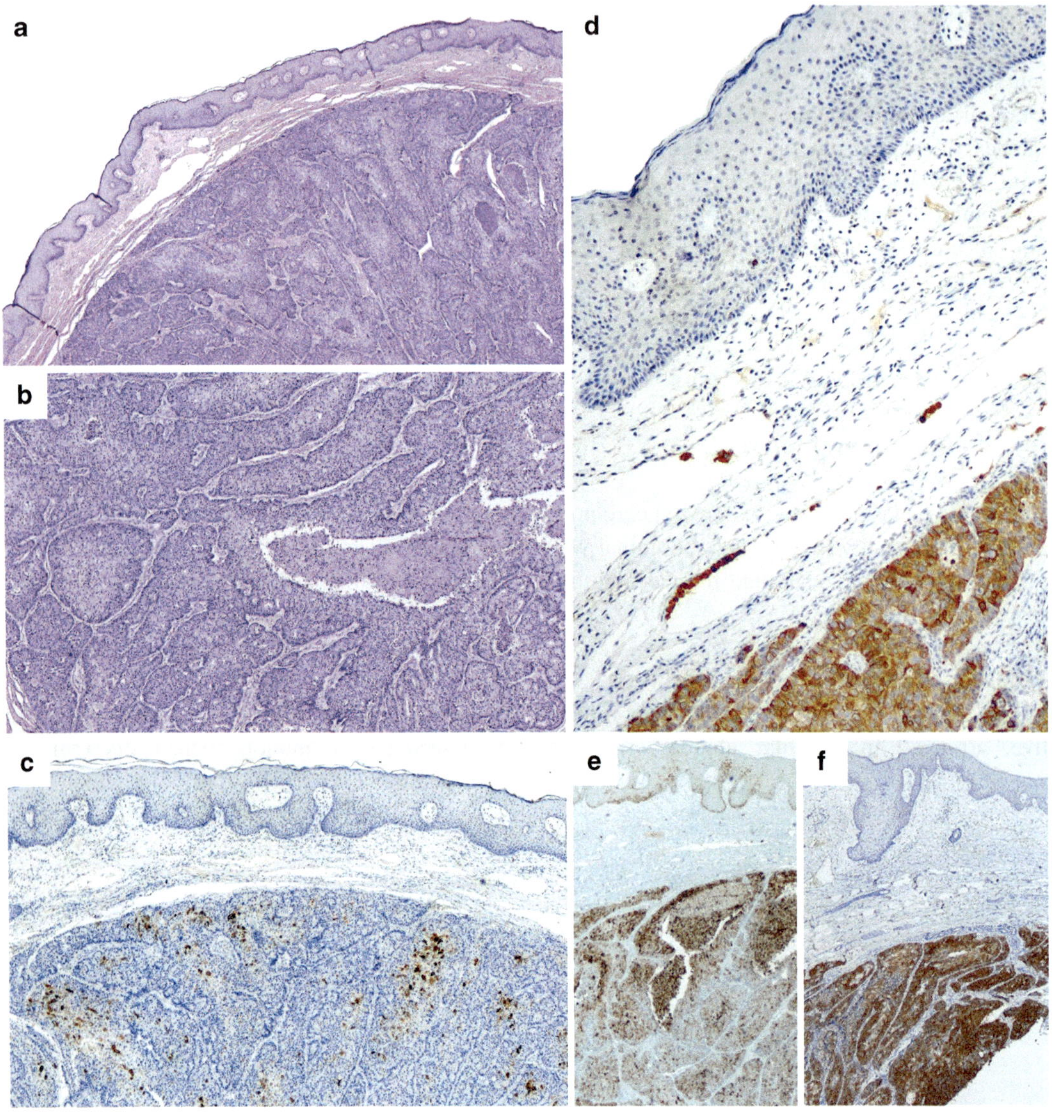

Fig. 28.7 Poorly differentiated colonic adenocarcinoma metastatic to the skin. (**a**) The atypical cells expand the dermis and preserve the overlying epidermis. (**b**) Solid and cystic neoplastic glands. Note the dirty or granular necrosis within the gland lumen. (**c**) The neoplastic cells show focal positivity for cytokeratin 20. (**d**) Strong staining of tumor cells for cytokeratin 7. Tumor cells within the lumina of small vessels also stained positively. (**e**) Epithelial membrane antigen (EMA) focal positivity. (**f**) Diffuse labeling of the tumor cells for villin. **a**, **b**: Hematoxylin and eosin stain. **c**–**f**: Immunohistochemistry. DAB chromogen

PMS2, MSH2, and MSH6). Loss of expression identifies microsatellite instability (MSI) and has diagnostic, prognostic, and therapeutic implications [12].

28.6.4.3 Molecular Pathology

Common mutations include KRAS and NRAS mutations, which predict resistance to anti-EGFR therapy, and BRAF V600E mutations, which are associated with poor prognosis and distinct clinicopathologic features.

Microsatellite instability (MSI) due to MMR deficiency may be identified by immunohistochemistry or molecular testing. Patients with MSI-high status are more likely to benefit from immune checkpoint inhibitors [12].

28.6.5 Cutaneous Metastases from Prostate Carcinoma

Prostate carcinoma rarely metastasizes to the skin. Cutaneous metastases, when present, usually involve the lower abdomen, genital region, and surgical scars (Fig. 28.8) [1, 2].

28.6.5.1 Histopathological Findings

In these rare cases, an infiltration of the dermis consisting of small, crowded, angulated glands or nests is observed (Fig. 28.9). Neoplastic cells show prominent nucleoli, scant to moderate cytoplasm, and variable mitotic activity. Rarely does the morphology differ, as in cases of plasmacytoid appearance, making diagnosis challenging (Fig. 28.10) [4, 6].

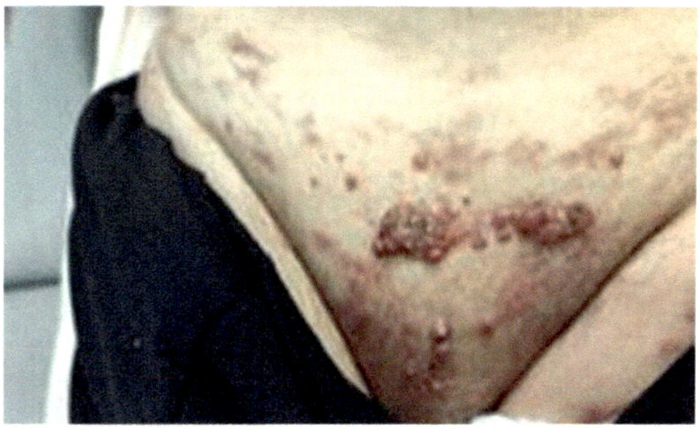

Fig. 28.8 Cutaneous metastases from prostate adenocarcinoma. Multiple firm, erythematous to violaceous papules and nodules, some coalescing into infiltrated plaques, are present on the lower abdomen and suprapubic region of an elderly male patient with advanced prostate carcinoma

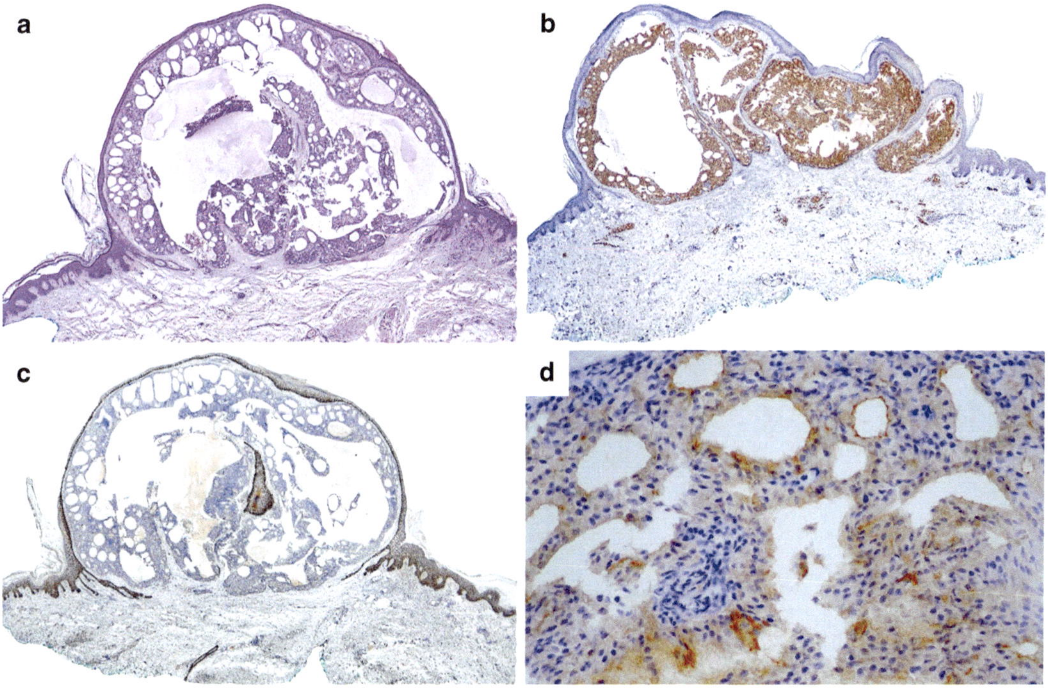

Fig. 28.9 Cutaneous metastasis from acinar adenocarcinoma of the prostate. (**a**) The tumor is relatively circumscribed and resembles, at low magnification, a primary dermal tumor showing nodulocystic and adenoid patterns. (**b**) Strong and diffuse nuclear positivity of NKX3.1, a prostatic tumor suppressor gene in neoplastic cells. (**c**) P63: absence of staining in tumor cells, whereas the internal controls (keratinocytes and ductal cells) are strongly positive. (**d**) Positive staining for prostate-specific antigen (PSA). **a**: Hematoxylin and eosin stain. **b–d**: Immunohistochemistry. DAB chromogen

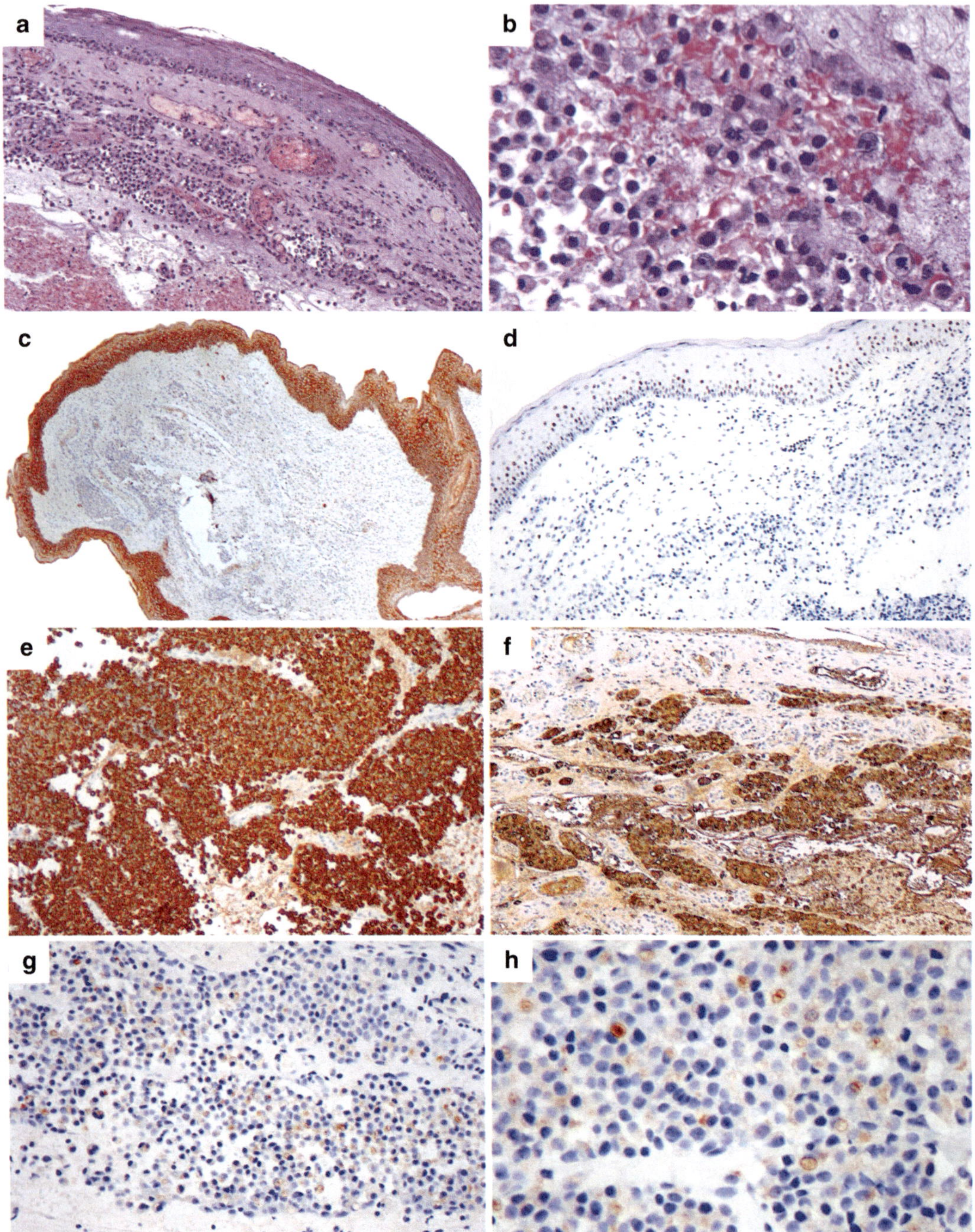

Fig. 28.10 Glans penis metastasis from plasmacytoid acinar adenocarcinoma of the prostate. (**a**) Carcinomas invade the lamina propria. (**b**) The tumor cells have a prominent plasmacytoid appearance. (**c**) E-cadherin was lost in the tumor compared to intact staining in the overlying epithelium. (**d**) GATA3: absence of staining in tumor cells. (**e**) Tumor is diffusely positive for cytokeratin 8/18. (**f**) PSAP immunoreactivity is present in tumor cells. (**g**, **h**) PSA was expressed in a fraction of tumor cells. **a**, **b**: Hematoxylin and eosin stain, **c**–**h** Immunohistochemistry. DAB chromogen

28.6.5.2 Immunohistochemical Profile

Cytokeratins CK7 and CK20 are typically not expressed in prostate cancer. NKX3.1 is the most sensitive and specific marker, demonstrating strong nuclear expression. PSA and PSAP are specific markers, but their expression may be reduced or absent in high-grade tumors. Androgen receptor expression further supports prostatic differentiation [11].

28.6.5.3 Molecular Pathology

The most characteristic genetic alteration that supports prostatic lineage is the TMPRSS2–ERG gene fusion. Loss of PTEN and alterations in DNA damage repair genes, including BRCA2, are common in advanced disease and have prognostic and therapeutic implications [11].

28.6.6 Cutaneous Metastases from Renal Cell Carcinoma

Skin metastases from renal cell carcinoma (RCC) are not common, and they often appear as red dermal nodules, including the scalp, face, and trunk [1, 2, 4].

28.6.6.1 Histopathological Findings

Clear cell carcinoma is the predominant histologic type of renal cell carcinoma metastasizing in the skin. The lesions consist of nests, alveolar sheets, or trabeculae of clear cells separated by a delicate sinusoidal vascular network. Tumor cells have abundant clear cytoplasm (lipid/glycogen), distinct cell borders, and variable nuclear atypia (Fig. 28.11) [4, 11]. More rarely, metastatic papillary RCC shows papillary structures with foamy macrophages, while chromophobe RCC may show solid architecture with pale eosinophilic cytoplasm and perinuclear halos [11].

28.6.6.2 Immunohistochemical Profile

Most RCC metastases express PAX8 (nuclear) and frequently CD10, indicating renal lineage. The RCC marker may be positive, and CAIX is typically strong and diffuse in clear cell RCC. CK7 is usually negative in clear cell RCC (often positive in papillary RCC) [11].

28.6.6.3 Molecular Pathology

Inactivation of the VHL pathway is characteristic for clear cell RCC, frequently associated with chromosome 3p loss, and dysregulation of hypoxia-inducible signaling [11, 16].

28.6.7 Cutaneous Metastases from Ovarian Carcinoma

Another uncommon primary origin of cutaneous metastases is ovarian carcinoma. They most frequently involve the abdominal wall, particularly the periumbilical region and surgical scars, and spread usually occurs through direct implantation or lymphatic routes [1, 2].

28.6.7.1 Histopathological Findings

The morphology depends on the histologic subtype of the primary tumor, most frequently high-grade serous carcinoma. Lesions are usually nodular or infiltrative, composed of nests, solid sheets, or papillary structures of atypical epithelial cells with marked pleomorphism within a fibrous or desmoplastic stroma. Neoplastic cells show high nuclear-to-cytoplasmic ratios, prominent nucleoli, and increased mitotic activity (Fig. 28.12). The presence of tumor necrosis and lymphovascular invasion is common. In some cases, psammoma bodies may be identified, supporting serous differentiation [4, 29].

28.6.7.2 Immunohistochemical Profile

Immunohistochemistry is essential for distinguishing ovarian carcinoma metastases from other CK7-positive carcinomas involving the skin. Tumors generally show a CK7-positive/CK20-negative immunophenotype [5]. PAX8 is a highly sensitive nuclear marker for ovarian carcinoma and is strongly expressed in most metastatic lesions. WT1 is a characteristic marker of high-grade serous carcinoma, and estrogen receptor (ER) expression is common, while

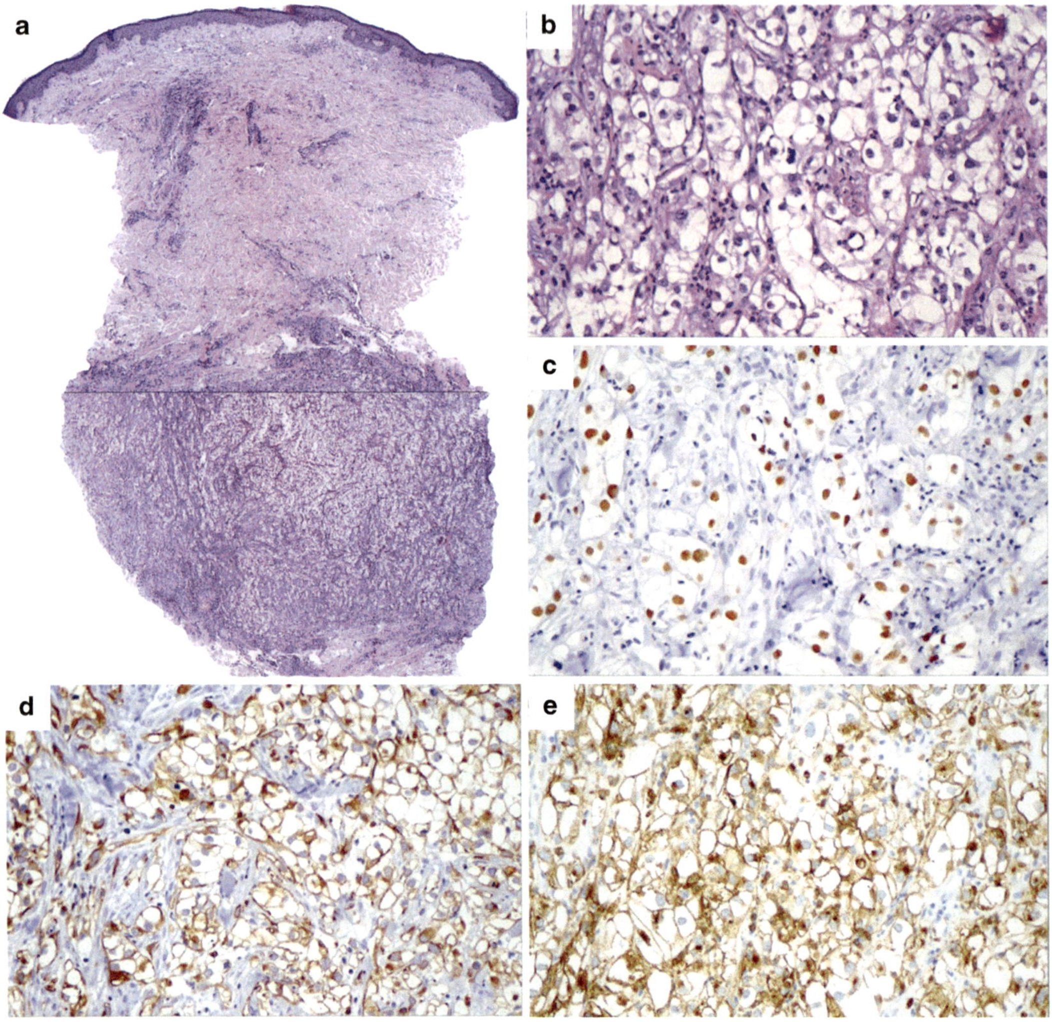

Fig. 28.11 Cutaneous metastasis from clear cell renal cell carcinoma. (**a**) Neoplastic nodule in deep dermis and subcutis from a clear cell neoplasm. (**b**) Tubules of clear glycogenated cells and a "chicken-wire" pattern of stromal vessels. (**c**) PAX8 diffuse nuclear expression in tumor cells. (**d**) Tumor is diffusely positive for pancytokeratin. E. Anti-CD10 antibody has intense reactivity against carcinoma cells. **a**, **b**: Hematoxylin and eosin stain. **c**–**e**: Immunohistochemistry. DAB chromogen

GATA3, TTF-1, and CDX2 are typically negative, helping exclude other epithelial lineages [5, 29].

28.6.7.3 Molecular Pathology

TP53 mutations are detected in high-grade serous carcinoma and underlie its aggressive clinical behavior. Alterations in repair genes, particularly BRCA1 and BRCA2, are frequent and have major therapeutic implications [29].

28.6.8 Cutaneous Metastases from Thyroid Carcinoma

Cutaneous metastases from thyroid carcinoma are extremely rare and usually occur in advanced disease. They are most frequently associated with papillary thyroid carcinoma (PTC) and follicular thyroid carcinoma (FTC), with occasional cases arising from anaplastic carcinoma. The prevalence of cutaneous metastases from thyroid pap-

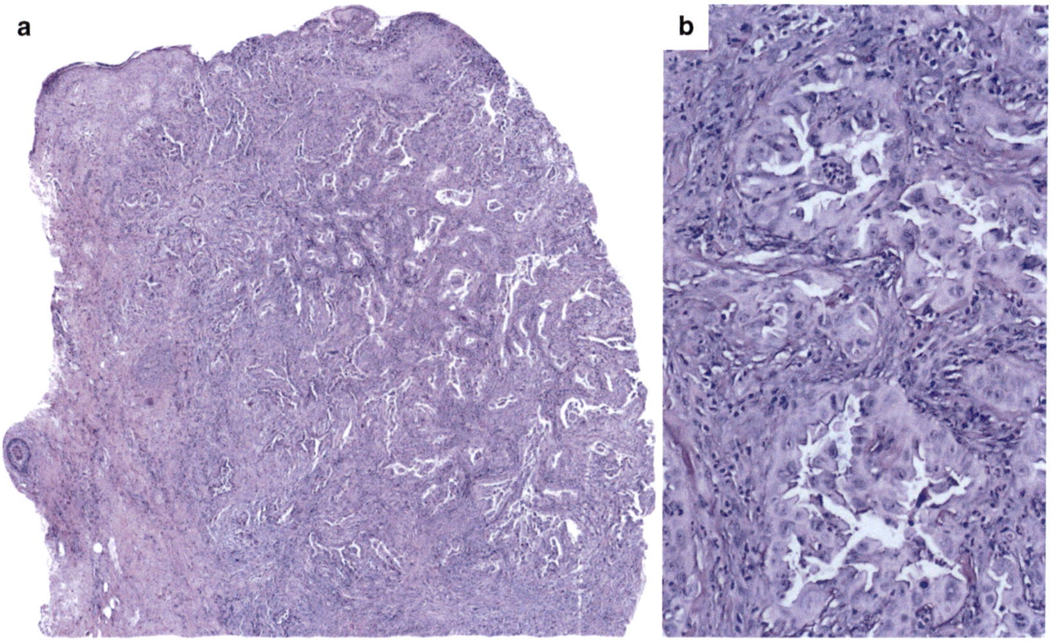

Fig. 28.12 Cutaneous metastasis from high-grade serous ovarian carcinoma. (**a**) Large neoplastic mass invading the dermis and focally the epidermis. (**b**) On high magnification, the tumor shows marked cytologic atypia, tufting, and detached cell clusters. **a**, **b**: Hematoxylin and eosin stain

illary carcinoma is 0.06–0.82%. Common sites include the scalp, face, neck, and upper trunk, consistent with hematogenous dissemination [1–3, 30, 31].

28.6.8.1 Histopathological Findings

Papillary thyroid carcinoma metastases show papillary, follicular, or solid architecture. The neoplastic cells manifest characteristic nuclear features, including nuclear enlargement, overlapping, grooves, and intranuclear pseudoinclusions (Fig. 28.13). Psammoma bodies are a common finding and support papillary differentiation [31].

Metastases from follicular thyroid carcinoma are composed of follicles or solid nests of tumor cells lacking the characteristic papillary nuclear features. Poorly differentiated and anaplastic carcinomas demonstrate solid growth, marked cytologic atypia, high mitotic activity, and necrosis [30].

28.6.8.2 Immunohistochemical Profile

A specific marker for differentiated thyroid carcinoma that is usually retained in metastatic PTC and FTC is thyroglobulin. TTF-1 shows nuclear positivity in most thyroid carcinomas but lacks specificity, as it is also expressed in lung carcinoma. PAX8 is frequently expressed and supports thyroid lineage, particularly in cases with reduced thyroglobulin expression. In anaplastic thyroid carcinoma, thyroglobulin is often negative, whereas PAX8 may remain positive and assist in diagnosis [31].

28.6.8.3 Molecular Pathology

BRAF V600E mutations are common in papillary thyroid carcinoma, and their frequency varies depending on the different subtypes of PTC, with the highest prevalence seen in tall cell PTC [30]. In cases of follicular tumors, RAS mutations are more frequently detected.

Anaplastic thyroid carcinoma develops after the occurrence of multiple alterations. The initial events are mostly RAS and BRAF p.V600E mutations, whereas the late events include, primarily, TP53 and TERT promoter mutations [31].

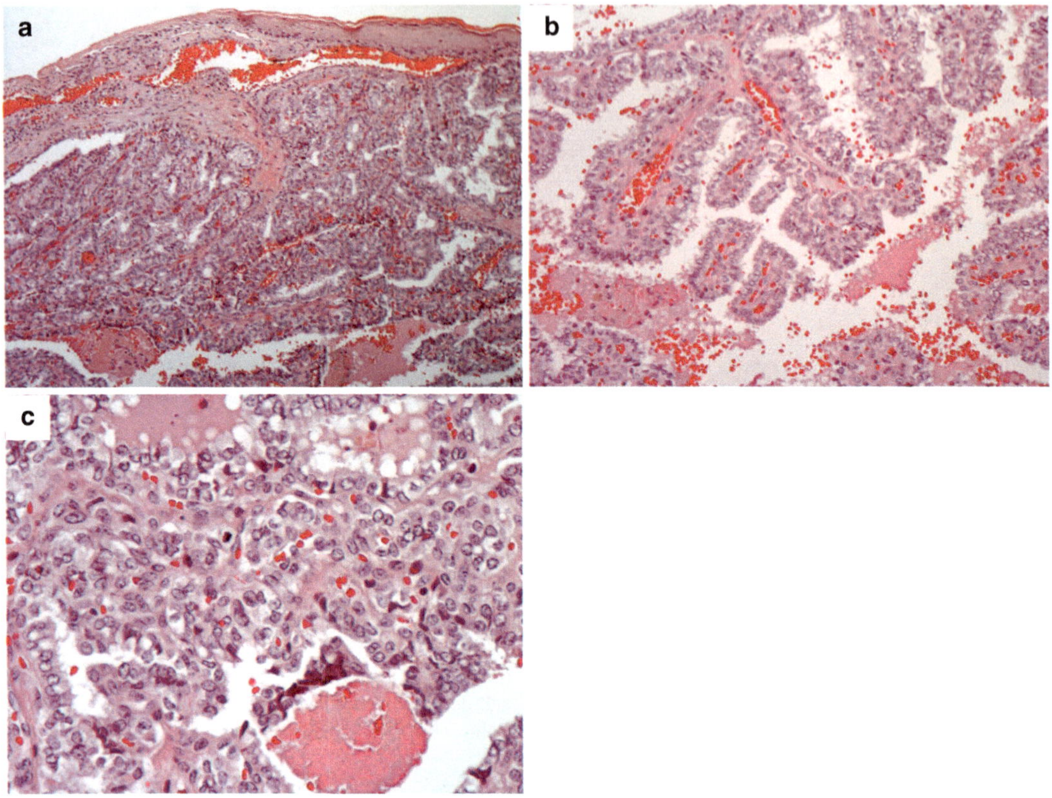

Fig. 28.13 Cutaneous metastasis from papillary thyroid carcinoma (PTC). (**a**) The carcinoma invades the dermis. (**b**) The neoplastic papillae are lined by one or several layers of tumor cells with crowded oval nuclei. (**c**) High magnification shows the hallmark nuclear features of classic PTC. **a**–**c**: Hematoxylin and eosin stain

28.6.9 Cutaneous Metastases from Urothelial Carcinoma

28.6.9.1 Histopathological Findings

Cutaneous metastases from urothelial carcinoma can grow as nests, cords, or sheets of atypical epithelial cells and frequently show lymphovascular invasion (Fig. 28.14) [1, 2]. The histological appearance is similar to that of the primary tumor and may include plasmacytoid, micropapillary, sarcomatoid, squamous, or glandular differentiation, mimicking primary cutaneous or other metastatic carcinomas [1, 11].

28.6.9.2 Immunohistochemical Profile

Pathologists use an immunohistochemical panel that includes GATA3, uroplakin II, uroplakin III, and p40 or p63 [3–5]. GATA3 is sensitive for UC but lacks specificity, as it can be expressed in breast carcinoma and some cutaneous adnexal tumors [4]. Uroplakins II and III are specific proteins in the urothelium and specific markers for urothelial differentiation, though less sensitive. p40 or p63 expression supports basal/urothelial differentiation, especially in poorly differentiated tumors. CK7 is frequently positive, CK20 expression is variable, and broad-spectrum cytokeratins are usually expressed [11].

28.6.9.3 Molecular Pathology

The most common alterations in urothelial carcinoma are mutations in the TERT promoter region. Evaluation of FGFR3 alterations is essential in advanced disease, as it can identify patients eligible for treatment with anti-FGFR agents. Patients with mutations in ERCC2 and other DNA damage repair genes seem to benefit from cisplatin-based chemotherapy. PDL1 expression

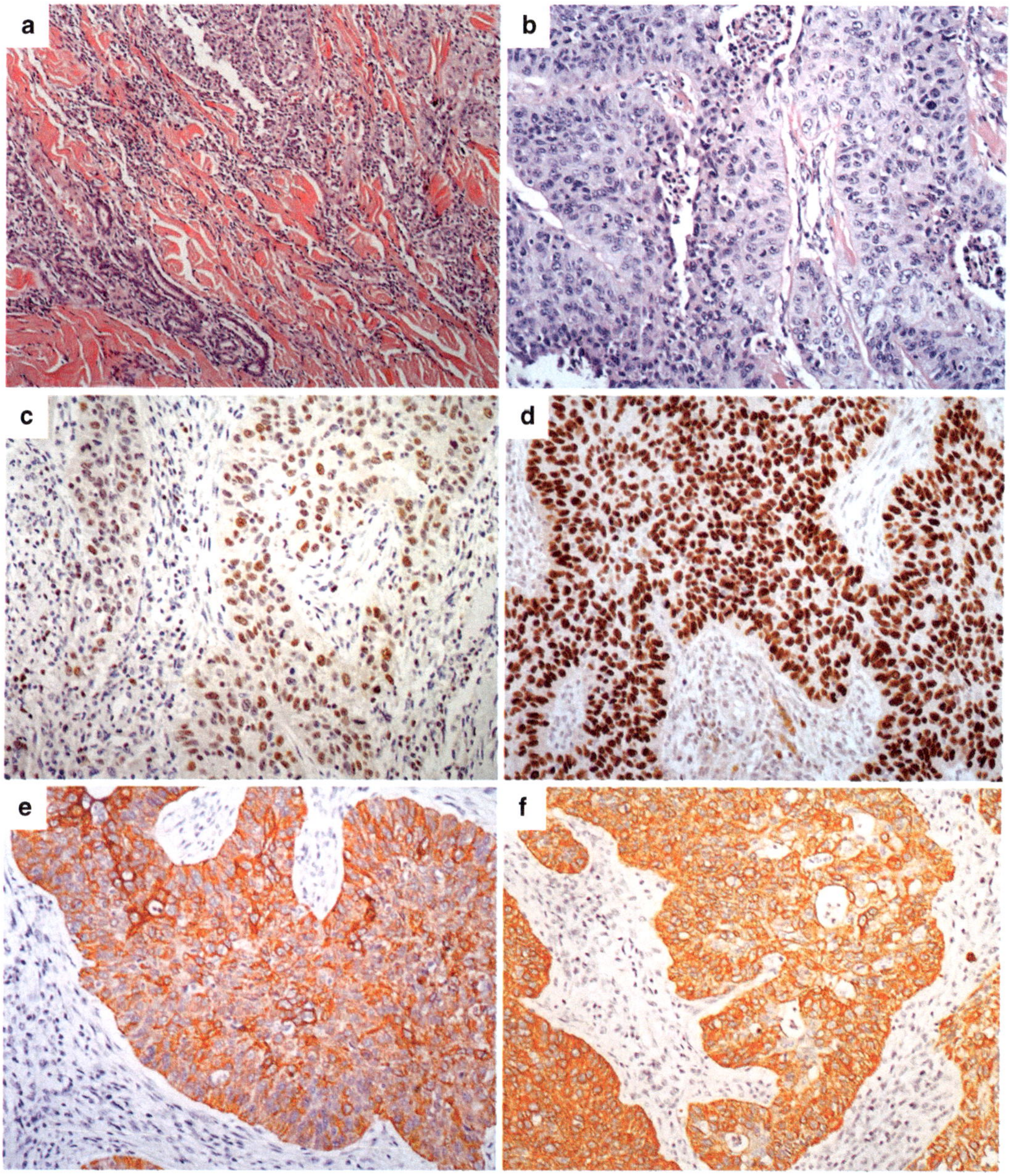

Fig. 28.14 Cutaneous metastasis from high-grade urothelial carcinoma. (**a**) The tumor invades the deep dermis. Note the eccrine glands in the lower left part of the figure. (**b**) The carcinoma cells show nuclear atypia and high mitotic activity. (**c**) GATA3 immunoreactivity was present in tumor cells. (**d**) p63 diffuse nuclear positivity. (**e**) Diffuse labeling of the tumor cells for cytokeratin 7. (**f**) High-molecular-weight cytokeratins were diffusely present in tumor cells. **a**, **b**: Hematoxylin and eosin stain. **c**–**f**: Immunohistochemistry. DAB chromogen

and microsatellite instability/mismatch repair deficiency are used as predictors of response to immunotherapy [11, 32].

28.6.10 Cutaneous Metastases from Uterine Carcinoma

Cutaneous metastases from uterine malignant neoplasms are rare, with a limited number of cases reported in the literature, usually suggesting advanced disease, and they may develop months to years following the initial diagnosis (Fig. 28.15). The lesions often involve the abdominal wall, the vulvar/perineal region, and surgical scars, and may appear as nodules, plaques, or erythematous lesions [33, 34].

28.6.10.1 Histopathological Findings

The morphology of metastases resembles the primary neoplasm. Endometrioid adenocarcinoma is the most common uterine malignancy metastasizing to skin, followed by high-grade lesions, serous carcinoma, clear cell carcinoma, carcinosarcoma, and squamous differentiation (particularly in cervical carcinoma) [29, 33, 34]. Tumor cells typically infiltrate the dermis and subcutis in irregular nests, cords, or sheets, frequently with lymphovascular invasion (Fig. 28.16). Tumor necrosis usually occurs in aggressive variants [29, 34].

28.6.10.2 Immunohistochemical Profile

Endometrial adenocarcinoma metastases show positivity for CK7, estrogen receptor (ER), progesterone receptor (PR), PAX8, and vimentin, while demonstrating CK20 negativity [5]. Metastases from serous carcinoma may express p53 and WT1 (Fig. 28.16). Expression of p63 and CK5/6 is observed, while cervical adenocarcinomas are typically positive for p16, reflecting HPV association [29].

28.6.10.3 Molecular Pathology

Common alterations in endometrial carcinoma include PTEN, PIK3CA, KRAS, ARID1A, and TP53 mutations. TP53 mutation and copy-number alterations are the characteristic findings

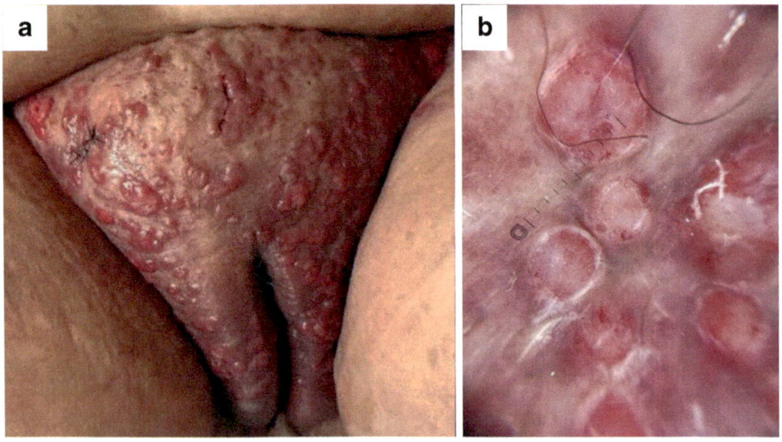

Fig. 28.15 Clinical and dermoscopic features of labial cutaneous metastases in a patient with a history of vaginal carcinoma. (**a**) Clinical presentation of several erythematous to violaceous, firm, and tender infiltrated nodules and plaques affecting the labia majora. These lesions appeared approximately one month ago in a 68-year-old female patient who had been treated with radiotherapy and chemotherapy for vaginal carcinoma and had a remote history of large intestinal carcinoma. (**b**) Dermoscopic examination in polarized light shows multiple pink to violaceous-colored nodules displaying a polymorphous vascular pattern consisting of serpentine and arborizing vessels arranged on a milky-red background, together with areas of ulceration and shiny white structures corresponding to dense tumor infiltration of the dermis. The overall findings are features of cutaneous metastases from vaginal carcinoma

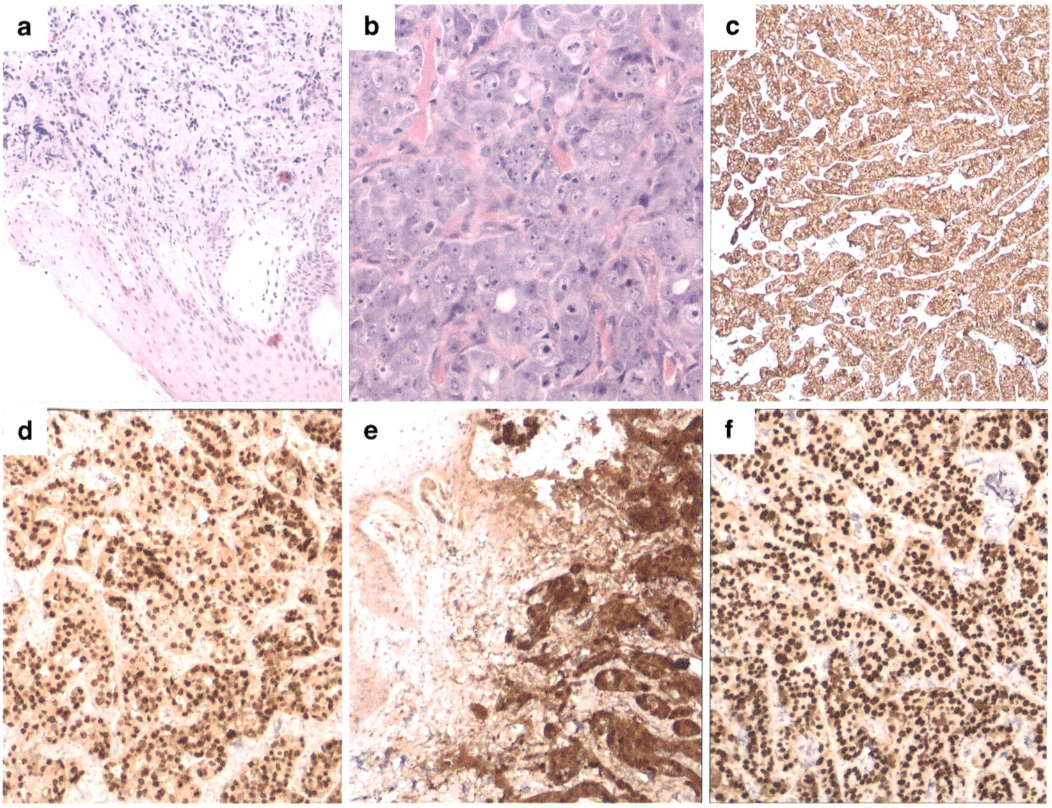

Fig. 28.16 (**a**) Skin invasion from serous carcinoma of the endometrium. (**b**) Markedly atypical tumor cells form glands with irregular luminal contours. Endometrial serous carcinoma demonstrating nuclear pleomorphism, prominent nucleoli, and increased mitotic activity. (**c**) Tumor cells showing positive cytoplasmic expression of CK7. (**d**) P16 nuclear and cytoplasmic expression. (**e**) Nuclear expression of PAX8. (**f**) Overexpression (intense and diffuse) nuclear expression of p53 is indicative of an underlying TP53 mutation. **a**, **b**: Hematoxylin and eosin stain. **c**–**f**: Immunohistochemistry. DAB chromogen

in serous carcinoma. Cervical carcinoma metastases frequently demonstrate nuclear signals in HR-HPV in situ hybridization [29].

We present the case of a 68-year-old woman admitted to the Dermatology Department with a four-week history of swelling and a diffuse eruption of painful, dome-shaped, umbilicated, erythematous papules and nodules over the mons pubis and labia (Fig. 28.15, panel A). She had a history of uterine cancer diagnosed 2 years earlier. Initial treatment included paclitaxel 160 mg/m^2 and carboplatin 520 mg, with the carboplatin dose calculated using an area under the curve (AUC) of 5 every 3 weeks, followed by dostarlimab 1000 mg administered intravenously every 6 weeks. She was receiving filgrastim at a daily dose of 0.5 MIU (5 μg/kg/day) via subcutaneous injection. Dermoscopy revealed translucent papules with central umbilication, whitish streaks, and occasional linear vessels on a shiny surface (Fig. 28.15, panel B). A skin biopsy confirmed cutaneous metastasis (Fig. 28.16). Dermoscopy may assist in clinical evaluation, while histopathologic confirmation remains essential for distinguishing metastatic lesions from infectious or other inflammatory dermatoses.

28.6.11 The Many Faces of Malignant Melanoma

28.6.11.1 Histopathological Findings

The broad morphologic spectrum of melanomas is associated with biologic heterogeneity and the subtype of the associated primary tumor. Although epidermotropic metastatic melanoma can resemble recurrent primary melanoma, lesions typically affect the dermis and subcutis, often sparing the epidermis. The growth patterns observed include infiltrative sheets that penetrate between collagen bundles to well-circumscribed nodular aggregates. Tumor cell morphology ranges from spindle-shaped, resembling sarcoma, to epithelioid, with abundant eosinophilic cytoplasm and noticeable nucleoli. In many cases, there is mixed morphology. Other histologic findings that are frequently observed include atypical mitoses, coarse chromatin, and nuclear pleomorphism. Brisk mitotic figures indicate high proliferative activity (Fig. 28.17) [35, 36].

Although melanin pigment may be noticeable, metastases may also be amelanotic, complicating recognition. The presence of numerous melanophages in the stroma and intracytoplasmic dusty brown melanin granules helps confirm the diagnosis. Extensive necrosis is a common finding, usually in rapid growth lesions. Particularly in metastases from desmoplastic melanomas, a desmoplastic stroma may be present; these lesions can entrap nerves (neurotropism), making diagnosis difficult because they may resemble neural neoplasms or scar tissue. Vascular and lymphatic invasion is common. Tumor nodules within two centimeters of the primary site are referred to as satellitosis [35, 36].

28.6.11.2 Immunohistochemical Profile

Immunohistochemical analysis is obligatory to confirm melanocytic lineage, particularly in amelanotic or poorly differentiated metastases. The markers used in daily routine are S100, SOX10, HMB-45, and Melan-A. S100 shows high sensitivity, while SOX-10, HMB-45, and Melan-A are more specific and less sensitive. In desmoplastic melanoma, loss of HMB-45 and Melan-A is not uncommon, so S100 and SOX10 are preferred. In some situations, PRAME expression may favor melanoma over benign nevus. For differentiating metastatic melanoma from metastatic carcinoma, cytokeratin is helpful. A broad immunopanel comprising cytokeratins, melanocytic markers, and lineage-specific markers is advised when necessary [5, 35–37].

28.6.11.3 Molecular Pathology

The most frequent alterations occur in BRAF, NRAS, KIT, and GNAQ/GNA11, with distributions influenced by melanoma subtype, anatomic site, and UV exposure. Their identification is essential in metastatic disease, guiding treatment selection and potential enrollment in targeted therapy trials [5, 38].

BRAF Mutations

BRAF mutations occur in ~50% of melanomas, particularly those arising in intermittently sun-exposed skin. They show characteristic UV mutational signatures and tend to present in younger patients. The most common variant, V600E, constitutively activates the MAPK/ERK pathway, promoting proliferation and survival.

Targeted therapy with selective BRAF inhibitors (vemurafenib and dabrafenib) and combined BRAF/MEK inhibition significantly improves outcomes in metastatic or unresectable melanoma. Current clinical guidelines recommend BRAF mutation testing in patients with distant metastasis, unresectable regional metastasis, or high-risk stage III disease. Testing metastatic tissue is preferred due to high concordance with primary lesions [35, 38].

NRAS Mutations

NRAS mutations occur in 15–20% of melanomas and activate the MAPK pathway through mechanisms distinct from BRAF. These mutations are typically mutually exclusive with BRAF alterations and define a clinically meaningful subgroup. Although no approved targeted inhibitors currently exist, novel MEK-based and immunotherapy-combined strategies remain under investigation. NRAS status is clinically useful in guiding therapy selection in BRAF-wild-type melanoma [35, 38].

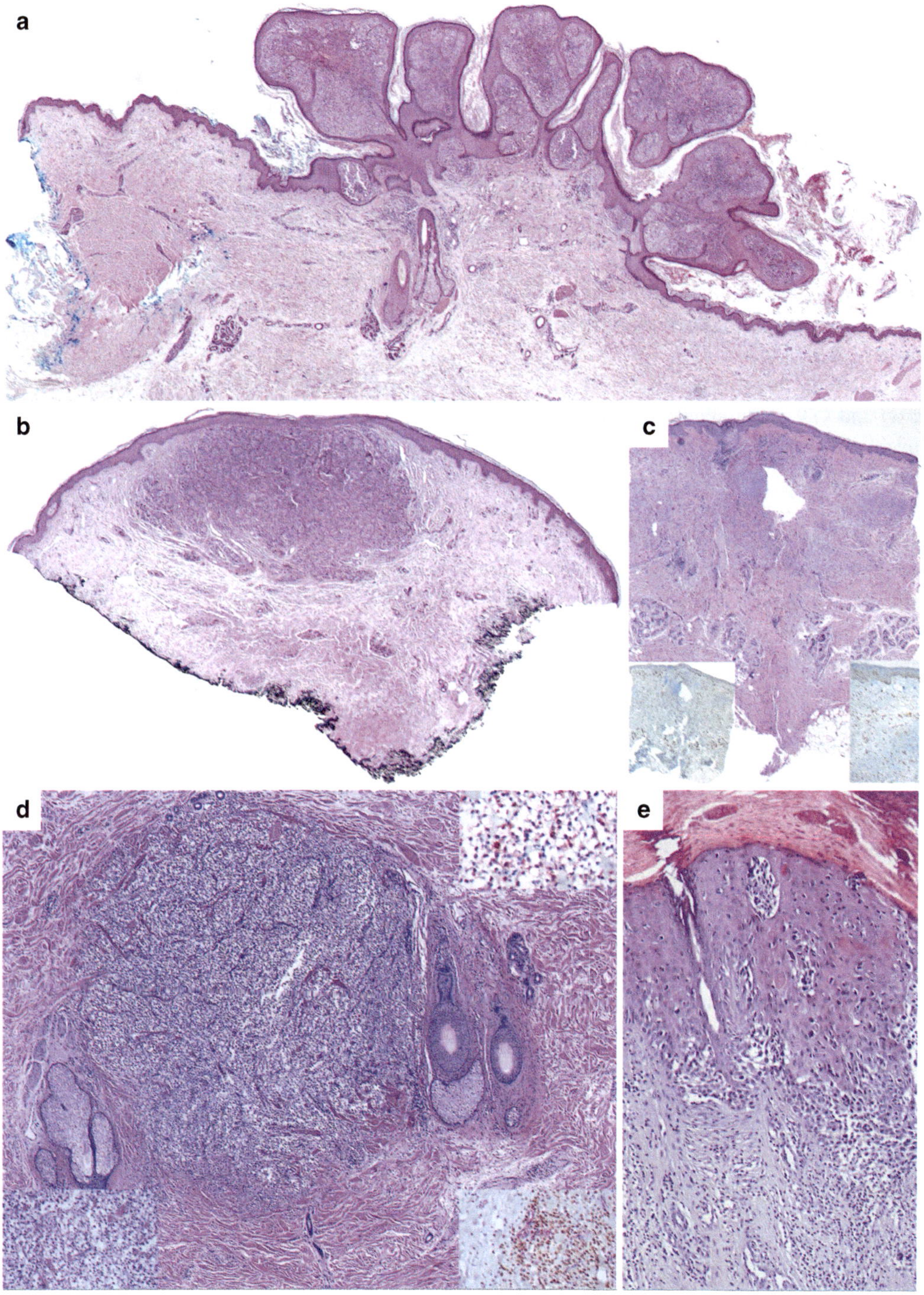

Fig. 28.17 The many faces of malignant melanoma (MM) cutaneous metastases. (**a**) Melanoma metastasis resembling verruciform nevus or primary nevoid MM. (**b**) MM metastasis simulating a dermal nevus. (**c**) Spindle cell metastatic melanoma resembling mesenchymal proliferations. Left bottom inset: IHC for SOX10; left right inset: IHC for PRAME. (**d**) Nodular deep dermal metastasis with clear cells mimicking clear cell carcinoma. Left bottom inset: high magnification of melanoma cells; Upper right inset: double IHC for Melan A (red chromogen, cytoplasmic stain) and the mitotic marker pHH3 (DAB-brown chromogen, nuclear stain); Lower right inset: double IHC for endothelial marker CD31 (red chromogen, cytoplasmic stain) and SOX10 (DAB-brown chromogen, nuclear stain). (**e**) Metastatic acral melanoma with epidermotropism. **a**–**e**: Hematoxylin and eosin stain. IHC: Immunohistochemistry

c-KIT Mutations

KIT mutations and amplifications are less frequent overall but enriched in acral, mucosal, and chronically sun-damaged melanomas, representing a biologically distinct subset. A stepwise diagnostic approach is recommended: test for BRAF/NRAS mutations first, followed by KIT analysis in negative cases. KIT-directed inhibitors demonstrate benefit in selected patients and continue to be explored, underscoring their relevance in personalized therapy [35, 38].

GNAQ/GNA11 Mutations

GNAQ and GNA11 mutations are characteristic of uveal melanoma, defining a separate molecular entity. In rare non-uveal melanomas, they exhibit lower UV mutational burden and tend to metastasize via lymphatics rather than hematogenous spread, unlike uveal primaries. Response to immune checkpoint inhibitors is generally limited, emphasizing the need for alternative therapeutic approaches [34, 35].

28.7 Differential Diagnosis

Metastatic melanoma may mimic a variety of malignancies, including metastatic poorly differentiated carcinoma (especially amelanotic melanoma), metastatic sarcoma or MPNST (spindle cell morphology), metastatic clear cell tumors (renal cell carcinoma), and hematolymphoid malignancies (large cell lymphoma). In challenging cases, clinical history in combination with imaging, morphology, and immunohistochemical and molecular analysis is required [5, 35].

References

1. Gschnell M, Volberg C, Hauser C, Krönig L. Cutaneous metastases: from epidemiology to therapy. JDDG Journal der Deutschen Dermatologischen Gesellschaft. 2024;22(7):974–93.
2. Souza B, Miyashiro D, Pincelli MS, Sanches JA. Cutaneous metastases from solid neoplasms—literature review. An Bras Dermatol. 2023;98(5):571–9.
3. Kwon HM, Kim GY, Shin DH, Bae YK. Clinicopathologic features of cutaneous metastases from internal malignancies. J Pathol Transl Med. 2021;55(4):289–97.
4. Starace M, Cedirian S, Rapparini L. Clinical aspects of cutaneous metastasis from non-cutaneous primary tumors. Cancer. 2025;17(19):3126.
5. Prieto V.G., Requena L., Zalaudek I., Ko J.S. Metastases to skin. In: WHO Classification of Tumours Editorial Board. Skin tumours [Internet; beta version ahead Of print]. Lyon (France): International Agency for Research on Cancer; 2023 [cited December 14]. (WHO classification of tumours series, 5th ed.; vol. 12). Available from: https://tumourclassification.iarc.who.int/chapters/64.
6. Tinca AC, Lazar BA, Cozac-Szőke AR, Radu GN, Simion SP, Chiorean DM, et al. Cutaneous metastases—histological particularities of multifaceted entities. Dermatopathology. 2025;12(2):14.
7. Hoon Tan P, Ellis I, Allison K, Brogi E, Fox SB, Lakhani S, et al. The 2019 WHO classification of tumours of the breast. Histopathology. 2020;77(2).
8. Nicholson AG, Tsao MS, Beasley MB, Borczuk AC, Brambilla E, Cooper WA, et al. The 2021 WHO classification of lung tumors: impact of advances since 2015. J Thoracic Oncol [Internet]. 2021 Nov 19;17(3):S1556-0864(21)033165.
9. Chu P, Wu E, Weiss LM. Cytokeratin 7 and cytokeratin 20 expression in epithelial neoplasms: a survey of 435 cases. Modern Pathol [Internet]. 2000;13(9):962–72.
10. Krämer A, Pauli C, Prall OWJ. Cancer of unknown primary site. In: WHO Classification of Tumours Editorial Board. Skin tumours [Internet; beta version ahead of print]. Lyon (France): International Agency for Research on Cancer; 2023 [cited 2025 December 14]. (WHO classification of tumours series, 5th ed.; vol. 12). Available from: https://tumourclassification.iarc.who.int/chapters/64.
11. Netto GJ, Amin MB, Berney DM, Compérat EM, Gill AJ, Hartmann A, et al. The 2022 World Health Organization classification of tumors of the urinary system and male genital organs—part B: prostate and urinary tract tumors. Eur Urol. 2022;82(5):469.
12. Nagtegaal ID, Odze RD, Klimstra D, Paradis V, Rugge M, Schirmacher P, et al. The 2019 WHO classification of tumours of the digestive system. Histopathology. 2019;76(2):182–8.
13. Gurel B, Ali TZ, Montgomery EA, Begum S, Hicks J, Goggins M, et al. NKX3.1 as a marker of prostatic origin in metastatic tumors. Am J Surg Pathol. 2010;34(8):1097–105.
14. Krämer A, Bochtler T, Pauli C, Baciarello G, Delorme S, Hemminki K, et al. Cancer of unknown primary: ESMO Clinical Practice Guideline for diagnosis, treatment and follow-up. Ann Oncol. 2023;34(3):228–46.
15. Lindeman NI, Cagle PT, Beasley MB, Chitale DA, Dacic S, Giaccone G, et al. Molecular testing guideline for selection of lung cancer patients for EGFR and ALK tyrosine kinase inhibitors: guideline from the College of American Pathologists, International Association for the Study of Lung Cancer, and

Association for Molecular Pathology. J Thorac Oncol. 2013;8(7):823–59.
16. Kotoula V, Bobos M, Vassilakopoulou M, Tsolaki E, Chrisafi S, Psyrri A, et al. Intact or broken-apart RNA. Appl Immunohistochem Mol Morphol. 2014;23(1):60–70.
17. Gravalos C, Jimeno A. HER2 in gastric cancer: a new prognostic factor and a novel therapeutic target. Ann Oncol. 2008;19(9):1523–9.
18. Cimino-Mathews A, Subhawong AP, Illei PB, Sharma R, Halushka MK, Vang R, et al. GATA3 expression in breast carcinoma: utility in triple-negative, sarcomatoid, and metastatic carcinomas. Hum Pathol. 2013;44(7):1341–9.
19. Tozbikian GH, Zynger DL. A combination of GATA3 and SOX10 is useful for the diagnosis of metastatic triple-negative breast cancer. Hum Pathol. 2019;85(85):221–7.
20. Rakha EA, El-Sayed ME, Powe DG, Green AR, Habashy H, Grainge MJ, et al. Invasive lobular carcinoma of the breast: response to hormonal therapy and outcomes. Eur J Cancer. 2008;44(1):73–83.
21. Mosele F, Stefanovska B, Lusque A, Dien AT, Garberis I, Droin N, et al. Outcome and molecular landscape of patients with PIK3CA-mutated metastatic breast cancer. Ann Oncol. 2020;31(3):377–86.
22. Lookingbill DP, Spangler N, Helm KF. Cutaneous metastases in patients with metastatic carcinoma: a retrospective study of 4020 patients. J Am Acad Dermatol. 1993;29(2 Pt 1):228–36.
23. Sharma G, Kumar P, Veerwal H, Singh P, Gupta S, Dhingra V. Cutaneous metastases as initial presentation of lung carcinoma. Cureus. 2021;13(5).
24. Bobos M, Hytiroglou P, Kostopoulos I, Karkavelas G, Papadimitriou CS. Immunohistochemical distinction between Merkel cell carcinoma and small cell carcinoma of the lung. Am J Dermatopathol. 2006;28(2):99–104.
25. Bergethon K, Shaw AT, Ignatius Ou SH, Katayama R, Lovly CM, McDonald NT, et al. ROS1 rearrangements define a unique molecular class of lung cancers. J Clin Oncol. 2012;30(8):863–70.
26. Yao GL, Tao YJ, Fan YG. Cutaneous metastasis from gastric cancer: manifestation, diagnosis, treatment and prognosis. Eur J Surg Oncol. 2024;50(2):107939.
27. Laurén P. The two histological main types of gastric carcinoma: diffuse and so-called intestinal-type carcinoma. Acta Pathologica Microbiologica Scandinavica. 1965;64(1):31–49.
28. Werling RW, Yaziji H, Bacchi CE, Gown AM. CDX2, a highly sensitive and specific marker of adenocarcinomas of intestinal origin. Am J Surg Pathol. 2003;27(3):303–10.
29. Höhn AK, Brambs CE, Hiller GGR, May D, Schmoeckel E, Horn LC. 2020 WHO classification of female genital tumors. Geburtshilfe Frauenheilkd. 2021;81(10):1145–53.
30. Reusser NM, Holcomb M, Rosen T, Orengo IF. Cutaneous metastasis of papillary thyroid carcinoma to the neck: a case report and review of the literature. Dermatol Online J. 2015;21(2).
31. Basolo F, Macerola E, Poma AM, Torregrossa L. The 5th edition of WHO classification of tumors of endocrine organs: changes in the diagnosis of follicular-derived thyroid carcinoma. Endocrine 2023;80(3).
32. Ross JS, Wang K, Al-Rohil RN, Nazeer T, Sheehan CE, Otto G, et al. Advanced urothelial carcinoma: next-generation sequencing reveals diverse genomic alterations and targets of therapy. Mod Pathol. 2014;27(2):271–80.
33. Massi G, LeBoit PE. Histological diagnosis of nevi and melanoma. Springer; 2014.
34. Hu S, Chen G, Lu Y, Wu C, Lan C. Cutaneous metastases from different internal malignancies: a clinical and prognostic appraisal. J Eur Acad Dermatol Venereol. 2008;22(6):735–40.
35. Shain AH, Bastian BC. Author correction: from melanocytes to melanomas. Nat Rev Cancer. 2020;20(6):355.
36. BOBOS M. Histopathologic classification and prognostic factors of melanoma: a 2021 update. Italian J Dermatol Venereol 2021;156(3).
37. Long GV, Menzies AM, Nagrial AM, Haydu LE, Hamilton AL, Mann GJ, et al. Prognostic and Clinicopathologic associations of oncogenic BRAF in metastatic melanoma. J Clin Oncol. 2011;29(10):1239–46.
38. Kim HJ, Kim YH. Molecular frontiers in melanoma: pathogenesis, diagnosis, and therapeutic advances. Int J Mol Sci. 2024;25(5):2984.

Part XVI

Imaging Techniques in Cutaneous Metastasis

Imaging Techniques in Cutaneous Metastasis

29

Nikolaos Galanakis

Abstract

Cutaneous metastases, defined as the spread of internal malignancies to the skin, are rare but a clinically significant manifestation of systemic cancer. Their presence often correlates with poor prognosis and advanced disease stage. While histopathological confirmation remains the definitive diagnostic modality, imaging techniques have emerged as critical adjuncts for early detection, characterization, and follow-up of cutaneous metastases. This chapter provides a comprehensive overview of the role of ultrasound, computed tomography, magnetic resonance imaging, single-photon emission computed tomography, and positron emission tomography in the evaluation of cutaneous metastases, focusing on their utility, diagnostic features, and integration into oncologic workflows.

Keywords

Ultrasound · Computed tomography · Magnetic resonance imaging · Positron emission tomography · Single-photon emission computed tomography

N. Galanakis (✉)
Medical School, University of Crete, Heraklion, Greece

29.1 Introduction

Cutaneous metastases, while relatively rare compared to other forms of metastases, can significantly impact the prognosis and management of cancer patients. Cutaneous metastases occur in approximately 0.7% to 10% of all patients with malignancies, depending on the type of cancer and its stage. These metastases tend to present later in the disease and are often indicative of advanced, disseminated cancer. Breast cancer is the most common malignancy associated with cutaneous metastasis. Breast cancer-related cutaneous metastases are most often seen in patients with poorly differentiated, metastatic disease. Lung cancer is the second most frequent source of cutaneous metastasis, especially small cell lung cancer (SCLC). Cutaneous involvement in patients with lung cancer often correlates with a poor prognosis. Other common sources include colorectal cancer and melanoma. Cutaneous metastases are more common in older adults, typically over 50 years of age, which correlates with the increasing incidence of cancer in this population. However, in some types of cancer, like melanoma, younger individuals may also be affected. Cutaneous metastasis typically occurs late in the disease process, often after metastases to internal organs, lymph nodes, and bones. However, in some cases, cutaneous involvement can be the first sign of metastatic spread. In these cases, early identification and treatment may improve patient

D. Koumaki et al. (eds.), *Cutaneous Metastases*, https://doi.org/10.1007/978-3-032-26764-1_29

outcomes by detecting systemic spread before it becomes clinically apparent. These metastases may present as nodules, plaques, or inflammatory lesions and are often mistaken for benign dermatologic conditions. While histopathological confirmation remains the definitive diagnostic modality, imaging techniques have emerged as critical adjuncts for early detection, characterization, and follow-up of cutaneous metastases. Imaging is indispensable not only in supporting clinical suspicion but also in determining the extent of disease and guiding subsequent diagnostic or therapeutic interventions. This chapter provides a comprehensive overview of the role of ultrasound, computed tomography (CT), magnetic resonance imaging (MRI), single-photon emission computed tomography (SPECT), and positron emission tomography (PET) in the evaluation of cutaneous metastases, focusing on their utility, diagnostic features, clinical applications, advantages, and limitations in a comparative and integrative context [1–12].

29.2 Ultrasound

Ultrasound is an accessible, non-invasive imaging modality well-suited for evaluating superficial structures, including the skin and subcutaneous tissues. High-frequency linear transducers (10–20 MHz) provide excellent resolution for the assessment of dermal and subdermal abnormalities [13].

29.2.1 Imaging Features

Cutaneous metastases typically appear as hypoechoic, well-circumscribed or irregular nodules within the dermis or subcutaneous fat. Their margins are generally poorly defined; however, there are also lesions with well-defined margins. They may exhibit heterogeneous internal echotexture and posterior acoustic enhancement. Color Doppler imaging often reveals increased vascularity with multiple peripheral poles or internal vessels, which can aid in differentiating malignant from benign lesions (Fig. 29.1). Avascular and hypovascular patterns in cutaneous metastases are rare and may be associated with small lesion size, necrosis, or small vessels that are difficult to detect with available equipment. Elastography is another advanced ultrasound-based technique that provides qualitative and quantitative information about tissue stiffness by measuring its response to mechanical stress. Two primary types of elastography are employed in clinical practice: strain elastography and shear wave elastography. Both modalities assess the biomechanical properties of tissues, which can differentiate benign from malignant lesions based on their relative elasticity. Malignant lesions, including metastatic lesions, tend to be stiffer than surrounding normal dermis or benign lesions due to increased cellular density, stromal fibrosis, and desmoplastic response [13–22].

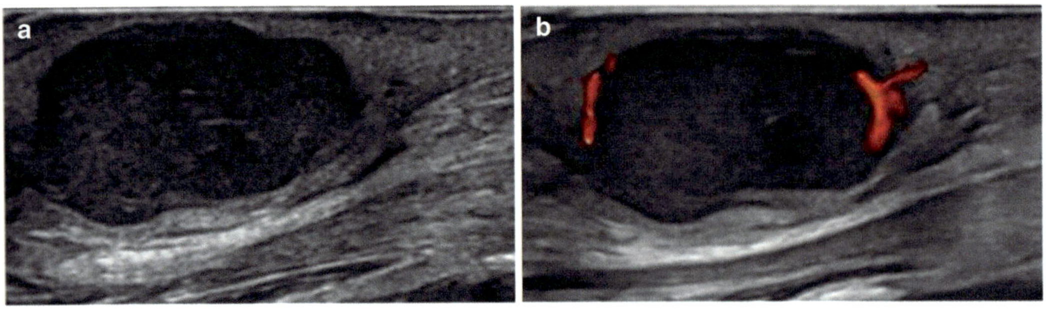

Fig. 29.1 A female patient with known metastatic lung adenocarcinoma. (**a**) Gray-scale ultrasound demonstrates a well-circumscribed, hypoechoic, heterogeneous lesion within the subcutaneous tissue of the anterior thoracic wall, consistent with cutaneous metastasis. (**b**) Color Doppler imaging reveals increased vascularity with multiple peripheral vascular poles

29.2.2 Advantages and Disadvantages

Ultrasound is valuable for the initial evaluation of suspicious superficial lesions. It allows detailed visualization of the epidermis, dermis, and subcutaneous fat, enabling precise localization and morphological characterization of superficial metastatic nodules. The addition of Doppler imaging provides valuable information on intralesional vascularity, which can aid in differential diagnosis. Furthermore, the modality permits real-time assessment and dynamic evaluation, making it particularly advantageous for guiding interventional procedures such as fine-needle aspiration and core biopsy. As a non-invasive, radiation-free, and relatively low-cost technique, ultrasound is ideally suited as the first-line diagnostic tool for evaluation of suspicious palpable cutaneous lesions, particularly in vulnerable populations such as pediatric and pregnant patients.

Nevertheless, ultrasound is not without limitations. Its utility is significantly reduced in the evaluation of deep-seated lesions, particularly in obese patients or when metastases extend beyond the subcutaneous fat. Artifacts from overlying structures and difficulty in distinguishing inflammation from malignancy can pose diagnostic challenges. Additionally, the technique is highly operator dependent, and diagnostic accuracy is contingent upon the skill and experience of the examiner. Moreover, contrast resolution is lower in comparison with CT and MRI, making it difficult to reliably differentiate various soft-tissue pathologies in complex clinical scenarios [13–23].

29.3 Computed Tomography (CT)

Computed tomography imaging remains a cornerstone in oncology and is widely used for staging and surveillance. The modality provides high spatial resolution, rapid image acquisition, and broad anatomical coverage, making it invaluable for systemic assessment. Although not specifically designed for cutaneous evaluation, CT can effectively identify metastatic lesions involving the skin and subcutaneous tissues, especially in the context of known malignancy [24].

29.3.1 Imaging Features

On CT, cutaneous metastases typically appear as iso- to hyperdense soft-tissue nodules compared to the surrounding subcutaneous fat. They often demonstrate irregular or ill-defined margins, reflecting the infiltrative nature of malignant spread. After intravenous administration of iodinated contrast agents, cutaneous metastases usually show heterogeneous or peripheral enhancement, although enhancement patterns may vary depending on the lesion's size, vascularity, and degree of necrosis. Calcifications, ulceration, or overlying skin thickening may also be present. CT is especially useful in evaluating the involvement of adjacent anatomical structures, including the underlying fascia, skeletal system, lymph nodes, and visceral organs [9, 11] (Fig. 29.2 and 29.3).

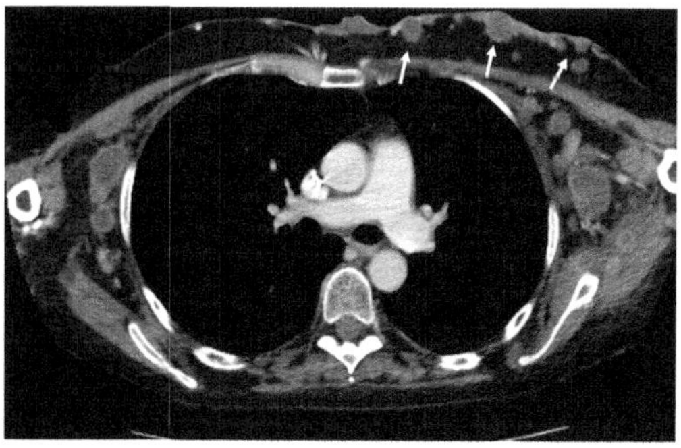

Fig. 29.2 A female patient with a history of breast cancer. Contrast-enhanced computed tomography reveals multiple isodense soft-tissue nodules (arrows) located within the dermis and subcutaneous fat of the anterior thoracic wall, consistent with cutaneous metastases. Associated findings include overlying skin thickening and stranding of the subcutaneous fat, indicative of inflammatory or neoplastic infiltration

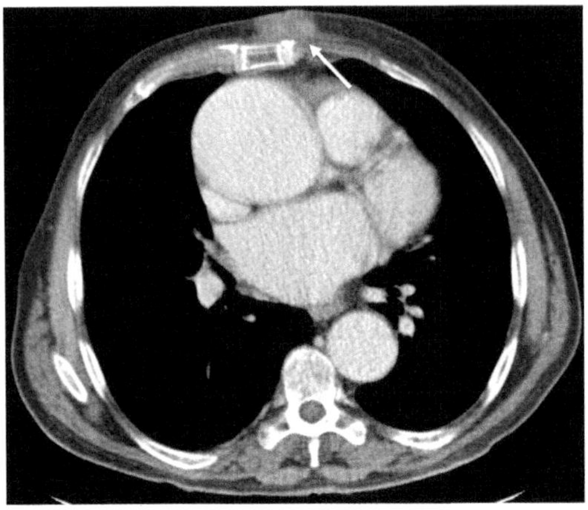

Fig. 29.3 A male patient with prostate cancer. Contrast-enhanced computed tomography reveals a solitary, lobulated, hyperdense soft-tissue lesion within the subcutaneous fat anterior to the sternum (arrow). The lesion demonstrates contrast enhancement, suggestive of cutaneous metastasis

29.3.2 Advantages and Disadvantages

CT offers several advantages, including fast image acquisition, reproducibility, and compatibility with staging protocols. CT provides a broad anatomical field of view, allowing simultaneous assessment of primary tumors and regional and distant metastases. This is particularly useful in patients with suspected widespread disease or atypical metastatic spread. The modality's ability to detect clinically occult lesions is important for early intervention and treatment planning. Furthermore, CT enables precise anatomical localization and three-dimensional reconstructions, which are valuable for surgical mapping, radiation therapy planning, and interventional procedures.

However, the use of ionizing radiation remains a significant limitation, especially in younger patients or those requiring serial imaging for disease surveillance. The cumulative radiation dose may raise concerns in these populations. Additionally, CT provides relatively limited soft-tissue contrast resolution when compared to MRI, which may reduce sensitivity for characterizing lesion composition or detecting subtle tissue invasion. The modality may also be less effective in identifying small, early-stage, intradermal lesions, particularly in areas with complex anatomy such as the face, scalp, or digits. Finally, although CT can detect the presence and extent of a lesion, it cannot reliably differentiate between benign and malignant skin nodules based solely on imaging features, necessitating histological confirmation in ambiguous cases [9, 25, 26].

29.4 Magnetic Resonance Imaging (MRI)

MRI offers superior contrast resolution and multiplanar capabilities, making it well-suited for the assessment of soft-tissue lesions, including those affecting the skin and subcutaneous compartments, especially in anatomically complex regions such as the face, perineum, or extremities [27].

29.4.1 Imaging Features

Cutaneous metastases typically demonstrate intermediate to low signal intensity on T1-weighted sequences and high signal intensity on T2-weighted and Short Tau Inversion Recovery (STIR) sequences due to their high water content and increased cellularity. On fat-suppressed sequences, metastases often become more conspicuous against the suppressed background signal of subcutaneous fat. Advanced MRI techniques such as diffusion-weighted imaging (DWI) and apparent diffusion coefficient (ADC) mapping may provide additional functional information, as malignant lesions often demonstrate restricted diffusion. Following the administration of gadolinium-based contrast agents, cutaneous metastases usually exhibit moderate to intense enhancement, which may be homogeneous or heterogeneous depending on the degree of necrosis, fibrosis, or vascularity within the lesion. The contrast enhancement helps to delineate the lesion from adjacent normal tissue and is particularly useful to depict ill-defined tumor margins, perilesional edema, and infiltration into surrounding structures [27–30].

29.4.2 Advantages and Disadvantages

MRI offers several key advantages over other imaging modalities in the evaluation of cutaneous metastases. Its superior soft-tissue contrast resolution enables the detection of small or infiltrative lesions that may be overlooked on CT or ultrasound, particularly in regions with complex anatomy such as the head and neck, pelvis, and extremities. The multiplanar imaging capability allows accurate visualization of lesion extent in coronal, sagittal, and axial planes, which supports comprehensive treatment planning. It is also valuable for assessing extension into muscle, fascia, and neurovascular bundles, as well as for detecting perineural spread, features critical for accurate staging, prognosis, and preoperative planning. MRI is particularly beneficial in pediatric, pregnant, or radiation-sensitive patients, as it does not employ ionizing radiation. Moreover, MRI techniques such as DWI, perfusion imaging, and MR spectroscopy are increasingly used for their potential to differentiate malignant from benign lesions, monitor treatment response, and provide prognostic biomarkers.

Despite its numerous advantages, MRI is not without limitations. The modality is more expensive and less widely available compared to ultrasound or CT, which may restrict access in everyday clinical practice. MRI requires longer acquisition times, making it more susceptible to motion artifacts, especially in uncooperative or claustrophobic patients. Contraindications to MRI include the presence of non-MRI-compatible implants, pacemakers, or ferromagnetic foreign bodies, which must be carefully assessed prior to imaging. Additionally, the use of gadolinium-based contrast agents carries a small risk for nephrogenic systemic fibrosis in patients with severe renal impairment, although the risk has been significantly reduced with modern agents [10, 11, 30–32].

29.5 Single-Photon Emission Computed Tomography (SPECT) and Positron Emission Tomography (PET)

Single-photon emission computed tomography (SPECT) and positron emission tomography (PET), particularly when combined with computed tomography (SPECT/CT and PET/CT), are functional imaging modalities that enable whole-body assessment of metabolic activity and molecular processes associated with malignancy. While not typically used as first-line modalities for evaluating cutaneous lesions, SPECT and PET imaging are increasingly utilized in the staging and surveillance of patients with known malignancies, particularly when cutaneous metastases are present alongside systemic disease [33].

29.5.1 Imaging Features

In PET imaging, 18F-fluorodeoxyglucose (18F-FDG) is the most commonly used radiotracer. Cutaneous metastases typically appear as foci of increased FDG uptake due to their high metabolic activity. Lesions may vary in intensity depending on tumor type, size, and biological behavior. Hypermetabolic cutaneous nodules may be visible in the skin or subcutaneous tissues, sometimes preceding clinical detection. PET is especially helpful in identifying multifocal or disseminated skin involvement in malignancies such as melanoma, breast, or lung cancer. Fusion PET/CT imaging provides both metabolic and anatomical information, allowing for precise localization and characterization of lesions (Fig. 29.4). SPECT imaging, while less com-

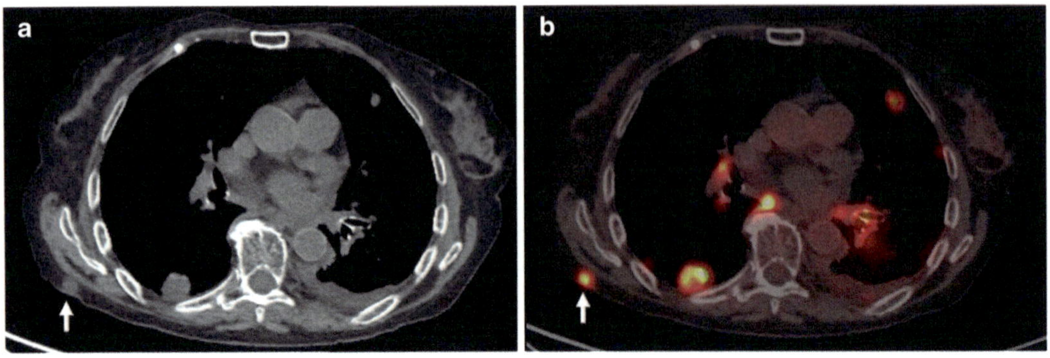

Fig. 29.4 A female patient with known metastatic colorectal cancer. (**a**) Computed tomography demonstrates a soft-tissue lesion in the posterior thoracic wall, consistent with a cutaneous metastasis. (**b**) Corresponding 18F-fluorodeoxyglucose (18F-FDG) PET imaging reveals increased radiotracer uptake within the lesion, indicating high metabolic activity and supporting its malignant nature

monly used for cutaneous assessment, can detect radiotracer uptake associated with certain tumor types using agents such as 99mTc-labeled compounds. In cases where PET is unavailable, SPECT offers valuable information, particularly when using tracers specific to tumor subtypes [33–35].

29.5.2 Advantages and Disadvantages

The main advantage of PET and, to a lesser extent, of SPECT lies in their ability to detect metabolically active lesions throughout the entire body in a single imaging session, making it a powerful tool for cancer staging, treatment monitoring, and recurrence detection. In the cases of cutaneous metastases, PET/CT can identify both clinically apparent and occult lesions and assess their relationship with systemic disease, helping to distinguish between isolated cutaneous spread and widespread metastatic burden, which is critical for prognosis and therapeutic decision-making. In addition to FDG-PET, other PET tracers such as 68Ga-DOTATATE (for neuroendocrine tumors), 18F-NaF (for bone metastases), and 18F-FES (for estrogen receptor-positive breast cancer) can also be used and may further enhance the role of PET imaging in oncology. SPECT and PET are also useful in therapy response evaluation, as metabolic changes on follow-up imaging often precede anatomical changes seen on MRI or CT. A decrease in FDG uptake following treatment is generally associated with therapeutic efficacy, while persistent or increased uptake may suggest residual disease or progression.

Despite its high sensitivity, PET imaging is limited by relatively low spatial resolution, which can hinder the detection of very small or superficial cutaneous metastases, especially in areas with high physiological FDG uptake such as the head and neck region. False-positive findings may occur due to inflammation, infection, or post-surgical changes, and histopathologic correlation remains essential for definitive diagnosis. The use of ionizing radiation, both from the PET radiotracer and the accompanying CT scan, is a consideration in younger or radiation-sensitive patients. Moreover, PET imaging is expensive and not widely available, and its use is generally reserved for patients with known malignancy rather than for primary assessment of isolated cutaneous lesions. SPECT offers lower sensitivity and resolution compared to PET but may still provide useful adjunctive information depending on tracer availability and tumor biology [35–38].

29.6 Conclusion

The integration of imaging into the evaluation of cutaneous metastases requires a multidisciplinary approach. Each imaging modality offers unique advantages that can be utilized based on lesion characteristics, patient profile, and clinical context (Table 29.1). Ultrasound provides a rapid, safe, and cost-effective approach for evaluating superficial lesions, particularly in vulnerable populations. CT is useful for assessing deeper anatomical involvement and integrating skin findings into systemic disease staging. MRI excels in soft-tissue characterization and mapping of lesion extent in anatomically complex areas. Finally, SPECT and PET-CT offer functional information and are particularly useful for detecting clinically occult lesions or widespread metastatic disease.

Future developments in imaging of cutaneous metastases are focused on enhancing diagnostic accuracy, tissue characterization, and personalized management. Radiomics and artificial intelligence (AI) are increasingly integrated into CT, MRI, and ultrasound workflows, enabling automated lesion detection and prediction of tumor behavior through quantitative imaging biomarkers. Hybrid imaging modalities such as PET/MRI combine metabolic and anatomical information with reduced radiation exposure, showing promise in evaluating metastases in complex anatomical regions. In ultrasound, advancements like contrast-enhanced ultrasound (CEUS) and elastography improve lesion differentiation and biopsy guidance. Furthermore, the development of targeted radiotracers (e.g., PSMA, HER2) may allow a more specific detection of metastases from certain primary tumors.

An optimized, patient-centered approach often involves a multimodal imaging strategy, combining the strengths of each technique to achieve accurate diagnosis and guide individualized treatment. Close collaboration between dermatologists, radiologists, and oncologists remains essential for the effective management of patients with cutaneous metastatic disease.

Table 29.1 Comparative Overview of imaging modalities for cutaneous metastases

Modality	Imaging features	Advantages	Limitations
Ultrasound	Hypoechoic nodules Poorly defined margins Increased vascularity on Doppler Increased stiffness on elastography	Non-invasive Radiation-free High-resolution for superficial structures Real-time guidance for biopsy	Operator dependent Limited penetration in obese patients or deep lesions Lower tissue contrast
Computed tomography)	Iso- to hyperdense nodules Variable contrast enhancement Skin thickening Calcifications	Fast acquisition High spatial resolution Integrates with whole-body staging protocols	Radiation exposure Lower tissue contrast than MRI Less effective in small/superficial lesions
Magnetic resonance imaging	Intermediate/low T1signal High T2 signal Variable gadolinium enhancement	Superior tissue contrast Multiplanar imaging No radiation Detects deep, fascial, or perineural spread	Expensive Longer scan duration Contraindicated in selected patients Susceptible to motion artifacts
Single-photon emission computed tomography /Positron emission tomography	Focal uptake in metabolically active lesions	Whole-body functional imaging High sensitivity for occult/systemic disease Detects early metastases	Radiation exposure Lower spatial resolution High cost Limited availability

References

1. Akcali C, Zincirkeser S, Erbagcý Z, et al. Detection of metastases in patients with cutaneous melanoma using FDG-PET/CT. J Int Med Res. 2007;35(4):547–53.
2. Alcaraz I, Cerroni L, Rütten A, Kutzner H, Requena L. Cutaneous metastases from internal malignancies: a clinicopathologic and immunohistochemical review. Am J Dermatopathol. 2012;34(4):347–93.
3. Alfageme Roldán F. Elastography in dermatology [Elastografía en dermatología]. Actas Dermosifiliogr. 2016;107(8):652–60.
4. Almuhanna N, Wortsman X, Wohlmuth-Wieser I, Kinoshita-Ise M, Alhusayen R. Overview of ultrasound imaging applications in dermatology. J Cutan Med Surg. 2021;25(5):521–9.
5. Becker-Weidman D, Mhuircheartaigh JN, Mortele KJ. The skinny on skin: MRI features of cutaneous and subcutaneous lesions detected on body MRI studies. Abdom Radiol (NY). 2018;43(10):2823–50.
6. Cha J, Kim S, Wang J, Yun M, Cho A. Evaluation of ^{18}F-FDG PET/CT parameters for detection of lymph node metastasis in cutaneous melanoma. Nucl Med Mol Imaging. 2018;52(1):39–45.
7. Cuenca-Barrales C, Aguayo-Carreras P, Bueno-Rodriguez A, Ruiz-Villaverde R. Ultrasound in the evaluation of cutaneous metastases of internal tumors [Estudio ecográfico de metástasis cutáneas de origen visceral]. Actas Dermosifiliogr (Engl Ed). 2019;110(6):506–9.
8. Dasgeb B, Morris MA, Mehregan D, Siegel EL. Quantified ultrasound elastography in the assessment of cutaneous carcinoma. Br J Radiol. 2015;88(1054):20150344.
9. Dinnes J, Ferrante di Ruffano L, Takwoingi Y, et al. Ultrasound, CT, MRI, or PET-CT for staging and re-staging of adults with cutaneous melanoma. Cochrane Database Syst Rev. 2019;7(7):CD012806.
10. Dobre EG, Surcel M, Constantin C, et al. Skin cancer pathobiology at a glance: a focus on imaging techniques and their potential for improved diagnosis and surveillance in clinical cohorts. Int J Mol Sci. 2023;24(2):1079.
11. Franklin C, Wetter A, Baba HA, et al. Computed tomography-guided biopsy of radiologically unclear lesions in advanced skin cancer: a retrospective analysis of 47 cases. Eur J Cancer. 2021;150:119–29.
12. Habermehl G, Ko J. Cutaneous metastases: a review and diagnostic approach to tumors of unknown origin. Arch Pathol Lab Med. 2019;143(8):943–57.
13. Horton L, Fakhoury JW, Manwar R, et al. Review of non-invasive imaging technologies for cutaneous melanoma. Biosensors (Basel). 2025;15(5):297.
14. Gan J, Nourzaie R, Doolan BJ, Connor S. CT and MRI of head and neck cutaneous lesions. BJR Open. 2023;5(1):20230006. Published 2023 Jun 13
15. Giovagnorio F, Andreoli C, De Cicco ML. Color Doppler sonography of focal lesions of the skin and subcutaneous tissue. J Ultrasound Med. 1999;18(2):89–93.
16. Kamińska-Winciorek G, Pilśniak A, Piskorski W, Wydmański J. Skin metastases in the clinical and dermoscopic aspects. Semin Oncol. 2022;49(2):160–9.
17. Kawaguchi M, Kato H, Noda Y, et al. Imaging findings of malignant skin tumors: radiological-pathological correlation. Insights Imaging. 2022;13(1):52.
18. Kim YJ, Kim HS, Lee JH, Yoon YC. Ultrasound and CT findings of subcutaneous metastases in trunk and pelvis: a comprehensive analysis. Skeletal Radiol. 2024;53(12):2665–75.
19. Krarup MMK, Fischer BM, Christensen TN. New PET tracers: current knowledge and perspectives in lung cancer. Semin Nucl Med. 2022;52(6):781–96.
20. Kwon HM, Kim GY, Shin DH, Bae YK. Clinicopathologic features of cutaneous metastases from internal malignancies. J Pathol Transl Med. 2021;55(4):289–97.
21. Lange S, Mędrzycka-Dąbrowska W, Zorena K, et al. Nephrogenic systemic fibrosis as a complication after gadolinium-containing contrast agents: a rapid review. Int J Environ Res Public Health. 2021;18(6):3000.
22. Libson K, Sheridan C, Carr DR, Shahwan KT. Use of imaging in cutaneous squamous cell carcinoma to detect high-risk tumor features, nodal metastasis, and distant metastasis: a systematic review. Dermatologic Surg. 2024;50(8):705–9.
23. Mandava A, Ravuri PR, Konathan R. High-resolution ultrasound imaging of cutaneous lesions. Indian J Radiol Imaging. 2013;23(3):269–77.
24. Metser U, Tau N. Benign cutaneous and subcutaneous lesions on FDG-PET/CT. Semin Nucl Med. 2017;47(4):352–61.
25. Morris MA, Ring CM, Managuli R, et al. Feature analysis of ultrasound elastography image for quantitative assessment of cutaneous carcinoma. Skin Res Technol. 2018;24(2):242–7.
26. Pathak P, Wondimu B, Jalilianhasanpour R, Pooyan A, Matesan MC, Mansoori B. Skin malignancies: imaging review with radiologic-histopathologic correlation. Radiographics. 2023;43(12):e230093.
27. Patten RM, Shuman WP, Teefey S. Subcutaneous metastases from malignant melanoma: prevalence and findings on CT. AJR Am J Roentgenol. 1989;152(5):1009–12.
28. Russo GM, Russo A, Urraro F, Cioce F, Gallo L, Belfiore MP, Sangiovanni A, Napolitano S, Troiani T, Verolino P, et al. Management of non-melanoma skin cancer: radiologists challenging and risk assessment. Diagnostics. 2023;13(4):793.
29. Sariya D, Ruth K, Adams-McDonnell R, et al. Clinicopathologic correlation of cutaneous metastases: experience from a cancer center. Arch Dermatol. 2007;143(5):613–20.
30. Souza BCE, Miyashiro D, Pincelli MS, Sanches JA. Cutaneous metastases from solid neoplasms - literature review. An Bras Dermatol. 2023;98(5):571–9.

31. Stefanowska J, Zakowiecki D, Cal K. Magnetic resonance imaging of the skin. J Eur Acad Dermatol Venereol. 2010;24(8):875–80.
32. Tanaka T, Kamata M, Fukaya S, et al. Usefulness of real-time elastography for diagnosing lymph node metastasis of skin cancer: does elastography potentially eliminate the need for sentinel lymph node biopsy in squamous cell carcinoma? J Eur Acad Dermatol Venereol. 2020;34(4):754–61.
33. Trotter J, Pantel AR, Teo BK, et al. Positron emission tomography (PET)/computed tomography (CT) imaging in radiation therapy treatment planning: a review of PET imaging tracers and methods to incorporate PET/CT. Adv Radiat Oncol. 2023;8(5):101212.
34. Vandenberghe S, Marsden PK. PET-MRI: a review of challenges and solutions in the development of integrated multimodality imaging. Phys Med Biol. 2015;60(4):R115–54.
35. Williams LS, Mancuso AA, Mendenhall WM. Perineural spread of cutaneous squamous and basal cell carcinoma: CT and MR detection and its impact on patient management and prognosis. Int J Radiat Oncol Biol Phys. 2001;49(4):1061–9.
36. Wortsman X, Wortsman J. Clinical usefulness of variable-frequency ultrasound in localized lesions of the skin. J Am Acad Dermatol. 2010;62(2):247–56.
37. Wortsman X. Ultrasound in skin cancer: why, how, and when to use it? Cancers (Basel). 2024;16(19):3301.
38. Zemtsov A, Lorig R, Ng TC, et al. Magnetic resonance imaging of cutaneous neoplasms: clinicopathologic correlation. J Dermatol Surg Oncol. 1991;17(5):416–22.

Part XVII

Management of Cutaneous Metastasis

30 Treatment of Cutaneous Metastasis

Ariadna Ortiz-Brugués

Abstract

Treatment of cutaneous metastasis depends on the type of tumour, the localization and extension of the lesions, the general health condition and patient comorbidities. Depending on these factors, currently available treatment options include local and systemic therapeutic options. Local therapies include surgery, radiotherapy, intralesional and topical treatment, as well as local therapeutic procedures. Systemic therapies mainly include chemotherapy, targeted therapies and immune checkpoint inhibitors. Palliative care should be performed by a multi-disciplinary team.

Keywords

Cutaneous metastasis treatment · Surgery · Radiotherapy · Electrochemotherapy · Limb perfusion · Talimogene laherparepvec · Imiquimod · Daromun · Immune checkpoint inhibitors · Palliative care

Treatment of cutaneous metastasis depends on the type of tumor, the localization and extension of the lesions, the general health condition, and patient comorbidities [1]. Depending on these factors, currently available treatment options include local and systemic therapeutic options.

30.1 Local Treatments

1. **Surgery**: complete excision of cutaneous metastasis with control of resection margins should be considered in cases of localized, anatomically accessible lesions, in the absence of distant metastasis. Potential functional deficits should also be taken into account.

The aim of surgery in cutaneous metastasis is a curative approach. Eventually, it could be discussed in the palliative setting, in case of painful necrotizing lesions [1, 2]. Excision and removal of metastases may be warranted to enhance the patient's quality of life, but excision of select metastases does little to increase survival.

2. **Radiotherapy**: the use of ionizing radiation has demonstrated a good response in cutaneous metastasis of melanoma [3], breast cancer [4], urothelial carcinoma, and renal cell carcinoma [5, 6], with smaller lesions showing a better response and longer-lasting remission. Superficial tumors are usually irradiated with fast electrons, and deep tumors with photons [3]. Hyperthermia can increase the complete response rate to 62% when added to radiotherapy [7].

A. Ortiz-Brugués (✉)
Skin Cancer Unit, Dermatology Department, Hospital Clínic, Barcelona, Spain

D. Koumaki et al. (eds.), *Cutaneous Metastases*, https://doi.org/10.1007/978-3-032-26764-1_30

Radiotherapy can also be discussed in patients with a resection of melanoma metastases and microscopic tumor at the margin, when additional surgery is not adequate [8].

Skin metastases may cause pain due to the space-occupying effect, resulting in bleeding and malodour due to tumor infiltration or degradation. In the palliative setting, short-wavelength radiation therapy using superficial electron beam therapy may be helpful for painful lesions. Of note, the analgesic effect of radiotherapy does not require complete regression of metastases [9].

The most frequent adverse events that are reported are erythema and fibrosis [10].

3. **Intralesional Therapies:**

   3.1 *Electrochemotherapy:* it combines electroporation, a mechanism that allows the cell membrane to become permeable through the application of electrical pulses, and the administration of chemotherapeutic agents intravenously or intratumorally. Treatment will be conducted under local or general anesthesia depending on the size, number, and localization of cutaneous metastases [11]. Electrochemotherapy may be indicated in the palliative setting to control advanced inoperable cutaneous metastases, as well as primary tumors [12].

   Local side effects include bleeding, necrosis, infection, and muscle pain [13].

   Calcium electroporation is non-inferior to classical electrochemotherapy with bleomycin and cisplatin and should, therefore, be considered an option [14]. Finally, the association of electrochemotherapy with immunotherapy has been successfully tested in several retrospective analyses and case reports [15, 16].

   3.2 *Isolated limb perfusion*: it consists of the vascular isolation and perfusion with chemotherapy agents (usually the alkylating agent melphalan), alone or in combination with recombinant human tumor necrosis factor-α, with tissue hyperthermia at 39–40 °C. They are administered throughout a canulated artery and vein using an extracorporeal bypass circuit, permitting a much higher concentration that would not be tolerated systemically [17]. TNF-α is a cytokine with antitumor effects probably mediated by a specific action against tumor blood vessels, enhancing the cytotoxic effect of melphalan [18].

   This complex technique could be considered in patients with multiple melanoma metastases and rapid recurrence, limited to the arm or leg [19]. The combination of both therapeutic agents results in a significantly higher response (46.5% vs. 68.9%) [20]. However, there are no differences regarding progression-free survival and overall survival [21].

   Other combination therapies are melphalan plus D-actinomycin, an antineoplastic antibiotic, with an OR of 87.65% and a CR of 76% [22], and melphalan plus dacarbazine, with an OR of 90.80% and a CR of 73.40% [23].

   Loco-regional toxicities include erythema, overheating, blisters, desquamation, lymphedema, followed by muscle atrophy or fibrosis, limb malfunction, neuropathy, pain, and recurrent infection [24], and compartment syndrome losing the whole extremity. Systemic toxicities may comprise rhabdomyolysis or cardiac stress when using TNF-α [1].

   3.3 *Isolated Limb Infusion*: it is a minimally invasive technique for the administration of high-dose melphalan alone or in combination with actinomycin-D to the extremities of patients presenting locally advanced or in-transit metastasis [25]. On contrary to isolated limb perfusion, catheters are placed percutaneously [26].

   Melphalan induces a pro-inflammatory microenvironment, inhibiting regulatory T cells; also directly inhibiting the DNA replication of melanoma cells [27]. Actinomycin-D inhibits the transcription of DNA by RNA polymerase and controls topoisomerase II activity. The combination of both agents is considered to enhance response rates with low toxicity rates compared to isolated limb perfusion [28]. Therefore, it may be the best option for treating elderly and frail patients, who cannot tolerate other treatments [29].

In the last few years, the association of systemic immunotherapy with local chemotherapy through isolated limb infusion has increased the responses in locoregional melanoma [30].

3.4 *Interleukin-2*: intralesional interleukin-2 results in tumor lysis and apoptosis via formation of lymphokine-activated killer cells, with an improved tolerance compared to the systemic administration [1]. In a phase II trial, complete response was observed in 85% of patients, and 6% had partial response [31]. Toxicities include local reactions, flu-like symptoms, fatigue, and, occasionally, gastrointestinal symptoms [32].

Furthermore, few case reports have analyzed the role of interferon- β, which could be an option to improve the quality of life in patients with in-transit melanoma metastasis refractory to immune checkpoint inhibitors [33].

3.5 *Talimogene laherparepvec (T-VEC)*: it is the first engineered oncolytic herpes simplex virus type 1 (HSV-1) intra-lesionally administered that duplicates in the tumor mass, causing the lysis of tumor cells, presenting tumor-derived antigens to CD8+ T-cells, and enhancing anti-tumor immunity [34].

In a phase III trial with melanoma patients in stage IIIB–IV, a response rate of 26.4% with 10.8% complete remissions was shown [35]. The combination with the PD-1 inhibitor pembrolizumab showed no significant improvement in progression-free survival or overall survival [36].

Of note, the efficacy of T-VEC is not confined only to injected lesions, but extends also through an abscopal effect on metastasis in distant sites [37]. A good response to the intralesional therapy with T-VEC has also been reported for squamous cell carcinoma, Merkel cell carcinoma, cutaneous lymphoma, and sarcoma [38].

The toxicity of T-VEC is usually mild and tolerable, with the most common toxicities being oedema and erythema at injection sites, chills, fever, and fatigue [39]. It is approved for patients with unresectable malignant melanoma with local or distant metastases without bone, brain, lung, or visceral metastases [1].

4. **Topical Therapies**

4.1 *Imiquimod:* it is a Toll-like receptor (TLR) 7 and 8 agonist that stimulates dendritic cells, activating Th1 cellular immune response and stimulating the activity of tumor-specific cytotoxic CD8+ T cells [40]. It is applied 5 times a week under occlusion during 8 to 22 weeks, showing complete remission in up to 82.3% of patients [41].

A phase I/II trial consisting of daily application of imiquimod for 4 weeks followed by intralesional interleukin-2 one to three times a week demonstrated response rates of 50%, including 40.7% of complete response [42]. In a case series of 20 patients with cutaneous melanoma metastases treated by imiquimod cryotherapy, 40% reported a complete response and 25% had a partial response [43]. Finally, a combination of imiquimod plus monobenzone was studied in a phase II trial, showing regression of cutaneous metastases in up to 52% of patients [44].

Therefore, imiquimod alone or in association with other drugs can be considered an option for the treatment of cutaneous metastases, including in a palliative setting [45].

4.2 *5-fluorouracil*: it is an anti-metabolite that induces the apoptosis of cancer cells through the inhibition of DNA synthesis [25]. It seems to be more effective when applied in combination. In this way, topical application of 5-fluorouracil in the morning and imiquimod at night has shown positive results, with more than

40% complete response and 55% of partial response [46] .

4.3 *Diphencyprone:* it is a contact sensitizer that should be considered for patients with skin metastases refractory to other therapies, showing up to 46% of complete response and 38% of partial response [47]. Application of a 2% dinitrochlorobenzene solution significantly increases the effectiveness of intravenous dacarbazine, with response rates up to 62% [48]. Moreover, diphencyprone with systemic immunotherapy has been tested with promising results [49, 50] .

5. **Local Therapeutic Procedures:**

5.1 *Cryotherapy*: it is the use of nitrogen evaporation at 195.8 °C with the formation of extracellular and intracellular ice crystals and secondary cell death. It also causes a disturbed microcirculation, resulting in tissue anoxia and additional necrosis [1].

Patients with metastatic malignant melanoma treated with cryotherapy have a mean remission time of 36 months and improved quality of life [51].

5.2 *CO2 laser ablation:* it results in ablation of the epidermal and upper dermal skin layers. In patients treated with melanoma metastases, complete clinical remission was shown in 62.5% of cases [52]. Similar to cryotherapy, ablative laser therapy is a safe and effective option for palliative treatment of skin metastases derived from melanoma, especially for small superficial metastases [1].

5.3 *Photodynamic therapy*: it consists of the use of topical photosensitizing substances that accumulate in the epidermis and are activated by exposure to light. This leads to the production of reactive oxygen species, resulting in cell damage and cell death [1]. Photodynamic therapy has demonstrated the complete remission of cutaneous metastases in 75.9% of cases [53].

6. **Systemic Therapies**

6.1 *Chemotherapy*: no specific chemotherapy has been shown to be the most effective for the treatment of cutaneous metastases [2]. Observations are limited to case reports, such as a patient with cutaneous metastases from pancreatic cancer treated with gemcitabine [54] and a patient with cutaneous metastases from urothelial carcinoma of the bladder treated with cyclophosphamide, methotrexate, and 5-fluorouracil [55]. Cutaneous metastases of lung cancer have been treated with cisplatin, cyclophosphamide, adriamycin, mitomycin, interferon-beta, etoposide, and carboplatin [56]. Case reports of cutaneous metastases from cancers of unknown origin treated with cisplatin, gemcitabine, vinorelbine, and paclitaxel have also been reported [57, 58].

6.2 *Targeted therapies:* Palbociclib, a cyclin-dependent kinases 4/6 (CDK4/6) inhibitor that induces G1 phase cell cycle arrest, is used in combination with aromatase inhibitors to treat metastatic and adjuvant breast cancer. One patient with cutaneous metastases of breast cancer achieved a complete response with palbociclib and letrozole, maintaining this response for 24 months [59].

Gefitinib, a first-generation EGFR tyrosine kinase inhibitor, is effective in EGFR-mutated metastatic lung adenocarcinoma. One patient with cutaneous metastases of lung adenocarcinoma patient achieved a complete response, with all skin lesions resolving within two months of gefitinib treatment, and maintained this response for 13 months [59].

6.3 *Breast cancer*:

6.3.1 *Eribulin*: in an observational study, 26% of patients with cutaneous breast cancer metastases treated with eribulin showed a complete response, 22% had a partial response, 39% stable disease, and

13% no response. There was an improvement of symptoms, infiltration, and ulceration [60] .

6.3.2 *Miltefosine*: in a randomized study, the application of 6% miltefosine solution to cutaneous breast cancer metastases achieved good control compared to placebo [61].

6.3.3 *ErbB2/HER2*: finally, 4/10 patients with SM from breast or colon cancer treated with intratumoral injections of recombinant single-chain antibodies targeted to ErbB2/HER2 showed a complete response [62].

6.4 *Melanoma*:

6.4.1 *Immune checkpoint inhibitors*: a retrospective study with patients presenting in transit metastasis showed that treatment with programmed cell death protein 1 (PD-1) inhibitor (pembrolizumab or nivolumab) demonstrated 58% of overall response, anti-CTLA4 (ipilimumab) had 38% response, while anti-PD-1 and anti-CTLA-4 showed 40% of response [63]. Another retrospective study evaluated the efficacy of the PD-1 inhibitor and/or CTLA-4 inhibitor according to the RECIST criteria, with an overall response rate of 56% [64]. According to the latest guidelines of the European Society of Medical Oncology, patients with unresectable satellite, in-transit metastases should be treated with systemic therapy, preferentially anti-PD-1, as these patients are at risk for developing distant metastasis [8].

6.4.2 *ECT and checkpoint inhibitors*: the combination of ECT and pembrolizumab achieved a higher response rate in cutaneous melanoma metastases than treatment with pembrolizumab alone (78% and 39%, respectively) [65]. Moreover, patients had a longer progression-free and overall survival in the group with pembrolizumab plus electrochemotherapy than in the group with pembrolizumab monotherapy [65].

6.4.3 *T-VEC and checkpoint inhibitors*: T-VEC with ipilimumab was studied in patients with advanced melanoma (stage IIIB–IV) with a response rate of 50% [66]. In another trial, patients with stage IIIB-IV melanoma were randomized to T-VEC plus ipilimumab versus ipilimumab alone, with a higher response rate in the combination group [66]. In the neoadjuvant setting, T-VEC with pembrolizumab is studied in patients with resectable stage III cutaneous melanoma with clinically palpable lymph node metastases [1].

6.4.4 *Daromun*: it is a combination of two antibody-cytokine fusions (L19-IL2 and L19-TNF) targeting the extra domain-B of fibronectin. A phase 2 study demonstrated that intralesional daromun induced responses in both injected and distant uninjected lesions in stage III/IV melanoma patients [67]. In a phase 3 study, patients were randomized to receive daromun followed by surgery or surgery alone [68]. Pathological complete response was observed in 21% of patients in the treatment arm. Toxicity was primarily low-grade.

6.5 *Merkel cell carcinoma*: intratumoral G100, an agonist of toll-like receptor 4, shows promising results in patients with locoregional tumors [1].

T-VEC prior to surgery and/or radiotherapy is investigated as monotherapy or in combination with immune checkpoint inhibitors in patients with localized or locally advanced Merkel cell carcinoma [69]. In addition, a single report of a patient with multifocal recurrence of Merkel cell carcinoma treated with T-VEC monotherapy showed a complete response [70].

Finally, vaccines targeting tumor-associated antigens or viral oncoproteins are also being developed [69].

6.6 *Squamous cell carcinoma*: current trials include combinations of checkpoint inhibition and EGFR inhibition, intralesional administration of PD-1 inhibitors in locally advanced squamous cell carcinoma, and the combination of an anti-PD1 antibody with RP1, an oncolytic herpes simplex virus [1].

7. **Palliative Care**

The care of palliative patients with cutaneous metastases should be performed by a multidisciplinary team, continuously re-evaluating the wishes of the patient and their closest ones.

The palliative treatment of cutaneous metastases includes adequate management of the pain, pruritus, possible bacterial superinfection, and, in some cases, the unpleasant smell that these lesions can produce [71–74]. Therefore, they are often associated with high psychological burden and reduced quality of life. Accordingly, the care of these patients requires a high level of empathy, sensitivity, communicative and professional competence [1].

Consultation with a wound expert for assessment and treatment is recommended. Analgesic therapy should be performed in consensus with palliative healthcare professionals. Local treatment procedures (for example, radiotherapy) may also be discussed. Finally, psychosocial problems of patients or relatives should be actively addressed by the treatment team, and specialist support by psycho-oncologists should be offered [1].

References

1. Gschnell M, Volberg C, Hauser C, Krönig L. Cutaneous metastases: from epidemiology to therapy. J Dtsch Dermatol Ges. 2024;22(7):974–93.
2. Fernández-Antón Martínez MC, Parra-Blanco V, Avilés-Izquierdo JA, Suárez-Fernández RM. Cutaneous metastases of internal tumors. Actas Dermosifiliogr. 2013;104(10):841–53.
3. Seegenschmiedt MH, Keilholz L, Altendorf-Hofmann A, et al. Long term results following radiation therapy of locally recurrent and metastatic malignant melanoma. Hautarzt. 1999;50(8):572–9.
4. Fritz P, Hensley FW, Berns C, et al. Long-term results of pulsed irradiation of skin metastases from breast cancer. Effectiveness and sequelae. Strahlenther Onkol. 2000;176(8):368–76.
5. Block CA, Dahmoush L, Konety BR. Cutaneous metastases from transitional cell carcinoma of the bladder. Urology. 2006;67(4):846.e15–7.
6. Gay HA, Cavalieri R, Allison RR, Finley J Jr, Quan WD Jr. Complete response in a cutaneous facial metastatic nodule from renal cell carcinoma after hypofractionated radiotherapy. Dermatol Online J. 2007;13(4)
7. Overgaard J, Gonzalez Gonzalez D, Hulshof MC, et al. Randomised trial of hyperthermia as adjuvant to radiotherapy for recurrent or metastatic malignant melanoma. European Society for Hyperthermic Oncology. Lancet. 1995;345(8949):540–3.
8. Amaral T, Ottaviano M, Arance A, et al. Cutaneous melanoma: ESMO clinical practice guideline for diagnosis, treatment and follow-up. Ann Oncol. 2025;36(1):10–30.
9. Fenig E, Eidelevich E, Njuguna E, et al. Role of radiation therapy in the management of cutaneous malignant melanoma. Am J Clin Oncol. 1999;22:184–6.
10. Olivier KR, Schild SE, Morris CG, et al. A higher radiotherapy dose is associated with more durable palliation and longer survival in patients with metastatic melanoma. Cancer. 2007;110:1791–5.
11. Reinhold U. Electrochemotherapy of skin tumors. Hautarzt. 2011;62(7):549–58.
12. Mir LM, Belehradek M, Domenge C, et al. Electrochemotherapy, a new antitumor treatment: first clinical trial. C R Acad Sci III. 1991;313(13):613–8.
13. Gehl J, Sersa G, Matthiessen LW, et al. Updated standard operating procedures for electrochemotherapy of cutaneous tumours and skin metastases. Acta Oncol. 2018;57(7):874–82.
14. Ágoston D, Baltás E, Ócsai H, et al. Evaluation of calcium electroporation for the treatment of cutaneous metastases: a double blinded randomised controlled phase II trial. Cancer. 2020;12(1):179.
15. Mozzillo N, Simeone E, Benedetto L, et al. Assessing a novel immuno-oncology-based combination therapy: ipilimumab plus electrochemotherapy. Onco Targets Ther. 2015;4:e1008842.
16. Heppt MV, Eigentler TK, Kahler KC, et al. Immune checkpoint blockade with concurrent electrochemotherapy in advanced melanoma: a retrospective multicenter analysis. Cancer Immunol Immunother. 2016;65:951–9.
17. Sevilla-Ortega L, Ferrandiz-Pulido L, Palazon-Carrion N, et al. Role of isolated limb perfusion in the era of targeted therapies and immunotherapy in melanoma. A systematic review of the literature. Cancers. 2021;13(21):5485.
18. Eggermont AM. The success of TNF alpha in isolated limb perfusion for irresectable extremity soft tissue

sarcomas, melanoma and carcinomas: observations in patients and preclinical perfusion models. Gan Kagaku Ryoho Cancer Chemother. 1996;23:1357–70.
19. Creech O Jr, Krementz ET, Kokame GM. Chemotherapy for cancer by perfusion. Rev Surg. 1962;19:149–58.
20. Moreno-Ramirez D, Cruz-Merino L, Ferrandiz L, et al. Isolated limb perfusion for malignant melanoma: systematic review on effectiveness and safety. Oncologist. 2010;15(4):416–27.
21. Hoekstra HJ, Veerman K, van Ginkel RJ. Isolated limb perfusion for in-transit melanoma metastases: melphalan or TNF melphalan perfusion? J Surg Oncol. 2014;109:338–47.
22. Kroon HM, Huismans AM, Kam PC, Thompson JF. Isolated limb infusion with melphalan and actinomycin D for melanoma: a systematic review. J Surg Oncol. 2014;109:348–51.
23. Edwards MJ, Boddie AW Jr, Ames FC, McBride CM. Isolated limb perfusion for stage I melanoma of the extremity: a comparison of melphalan and dacarbazine (DTIC). South Med J. 1989;82:985–9.
24. Vrouenraets BC, Klaase JM, Kroon BB, van Geel BN, Eggermont AM, Franklin HR. Long-term morbidity after regional isolated perfusion with melphalan for melanoma of the limbs. The influence of acute regional toxic reactions. Arch Surg. 1995;130:43–7.
25. Di Raimondo C, Lozzi F, Di Domenico PP, Campione E, Bianchi L. The diagnosis and management of cutaneous metastases from melanoma. Int J Mol Sci. 2023;24(19):14535.
26. Kroon HM, Huismans A, Waugh RC, Kam PC, Thompson JF. Isolated limb infusion: technical aspects. J Surg Oncol. 2014;109:352–6.
27. Kuczma M, Ding ZC, Zhou G. Immunostimulatory effects of melphalan and usefulness in adoptive cell therapy with antitumor CD4+ T cells. Crit Rev Immunol. 2016;36:179–91.
28. Lindner P, Doubrovsky A, Kam PC, Thompson JF. Prognostic factors after isolated limb infusion with cytotoxic agents for melanoma. Ann Surg Oncol. 2002;9:127–36.
29. Kroon HM, Thompson JF. Isolated limb infusion: a review. J Surg Oncol. 2009;100:169–77.
30. Carr MJ, Sun J, Kroon HM, Miura JT, Beasley GM, Farrow NE, et al. Oncologic outcomes after isolated limb infusion for advanced melanoma: an international comparison of the procedure and outcomes between the United States and Australia. Ann Surg Oncol. 2020;27:5107–18.
31. Radny P, Caroli UM, Bauer J, et al. Phase II trial of intralesional therapy with interleukin-2 in soft-tissue melanoma metastases. Br J Cancer. 2003;89(9):1620–6.
32. Weide B, Derhovanessian E, Pflugfelder A, et al. High response rate after intratumoral treatment with interleukin-2: results from a phase 2 study in 51 patients with metastasized melanoma. Cancer. 2010;116(17):4139–46.
33. Takahara Y, Kan T, Teshima Y, et al. Malignant melanoma with in-transit metastases refractory to programmed cell death-1 inhibitor successfully treated with local interferon-beta injections: a case report. Mol Clin Oncol. 2021;15:212.
34. Kohlhapp FJ, Kaufman HL. Molecular pathways: mechanism of action for Talimogene Laherparepvec, a new oncolytic virus immunotherapy. Clin Cancer Res. 2016;22:1048–54.
35. Andtbacka RHI, Collichio F, Harrington KJ, et al. Final analyses of OPTIM: a randomized phase III trial of talimogene laherparepvec versus granulocyte-macrophage colony-stimulating factor in unresectable stage III–IV melanoma. J Immunother Cancer. 2019;7(1):145.
36. Chesney JA, Ribas A, Long GV, et al. Randomized, double-blind, placebo-controlled, global phase III trial of talimogene laherparepvec combined with pembrolizumab for advanced melanoma. J Clin Oncol. 2023;41(3):528–40.
37. Andtbacka RH, Ross M, Puzanov I, et al. Patterns of clinical response with talimogene laherparepvec (T-VEC) in patients with melanoma treated in the OPTIM phase III clinical trial. Ann Surg Oncol. 2016;23:4169–77.
38. Salloum A, Koblinski J, Bazzi N, Zeitouni NC. Talimogene laherparepvec in non-melanoma cancers. J Clin Aesthet Dermatol. 2021;14(11):18–25.
39. Zhang T, Jou TH, Hsin J, et al. Talimogene laherparepvec (T-VEC): a review of the recent advances in cancer therapy. J Clin Med. 2023;12:1098.
40. Hanna E, Abadi R, Abbas O. Imiquimod in dermatology: an overview. Int J Dermatol. 2016;55:831–44.
41. Sisti A, Sisti G, Oranges CM. Topical treatment of melanoma skin metastases with imiquimod: a review. Dermatol Online J. 2015;21(2)
42. Green DS, Bodman-Smith MD, Dalgleish AG, Fischer MD. Phase I/II study of topical imiquimod and intralesional interleukin-2 in the treatment of accessible metastases in malignant melanoma. Br J Dermatol. 2007;156(2):337–45.
43. Rivas-Tolosa N, Ortiz-Brugues A, Toledo-Pastrana T, et al. Local cryosurgery and imiquimod: a successful combination for the treatment of locoregional cutaneous metastasis of melanoma: a case series. J Dermatol. 2016;43:553–6.
44. Teulings HE, EPM T, Willemsen KJ, et al. Anti-melanoma immunity and local regression of cutaneous metastases in melanoma patients treated with monobenzone and imiquimod; a phase 2 a trial. Onco Targets Ther. 2018;7:e1419113.
45. Scarfi F, Patrizi A, Veronesi G, et al. The role of topical imiquimod in melanoma cutaneous metastases: a critical review of the literature. Dermatol Ther. 2020;33:e14165.
46. Florin V, Desmedt E, Vercambre-Darras S, Mortier L. Topical treatment of cutaneous metastases of malignant melanoma using combined imiquimod and 5-fluorouracil. Investig New Drugs. 2012;30:1641–5.

47. Damian DL, Saw RP, Thompson JF. Topical immunotherapy with diphencyprone for in transit and cutaneously metastatic melanoma. J Surg Oncol. 2014;109:308–13.
48. Terheyden P, Kortüm AK, Schulze HJ, et al. Chemoimmunotherapy for cutaneous melanoma with dacarbazine and epifocal contact sensitizers: results of a nationwide survey of the German Der matologic Co-operative Oncology Group. J Cancer Res Clin Oncol. 2007;133(7):437–44.
49. Gulati N, Carvajal RD, Postow MA, Wolchok JD, Krueger JG. Definite regression of cutaneous melanoma metastases upon addition of topical contact sensitizer diphencyprone to immune checkpoint inhibitor treatment. Exp Dermatol. 2016;25:553–4.
50. Fujimura T, Furudate S, Kakizaki A, et al. Contact immunotherapy enhances the therapeutic effects of nivolumab in treating in-transit melanoma: two cases reports. J Dermatol. 2016;43:686–9.
51. John HE, Mahaffey PJ. Laser ablation and cryotherapy of melanoma metastases: cryotherapy/laser ablation. J Surg Oncol. 2014;109(4):296–300.
52. Kandamany N, Mahaffey P. Carbon dioxide laser ablation as first-line management of in-transit cutaneous malignant melanoma metastases. Lasers MedSci. 2009;24(3):411–4.
53. Spratt DE, Gordon Spratt EA, Wu S, et al. Efficacy of skin-directed therapy for cutaneous metastases from advanced cancer: a meta-analysis. J Clin Oncol. 2014;32(28):3144–55.
54. Florez A, Roson E, Sanchez-Aguilar D, Peteiro C, Toribio J. Solitary cutaneous metastasis on the buttock: a disclosing sign of pancreatic adenocarcinoma. Clin Exp Dermatol. 2000;25:201–3.
55. Rosati G, Rossi A, Germano D, Piccirillo A, De Santis D, Manzione L. Responsiveness of skin metastases to CMF in a patient with urothelial carcinoma of the bladder: a case report. Tumori. 2003;89:85–7.
56. Kim HK, Kang SH, Kim WS, et al. Scalp metastasis from an adenocarcinoma of the lung mimicking a cystic mass: case report and literature review. Arch Craniofac Surg. 2022;23(5):237–40.
57. Massard C, Voigt JJ, Laplanche A, et al. Carcinoma of an unknown primary: are EGF recep tor, Her-2/neu, and c-Kit tyrosine kinases potential targets for therapy. Br J Cancer. 2007;97:857–61.
58. Palmeri S, Lorusso V, Palmeri L, et al. Cisplatin and gemcitabine with either vinorelbine or paclitaxel in the treatment of carcinomas of unknown primary site: results of an Italian multicenter, randomized, phase ii study. Cancer. 2006;107:2898–905.
59. Arshad M, Paul AJ, Kumar R. Skin metastasis from solid tumors: is targeted therapy making an impact? Cureus. 2024;16(11):e74362.
60. La Verde N, Moretti A, Farina G, et al. Eribulin in cutaneous breast cancer metastasis treatment: clinical activity and symptom control. Future Oncol. 2013;9(12):1841–8.
61. Leonard R, Hardy J, van Tienhoven G, et al. Randomized, double-blind, placebo controlled, multicenter trial of 6% miltefosine solution, a topical chemotherapy in cutaneous metastases from breast cancer. J Clin Oncol. 2001;19:4150–9.
62. Azemar M, Djahansouzi S, Jager E, et al. Regression of cutaneous tumor lesions in patients intratumorally injected with a recombinant single chain antibody-toxin targeted to ErbB2/HER2. Breast Cancer Res Treat. 2003;82:155–64.
63. Nan-Tie E, Lai-Kwon J, Rtshiladze MA, et al. Efficacy of immune checkpoint inhibitors for in-transit melanoma. J Immunother Cancer. 2020;8:e000440.
64. Holmberg CJ, Ny L, Hieken TJ, et al. The efficacy of immunecheckpoint blockade for melanoma in-transit with or without nodal metastases—a multicenter cohort study. Eur J Cancer. 2022;169:210–22.
65. Campana LG, Peric B, Mascherini M, et al. Combination of pembrolizumab with electrochemotherapy in cutaneous metastases from melanoma: a comparative retrospective study from the InspECT and Slovenian Cancer Registry. Cancers (Basel). 2021;13(17):4289.
66. Zawit M, Swami U, Awada H, et al. Current status of intralesional agents in treatment of malignant melanoma. Ann Transl Med. 2021;9(12):1038.
67. Garbe C, Amaral T, Peris K, et al. European consensus-based interdisciplinary guideline for melanoma. Part 2: treatment—update 2024. Eur J Cancer. 2025;215:115153.
68. Hauschild A, Hassel JC, Ziemer M, et al. Phase 3 study (PIVOTAL) of neoadjuvant intralesional daromun vs. immediate surgery in fully resectable melanoma with regional skin and/or nodal metastases. J Clin Oncol. 2024;42:LBA9501.
69. Ricco G, Andrini E, Siepe G, et al. Multimodal strategy in localized Merkel cell carcinoma: where are we and where are we heading? IntJ MolSci. 2021;22(19):10629.
70. Casale F, Tchanque-Fossuo C, Stepenaskie S, Durkin J. Complete response of Merkel cell carcinoma with talimogene laherparepvec (TVEC) monotherapy. Dermatol Online J. 2022;28(1)
71. Borgermann C, Vom Dorp F, Krege S, Rübben H. The management of cutaneous metastases. Urologe A. 2007;46:56–8.
72. Pogatzki-Zahn E, Marziniak M, Schneider G, Luger TA, Ständer S. Chronic pruritus: targets, mechanisms and future therapies. Drug News Perspect. 2008;21:541–51.
73. Alexander S. Malignant fungating wounds: managing pain, bleeding and psychosocial issues. J Wound Care. 2009;18:418–25.
74. Stephen Haynes J. An overview of caring for those with palliative wounds. Br J Community Nurs. 2008;13:6–8.

Quality of Life in Patients with Cutaneous Metastases

31

Pavel V. Chernyshov

Abstract

Skin metastases have a strong negative influence on the overall QoL and are often associated with a poor prognosis. There is a lack of literature on QoL in patients with cutaneous metastases. Similar to other skin cancers, general measures may not always be sensitive enough to measure the total impact of cutaneous metastases on patients' lives. Cancer-specific instruments (e.g., EORTC QLQ-C30 and FACT-G) should be primarily used to assess HRQoL in patients with skin metastases. Treatment, especially palliative, should be primarily focused on QoL improvement.

Keywords

Cutaneous metastases · Quality of life · Oncology · Treatment · Questionnaires

About 10% of patients with metastatic disease have cutaneous metastases. In many of them, the skin metastases are the first sign of extranodal metastatic disease [1]. The diagnosis of metastatic cancer in an unknown primary is associated with a poor prognosis [2, 3]. A literature review on management of cutaneous metastases published in 2007 stated that the therapy occurs mostly with palliative intention, and the QoL of the patient should take first priority. For local tumor control and wound care, metastasis surgery and radiotherapy were recommended [4]. There is no established treatment for cutaneous metastases. Response to skin-directed therapy for cutaneous metastases is high but heterogeneous across treatment modalities, with low rates of recurrence post-treatment. Treatment was generally well tolerated and conferred improvements in QoL [5]. There is a scarcity of literature on cutaneous metastases, particularly on the patient experience of living with cutaneous metastases. This may indicate that the influence on QoL, caused by cancer that has spread to the skin, could be underestimated [6]. Skin metastases have a strong negative influence on the overall QoL [7]. Similar to other skin cancers, general measures may not always be sensitive enough to measure the total impact of cutaneous metastases on patients' lives. In cutaneous metastases of unknown primary, the impact of fears related to cancer may be missed when assessing QoL using generic or dermatology-specific instruments. On the other hand, in the late stages, patients' HRQoL may be severely affected by "non-skin" problems. Symptoms caused by disease progression may overshadow those caused by skin problems [8]. It is recommended, therefore, to primarily use cancer-specific HRQoL instru-

P. V. Chernyshov (✉)
Department of Dermatology and Venereology, National Medical University, Kiev, Ukraine

D. Koumaki et al. (eds.), *Cutaneous Metastases*, https://doi.org/10.1007/978-3-032-26764-1_31

ments. Dermatology-specific and generic HRQoL instruments may be used together with cancer-specific instruments to assess the total impact on a patient's life [8]. A review that focused on the two most widely used cancer-specific HRQoL instruments, the European Organisation for the Research and Treatment of Cancer Quality of Life Questionnaire Core 30 (EORTC QLQ-C30)) and the Functional Assessment of Cancer Therapy -General (FACT-G), did not recommend the use of one questionnaire over the other [9]. The characteristics of the cancer-specific instruments EORTC QLQ-C30 and FACT-G are presented in Table 31.1. Lo et al. [10] used a generic McGill QoL questionnaire to study HRQoL in patients with malignant fungating wounds. Participants were recruited from the palliative care, hospice, outpatient clinic, and oncology units. Malignant fungating wounds had a profound impact on patients' lives. The participants' age, dressing change frequency, pain, wound dressing comfort, wound symptoms, bleeding, and malodour had statistically significant negative correlations with QoL scores. Multiple regression analysis showed that age, malodour, pain issues, and psychological issues explained 87% of the total variance in QoL. Reingold et al. used the dermatology-specific HRQoL instrument, Skindex-16, to assess HRQoL of patients with cutaneous metastases before and after treatment with palliative radiotherapy [11]. Despite the overall HRQoL having a non-significant positive change in mean scores after palliative radiotherapy, the emotional scale of Skindex-16 had a significant improvement. Vestergaard et al. used interviews to collect data on QoL in patients treated with calcium electroporation for cutaneous metastases [6]. The qualitative interview was semi-structured with open-ended questions. The guide allowed change during the interview to ensure a focus on unexplored topics. The questions examined patients' emotional and physical well-being with emphasis on symptoms related to their cutaneous metastases before and after the treatment. The authors of that study considered that the HRQoL of patients improved after the treatment. An increase in HRQoL correlated with successful treatment and symptom relief. Pain relief led to better sleep and improved energy. All patients reported being able to resume activities that they had been unable to do due to pain, discomfort, cosmetic distress, or bleeding.

In general, the ultimate aim of therapy is to eradicate a disease in an individual and return the person's life to normal. But until the day comes when this has been achieved for every disease and for every patient, there will be a need to support and assist many patients in additional non-pharmaceutical ways. So the question that needs to be answered, while we await further advances in our drug-based armamentarium, is how we can improve patients' QoL beyond drugs. A working group was formed from members of the European Academy of Dermatology and Venereology Task Force on QoL and Patient-Oriented Outcomes. Participants suggested the ways in which they considered patients' QoL may be improved beyond medicines [25]. The following approaches were identified: external services (corrective make-up, climatotherapy, and balneotherapy); psychological (psychological intervention, cognitive therapy, and hypnosis); and lifestyle (lifestyle behavioral changes, religion and spirituality, and music). All these approaches were reported in cancer patients. However, most have a very poor evidence base.

The number of clinical cases of patients with cutaneous metastases contains information on HRQoL of the patients that was not, however, assessed by any instrument. Thus, Takeda et al. considered that resection of cutaneous metastasis of malignant tumors may be effective in preserving QoL even in a 100-year-old elderly patient and should be considered as an indication [12]. A chemotherapeutic treatment with gemcitabine and cisplatin resulted in the stabilization of the renal and metastatic lesions with an improvement in the QoL of the 59-year-old male patient with a subcutaneous nodule on the upper chest extending to the jugular region [13]. Luo et al., in their clinical case, reported that the rational use of individualized comprehensive treatment methods and appropriate timing of genetic testing are very important for patients with lung adenocarcinoma to prolong their survival time and improve their

Table 31.1 Brief description, scoring system, recall period, and information on validation of the most frequently used cancer-specific HRQoL instruments

Instrument title	Type	Brief description	Scoring	Recall period	Validity
The European Organisation for Research and Treatment of Cancer Core Questionnaire (EORTC QLQ-C30)	Cancer-specific	30 items (version 3.0) Five functional scales: Physical, Role, Cognitive, Emotional, Social functioning. A global QoL measure. Three symptom scales 6 single items	All of the scales and single-item measures range in score from 0 to 100. A high scale score represents a higher response level	The recall period for all but the physical functioning scale is 1 week (no recall period for physical functioning)	Test-retest reliability Internal Consistency Construct validity Responsiveness
The Functional Assessment of Cancer Therapy – General (FACT-G)	Cancer-specific	27 items (version 4) Four subscales: Physical Well-being (7 items), Social/family Well-being (7 items), Emotional Well-being (6 items), Functional Well-being (7 items)	5-point Likert scale ranging from 0 (Not at all) to 4 (Very much). Questions are phrased so that higher numbers indicate a better health state, leading to some items being reverse-scored. Scoring the FACT-G is performed through a simple sum of item scores. Higher numbers indicate a better QoL	Last 7 days	Test-retest reliability Internal Consistency Construct validity Responsiveness

QoL [14]. Nisi et al. reported a case of cutaneous upper lip metastasis from an adenocarcinoma of the gastrooesophageal junction in a 72-year-old white man, which was excised and the defect repaired with a transposition flap from the cheek [15]. Authors concluded that despite the prognosis of such lesions is poor, and the incidence of other synchronous secondary localisations is high in these cases, prompt treatment preserves the functionality and aesthetic appearance of the region, ensuring a good QoL. Masumoto and Fujiwara used the topical application of Mohs paste in a 71-year-old man with cutaneous metastasis of urothelial carcinoma, which resulted in dramatic improvement of the pain and exudate, thereby improving the patient's QoL to a level enabling discontinuation of narcotic drug therapy for cancer-related pain [16]. Kanayama et al. reported a Sister Mary Joseph nodule (SMJN) in the umbilicus of a 58-year-old female, previously diagnosed with right breast cancer 17 years ago, who underwent breast-conserving surgery, adjuvant radiotherapy, and endocrine therapy. The patient underwent extensive excision of the umbilical tumor and immediate abdominal wall reconstruction. Endocrine therapy was continued postoperatively. Five years later, no local recurrence was observed, and the patient continued to work full-time, achieving over 9 years of survival following SMJN diagnosis. The authors considered that their findings underscore the significance of adopting a multimodal treatment approach comprising timely and wide excision along with adjunctive therapy and that this approach can control the disease, prolong survival, and improve QoL in patients with SMJN [17]. Oike reported a case of a 70-year-old male with non-small cell lung cancer who was referred to the radiation oncology unit for treatment of a cutaneous metastatic tumor in the left arm. The tumor was nonresponsive to platinum-based chemotherapy and was considered unresectable. The patient was distressed by the disfigurement. Treatment with photon radiotherapy led to complete remission with no adverse effects. Authors concluded that radiotherapy for cutaneous metastatic tumors in the limbs may lead to QoL improvement [18]. Nicholson et al. reported a 62-year-old man presented with a 6-week history of shortness of breath, weight loss, and painful swelling of the great toe [19]. Biopsies of the toe swelling and bronchi both showed squamous cell carcinoma, confirmed radiologically as stage IV lung cancer. The authors concluded that cutaneous metastases and those in the digits indicate a very poor prognosis. Their prompt diagnosis and management can dramatically improve a patient's QoL and should be strived for. Falbo et al. reported a case of a solitary large skin lesion as an early manifestation of a lung adenocarcinoma [20]. The authors concluded that albeit not having a proven positive effect on survival or a curative role, mainly for lack of a sufficiently large group of patients, surgical resection can be beneficial in terms of QoL and pain reduction. D'Aniello et al. reported a case of cutaneous metastatic small cell lung carcinoma of the upper lip in a 73-year-old man, which was excised, and the defect was repaired with a single advancement flap from the cheek. The authors recognized that the prognosis of such lesions is poor and the incidence of other metastases elsewhere is high and considered that the aim of treatment was to give the patient optimal QoL for the short time left [21]. The combined application of cryosurgery and hyperthermia resulted in a greatly improved QoL of a 70-year-old woman with skin metastasis from breast cancer [22]. Lido et al. reported a case of a 54-year-old Caucasian woman with a 6-month history of a large and painful lesion on her hypogastric region, extending up to the pubic area. The lesion was ulcerated, malodorous, and bleeding. The patient received intravenous bleomycin under general anesthesia, followed by electroporation on the tumoral lesion. The authors observed a complete response in peripheral and smaller nodules, with a partial response in the biggest ones, and concluded that palliative treatment improved patients' QoL, reducing pain, smelliness, and bleeding [23].

Caracò et al., in their study on 60 patients with relapsed and refractory metastases of cutaneous melanoma treated with electrochemotherapy and intravenous injection of bleomycin, concluded that electrochemotherapy is a reliable and effective procedure that provides long-term benefit in terms of curative and palliative treatment for unresectable cutaneous lesions without adversely impacting the QoL of patients. However, patients' QoL in that study was not assessed by any HRQoL instrument [24].

The statement of Reingold et al. [10] that any improvement in HRQoL is meaningful in patients treated with palliative intent is also true for patients with cutaneous metastases.

In general, the ultimate aim of therapy is to eradicate a disease in an individual and return the person's life to normal. But until the day comes when this has been achieved for every disease and for every patient, there will be a need to support and assist many patients in additional non-pharmaceutical ways. So the question that needs to be answered, while we await further advances in our drug-based armamentarium, is how we can improve patients' QoL, beyond drugs. A working group was formed from members of the European Academy of Dermatology and Venereology Task Force on QoL and Patient-Oriented Outcomes. Participants suggested the ways in which they considered patients' QoL may be improved beyond medicines [25]. The following approaches were identified: external services (corrective make-up, climatotherapy, and balneotherapy); psychological (psychological intervention, cognitive therapy, and hypnosis); and lifestyle (lifestyle behavioral changes, religion and spirituality, and music). All these approaches were reported in cancer patients. However, most have a very poor evidence base.

31.1 Conclusion

Skin metastases have a strong negative influence on the overall QoL and are often associated with a poor prognosis. There is a lack of literature on QoL in patients with cutaneous metastases. Cancer-specific instruments (e.g., EORTC QLQ-C30 and FACT-G) should be primarily used to assess HRQoL in patients with skin metastases. Treatment, especially palliative, should be primarily focused on QoL improvement.

Conflict of Interest Author reported no conflicts of interests.

References

1. Lookingbill D, Spangler N, Helm KF. Cutaneous metastases in patients with metastatic carcinoma: a retrospective study of 4020 patients. J Am Acad Dermatol. 1993;29:228–36.
2. Carroll MC, Fleming M, Chitambar CR, Neuburg M. Diagnosis, workup, and prognosis of cutaneous metastases of unknown primar origin. Dermatologic Surg. 2002;28:533–5.
3. Azam M, Shoukfeh R, Fried S, et al. Cutaneous metastasis of gastric cancer is associated with a poor prognosis: a systematic review. Int J Dermatol. 2024;63(2):e49–51.
4. Börgermann C, Vom Dorp F, Krege S, Rübben H. Management kutaner Metastasen [The management of cutaneous metastases]. Urologe A. 2007;46(1):56–8.
5. Spratt DE, Gordon Spratt EA, Wu S, et al. Efficacy of skin-directed therapy for cutaneous metastases from advanced cancer: a meta-analysis. J Clin Oncol. 2014;32(28):3144–55.
6. Vestergaard K, Vissing M, Gehl J, Lindhardt CL. Qualitative investigation of experience and quality of life in patients treated with calcium electroporation for cutaneous metastases. Cancers (Basel). 2023;15(3):599.
7. Shimozuma K, Sonoo H, Ichihara K. Analysis of the factors influencing the quality of life of patients with advanced or recurrent breast cancer. Surg Today. 1995;25(10):874–82.
8. Chernyshov PV, Lallas A, Tomas-Aragones L, et al. Quality of life measurement in skin cancer patients: literature review and position paper of the European academy of dermatology and venereology task forces on quality of life and patient oriented outcomes, melanoma and non-melanoma skin cancer. J Eur Acad Dermatol Venereol. 2019;33(5):816–27.
9. Luckett T, King MT, Butow PN, et al. Choosing between the EORTC QLQ-C30 and FACT-G for measuring health-related quality of life in cancer clinical research: issues, evidence and recommendations. Ann Oncol. 2011;22:2179–90.
10. Lo SF, Hayter M, Hu WY, Tai CY, Hsu MY, Li YF. Symptom burden and quality of life in patients with malignant fungating wounds. J Adv Nurs. 2012;68(6):1312–21.
11. Reingold RE, Corbett BE, Blank NR, et al. Quality of life before and after treatment of cutaneous metastases with palliative radiotherapy. Am Acad Dermatol. 2022;87(4):868–70.
12. Takeda E, Toyoda Y, Yamamoto H, et al. A case of surgery for skin metastasis of papillary thyroid carcinoma in a very elderly patient to improve the quality of life. Gan To Kagaku Ryoho. 2023;50(13):1441–3.

13. Paolino G, Lido P, Bei R, Polisca P. Undifferentiated metastatic renal cell carcinoma presenting as a cutaneous nodular lesion. Turk J Urol. 2015;41(4):228–30.
14. Luo B, Rao L, Ma F, Liu X. Individualized comprehensive treatment for lung adenocarcinoma with multiple skin and bilateral breast metastasis: a case report. Zhong Nan Da Xue Xue Bao Yi Xue Ban. 2020;45(1):102–8.
15. Nisi G, Grimaldi L, Brandi C, et al. Cutaneous metastasis of the superior lip from adenocarcinoma of the gastro-oesophageal junction. A case report. Chir Ital. 2007;59(6):883–6.
16. Masumoto H, Fujiwara S. Cutaneous metastasis of urotherial carcinoma for which Mohs paste was useful: a case report. Nihon Hinyokika Gakkai Zasshi. 2017;108(1):41–4.
17. Kanayama K, Tanioka M, Hattori Y, et al. Long-term survival of the Sister Mary Joseph nodule originating from breast cancer: a case report. World J Clin Cases. 2023;11(34):8205–11.
18. Oike T, Adachi A, Shirai K, Ohno T. Unresectable cutaneous metastatic tumor in the arm that underwent complete remission after radiotherapy. Clin Case Reports. 2020;8(12):3542–4.
19. Nicholson S, Mohamed I, Tahir A, Antunes G. Primary lung cancer presenting as metastasis to the big toe. J Surg Case Rep. 2011;2011(12):5.
20. Falbo F, Krizzuk D, Urciuoli P, et al. Lung tumor skin metastasis: case report of a solitary cutaneous ulcerated lesion as initial manifestation of lung carcinoma. Case Rep Oncol. 2022;15(3):1034–8.
21. D'Aniello C, Brandi C, Grimaldi L. Cutaneous metastasis from small cell lung carcinoma. Case report. Scand J Plast Reconstr Surg Hand Surg. 2001;35(1):103–5.
22. Hachisuka J, Doi K, Furue M. Combination cryosurgery with hyperthermia in the management of skin metastasis from breast cancer: a case report. Int J Surg Case Rep. 2012;3(2):68–9.
23. Lido P, Paolino G, Feliziani A, et al. Cutaneous metastasis of unknown primary presenting as massive and invasive abdominal lesion: an elective approach with electrochemotherapy. An Bras Dermatol. 2015;90(6):879–82.
24. Caracò C, Mozzillo N, Marone U, et al. Long-lasting response to electrochemotherapy in melanoma patients with cutaneous metastasis. BMC Cancer. 2013;13:564.
25. Finlay AY, Chernyshov PV, Tomas Aragones L, et al. Methods to improve quality of life, beyond medicines. Position statement of the European Academy of Dermatology and Venereology Task Force on Quality of Life and Patient Oriented Outcomes. J Eur Acad Dermatol Venereol. 2021;35(2):318–28.

Prognosis of Cutaneous Metastasis 32

Marios Papadakis

Abstract

The development of cutaneous metastases is widely recognized as an adverse prognostic sign, most often reflecting disseminated disease and limited survival prospects. Although the frequency, clinical appearance, and outcome vary according to the primary tumor type, the presence of secondary skin lesions generally denotes an advanced stage with restricted therapeutic options.

Demographic parameters such as age and gender distribution, along with clinical features including the timing of cutaneous involvement (before or after the diagnosis of the primary tumor), multiplicity of lesions, and degree of histologic differentiation, further contribute to prognostic assessment. Importantly, extracutaneous metastatic spread is commonly observed in conjunction with cutaneous lesions. Median overall survival after the diagnosis of cutaneous metastases remains poor across most tumor entities, although variations exist depending on the tumor origin and biological aggressiveness. Prognostic and treatment-related factors, such as responsiveness to systemic therapy, tumor burden, and pattern of dissemination, also influence survival outcomes.

To provide a comprehensive overview, the following chapter collates demographic, clinical, and prognostic features across different primary tumor categories, accompanied by the appropriate references.

Keywords

Prognosis · Survival · Primary tumor · Extracutaneous metastasis · Histologic differentiation

The prognosis of cutaneous metastases depends largely on the primary tumor type, tumor biology, and the presence of systemic disease. In most malignancies, the detection of skin metastases indicates advanced-stage disease and correlates with reduced survival. However, prognosis varies across tumor entities and may be influenced by factors such as lesion number, tumor differentiation, and the presence of extracutaneous metastases. Table 32.1 summarizes the principal demographic, clinical, and prognostic characteristics reported for the most relevant primary tumors associated with cutaneous metastases.

Melanoma represents one of the most frequent malignancies associated with cutaneous metastatic spread. Metastases most commonly involve

M. Papadakis (✉)
University of Ioannina, Ioannina, Greece
e-mail: marios_papadakis@uoi.gr

D. Koumaki et al. (eds.), *Cutaneous Metastases*, https://doi.org/10.1007/978-3-032-26764-1_32

Table 32.1 Demographic, clinical, and prognostic features of cutaneous metastases for the most important primary tumor categories

Primary tumor	Mean age (y)	Male gender	Most common metastasis location	Moderately/poorly differentiated tumors	Multiple metastases	Metastasis diagnosed prior to tumor (% of cases)	Presence of extracutaneous metastases	Median overall survival	Prognostic and treatment-related factors	ReferenceS
Skin cancer										
Melanoma	64	48%	Lower extremity (45%), locoregional (80%)	Not reported	Frequent	2–8%	12%	Not reported	Metastasectomy can prolong survival in up to 40% of cases	Di Raimondo et al. [10] Kostaki et al. [15] Savoia et al. [24]
Head & neck cancer										
Squamous cell cancer	64	74%	Neck (63%)	94%	68%	Not reported	37%	7 months	*Treatment:* Local excision	Stanisce et al. [27] Yoskovitch et al. [33]
Thyroid cancer	63	45%	Scalp (35%)	Mostly well differentiated	Not reported	24% synchronous manifestation	73%	13 months	*Treatment:* Surgical excision in cases of localized lesions, followed by either radioactive iodine or radiation	Sciscent et al. [25]
Thoracic cancer										
Lung cancer	60	Not reported	Scalp, Head & Neck, chest wall	Mostly moderately differentiated.	Not reported	20–60%	Not reported	8.5 months	*Negative prognostic factors:* Nonresectability, small-cell tumors, multiple lesions. *Chemotherapy:* For cases with multiple or internal metastases. *Metastasectomy:* Improves prognosis when performed in patients with Distant solitary skin metastasis. *Radiation:* Usually not effective but may be implemented palliatively in bleeding/painful lesions	Bobba et al. [5] Alcaraz et al. [1] Mollet et al. [17]

Breast cancer	74		Chest wall	Often, very poorly differentiated	Not reported	3%	57%	Mortality >70% the first 12 months	Treatment: Systemic, based on the molecular type (HR-positive, HER2-positive, TN)	González--Martínez et al. [12] Choate et al. (2019)
Gastrointestinal cancer										
Hepato--biliary cancer	60	77%	Scalp (37%)	47%	40%	27%	43%	4 months	Negative prognostic factors: Male gender (2,5 vs. 10 months) and single metastasis (2,3 vs. 7 months) *No association:* Patient age and cutaneous metastatic site	Cazzato et al. [7] Liu et al. (2015)
Gastric cancer	60	72%	Thoraco--abdominal wall (57–63%)	98%	61%	41%	65%	6 months	Possible benefit through surgery in cases of local skin metastasis with no extracutaneous metastasis	Yao et al. [31] Azam et al. [2] Zhang et al. [35]
Colorectal cancer	58	69%	*Overall*: abdominal wall (70%) *Rectal cancer:* Perineum (57%)	50%	31%	*Overall: 52%* Rectal cancer: 4%** (*synchronous manifestation)	*Overall:* 33% *Rectal cancer:* 57%	8.5 months	*Overall:* No standardized treatment, wide excision, and reconstruction have been reported. *Rectal cancer:* High CEA levels before treatment are a negative prognostic factor for both primary tumors and skin metastases	Parente et al. [21] Tokarski et al. [29] Zelenova et al. [34]
Pancreatic cancer	63	49%–62%	Head & Neck (33%)	78%	32%	58%	74%	5 months	Treatment strategies, e.g., surgery, radiation, chemotherapy, or a combination may improve survival time from 3.0 to 8.3 months	Cassalia et al. [6] Zhou et al. [36]

(continued)

Table 32.1 (continued)

Primary tumor	Mean age (y)	Male gender	Most common metastasis location	Moderately/ poorly differentiated tumors	Multiple metastases	Metastasis diagnosed prior to tumor (% of cases)	Presence of extracutaneous metastases	Median overall survival	Prognostic and treatment-related factors	ReferenceS
Gynecologic cancer										
Ovarian cancer	68		abdominal wall	100%	Not reported	Extremely rare	100%	2.5 months	*Treatment:* Surgery for solitary lesions	Otsuka [20]
Cervical cancer	55		Scalp, lower abdominal wall, vulva	100%%	33%	Not reported	Not reported	5–6 months	*Treatment:* Surgery with or without radiotherapy for solitary lesions	Dai et al. [9] Popovic et al. [22] Shen et al. [26]
Endometrial cancer	61		Skull, vulva	Not reported	33%	Not reported	57%	4 months	*Negative prognostic factor:* A positive p53 expression rate of ≥50%. *Treatment:* Local excision for solitary lesions. Chemotherapy and radiotherapy are popular but often ineffective	Nienhaus et al. [18] Fan et al. [11]
Urologic Cancer										
Prostate cancer	66		Perineum (scrotal, inguinal, suprapubic)f, chest wall	Not reported	71%	18%	67%	8 months	No special treatment	Udupa et al. [30]
Renal cancer	61	74%	Head, chest wall, abdominal wall	Not reported	Not reported	53%	Not reported	11 months	No special treatment	Ohlsson et al. [19] Choate et al. (2019)
Bladder cancer	66	85%	abdominal wall (25%), chest wall (20%)	Not reported	Mostly solitary lesions	7%, 24% synchronous manifestation	Not reported	<12 months	*Treatment:* Not reported 38%, chemotherapy alone 17%, radiotherapy 15%, no treatment 10%, surgery for the organ with affected skin 8%	Bazzi et al. [3] Izzo et al. [14]

Primary tumor	Mean age (y)	Male gender	Most common metastasis location	Moderately/poorly differentiated tumors	Multiple metastases	Metastasis diagnosed prior to tumor (% of cases)	Presence of extracutaneous metastases	Median overall survival	Prognostic and treatment-related factors	ReferenceS
Hematological malignancies										
Leukemia cutis	46	65%	Trunk	Not reported	87%	2%, 23–44% synchronous manifestation	Virtually all patients will develop systemic disease	5–7 months	*Risk factors*: Exposure to benzene, ionizing radiation, alkylating agents, and viruses *Negative prognostic factors:* AML, T-cell prolymphocytic leukemia, and Richter syndrome	Bhutani et al. [4] Grunwald et al. [13] Robak et al. [23] Starace et al. [28] Yook et al. [32]

the lower extremities, and the majority occur in a locoregional distribution. In approximately 2–8% of cases, skin metastases precede the diagnosis of the primary melanoma. Prognosis varies considerably depending on disease burden. Surgical removal of isolated lesions may improve outcomes in selected patients, and metastasectomy has been reported to prolong survival in up to 40% of cases [10, 15, 24].

Cutaneous metastases from head and neck squamous cell carcinoma show a marked male predominance. The neck represents the most frequent metastatic site. Most tumors demonstrate moderate or poor differentiation, and multiple lesions occur in a majority of patients. The reported median overall survival is approximately 7 months. Local surgical excision is the most frequently described therapeutic approach [27, 33].

In thyroid carcinoma, the scalp represents the most common location of cutaneous metastases. Most tumors are well differentiated. Skin metastases occur synchronously with the primary tumor in approximately one-quarter of cases. Median overall survival has been reported at approximately 13 months [25].

Among thoracic malignancies, lung cancer frequently produces cutaneous metastases. Lesions typically involve the scalp, head and neck region, or chest wall. In 20–60% of cases, cutaneous metastases precede the diagnosis of the primary lung tumor. The reported median overall survival is approximately 8.5 months. Poor prognostic factors include unresectable disease, small-cell histology, and multiple lesions. Systemic chemotherapy is commonly used in patients with disseminated disease, whereas metastasectomy may improve prognosis in selected patients with solitary lesions. Radiotherapy generally serves a palliative role, particularly in symptomatic lesions [1, 5, 17].

Breast carcinoma represents one of the most common sources of cutaneous metastases. The chest wall is the most frequent site of involvement. Tumors are often poorly differentiated, and mortality exceeds 70% within the first year after the diagnosis of cutaneous metastases. Treatment is primarily systemic and depends on the molecular subtype of the tumor, including hormone receptor–positive, HER2-positive, and triple--negative disease [12, 8].

Among gastrointestinal malignancies, hepatobiliary cancers demonstrate a strong male predominance. The scalp represents the most common metastatic site. Multiple lesions occur in about 40% of patients. Median survival is approximately 4 months. Male sex and the presence of solitary cutaneous metastasis have been associated with worse survival, whereas patient age and the specific skin location appear to have no significant prognostic impact [7, 16].

Cutaneous metastases from gastric carcinoma most frequently involve the thoracoabdominal wall. Poorly differentiated tumors are common, and multiple lesions occur in the majority of patients. The reported median survival is about 6 months. Surgical treatment may offer benefit in selected patients with localized cutaneous metastases and no visceral involvement [2, 31, 35].

Colorectal carcinoma may also produce cutaneous metastases. The abdominal wall represents the most frequent location, whereas rectal cancers often metastasize to the perineal region. Approximately one-third of patients develop multiple lesions. Median overall survival has been reported at approximately 8.5 months. No standardized treatment strategy exists. Wide surgical excision and reconstruction have been described in selected cases. In rectal carcinoma, elevated pre-treatment carcinoembryonic antigen (CEA) levels represent a negative prognostic factor for both the primary tumor and the associated cutaneous metastases [21, 29, 34].

Pancreatic carcinoma produces cutaneous metastases with a particularly unfavorable prognosis. Lesions frequently involve the head and neck region. Extracutaneous metastases occur in nearly three-quarters of patients. Median survival is approximately 5 months. Combined treatment strategies, including surgery, radiotherapy, chemotherapy, or multimodal approaches, may extend survival from roughly 3 to 8 months in selected patients [6, 36].

Among gynecologic malignancies, ovarian carcinoma frequently metastasizes to the abdominal wall. Tumors are usually poorly differentiated, and systemic dissemination is common. Median survival has been reported at approximately 2.5 months. Surgical excision may be considered for isolated lesions [20].

Cutaneous metastases from cervical carcinoma may involve the scalp, lower abdominal wall, or vulva. Approximately one-third of patients present with multiple lesions. Median survival ranges from 5 to 6 months. Surgical excision, with or without radiotherapy, represents the most frequently described treatment for solitary lesions [9, 22, 26].

Endometrial carcinoma may produce cutaneous metastases involving the skull or vulva. Extracutaneous metastases occur in more than half of cases. Median survival is approximately 4 months. High p53 expression (≥50%) has been associated with worse prognosis. Local excision may be performed for isolated lesions, although chemotherapy and radiotherapy often show limited effectiveness [11, 18].

Among urologic malignancies, prostate carcinoma metastasizes to the skin primarily in the perineal region, including the scrotal, inguinal, and suprapubic areas, as well as the chest wall. Multiple lesions occur in most patients, and extracutaneous metastases are common. Median survival has been reported at approximately 8 months [30].

Renal cell carcinoma frequently produces cutaneous metastases involving the head, chest wall, or abdominal wall. In more than half of cases, skin metastases precede the diagnosis of the primary tumor. Median survival is approximately 11 months [8, 19].

Bladder carcinoma rarely metastasizes to the skin but typically indicates advanced disease. Lesions most commonly occur on the abdominal or chest wall and are often solitary. Reported survival rarely exceeds 12 months. Treatment strategies vary and include chemotherapy, radiotherapy, and surgical approaches [3, 14].

Hematologic malignancies may also present with cutaneous involvement. Leukemia cutis often manifests with multiple nodular lesions on the trunk. Nearly all patients develop systemic disease during the course of the illness. Median survival ranges between 5 and 7 months. Poor prognostic factors include acute myeloid leukemia, T-cell prolymphocytic leukemia, and Richter syndrome. Environmental and therapeutic exposures such as benzene, ionizing radiation, alkylating agents, and viral infections represent recognized risk factors [4, 13, 23, 28, 32].

References

1. Alcaraz I, Cerroni L, Rütten A, Kutzner H, Requena L. Cutaneous metastases from internal malignancies: a clinicopathologic and immunohistochemical review. Am J Dermatopathol. 2012;34(4):347–93.
2. Azam M, Shoukfeh R, Fried S, Rehman S, Rehman W, Rehman R, Mehregan D. Cutaneous metastasis of gastric cancer is associated with a poor prognosis: a systematic review. Int J Dermatol. 2024;63(2):e49–51. https://doi.org/10.1111/ijd.16839.
3. Bazzi N, Jaber S, Saad WA, Al Hassan S, Dbouk S, Alhousseini A. Cutaneous metastasis of bladder cancer: a systematic review. Cureus. 2024;16(11):e74439. https://doi.org/10.7759/cureus.74439.
4. Bhutani M, Shahid Z, Schnebelen A, Alapat D, Usmani SZ. Cutaneous manifestations of multiple myeloma and other plasma cell proliferative disorders. Semin Oncol. 2016;43(3):395–400.
5. Bobba RK, Odem JL, Doll DC, Perry MC. Skin metastases in non-small cell lung cancer. Am J Med Sci. 2012;344(1):59–62. https://doi.org/10.1097/MAJ.0b013e31823e5ec1.
6. Cassalia F, Bolzon A, Ponzano M, Ventura L, Danese A, Del Fiore P, Belloni Fortina A, Jovine E, Perri G, Cillo U, Marchegiani G. The importance of reading the skin: cutaneous metastases of pancreatic cancer, a systematic review. J Clin Med. 2023;13(1):104. https://doi.org/10.3390/jcm13010104.
7. Cazzato G, Colagrande A, Cimmino A, De Marco A, Romita P, Foti C, Resta L, Ingravallo G. Cutaneous metastases from primary liver cancers: the need for knowledge and differential diagnosis. Life (Basel). 2021;11(6):559. https://doi.org/10.3390/life11060559.
8. Choate EA, Nobori A, Worswick S. Cutaneous Metastasis of Internal Tumors. Dermatol Clin. 2019;37(4):545–554
9. Dai Y, Zhang Y, Ke X, Liu Y, Zang C. Cutaneous metastasis from cervical cancer to the scalp and trunk: a case report and review of the literature. J Med Case Rep. 2023;17(1):435. https://doi.org/10.1186/s13256-023-04171-x.
10. Di Raimondo C, Lozzi F, Di Domenico PP, Campione E, Bianchi L. The diagnosis and management of cutaneous metastases from melanoma. Int J Mol Sci. 2023;24(19):14535. https://doi.org/10.3390/ijms241914535.
11. Fan Y, Deng H, Tian L, Wang J. Cutaneous metastases of endometrial carcinoma: report

of an unusual case and literature review. Arch Gynecol Obstet. 2021;304(5):1127–33. https://doi.org/10.1007/s00404-021-06165-w.
12. González-Martínez S, Pizarro D, Pérez-Mies B, Caniego-Casas T, Curigliano G, Cortés J, Palacios J. Clinical, pathological, and molecular features of breast carcinoma cutaneous metastasis. Cancers (Basel). 2021;13(21):5416. https://doi.org/10.3390/cancers13215416.
13. Grunwald MR, McDonnell MH, Induru R, Gerber JM. Cutaneous manifestations in leukemia patients. Semin Oncol. 2016;43(3):359–65. https://doi.org/10.1053/j.seminoncol.2016.02.020.
14. Izzo P, Izzo L, Lai S, D'Onghia G, Giancontieri P, Gabriele R, Polistena A, Sibio S, Costanzo ML, De Intinis C, Izzo S. Nodular cutaneous metastasis of the leg in advanced urothelial bladder carcinoma: a case report and systematic literature review. Front Oncol. 2023;13:1216725. https://doi.org/10.3389/fonc.2023.1216725.
15. Kostaki M, Plaka M, Moustaki M, Befon A, Champsas G, Kypreou K, Chardalia V, Chasapi V, Polydorou D, Stratigos A. Cutaneous melanoma metastases: clinical and dermoscopic findings. J Eur Acad Dermatol Venereol. 2023;37(5):941–4. https://doi.org/10.1111/jdv.18701.
16. Liu M, Liu BL, Liu B, Guo L, Wang Q, Song YQ, Dong LH. Cutaneous metastasis of cholangiocarcinoma. World J Gastroenterol. 2015;21(10):3066–71
17. Mollet TW, Garcia CA, Koester G. Skin metastases from lung cancer. Dermatol Online J. 2009;15(5):1.
18. Nienhaus A, Rajakulendran R, Bernad E. Cutaneous metastasis of endometrial cancer and long-term survival: a scoping review and our experience. Diagnostics (Basel). 2023;13(15):2603. https://doi.org/10.3390/diagnostics13152603.
19. Ohlsson R, Geertsen L, Berge Stuveseth S, Lund L. Cutaneous metastases in renal cell carcinoma: a systematic review and a case report. Scand J Urol. 2019;53(1):9–13. https://doi.org/10.1080/21681805.2019.1585473.
20. Otsuka I. Cutaneous metastases in ovarian cancer. Cancers (Basel). 2019;11(9):1292. https://doi.org/10.3390/cancers11091292.
21. Parente P, Ciardiello D, Reggiani Bonetti L, Famiglietti V, Cazzato G, Caramaschi S, Attino V, Urbano D, Di Maggio G, Ingravallo G. Cutaneous metastasis from colorectal cancer: making light on an unusual and misdiagnosed event. Life (Basel). 2021;11(9):954. https://doi.org/10.3390/life11090954.
22. Popovic A, Bojic MD, Bojic M, Vukmirovic F, Juskovic A. Cutaneous metastases of cervical cancer: a rare entity and possible mechanisms of dissemination. Postepy Dermatol Alergol. 2024;41(1):136–8.
23. Robak E, Braun M, Robak T. Leukemia cutis-the current view on pathogenesis, diagnosis, and treatment. Cancers (Basel). 2023;15(22):5393. https://doi.org/10.3390/cancers15225393.
24. Savoia P, Fava P, Nardò T, Osella-Abate S, Quaglino P, Bernengo MG. Skin metastases of malignant melanoma: a clinical and prognostic survey. Melanoma Res. 2009;19(5):321–6. https://doi.org/10.1097/CMR.0b013e32832ac775.
25. Sciscent BY, Eberly HW, Goyal N, Goldenberg D. Thyroid cancer with cutaneous metastases. Ear Nose Throat J. 2024:1455613241239533. https://doi.org/10.1177/01455613241239533.
26. Shen Y, Jin X, Zhu Y, He C. Clinical analysis of patients with skin metastasis of cervical squamous cell carcinoma. Chin Clin Oncol. 2024;13(3):35. https://doi.org/10.21037/cco-24-60.
27. Stanisce L, Comess SR, Chai R, Khan MN, Brandwein-Weber M, Urken ML. Dermal metastasis from head and neck squamous cell carcinoma: systematic review and pooled analysis. Laryngoscope. 2025;
28. Starace M, Cedirian S, Rapparini L. Clinical aspects of cutaneous metastasis from non-cutaneous primary tumors. Cancers (Basel). 2025;17(19):3126.
29. Tokarski E, Conan PL, Picchi H, Malgras B, Peroux E, Ezanno AC. Prognostic implications of cutaneous metastases in colorectal cancer: a comprehensive systematic review and meta-analysis. Cancer Med. 2025;14(18):e71197.
30. Udupa M, Qian SY, Udupa S, Pehr K. Clinical presentations and outcomes of cutaneous metastases from prostate cancer: a systematic review. J Am Acad Dermatol. 2025:S0190-9622(25)02219–4. https://doi.org/10.1016/j.jaad.2025.05.1430.
31. Yao GL, Tao YJ, Fan YG. Cutaneous metastasis from gastric cancer: manifestation, diagnosis, treatment and prognosis. Eur J Surg Oncol. 2024;50(2):107939. https://doi.org/10.1016/j.ejso.2023.107939.
32. Yook HJ, Son JH, Kim YH, Han JH, Lee JH, Park YM, Chung NG, Kim HJ, Bang CH. Leukaemia cutis: clinical features and outcomes of 56 patients. Acta Derm Venereol. 2022;102:adv00647. https://doi.org/10.2340/actadv.v102.1123.
33. Yoskovitch A, Hier MP, Okrainec A, Black MJ, Rochon L. Skin metastases in squamous cell carcinoma of the head and neck. Otolaryngol Head Neck Surg. 2001;124(3):248–52. https://doi.org/10.1067/mhn.2001.113036.
34. Zelenova E, Belysheva T, Sofronov D, Semenova V, Radjabova G, Vishnevskaya Y, Kletskaya I, Sharapova E, Karasev I, Romanov D, Denieva M, Petrochenko N, Valiev T, Nasedkina T. Cutaneous metastasis of rectal cancer as a diagnostic challenge: a clinical case and literature review. Diagnostics (Basel). 2024;14(21):2420. https://doi.org/10.3390/diagnostics14212420.
35. Zhang LW, Wang WJ, Chen T, Xu RH. Cutaneous metastasis from gastric carcinoma. Cleve Clin J Med. 2023;90(9):533–4.
36. Zhou HY, Wang XB, Gao F, Bu B, Zhang S, Wang Z. Cutaneous metastasis from pancreatic cancer: a case report and systematic review of the literature. Oncol Lett. 2014;8(6):2654–60. https://doi.org/10.3892/ol.2014.2610.

Part XVIII

Advances in Research and Future Directions in Cutaneous Metastasis

Imaging and Diagnostic Techniques in Cutaneous Metastases

33

Georgios Evangelou

Abstract

Conventional imaging techniques, including CT, MRI, ultrasound, Doppler sonography, and ^{18}F-FDG PET/CT, are commonly employed in oncology to stage and monitor disease progression and to assess treatment response. Their increased sensitivity and specificity have enabled the detection of early skin lesions or underlying tumors that may indicate metastatic disease. These methods are widely used to identify skin metastasis from various cancers such as lung, breast, mesothelioma, neuroendocrine tumors, and colorectal cancers. Such findings often prompt additional diagnostic tests and histopathological confirmation. Continued use of these techniques is vital for improving cancer monitoring and detecting unusual skin metastatic presentations at an early stage.

Keywords

Cutaneous metastases · Imaging techniques · Ultrasound Doppler sonography · Reflectance confocal microscopy · Optical coherence tomography

G. Evangelou (✉)
Consultant Dermatologist University Hospital of Crete, Crete, Greece

33.1 Ultrasound Doppler Sonography

Ultrasound and Doppler sonography have long been recognized as vital diagnostic tools for assessing superficial and subcutaneous lesions. Numerous case reports and reviews by experienced radiologists highlight their usefulness in detecting skin abnormalities that may indicate underlying malignancy. As a non-invasive, economical, and easily accessible imaging modality, ultrasonography is particularly effective for examining firm, painless nodules located within the dermis or subcutaneous tissue [1].

The addition of color Doppler imaging markedly improves diagnostic capabilities by enabling the evaluation of vascular features, which are key indicators in distinguishing between benign and malignant lesions. Doppler assessment can show increased vascular flow, often linked to tumor-induced neovascularization.

However, the accuracy of this technique depends heavily on the operator's skill and can be subjective, especially in less typical cases such as cutaneous metastases. Therefore, diagnostic interpretation must be integrated with clinical findings and relies considerably on the radiologist's expertise [2].

A useful framework for interpreting vascular patterns was proposed by Giovagnorio et al., who classified lesions based on Doppler features. Avascular patterns generally suggest benign pro-

D. Koumaki et al. (eds.), *Cutaneous Metastases*, https://doi.org/10.1007/978-3-032-26764-1_33

Table 33.1 Doppler vascular patterns in cutaneous lesions (adapted from Giovagnorio et al.)

Vascular pattern	Doppler characteristics	Interpretation
Avascular	No detectable flow	Likely benign
Hypovascular	Scattered low-velocity peripheral flow	Possibly benign
Hypervascular (peripheral)	High-velocity flow localized to the lesion periphery	Suggestive of malignancy
Hypervascular (internal)	Chaotic, multidirectional flow within the lesion core	Strong suspicion of metastasis
Rim vascularity	Vascular ring around the necrotic lesion core	Indicative of rapid tumor growth

cesses, while hypervascular lesions—particularly those with peripheral or internal flow—are more suspicious for metastases [3] (Table 33.1).

These vascular patterns often mirror the angiogenic processes characteristic of malignant tumors, which promote the development of fragile, irregular vessels. In more advanced lesions, rapid tumor growth may cause central necrosis due to inadequate blood supply, resulting in a peripheral rim of vascularity.

Efforts to link lesion size with detectable vascularity on Doppler imaging have yielded inconsistent results. Some studies suggest a diagnostic threshold of 0.7–0.9 cm, below which vascular signals may be minimal or absent, complicating assessment. Others recommend a higher cutoff around 1.5–1.8 cm, citing better detection in larger nodules. These differences highlight the limitations of relying solely on ultrasonography and emphasize the importance of a multimodal diagnostic approach.

Although ultrasound is a practical and efficient first-line tool for identifying potentially malignant lesions, it may not provide a definitive diagnosis. In such cases, advanced imaging techniques—such as MRI, CT, or ^ 18 F- FDG PET/CT—are often necessary to obtain detailed anatomical and functional information, supporting both detection and accurate staging of metastatic disease.

33.2 Magnetic Resonance Imaging (MRI)

Magnetic Resonance Imaging (MRI) is particularly valuable for assessing deep-seated tumor lesions and their extension into underlying soft tissues. MRI's effectiveness is further enhanced when using T1- and T2-weighted sequences, along with contrast agents, providing excellent visualization of the vascular architecture and tissue composition. The contrast enhancement highlights abnormal neovascularization, allowing radiologists to distinguish malignant infiltration from benign processes with high sensitivity, thereby reassuring them of its effectiveness in evaluating deep-seated tumor lesions.

While MRI excels in evaluating deeper tissue involvement, it is comparatively less effective for imaging lesions located in the superficial layers of the skin, such as the epidermis and upper dermis. In these cases, computed tomography (CT) scans often provide better spatial resolution and are more adept at characterizing cutaneous or subcutaneous lesions that are close to the surface. CT imaging can delineate lesion margins and detect subtle changes in soft tissue density, making it a valuable tool for evaluating more superficial suspicious skin nodules.

The decision to utilize either CT or MRI is dependent on the anatomical depth and on the clinical presentation, location, and depth of the lesion, aiming to maximize diagnostic yield. For superficial or dermal lesions, CT is often preferred due to its higher resolution for shallow structures. At the same time, MRI is reserved for cases where deeper infiltration or soft tissue extension is suspected. This tailored imaging approach enhances diagnostic accuracy and ensures optimal visualization of cutaneous metastases across varying tissue depths [4, 5] (Table 33.2).

Table 33.2 Comparative utility of imaging modalities in cutaneous metastases

Modality	Best for	Limitations	Imaging depth
Ultrasound/Doppler	Superficial nodules, vascularity	Operator-dependent, limited deep visualization	~5–10 mm
CT	Superficial-to-mid dermal lesions	Radiation exposure, lower soft tissue contrast	Full body
MRI	Deep infiltration, soft tissue evaluation	Less effective for epidermal lesions	Full body
^18F-FDG PET/CT	Functional imaging, whole-body screening	False positives in inflammation	Full body

33.3 18F-FDG PET/CT

18F-fluorodeoxyglucose positron emission tomography/computed tomography (18F-FDG PET/CT) represents a significant advancement in functional imaging, enabling the assessment of metabolic activity in tissues. This hybrid imaging technique combines the anatomical detail of CT with the metabolic sensitivity of PET, allowing early detection of malignancies based on glucose uptake—often before structural abnormalities are visible. In cases of suspected cutaneous metastases (CM), PET/CT can provide vital insights by detecting hypermetabolic lesions that may precede visible or palpable clinical signs [6].

Despite its potential, the specificity of 18F-FDG PET/CT in diagnosing CM remains a subject of ongoing discussion in the literature. While many studies report high diagnostic sensitivity and yield for metastatic skin lesions, others express concerns about their potential for false positives. Increased FDG uptake has been observed not only in malignant lesions but also in various benign dermatologic conditions. False-positive results have been reported in cases involving skin folds, actinic keratoses, chronic inflammatory dermatoses, and other skin disorders that can mimic malignancy both metabolically and morphologically. These atypical findings complicate interpretation and underscore the importance of correlating PET/CT results with clinical and histopathologic data [7, 8].

One of the most widely used quantitative measures in PET imaging is the maximum standardized uptake value (SUVmax), which indicates the extent of FDG accumulation within a lesion. Higher SUVmax values are generally linked to increased metabolic activity and often suggest malignancy. In suspected CM, a markedly elevated SUVmax may heighten clinical suspicion and justify further investigation. Moreover, PET/CT offers the significant advantage of evaluating lesions located in deeper tissues—beyond the reach of traditional imaging modalities such as ultrasound or dermoscopy—especially when lesion thickness exceeds 6–9 mm, a range where conventional techniques often struggle [9].

However, the limited number of published reports focusing specifically on the utility of 18F-FDG PET/CT in cutaneous metastasis limits the strength of the available evidence. Therefore, while PET/CT is a valuable addition in oncologic imaging, its role in the definitive diagnosis of CM should be approached with caution. A multidisciplinary approach that combines clinical assessment, histological confirmation, and appropriate imaging is essential for accurate diagnosis and effective management.

33.4 Reflectance Confocal Microscopy (RCM)

Reflectance confocal microscopy (RCM) is a non-invasive imaging technique that provides high-resolution, cellular-level images of the skin with an effective imaging depth of up to approximately 300 μm. This capability enables detailed visualization of the epidermis and upper dermis, including the reticular dermal layer, making RCM a valuable tool for identifying cell-to-cell architectural changes that may indicate malignancy. In contrast, optical coherence tomography (OCT) offers deeper tissue penetration, reaching depths of approximately 1000–2000 μm, though with reduced resolution compared to RCM.

When utilized in the evaluation of cutaneous metastases (CM), RCM can reveal key morphological features indicative of malignancy. These include clusters of large, polygonal or oval reflective cells with centrally located hyporeflective areas—features that are often interpreted as signs of metastatic infiltration. Additional findings, such as dense collagen bundles, dilated blood vessels, and infiltration by inflammatory cells, have been reported in the RCM literature as suggestive of a stromal response to neoplastic growth.

Although RCM has demonstrated precise diagnostic capability in non-melanocytic skin tumors such as basal cell carcinoma (BCC) and trichoepithelioma, reports documenting its successful use in detecting cutaneous metastases from internal solid tumors—such as bladder adenocarcinoma and breast cancer—remain limited. One of the primary limitations of RCM is its restricted imaging depth, which prevents reliable assessment of lesions located beneath the reticular dermis.

Consequently, deeply seated or marginally located metastatic lesions may be overlooked, especially if they are small or lack clear surface manifestations.

This limitation highlights the need for complementary use of imaging modalities, such as OCT or traditional biopsy, to ensure accurate detection and diagnosis of deeper or less conspicuous cutaneous metastases [10–12] (Table 33.3).

Table 33.3 Key confocal microscopy (RCM) features in cutaneous metastases

RCM feature	Interpretation
Reflective polygonal/oval cells	Atypical tumor cell clusters
Central hyporeflective area in cells	Nuclear displacement or cytoplasmic clearing
Dense collagen bundles	Stromal reaction to tumor infiltration
Enlarged, irregular blood vessels	Neovascularization
Inflammatory infiltrates	Stromal immune response to neoplastic cells

33.5 Optical Coherence Tomography (OCT)

Optical Coherence Tomography (OCT) is a non-invasive imaging technique that employs low-coherence light to produce high-resolution cross-sectional images of biological tissues. Although the published data on OCT specifically related to the detection of cutaneous metastases (CM) remains limited, its potential in oncologic dermatology is increasingly recognized. One of the key advantages of OCT lies in its ability to visualize structures at greater tissue depths compared to other non-invasive techniques such as reflectance confocal microscopy (RCM) [13].

OCT can image structures to a depth of approximately 1000–2000 μm, thereby extending its utility into the mid-to-deep dermis. However, this increase in depth comes at the expense of image resolution, making it less effective for fine morphological analysis compared to RCM. OCT is beneficial in detecting lesions located around 1000 μm in depth but tends to show reduced sensitivity for detecting smaller or deeper abnormalities beyond this threshold [14].

OCT has been shown to be effective in outlining the peripheral margins of suspicious lesions, making it a valuable tool for guiding biopsy procedures and improving diagnostic accuracy. Characteristic OCT features associated with CM may include grayish to dark nodular formations of varying sizes, surrounded by reactive stromal tissue. These structures are often accompanied by coarse, hyperreflective collagen bundles and enlarged, hyporeflective, tubular-shaped blood vessels, which may represent tumor-induced neovascularization and stromal remodeling [15].

Given its vertical imaging capability and ability to penetrate up to 1–2 mm into the dermis, OCT complements the high lateral resolution and superficial cellular detail offered by reflectance confocal microscopy (RCM). While OCT alone provides crucial information about lesion architecture and depth, the combination of OCT and RCM offers a synergistic approach to non-invasive CM diagnosis [16, 17].

The integration of these two modalities allows for a comprehensive evaluation—RCM contributing detailed horizontal reflectance at the cellular level, and OCT providing vertical depth information necessary for assessing lesion extent. Such a dual-modality strategy enhances pre-biopsy lesion characterization, potentially reducing unnecessary invasive procedures and optimizing sampling accuracy. Although further clinical validation is required, OCT, especially when used in conjunction with RCM, holds promise for improving early identification and evaluation of cutaneous metastases.

33.6 Dermoscopy

Dermoscopy has gained increasing recognition as a valuable diagnostic tool for the early assessment of cutaneous metastases (CM), especially when used before histological confirmation. However, the limited number of published dermoscopic case reports hampers the development of standardized diagnostic criteria. Most of the existing literature comprises isolated observations, which, while suggestive of underlying malignancy, do not offer definitive diagnostic benchmarks. Experienced clinicians using dermoscopy can gather important visual clues about the morphology and vascular features of suspicious lesions. When used systematically, this technique helps distinguish CM from benign skin lesions and other primary cutaneous neoplasms (see Sect. 1.3) [18–23].

33.7 Histopathological Evaluation of Cutaneous Metastases

Histopathological analysis is crucial in understanding the underlying mechanisms involved in the seeding and growth of cutaneous metastases (CM). As shown in a retrospective study by Fernandez-Flores, CM usually displays six distinct morphological patterns: nodular, infiltrative, diffuse, intravascular, and the top-heavy and bottom-heavy distributions. Among these, the infiltrative pattern is most often linked to breast cancer metastases, whereas colorectal carcinoma tends to show a nodular growth pattern [24] (Table 33.4).

Table 33.4 Histopathologic patterns of cutaneous metastases

Pattern	Typical primary tumor	Localization
Nodular	Colorectal carcinoma	Dermis/subcutis
Infiltrative	Breast carcinoma	Diffuse dermal spread
Diffuse	Melanoma, neuroendocrine tumors	Uniform dermal extension
Intravascular	Lung, gastric adenocarcinoma	Dermal vessels
Top-heavy	Lung, renal cell carcinoma	Upper dermis
Bottom-heavy	Breast, pancreatic carcinoma	Lower dermis/subcutis

Routine Hematoxylin and Eosin (H&E) staining, though fundamental in histopathology, often struggles to definitively identify the primary source of CM. This difficulty largely arises from the histologic resemblance between metastatic deposits and primary skin cancers, which presents significant diagnostic challenges. In some instances, identifying specific cell types—such as signet-ring cells—may suggest a gastrointestinal origin. Additional H&E features like focal vascular invasion or intraglandular neutrophilic infiltrates can also raise suspicion of metastatic disease. However, these signs are not always present, creating gaps in diagnostic certainty when such features are absent [25].

Epidermotropism—a key feature of some primary cutaneous malignancies—is quite rare in CMs, which explains their typical localization within the dermis or subcutis rather than the epidermis. This observation is supported by studies, including those by Yiping Gan et al. and Guanziroli et al., which consistently report minimal or no epidermal involvement in CM cases. The lack of epidermal infiltration likely accounts for the infrequent ulceration seen in CMs, contrasting with the more common ulceration observed in primary cutaneous malignancies [26–28].

Other frequently observed histological features in CM include vascular invasion, necrosis, and mild peritumoral inflammatory infiltrates. While these findings support malignancy, they are nonspecific and must be interpreted carefully within the clinical context.

To overcome these limitations, immunohistochemical (IHC) staining has become an essential tool in diagnosing CM. Comprehensive IHC panels enable more precise characterization of tumor origin and behavior, particularly in cases of metastatic carcinoma of unknown primary or when differentiating CM from adnexal tumors. Modern diagnostic approaches heavily depend on immunophenotyping to determine diagnosis and guide subsequent treatment decisions, especially in complex or ambiguous cases [29, 30].

Ultimately, combining H&E morphology with targeted immunohistochemistry is vital for resolving differential diagnostic challenges, especially in distinguishing CM from primary cutaneous malignancies. This integrated approach improves diagnostic accuracy and supports better-informed therapeutic management.

References

1. Scotto Di Santolo M, Sagnelli M, Mancini M, Scalvenzi M, Delfino M, Schonauer F, et al. High-resolution color-Doppler ultrasound for the study of skin growths. Arch Dermatol Res. 2015;307(7):559–66.
2. Toprak H, Kiliç E, Serter A, Kocakoç E, Ozgocmen S. Ultrasound and Doppler US in evaluation of superficial soft-tissue lesions. J Clin Imaging Sci. 2014;4:12.
3. Giovagnorio F, Andreoli C, De Cicco ML. Color Doppler sonography of focal lesions of the skin and subcutaneous tissue. J Ultrasound Med. 1999;18(2):89–93.
4. Ginat D, Lotfian G. Review of diagnostic radiology imaging modalities for evaluating skin lesions involving the head and neck. Med Res Arch [Internet]. 2024 [cited 2025 July 27];12(10). Available from: https://esmed.org/MRA/mra/article/view/5763
5. Shu H, Ma Q, Li A, Wang P, Gao Y, Yao Q, et al. Diagnostic performance of US and MRI in predicting malignancy of soft tissue masses: using a scoring system. Front Oncol. 2022;12:853232.
6. Boellaard R, Delgado-Bolton R, Oyen WJG, Giammarile F, Tatsch K, Eschner W, et al. FDG PET/CT: EANM procedure guidelines for tumour imaging: version 2.0. Eur J Nucl Med Mol Imaging. 2015;42(2):328–54.
7. Blumer SL, Scalcione LR, Ring BN, Johnson R, Motroni B, Katz DS, et al. Cutaneous and subcutaneous imaging on FDG-PET: benign and malignant findings. Clin Nucl Med. 2009;34(10):675–83.
8. Bingham BA, Hatef DA, Chevez-Barrios P, Blackmon SH, Kim MP. Increased FDG activity in a dermatofibroma in esophageal cancer patient. Clin Nucl Med. 2013;38(3):e140–2.
9. Weiss GJ, Korn RL. Interpretation of PET scans: do not take SUVs at face value. J Thorac Oncol. 2012;7(12):1744–6.
10. Hartmann D, Ruini C, Mathemeier L, Bachmann MR, Dietrich A, Ruzicka T, et al. Identification of *ex-vivo* confocal laser scanning microscopic features of melanocytic lesions and their histological correlates. J Biophotonics. 2017;10(1):128–42.
11. Iftimia N, Peterson G, Chang EW, Maguluri G, Fox W, Rajadhyaksha M. Combined reflectance confocal microscopy-optical coherence tomography for delineation of basal cell carcinoma margins: an *ex vivo* study. J Biomed Opt. 2016;21(1):016006.
12. Ilie M, Caruntu C, Lupu M, Lixandru D, Tampa M, Georgescu SR, et al. Current and future applications of confocal laser scanning microscopy imaging in skin oncology (Review). Oncol Lett [Internet]. 2019 [cited 2025 July 27]; Available from: http://www.spandidos-publications.com/10.3892/ol.2019.10066
13. Fujimoto JG, Pitris C, Boppart SA, Brezinski ME. Optical coherence tomography: an emerging technology for biomedical imaging and optical biopsy. Neoplasia. 2000;2(1–2):9–25.
14. Huang D, Swanson EA, Lin CP, Schuman JS, Stinson WG, Chang W, et al. Optical coherence tomography. Science. 1991;254(5035):1178–81.
15. Welzel J. Optical coherence tomography in dermatology: a review. Skin Res Technol. 2001;7(1):1–9.
16. Olsen J, Holmes J, Jemec GBE. Advances in optical coherence tomography in dermatology—a review. J Biomed Opt. 2018;23(04):1.
17. Mogensen M, Thrane L, Joergensen TM, Andersen PE, Jemec GBE. Optical coherence tomography for imaging of skin and skin diseases. Semin Cutan Med Surg. 2009;28(3):196–202.
18. Raika AE, Sidhoma E, Hasnere S. Dermoscopic findings in cases of cutaneous metastases. Open Dermatol J. 2022;16(1):e187437222112211.
19. Chernoff KA, Marghoob AA, Lacouture ME, Deng L, Busam KJ, Myskowski PL. Dermoscopic findings in cutaneous metastases. JAMA Dermatol. 2014;150(4):429.
20. Kelati A, Gallouj S. Dermoscopy of skin metastases from breast cancer: two case reports. J Med Case Rep. 2018;12(1):273.
21. Rubegni P, Lamberti A, Mandato F, Perotti R, Fimiani M. Dermoscopic patterns of cutaneous melanoma metastases. Int J Dermatol. 2014;53(4):404–12.
22. Soares GH, Lallas A, Lombardi M, Longo C, Moscarella E, Raucci M, et al. Cutaneous metastasis of renal carcinoma. J Am Acad Dermatol. 2015;72(1):S45–6.

23. Jaimes N, Halpern JA, Puig S, Malvehy J, Myskowski PL, Braun RP, et al. Dermoscopy: an aid to the detection of amelanotic cutaneous melanoma metastases. Dermatologic Surg. 2012;38(9):1437–44.
24. Fernandez-Flores A. Cutaneous metastases: a study of 78 biopsies from 69 patients. Am J Dermatopathol. 2010;32(3):222–39.
25. Sariya D, Ruth K, Adams-McDonnell R, Cusack C, Xu X, Elenitsas R, et al. Clinicopathologic correlation of cutaneous metastases: experience from a cancer center. Arch Dermatol [Internet]. 2007 May 1 [cited 2025 July 28];143(5). Available from: http://archderm.jamanetwork.com/article.aspx?doi=10.1001/archderm.143.5.613
26. Guanziroli E, Coggi A, Venegoni L, Fanoni D, Ercoli G, Boggio F, et al. Cutaneous metastases of internal malignancies: an experience from a single institution. Eur J Dermatol. 2017;27(6):609–14.
27. Guanziroli E, Coggi A, Venegoni L, et al. Cutaneous metastases: a retrospective study of 132 patients. Dermatol Pr Concept. 2018;8(3):238–44.
28. Gan EY, Chio MT, Tan WP. A retrospective review of cutaneous metastases at the N ational S kin C entre S ingapore. Australas J Dermatol. 2015;56(1):1–6.
29. Saeed S, Keehn CA, Morgan MB. Cutaneous metastasis: a clinical, pathological, and immunohistochemical appraisal. J Cutan Pathol. 2004;31(6):419–30.
30. Weimann ETDS, Botero EB, Mendes C, Santos MASD, Stelini RF, Zelenika CRT. Cutaneous metastasis as the first manifestation of occult malignant breast neoplasia. An Bras Dermatol. 2016;91(5 suppl 1):105–7.

Novel Therapeutic Strategies and Innovations in Cutaneous Metastasis

34

Georgios Evangelou

Abstract

Cutaneous metastases (CM) are a late stage of systemic malignancies and often indicate a poor prognosis. However, they occur in only a small percentage of cancer patients, ranging from 0.7% to 10% depending on the primary tumor type; their clinical significance cannot be overstated. They may present as the first sign of an internal malignancy or appear later in the course of the disease, often alongside widespread dissemination. Traditionally, treatment for CM has been largely palliative, reflecting the advanced stage of the disease at diagnosis. However, the past decade has seen significant innovation in therapeutic strategies that are revolutionising the management landscape. Driven by advances in molecular biology, immunology, nanotechnology, and personalized medicine, clinicians now have access to a broader and more effective arsenal against CM. New therapies not only target the lesion itself but also address the systemic nature of the disease, offering dual benefits in local control and overall disease burden. This chapter explores these evolving approaches, highlighting both clinically established treatments and experimental innovations poised to redefine the standard of care.

The therapeutic approach to CM is highly individualized and influenced by several clinical and patient-specific factors, including the anatomical location of the lesions, morphological characteristics of metastases, the histological type of the primary tumor, patient age, presence of comorbidities, and overall performance status. Based on these parameters, treatment plans may involve local therapies, systemic regimens, or a combination of both. These interventions, while frequently palliative in intent, can significantly reduce the lesion burden, control ulceration, and minimise associated complications such as bleeding, infection, or malodour (Hu et al. J Eur Acad Dermatol Venereol JEADV 22(6):735–40, 2008; Krathen et al. South Med J 96(2):164–7, 2003; Lookingbill et al. J Am Acad Dermatol 29(2):228–36, 1993, Gschnell et al. JDDG J Dtsch Dermatol Ges 22(7):974–93, 2024).

Keywords

Cutaneous metastases · Novel therapeutic strategies · Surgery · Radiotherapy · Electrochemotherapy · Bleomycin · Isolated limb perfusion · Imiquimod · EGFR inhibitors · HER2 targeted therapy · Immunotherapy · Oncolytic viral therapy · Nanomedicine · PDT · Theranostics · Gene therapy

G. Evangelou (✉)
Consultant Dermatologist University Hospital of Crete, Crete, Greece

D. Koumaki et al. (eds.), *Cutaneous Metastases*, https://doi.org/10.1007/978-3-032-26764-1_34

34.1 Surgical Management

Surgery remains a potentially curative option in selected cases of CM, especially when systemic dissemination is absent and complete (R0) resection is feasible. The decision to pursue surgical excision is guided by factors such as the number of metastases, their anatomical distribution, and the potential for functional or cosmetic compromise.

The primary objective is complete excision with histologically clear margins, which provides the best chance for local control. In patients with limited disease burden and good overall health, surgery can significantly delay recurrence and may be followed by adjuvant therapy tailored to the primary tumor type, in accordance with current oncologic guidelines. In all cases, surgical planning must balance oncologic efficacy with the preservation of function and form, especially when lesions are located near critical anatomical structures [5–7].

34.2 Radiotherapy

Radiotherapy remains an essential component in the management of CM, both for local control and palliative purposes. It works by delivering ionizing radiation that generates free radicals within malignant cells, leading to DNA damage and cell death. Among patients with melanoma-derived skin metastases, radiotherapy has shown favorable outcomes, particularly in smaller lesions, which tend to exhibit more prolonged remissions. The modality employed depends largely on tumor depth—fast electrons are suited for superficial lesions, while photon therapy is preferred for deeper tumor deposits.

Fractionation schedules vary by clinical goals and patient prognosis. Common regimens include 5 × 4 Gy, 10 × 3 Gy, and 20–25 × 2 Gy. Adjunctive hyperthermia, in which the affected area is heated to approximately 43 °C for 1 h, may enhance therapeutic response, with studies reporting complete remission in up to 62% of cases. Pulsed-dose-rate brachytherapy has also demonstrated efficacy, particularly in patients with cutaneous breast cancer metastases, with local control rates exceeding 85% after two treatment sessions spaced 4 weeks apart.

Radiotherapy has also been successfully used in isolated cases of cutaneous involvement from urogenital tumors, including renal and urothelial carcinomas. Its utility extends beyond tumor control, providing significant symptom relief. Pain, ulceration, bleeding, and foul odour—common in advanced CM—can be effectively mitigated using hypofractionated regimens. These regimens deliver higher doses per fraction (e.g., 3.0–8.0 Gy), enabling rapid palliation within a shortened treatment timeline.

Crucially, the analgesic effect of radiotherapy does not require complete tumor regression. Symptom relief can occur even after a single fraction as low as 8 Gy, with the maximum benefit usually seen 2–4 weeks after treatment. Long-lasting pain control is achieved in 60–80% of patients, with some experiencing relief for several months or even years. Given its favorable risk-benefit profile, radiotherapy remains an essential tool for both disease-modifying and supportive care in managing CM.

34.3 Electrochemotherapy

Electrochemotherapy (ECT) , first introduced in France in the late 1980, has since become a well-established modality in the palliative management of advanced or unresectable CM, and for certain primary skin tumors [8, 9].

The technique involves administering a chemotherapeutic agent—either intravenously or directly into the tumor—combined with the targeted application of short, high-voltage electric pulses. This process, called electroporation, temporarily enhances the permeability of cancer cell membranes by altering their transmembrane potential. The formation of temporary membrane pores enables increased intracellular uptake of the cytotoxic agent, greatly boosting its effectiveness. Notably, the effectiveness of bleomycin, when administered with electroporation, can increase by up to 8000 times, while cisplatin exhibits an 80-fold increase in cytotoxicity [8, 10–12].

The technique is typically performed following the *ESOPE protocol* (European Standard Operating Procedure for Electrochemotherapy), which standardizes the methodology across clinical settings [13].

Adverse effects of electrochemotherapy are typically mild and localized, such as temporary pain or superficial necrosis, occuring in 5–16% of patients. Systemic drugs may add risks like pulmonary toxicity (bleomycin) or gastrointestinal issues (cisplatin). Clinical results are encouraging across various tumor types, with objective response rates up to 85% and complete remission in about 74%. Lesion location affects efficacy, with the best outcomes on the trunk and limbs. Patients often experience swift symptom relief, improving their quality of life [14].

A new form of ECT called calcium electroporation (Ca-EP) is under nvestigation. Rather than using drugs, Ca-EP uses electroporation to deliver high calcium levels, disrupting cellular energy and leading to cell death. A phase II trial compared Ca-EP with bleomycin-based ECT, treating up to ten skin metastases per patient with both methods. After 6 months, Ca-EP was as effective, with fewer side effects like ulceration and hyperpigmentation, and no serious adverse events. These results suggest Ca-EP is a safe, affordable alternative to traditional electrochemotherapy. [15]

34.4 Ablative Treatments

34.4.1 Cryotherapy

Cryotherapy is the application of a cold agent, most commonly liquid nitrogen, which reaches temperatures of up to −195.8 °C to selectively destroy tumoral tissue through the formation of intracellular and extracellular ice crystals, disrupting microcirculation and inducing *local tissue ischemia and necrosis*.

Although listed as a therapeutic option in some melanoma guidelines, *cryotherapy for CM* remains underreported and supported by limited data. In one series, Grotmann et al. treated *30 patients with metastatic melanoma*, achieving a *mean remission duration of 36 months* and notable improvements in quality of life.

Cryotherapy is a low-risk, practical treatment option with few contraindications, especially for small or superficial lesions, and is characterized by simplicity and repeatability [16].

34.4.2 CO_2 Laser Ablation

The *CO_2 laser* is a traditional ablative laser system used in the treatment of superficial melanoma skin metastases. Emitting light at a wavelength of *10,600 nm*, the laser effectively vaporizes tissue within the epidermal and superficial dermal layers.

For metastases smaller than 1 cm, direct ablation is feasible. In larger lesions, the periphery is first treated, followed by mechanical removal of the central tissue. In a cohort study by Kandamany et al. involving *16 patients and 559* melanoma lesions, complete clinical remission was achieved in *62.5% of patients*, with responses maintained at 12 months follow-up.

Like cryotherapy, CO_2 laser therapy offers a minimally invasive, well tolerated approach to palliation in melanoma patients, particularly when dealing with numerous small, superficial metastases [4, 16–18].

34.5 Intralesional Treatments

(a) *Bleomycin* alone or in combination with electroporation enhances drug penetration and cytotoxicity [9, 11].
(b) *Cytokine-based therapies* like intralesional IL-2 or interferon-alpha stimulate T-cell infiltration and have shown benefit in melanoma CMs [19].
(c) *Isolated Hyperthermal Limb Perfusion (ILP)* is a sophisticated regional treatment technique especially suitable for patients with multiple, rapidly recurring melanoma metastases confined to a single limb (arm or leg). The procedure involves isolating the affected

limb's blood vessels, followed by extracorporeal perfusion with melphalan, with or without recombinant human tumor necrosis factor-alpha (rhTNF-α), under mild hyperthermic conditions (39–40 °C) to enhance drug effectiveness. A comprehensive review of over 2000 melanoma patients reported a median overall response rate of 90.35%, with a complete remission rate of 58.2%. The therapeutic benefit was notably higher when melphalan was combined with rhTNF-α, (68.9% response compared to 46.5% with melphalan alone). Local adverse effects may include erythema, blistering, desquamation, lymphedema, and, in severe cases, compartment syndrome, which could threaten limb viability. Systemic complications, especially when rhTNF-α is used, can include rhabdomyolysis and cardiac strain. Besides melanoma, ILP has established utility in treating soft tissue sarcomas and could theoretically be extended to other tumor types with metastatic involvement limited to a single limb, although this remains less common due to the procedure's complexity [20, 21].

(d) *Intralesional immunotherapy.*

This treatment modality involves the injection of immune stimulants and offers a targeted, low-toxicity strategy for cutaneous leions. Agents such as toll-like receptor (TLP) agonists (e.g imiquimod) or interleukins can recuit local immune responses and promote systemic antitumor immunity [22, 23].

34.6 Topical Treatments

(a) *Imiquimod* (a TLR-7 agonist) induces local immune activation and has been successfully used in CM from breast and melanoma primaries [24].
(b) *5-fluorouracil (5-FU)*, typically employed for actinic keratoses and superficial carcinomas, has shown anecdotal benefit in selected CM cases [25].
(c) *Miltefosin* is a phospholipid derivative with an unclear mechanism of action. It has been suggested that it competes with natural phospholipids in the cell membrane, thus inhibiting the biosynthesis of factors required for cell division, such as protein kinase C, phospholipase C, and phosphatidylcholine. It also interferes with the intracellular calcium ion concentration. It is administered by topical application of the solution on the cutaneous lesions in relation to breast cancer. Recommended dosing is once daily for 1 week, then twice daily thereafter. Local adverse reactions are usually mild, including erythema, xerosis, pruritus, exfoliation, and burning sensation. [26].
(d) *Contact sensitizers* like Diphencyprone is a contact sensitizer traditionally used as immunotherapy for alopecia areata and warts. It has been reported in two studies to be effective against cutaneous melanoma metastasis, with 37,5% complete and 24% partial responses, and 46% complete and 38% partial responses, respectively, suggesting that topical diphencyprone although not approved by the Food and Drug Administration (FDA) and the European Medicines Agency (EMA) could be considered for patients with cutaneous metastasis refractory to other treatments [7, 25, 26].

34.7 Targeted Systemic Therapies

Targeted therapies have transformed cancer treatment by blocking specific molecular pathways essential for tumor growth and survival. In the context of CM, these agents are often chosen based on the molecular features of the primary tumor, such as HER2 amplification in breast cancer or EGFR mutations in lung adenocarcinoma.

- EGFR inhibitors (e.g., erlotinib, gefitinib) have shown effectiveness in treating CM from non-small cell lung cancer.
- HER2-targeted agents (e.g., trastuzumab, lapatinib) are crucial in managing breast cancer metastases, including skin involvement.
- VEGF inhibitors like bevacizumab have been used to restrict tumor angiogenesis and may

decrease vascular support to cutaneous lesions. Emerging research indicates that these agents might also modify the tumour microenvironment to promote immune cell infiltration, thereby enhancing the effects of immunotherapy [27–31].

Emerging research indicates that these agents might also modify the tumor microenvironment to promote immune cell infiltration, thereby enhancing the effects of immunotherapy [27–31].

34.8 Immunotherapy

(a) *Immune checkpoint inhibitors* (PD-1, PD-L1,CTLA-4). Agents targeting PD-1, PD-L1, and CTLA-4 have demonstrated efficacy in treating metastatic melanoma and non-melanoma skin cancers. Their activity in CM from solid tumors like lung, renal, and bladder cancer is under active investigation.
(b) *Pembrolizumab* and *nivolumab* (anti-PD-1 antibodies) have shown promising results in reducing skin lesions and controlling systemic disease.
(c) The *combination of nivolumab and ipilimumab* (anti-CTLA-4) has demonstrated enhanced efficacy in some tumor types, though at the cost of increased toxicity [32–34].

34.9 Oncolytic Virus Therapy

Talimogene laherparepvec is the first FDA-approved oncolytic viral therapy for melanoma cutaneous metastasis, a genetically modified herpes simplex virus complex to selectively infect and lyse tumor cells whilst also stimulating an immune response. The combination of oncolytic viruses with checkpoint inhibitors is under intense investigation, offering the potential for synergistic tumor eradication [35, 36].

34.10 Nanomedicine and Drug Delivery Innovations

Nanocarriers such as liposomes, dendrimers, micelles, and solid lipid nanoparticles provide targeted delivery of chemotherapeutics, immunomodulators, or gene therapy vectors directly to tumor sites while reducing systemic toxicity. One of the main benefits of nanomedicine is the enhanced permeability and retention (EPR) effect, where nanoparticles accumulate in tumor tissues due to leaky blood vessels and poor lymphatic drainage. In CM, this effect allows high local drug levels with fewer off-target effects.
(a) *Liposomal doxorubicin (Doxil)* has been investigated for skin-involved breast cancer.
(b) *Paclitaxel-loaded nanoparticles* show promise in metastatic triple-negative breast cancer with cutaneous involvement.
(c) *Thermosensitive hydrogels* and *microneedle arrays* are also being explored for localized drug release in skin lesions [37–40].

34.11 Photodynamic Therapy

Photodynamic therapy (PDT) represents a non-invasive treatment modality that involves the administration of a photosensitizing agent followed by targeted light exposure. Upon activation, the agent generates reactive oxygen species that cause direct tumor cell death and local immune stimulation.

- For decades, PDT has been widely used in dermatology with topical photosensitizers such as aminolevulinic acid (ALA) or methyl aminolevulinate (MAL) for actinic keratosis, superficial basal cell carcinoma, and intraepidermal squamous cell carcinoma. However, PDT with ALA or MAL has also been explored in CM, particularly for superficial metastases or early-stage breast cancer lesions. A wide variety of systemic agents, such as porfimer sodium, Chlorin e6, AlPcS4, Verteporfin, and Photochlor (HPPH), have been used in lung and breast cancer, as well as in pulmonary metastasis, in humans and animal models. In addition, Temoporfin, Redaporfin, and IRDye700DX have been used in head and neck cancer. Temoporfin, 5_ALA, and Radoporfin have been used in prostate cancer. [41–43].

34.12 Theranostics and Precision Oncology

Theranostics—an emerging field that combines *diagnostic imaging and targeted therapy*—is gaining ground in metastatic oncology. Although still in early-phase development for CM, several platforms show promise. Radiolabeled antibodies or ligands targeting tumor-specific markers (e.g., HER2, PSMA) can be used for both imaging and delivering cytotoxic payloads. Molecular profiling of cutaneous lesions via biopsy or liquid biopsy can guide personalized treatment plans, particularly when primary tumor status is unclear or discordant from metastases.

CM provide a unique opportunity for serial sampling due to their accessibility. This makes the skin an ideal site for studying *tumor heterogeneity, treatment resistance*, and real-time therapeutic response. As such, CM may serve not only as a disease burden but also as a strategic site for *biomarker development* and *clinical trial entry* [44].

34.13 Emerging Technologies: Gene Therapy, CRISPR, and mRNA Platforms

Recent technological advances are opening new possibilities for next-generation treatments in cutaneous metastasis. Although most are still in the experimental phase, the potential benefits are promising.

Gene Therapy
Vectors delivering *tumor suppressor genes*, *proapoptotic factors*, or *immune-stimulating genes* directly into CM lesions are under investigation. Viral and non-viral delivery systems can be applied topically or via injection.

CRISPR/Cas9 Gene Editing
CRISPR technology is being investigated for in vivo tumor gene disruption. Early research has aimed to knock out genes, such as PD-L1 or oncogenic drivers, in CM. Although clinical applications are still in the early stages, the potential for targeted, mutation-specific correction remains substantial.

mRNA Therapeutics
Inspired by the success of mRNA vaccines, similar platforms are now being investigated in oncology. *mRNA-based intratumoral vaccines* encoding tumor antigens or immune activators are being tested in melanoma and may be extended to other tumors with cutaneous spread. These approaches aim to transform the tumor site into an antigen-presenting center that primes systemic immunity. [45–48]

Disclosure The author confirms that an AI-based language assistance tool was used solely for language polishing, grammatical refinement, and stylistic consistency. All scientific content, clinical concepts and academic judgment were entirely conceived, structured, and validated by the author. No AI tool was used for data generation, clinical decision-making, or scientific interpretation.

References

1. Hu SCS, Chen GS, Lu YW, Wu CS, Lan CCE. Cutaneous metastases from different internal malignancies: a clinical and prognostic appraisal. J Eur Acad Dermatol Venereol JEADV. 2008;22(6):735–40.
2. Krathen RA, Orengo IF, Rosen T. Cutaneous metastasis: a meta-analysis of data. South Med J. 2003;96(2):164–7.
3. Lookingbill DP, Spangler N, Helm KF. Cutaneous metastases in patients with metastatic carcinoma: a retrospective study of 4020 patients. J Am Acad Dermatol. 1993;29(2):228–36.
4. Gschnell M, Volberg C, Hauser C, Krönig L. Cutaneous metastases: from epidemiology to therapy. JDDG J Dtsch Dermatol Ges. 2024;22(7):974–93.
5. Stratigos AJ, Garbe C, Dessinioti C, Lebbe C, Van Akkooi A, Bataille V, et al. European consensus-based interdisciplinary guideline for invasive cutaneous

squamous cell carcinoma: Part 2. Treatment–Update 2023. Eur J Cancer. 2023;193:113252.
6. Huang S, Parekh V, Waisman J, Jones V, Yuan Y, Vora N, et al. Cutaneous metastasectomy: is there a role in breast cancer? A systematic review and overview of current treatment modalities. J Surg Oncol. 2022;126(2):217–38.
7. Di Raimondo C, Lozzi F, Di Domenico PP, Campione E, Bianchi L. The diagnosis and management of cutaneous metastases from melanoma. Int J Mol Sci. 2023;24(19):14535.
8. Giardino R, Fini M, Bonazzi V, Cadossi R, Nicolini A, Carpi A. Electrochemotherapy a novel approach to the treatment of metastatic nodules on the skin and subcutaneous tissues. Biomed Pharmacother. 2006;60(8):458–62.
9. Gehl J, Sersa G, Matthiessen LW, Muir T, Soden D, Occhini A, et al. Updated standard operating procedures for electrochemotherapy of cutaneous tumours and skin metastases. Acta Oncol. 2018;57(7):874–82.
10. Sersa G, Miklavcic D, Cemazar M, Rudolf Z, Pucihar G, Snoj M. Electrochemotherapy in treatment of tumours. Eur J Surg Oncol J Eur Soc Surg Oncol Br Assoc Surg Oncol. 2008;34(2):232–40.
11. Fiorentzis M, Kalirai H, Katopodis P, Seitz B, Viestenz A, Coupland SE. Electrochemotherapy with bleomycin and cisplatin enhances cytotoxicity in primary and metastatic uveal melanoma cell lines in vitro. Neoplasma. 2018;65(02):210–5.
12. Mir LM. Bases and rationale of the electrochemotherapy. Electrochemotherapy. 2006;4(11):38–44.
13. Marty M, Sersa G, Garbay JR, Gehl J, Collins CG, Snoj M, et al. Electrochemotherapy—an easy, highly effective and safe treatment of cutaneous and subcutaneous metastases: results of ESOPE (European Standard Operating Procedures of Electrochemotherapy) study. Eur J Cancer Suppl. 2006;4(11):3–13.
14. Cadossi R, Ronchetti M, Cadossi M. Locally enhanced chemotherapy by electroporation: clinical experiences and perspective of use of electrochemotherapy. Future Oncol. 2014;10(5):877–90.
15. Vissing M, Pervan M, Pløen J, Schnefeldt M, Rafaelsen SR, Jensen LH, et al. Calcium electroporation in cutaneous metastases—a non-randomised phase II multicentre clinical trial. Eur J Surg Oncol. 2023;49(9):106925.
16. John HE, Mahaffey PJ. Laser ablation and cryotherapy of melanoma metastases. J Surg Oncol. 2014;109(4):296–300.
17. Algarin YA, Pulumati A, Jaalouk D, Tan J, Zeitouni NC, Nouri K. The palliative role of lasers in the treatment of melanoma. Arch Dermatol Res. 2024;316(6):244.
18. Kandamany N, Mahaffey P. Carbon dioxide laser ablation as first-line management of in-transit cutaneous malignant melanoma metastases. Lasers Med Sci. 2009;24(3):411–4.
19. Radny P, Caroli UM, Bauer J, Paul T, Schlegel C, Eigentler TK, et al. Phase II trial of intralesional therapy with interleukin-2 in soft-tissue melanoma metastases. Br J Cancer. 2003;89(9):1620–6.
20. Olieman AFT. Hyperthermic isolated limb perfusion with tumor necrosis factor α, interferon gamma, and melphalan for locally advanced nonmelanoma skin tumors of the extremities: a multicenter study. Arch Surg. 1999;134(3):303.
21. Moreno-Ramirez D, Cruz-Merino L, Ferrandiz L, Villegas-Portero R, Nieto-Garcia A. Isolated limb perfusion for malignant melanoma: systematic review on effectiveness and safety. Oncologist. 2010;15(4):416–27.
22. Leventhal JS, Odell ID, Imaeda S, Maverakis E, King BA. Treatment of melanoma in-transit metastases with combination intralesional interleukin-2, topical imiquimod, and tretinoin 0.1% cream. JAAD Case Rep. 2016;2(2):114–6.
23. Green DS, Dalgleish AG, Belonwu N, Fischer MD, Bodman-Smith MD. Topical imiquimod and intralesional interleukin-2 increase activated lymphocytes and restore the Th1/Th2 balance in patients with metastatic melanoma. Br J Dermatol. 2008;159(3):606–14.
24. Nguyen NC, Chaar BT, Osman MM. Prevalence and patterns of soft tissue metastasis: detection with true whole-body F-18 FDG PET/CT. BMC Med Imaging. 2007;7(1):8.
25. Florin V, Desmedt E, Vercambre-Darras S, Mortier L. Topical treatment of cutaneous metastases of malignant melanoma using combined imiquimod and 5-fluorouracil. Investig New Drugs. 2012;30(4):1641–5.
26. Ragnarsson-Olding B, Djureen-Mårtensson E, Månsson-Brahme E, Hansson J. Loco-regional control of cutaneous metastases of malignant melanoma by treatment with miltefosine (Miltex®). Acta Oncol. 2005;44(7):773–7.
27. Tsai MH, Hsiao YP, Lin WL, Tseng SW. Steatocystoma multiplex as initial impression of non-small cell lung cancer with complete response to gefitinib. Chin J Cancer Res Chung-Kuo Yen Cheng Yen Chiu. 2014;26(1):E5–9.
28. Conlin AK, Chun BM, Borges VF, Moxon NM, Parris HJ, Walker LN, et al. Cutaneous responses in HER2+ metastatic breast cancer: a retrospective case series of a Phase 1b study of Tucatinib, an Oral HER2-specific inhibitor in combination with Capecitabine and/or Trastuzumab in third-line or later treatment. Curr Probl Cancer Case Rep. 2022;7:100170.
29. Giarratano T, Miglietta F, Giorgi CA, Tsvetkova V, Michieletto S, Evangelista L, et al. Exceptional and durable responses to TDM-1 after Trastuzumab failure for breast cancer skin metastases: potential implications of an immunological sanctuary. Front Oncol. 2018;8:581.
30. Yu J, Jin F, Zhu H, Kong L. A spectrum of cutaneous toxicities from erlotinib may be a robust clinical marker for non-small-cell lung therapy: a case report and literature review. Onco Targets Ther. 2015;8:943.

31. Cho J, Park Y, Lee JC, Jung WJ, Lee S. Case series of different onset of skin metastasis according to the breast cancer subtypes. Cancer Res Treat. 2014;46(2):194–9.
32. Pham JP, Staeger R, Joshua AM, Liu J, Da Silva IP, Dummer R, et al. An updated review of immune checkpoint inhibitors in cutaneous oncology: beyond melanoma. Eur J Cancer. 2025;214:115121.
33. Knight A, Karapetyan L, Kirkwood JM. Immunotherapy in melanoma: recent advances and future directions. Cancer. 2023;15(4):1106.
34. Munhoz RR, Nader-Marta G, De Camargo VP, Queiroz MM, Cury-Martins J, Ricci H, et al. A phase 2 study of first-line nivolumab in patients with locally advanced or metastatic cutaneous squamous-cell carcinoma. Cancer. 2022;128(24):4223–31.
35. Bommareddy PK, Patel A, Hossain S, Kaufman HL. Talimogene Laherparepvec (T-VEC) and other oncolytic viruses for the treatment of melanoma. Am J Clin Dermatol. 2017;18(1):1–15.
36. Pol J, Kroemer G, Galluzzi L. First oncolytic virus approved for melanoma immunotherapy. Onco Targets Ther. 2016;5(1):e1115641.
37. Zhu L, Qiao G, Gao H, Jiang A, Zhang L, Wang X. Enhancing melanoma therapy with hydrogel microneedles. Front Oncol. 2025;15:1590534.
38. Filho D, Guerrero M, Pariguana M, Marican A, Durán-Lara EF. Hydrogel-based microneedle as a drug delivery system. Pharmaceutics. 2023;15(10):2444.
39. Li JY, Feng YH, He YT, Hu LF, Liang L, Zhao ZQ, et al. Thermosensitive hydrogel microneedles for controlled transdermal drug delivery. Acta Biomater. 2022;153:308–19.
40. Franchina T, Adamo B, Ricciardi GRR, Caristi N, Agostino RM, Proto C, et al. Activity of pegylated liposomal doxorubicin in combination with gemcitabine in triple negative breast cancer with skin involvement: two case reports. Cancer Biol Ther. 2012;13(7):472–6.
41. Kim TE, Chang JE. Recent studies in photodynamic therapy for cancer treatment: from basic research to clinical trials. Pharmaceutics. 2023;15(9):2257.
42. Sachsenmaier SM, Traub F, Cykowska A, Riester R, Wülker N, Walter C, et al. Assessment of 5-aminolevulinic acid-mediated photodynamic therapy on bone metastases: an in vitro study. Biology. 2021;10(10):1020.
43. Rollakanti KR, Anand S, Maytin EV. Vitamin D enhances the efficacy of photodynamic therapy in a murine model of breast cancer. Cancer Med. 2015;4(5):633–42.
44. Jiao R, Allen KJH, Malo ME, Yilmaz O, Wilson J, Nelson BJB, et al. A Theranostic approach to imaging and treating melanoma with 203Pb/212Pb-labeled antibody targeting melanin. Cancer. 2023;15(15):3856.
45. Boehm DT, Landreth KM, Kilic ES, Lee KS, Misra B, Bobbala S, et al. Intratumoral administration of mRNA COVID-19 vaccine delays melanoma growth in mice. Sci Rep. 2025;15(1):5337.
46. Bidram M, Zhao Y, Shebardina NG, Baldin AV, Bazhin AV, Ganjalikhany MR, et al. mRNA-based cancer vaccines: a therapeutic strategy for the treatment of melanoma patients. Vaccine. 2021;9(10):1060.
47. Hromic-Jahjefendic A, Lundstrom K. Viral vector-based melanoma gene therapy. Biomedicines. 2020;8(3):60.
48. Klatzmann D, Herson S, Cherin P, Chosidow O, Baillet F, Bensimon G, et al. Gene therapy for metastatic malignant melanoma: evaluation of tolerance to intratumoral injection of cells producing recombinant retroviruses carrying the herpes simplex virus type 1 thymidine kinase gene, to be followed by ganciclovir administration. Laboratoire Immunologie B, Hôpital Pitié-Salpêtrière, Paris Cedex, France. Hum Gene Ther. 1996;7(2):255–67.

35 Advances in Prognosis: Biomarkers, Predictive Tools, and Future Directions

George I. Lambrou

Abstract

Tumor biology remains one of the most challenging research topics up-to-date. There are many more things that we still do not know and understand as compared to those we do know. Neoplasms can be considered as one of the more complex biological systems known to the scientific community, but also they consist a significant health care burden, due its devastating effects on the patient, as well as their loved ones. In addition, neoplasms, in the majority, still have a dismal prognosis and deprive the patient both from quality of life as well as from their dignity. Especially, the potential of tumor cells to migrate and create metastatic sites is one of the most difficult problems to be addressed. Therefore, it is imperative to understand both the mechanics of tumor ontogenesis and the mechanics of metastasis. In the present chapter, we will address some of the cutting-edge biological factors that can be used for disease prognosis, the potential tools, and the future directions.

G. I. Lambrou (✉)
Choremeio Research Laboratory, First Department of Pediatrics, School of Medicine, National and Kapodistrian University of Athens, Athens, Greece

University Research Institute of Maternal and Child Health & Precision Medicine, National and Kapodistrian University of Athens, Athens, Greece
e-mail: glamprou@med.uoa.gr

Keywords

Prognosis · Biomarkers · G-quadruplexes · miRNA · Long non-coding RNAs · Circular RNAs · Machine learning

35.1 Introduction

Despite all the efforts, research, and resources dedicated to the understanding of tumor biology, the disease still remains a tremendous challenge and an unresolved puzzle. Cancer remains a major global cause of mortality; the estimated incidence is predicted to double over the next decades [1].

At the same time, the prevalence of skin cancer has been on the rise over the last decades, where the major risk factor is considered the exposure to the sun's Ultraviolet (UV) radiation. At this point, I would like to draw attention to a probable paradox: total solar irradiance (TSI) has been found to be stable, or at least follow the same oscillatory pattern, since the 1950s and with more certainty until the first satellite measurements in 1978 [2].

Thus, it is possible that the increasing prevalence of skin cancer is not only due to exposure to solar irradiation, but also to the socioeconomic changes of humans. For example, shorter vacation times could lead to an intensification of UV exposure on human skin. In any case, skin cancer

D. Koumaki et al. (eds.), *Cutaneous Metastases*, https://doi.org/10.1007/978-3-032-26764-1_35

has taken on the characteristics of an epidemic, which should be dealt with, and the most important way is through prognosis.

Having addressed that paradox, cutaneous metastases are an almost completely different story. As it has been discussed in previous chapters, cutaneous metastases constitute a serious complication where tumor cells form a metastatic lesion to the skin. The main and critical question to be answered, in the case of such a diagnosis, is whether the tumor consists of a primary cutaneous neoplasm or a metastasis [3]. Taking into account the reported incidence of cutaneous metastases, it appears to take place in between 0.5% and 10.4% of all cases [3], with older reports referring to an 0.7% and 9.4% incident (which is a small difference, yet could be significant) [4].

For different tumor types, different incidences have been reported, yet it has been evident at least for the last 40 years that cutaneous metastases are a fact, and they should be considered in the mail anti-tumor clinical practice [5]. The first reported case of a cutaneous metastasis was reported by Martin and Hamilton (1896) [6]. Since that time, there have been more than 10,000 works concerning the topic (Fig. 35.1), indicating both the importance of the subject as well as its seriousness.

If I could put it in simple terms, the importance of cutaneous metastases comes from the simple fact that they appear on the skin and thus it is easier to detect, but more difficult to understand their biology, i.e., whether those are primary tumors or secondary tumors derived from an unknown primary tumor. Also, another challenging aspect is that some metastatic lesions may be clinically presented as benign, painless nodules, to which no attention is being drawn, at least at the first site [7]. Hence, cutaneous metastatic disease is not unusual, yet it is often "overlooked," and our knowledge is limited concerning its significance in diagnosis and prognosis [4].

Hence, it is possible that these lesions were/are there, but they were largely overlooked due to lack of available data. In simpler words, the clinical dermatologist could be the one who first makes a diagnosis on a possible tumorous disease rather than the specialist whose advice comes after the first neoplasmatic symptoms are present. Another significant aspect is that cutaneous metastases indicate a progressed stage of the disease, which makes prognosis dismal, since these metastases clinically appear in a time interval that ranges between two and 22 years [8].

From this clinical observation, another question arises: Is it possible to detect the potential or ability of a tumor to create cutaneous lesions before they even appear? One thing is certain: routine clinical examination (as well as self-examination) of apparent cutaneous anomalies could provide an early indicator of metastasis (or even the presence of a primary tumor site), which is easy to overlook but important to take into consideration.

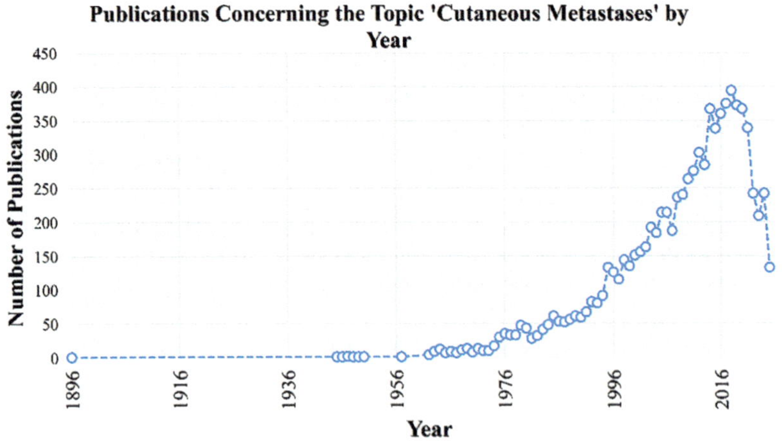

Fig. 35.1 The number of publications from 1896 to 2025 on the topic "Cutaneous Metastases"

In the present chapter, we will review some potentially cutting-edge advances for cutaneous metastases.

35.2 Biomarkers

The diagnosis of a systemic primary neoplasm, with cutaneous involvement, cannot always reliably be established solely on histopathologic criteria and related clinical characteristics [7]. The most immediate and fastest way to further investigate the metastatic nature of a primary tumor is immunohistochemistry. For example, for the identification of lymphoma-originated cutaneous metastasis, cytokeratins, Glycoprotein 100 (GP100), S-100, Prostate-Specific Antigen (PSA), Thyroid Transcription Factor (TTF), and estrogen/progesterone receptors (ER/PR) are utilized [5, 7].

Although these biomarkers have been known for years and have been utilized in differential diagnosis, new tools have surfaced, some of which we will review below. In particular, in the present section, we will address some cutting-edge topics related to the prognosis and outcome of tumors.

35.2.1 Circulating Tumor Cells

One of the most appraised and known mechanisms of metastasis is the presence of tumor cells in circulation, or circulating tumor cells. This has been known for many years, and at least during the last 40 years, research on the topic has intensified.

Circulating tumor cells pose some interesting challenges. For example, they are very rare and difficult to detect. In humans, a cell concentration of 1/ml is considered an indicator of poor prognosis. This is also the reason that investigating their role in tumor metastatic mechanisms is very difficult, even in animal models, where sometimes the complete blood content of the animal must be removed [9].

Another "frightening" property of circulating tumor cells is that they have been found to circulate in the blood for more than a decade before forming a new metastatic site [10]. An important factor for the development of a cutaneous metastatic site is the cell population present at that site. Circulating tumor cells appear to play an important role, with their chances of inoculating at another location increasing with the circulating cells' population [11].

Tumor cells from a primary site could reach the skin through circulation routes, where surgical injury could (unfortunately) play a beneficial factor for tumor cells [12]. As aforementioned, the detection of circulating tumor cells is a biomarker of poor prognosis for a plethora of tumors, such as breast cancer, colon cancer, and prostate cancer, as well as lung and ovarian cancer [12].

Unfortunately, cutaneous metastases can form after surgical incisions, even if these include the resection of a benign tumor and have helped to the circulation of malignant cells for whose presence was neglected [13]. Interestingly, it has been found that circulating tumor cells take advantage of the wound healing mechanisms, whose signal transduction pathways facilitate tumor cell growth and proliferation. In that machinery, an important "player" is the inflammatory response mechanism and, in particular, the cytokine signaling pathway [14].

However, one of the most crucial "assistants" of the metastatic machinery and of the circulating tumor cells is fibroblasts. Fibroblasts are probably the main cell type that strongly correlates with the formation of a favorable tumor microenvironment [15]. These Cancer-Associated Fibroblasts (CAF) host circulating tumor cells, providing the necessary stimuli for tumor growth, cell proliferation, and invasion, including the potential for angiogenesis.

35.2.2 G-Quadruplexes

Although not a very familiar topic, G-quadruplexes (G4) are gaining more and more attention in research, due to their important role in transcription and translation.

The definition of a G-quadruplex is described as a "Higher-order DNA and RNA structures formed from guanine-rich sequences. They are formed around a core of at least two stacked tetrads of hydrogen-bonded guanine bases. They can be formed from one, two, or four separate strands of DNA (or RNA) and can display a wide variety of topologies, which are a consequence of various combinations of strand direction, length, and sequence," held together with Hoogsteen hydrogen bonds [16] (MeSH Term ID: D054856) [17] (Fig. 35.2).

Initially, it was found that DNA forms "tetrads" due to a secondary structural property of guanines (Hoogsteen hydrogen bonds) in the DNA sequence [20–22]. Later on, it was also found that RNA can form tertiary G-quadruplexes, which opened new avenues to the understanding of RNA biology, but also tumor biology [23, 24]. Amazingly, recent experimental data have shown that G-quadruplexes can form in longer loops and also with three guanine molecules [25, 26]. This trait is not only unique to the mammalian genome, since it has been found that also bacteria and viruses can have genomic and transcriptomic regions, which can form G-quadruplexes [27, 28].

Further experimental evidence has shown that not only do G-quadruplexes play a significant role, but also that specific proteins can identify, bind, and unfold these structures [29]. In general, there are three protein families known for their ability to bind to G-quadruplexes: binding-related proteins, stabilizing-related proteins, and unwinding-related proteins. It can be concluded that alterations in these proteins lead to changes in the signal transduction pathways, consequently causing genomic and transcriptomic instability. The experimental data have led to the conclusion that the nucleotide tertiary structures could be potential therapeutic targets. Several approaches have been attempted with developed ligands intended to be used as therapeutic drugs [30].

As a consequence, the basic idea on how to exploit G-quadruplexes is based itself on their potential against tumors. The main strategy behind that idea had to do with the stabilization and/or formation of G-quadruplexes, which are believed to be aberrant in tumors. For example, in the majority of tumors (which exceed 85%), telomerase activity is up-regulated, allowing a kind of "immortality" for tumor cells and basically, without having telomeres being shortened [31]. Hence, an idea behind the use of G-quadruplexes is to enhance these structures at telomeres, which probably could lead to cell proliferation and division inhibition. There are already examples of such molecules, such as telomestatin and 2,6-diamidoanthraquinone derivatives [32].

Another important recent finding concerning G-quadruplexes is that they can affect and/or regulate the expression of certain oncogenes, for example, genes of the *MYC* family, *BCL2*, *KRAS*, and *KIT* [16]. A recent work has reported on the development of a novel quindoline derivative, which specifically targets the RNA G-quadruplex of *NRAS* mRNA [33], a gene known for its role in

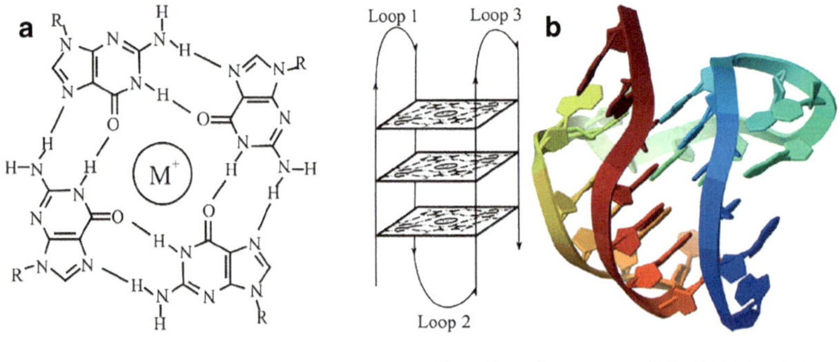

Fig. 35.2 A 2D (**a**) and 3D (**b**) structures of a G-quadruplex (Subfigure **a** was reproduced from https://en.wikipedia.org/wiki/G-quadruplex#/media/File:G-quadruplex.svg. (Accessed June 30th 2025) under the Creative Commons CC BY-SA 2.5 License https://creativecommons.org/licenses/by-sa/2.5/ [18]. Subfigure **b** was reproduced from the Protein Database (PDB) with Protein ID 2HY9 [19])

cutaneous melanoma and its metastases. The same strategy (yet, with another synthesized inhibitor) has been followed to stabilize promoters of other oncogenes (e.g., *cMYC*, again *BCL2*, and *KRAS*) in acute myeloid [34] and acute lymphoblastic leukemia [35].

Melanomas are a special case of tumors due to their aggressiveness. The overall survival of melanoma patients has improved greatly over the last years, but it still remains poor in cases of metastatic disease [16]. Melanomas also pose a challenge since they are known to have numerous mutations in key-regulating genes such as *TP53*, *BRCA1*, *BRCA2* [36], *NRAS*, *KRAS*, *RSK*, *BRAF* [37], and others. All those genes are known to possess promoter G-quadruplex structures, which get destabilized due to the mutational burden of these genes. Thus, stabilization of G-quadruplexes appears to be a very promising strategy for melanoma.

Below, we reproduce a table (Table 35.1) from a recent report, summarizing the potential G4 stabilizers, which have been used for the treatment of melanoma, including inhibiting its metastatic potential.

Despite the importance of this topic, that is, the properties and potential therapeutic and prognostic value of G-quadruplexes, there are not many studies, and there is a lot to learn from these amazing structures.

Table 35.1 A table from the literature summarizing the utilized G4 stabilizers for the treatment of melanoma

Ligand	Cell line	CE		
		I	II	III
5ME	B16F10$_{m}$			X
Ant1,5	SKMel-5$_{h}$, ROSS$_{h}$, A375$_{h}$, M14$_{h}$	X		
BRACO19	B16$_{m}$			
C8	B16$_{m}$			
C14 Derivate from TMPyP4; induces singlet oxygen ($^{1}O_2$) production	B78-H1$_{m}$		X	
c-exNDIs	A375$_{h}$, SK-MEL-2$_{h}$		X	
CORON	M14h, LOX IMVI$_{h}$, MALME-3M$_{h}$, SK-MEL-2$_{h}$, SK-MEL-28$_{h}$, SK-MEL-5$_{h}$, UACC-62$_{h}$	X	X	X
CX-3543 (Quarfloxin)	M14$_{h}$, MALME-3M$_{h}$, UACC-257$_{h}$, UACC-62$_{h}$		X	X
EMICORON	M14$_{h}$, LOX IMVI$_{h}$, MDA-MB-435$_{h}$, SK-MEL-2$_{h}$, SK-MEL-28$_{h}$, SK-MEL-5$_{h}$, UACC-62$_{h}$, UACC-257$_{h}$	X	X	X
IZCZ-0	A375$_{h}$		X	
IZCZ-3	A375$_{h}$		X	
IZTC-1	B16$_{m}$		X	
N,N′-bis(3,4-dihydroxbenzylidene)-1,2-diaminobenzene (crosslinker)	B16F1$_{m}$		X	
Naphthalene diimide derivatives (compound 2)	SKMEL-5$_{h}$	X		X
PhenDC3	A375$_{h}$			
Phenyl 1,2,3-triazole-thymidine ligands (L1, L2, L3)	B16F10$_{m}$	X		
PPL3C	M14$_{h}$	X		
Pyridostatin	A375$_{h}$			

(continued)

35.2.3 miRNAs, Long Non-Coding RNAs, and Circular RNAs

35.2.3.1 miRNAs

As we move down from the cellular to the molecular level, the most recent topic concerning the mechanics of cutaneous metastasis is the presence and role of miRNAs. We will not get into the details of the miRNA molecules, but we will certainly mention that those have been the most attractive biomarkers both for disease (i.e., tumors) diagnosis, prognosis, and therapy. Unfortunately, there is not much knowledge on the topic, and the role of miRNAs in cutaneous metastases still remains to be elucidated.

Table 35.1 (continued)

Ligand	Cell line	CE		
		I	II	III
RHPS4	$M14_h$, $PLF2_h$, $JR1_h$, $JR8_h$, $SBCL1_h$, SAN_h, LP_h, LM_h, $JR5_h$, $M14_h$	X		
TMPyP4	$B78\text{-}H1_m$		X	
Trans-resveratrol (tRES)	$M14_h$, $SKMEL\text{-}28_h$	X	X	
Trisubstituted naphthalimides (compounds VII, VIII and IX)	$M14_h$	X		

Legend: molecules with an "h" subscript indicate testing on human cell lines, and subscripts with "m" indicate testing on mouse cell lines. *CE* Cellular Effects. Under "CE," *I* indicates Telomere maintenance, *II* indicates Oncogene regulation, and *III* indicates Genome instability

A recent report investigated the potential role of miR-146a in melanoma progression and metastasis. In this report, it was found that miR-146a consisted of a dual-role molecule; on one hand, promoting melanoma cells' proliferation and on the other hand inhibiting metastasis [38].

It was found that miR-146 promoted cell growth through its direct targets Lunatic Fringe (*LFNG*) and *NUMB*, which participate in a larger cascade formed by the NOTCH/PTEN/Akt pathway. At the same time, metastatic machinery inhibition was found to take place through the down-regulation of *ITGAV* and *ROCK1* genes. In the same study, it was interestingly reported that miR-146a was upregulated in both the primary melanoma site, but also in the cutaneous metastatic site and yet was down-regulated in the circulating melanoma cells. This finding proposed a contradictory role for miR-146a, whose behavior changes depending on the local microenvironment [38]. In that sense, this molecule could pose a probable biomarker for disease prognosis. Having talked about the microenvironment and the role of fibroblasts, a recent report showed that there is a distinctive, differential profile of miRNA expression (Fig. 35.3) in CAFs, taken from primary and cutaneous metastatic breast cancer cells [39].

In this work, the experimental data concerned the investigation of the effects of estrogen on tumor fibroblasts taken from primary and metastatic breast cancer cells. It has been found that, depending on the origin of the fibroblasts, there was a distinctive expression profile for each category.

The most interesting finding though it was that 77 miRNAs participated in both mechanisms, which would be tumor cell proliferation at the primary site and facilitation of metastasis at the metastatic site [39]. More interesting was the finding that there were no common down-regulated miRNAs for both cell types, as well as no up-regulated and down-regulated at the same time in the case of the primary tumor and metastatic tumor fibroblasts. On the other hand, 22 miRNAs were found to be commonly up-regulated in both fibroblast types, and 55 had the exact opposite expression profile.

Similarly, other contemporary studies have shown that miRNAs play an important role in the potential of melanoma to procure metastases, for example, miR-182, which facilitates tumor migration and invasion, as well as miR-145, which is known as a regulator of cell migration and invasion [40].

The important message from this study is that miRNAs could make a significant and important biomarker for disease prognosis.

35.2.3.2 lncRNAs

Similar to miRNAs, long non-coding RNAs (lncRNA) are known to play a significant role in tumor biology, yet there are not many studies on their role in cutaneous metastases. Recent evidence has shown that more than 90% of the human transcriptome concerns transcripts that are not related to translation, i.e., will not give any proteins [41]. LncRNAs are defined as "non-protein coding RNAs, with transcripts longer than 200 base pairs." There is a close relation between lncRNAs and miRNAs. This type of RNA, similarly to other types of RNAs, is located either in the cytoplasm or the nucleus. Depending on their position, lncRNAs have different respec-

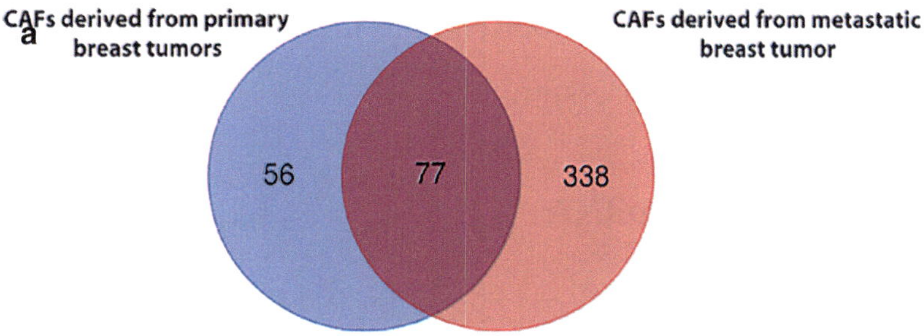

b **Joint regulated miRNAs in CAFs derived from primary and metastatic breast tumors**

CAFs derived from primary breast tumors ↑ CAFs derived from metastatic breast tumor ↑	22	hsa-miR-769-3p; hsa-miR-572; hsa-miR-548J; hsa-miR-1262; hsa-miR-630; hsa-miR-150-5p; hsa-miR-9-3p; hsa-miR-125a-3p; hsa-miR-30c-1-3p; hsa-miR-1201; hsa-miR-1184; hsa-miR-511-5p; hsa-miR-651-5p; hsa-miR-497-3p; hsa-let-7b-3p; hsa-miR-92b-5p; hsa-miR-375-3p; hsa-miR-541-3p; hsa-miR-144-5p; hsa-miR-504-5p; hsa-miR-101-5p; hsa-miR-326
CAFs derived from primary breast tumors ↑ CAFs derived from metastatic breast tumor ↓	0	
CAFs derived from primary breast tumors ↓ CAFs derived from metastatic breast tumor ↑	55	hsa-miR-449a; hsa-miR-1226-5p; hsa-miR-7-2-3p; hsa-miR-485-5p; hsa-miR-885-5p; hsa-miR-570-3p; hsa-miR-1291; hsa-miR-432-3p; hsa-miR-1247; hsa-miR-30e-3p; hsa-miR-888-5p; hsa-miR-135b-3p; hsa-miR-23b-5p; hsa-miR-198; hsa-miR-1276; hsa-let-7a-3p; hsa-miR-596; hsa-miR-378a-5p; hsa-miR-1255a; hsa-miR-302c-5p; hsa-miR-17-3p; hsa-miR-541-5p; hsa-miR-380-3p; hsa-miR-29b-2-5p; hsa-miR-342-5p; hsa-miR-1225-3p; hsa-miR-1253; hsa-miR-486-5p; hsa-miR-520d-3p; hsa-miR-571; hsa-miR-1294; hsa-miR-641; hsa-miR-1208; hsa-miR-1825; hsa-miR-24-1-5p; hsa-miR-622; hsa-miR-206; hsa-miR-623; hsa-miR-143-5p hsa-miR-218-2-3p; hsa-miR-372-3p; hsa-miR-200b-3p; hsa-miR-519a-3p; hsa-miR-216b-5p; hsa-miR-129-1-3p; hsa-miR-1256; hsa-miR-489-3p; hsa-miR-522-3p; hsa-miR-548b-5p; hsa-miR-486-3p; hsa-miR-518e-3p; hsa-miR-141-3p; hsa-miR-517c-3p; hsa-miR-1183; hsa-miR-1269
CAFs derived from primary breast tumors ↓ CAFs derived from metastatic breast tumor ↓	0	

Fig. 35.3 Recent experimental data manifested the differential role of miRNAs in primary and cutaneous metastatic breast cancer. In particular, this study showed the role of oestrogen in Cancer-Associated Fibroblasts (CAFs) and also their role in facilitating tumor migration. It appeared that 77 miRNAs were commonly participating in both categories of CAFs, i.e., those derived from the primary site as well as those derived from the metastatic site. (Reproduced from Vivaqua et al. (2019) [39], under the Creative Commons CC BY 4.0 License https://creativecommons.org/licenses/by/4.0/)

tive roles. Cytoplasmatic lncRNAs compete with miRNAs for binding to mRNAs complementary to each other, while during tumorigenesis, aberrantly expressed lncRNAs override miRNAs' ability for inhibition, leading to over-expression of oncogenes or under-expression of tumor suppressor genes [42] (Fig. 35.4).

To the best of our knowledge, there are no known biomarkers for disease prognosis, progression, and therapy. However, several reports have addressed that problem, with an increasing number of scientific works, indicating the role of lncRNA, in tumor invasiveness and aggressiveness.

For example, a very recent report, using next-generation transcriptomic sequencing, has shown that there is a lncRNA "signature" for the prognosis and disease progression of squamous cell carcinoma, including its ability to metastasize [43]. More interestingly, another report has identified lncRNA-45 as an important factor for the ability of breast cancer to metastasize, poten-

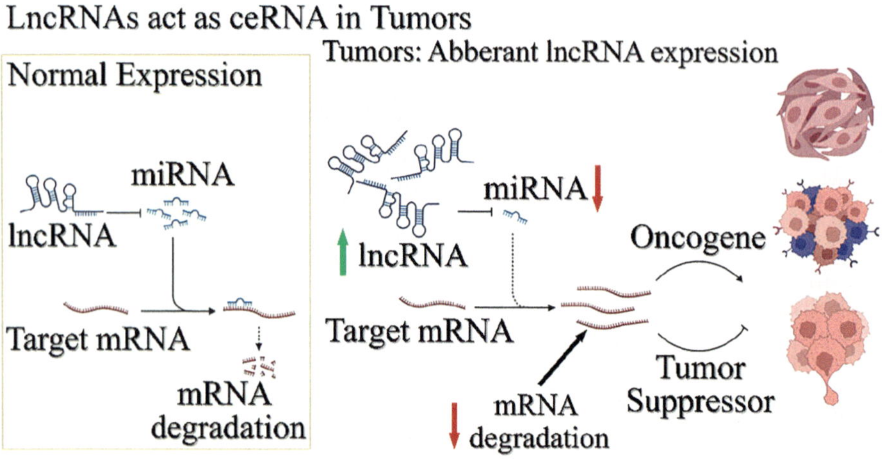

Fig. 35.4 The inter-relationship between lncRNAs and miRNAs. Under normal conditions, lncRNAs compete with miRNAs, which leads to mRNA degradation (left). In the case of aberrant functionality, the over-expression of specific lncRNAs leads to the down-regulation of competing miRNAs, leading subsequently to the preservation of mRNAs that could lead to the activation of oncogenes (right). (Adopted from Liu & Li (2022) [42], under the Creative Commons CC BY 4.0 License https://creativecommons.org/licenses/by/4.0/)

tially also to the skin, which appears to take place through the regulation of the mTOR pathway [44].

Another recent report identified *HOTTIP* and *LINC00543* as potential biomarkers for metastatic squamous cell carcinoma, both cutaneously as well as internally (lungs) [45]. Another recent study identified 27 lncRNAs, among them *ZNF252P-AS1*, *MIAT*, *FAM13A-AS1*, *LINC-PINT*, *LINC00893*, *AGAP2-AS1*, *OIP5-AS1*, and *SEMA6A-AS1*, which were found to directly enhance the ability of melanoma to give cutaneous metastases [46]. Also, an lncRNA, *LINC00893*, was found to be significantly down-regulated in melanoma, which probably enhanced its ability to form cutaneous metastases. Another lnc identified as a potential biomarker was *SMG7-AS1*, which was found to be overexpressed in squamous cell carcinoma and contributed to the tumor's metastatic machinery [47].

Similarly, another work evaluated the potential of lncRNAs for being key players in breast cancer metastases (although not cutaneous, but probably also contributing to) and found that lncRNAs and miRNAs form a complex network, whose hub molecules appeared to be two transcription factors, ETS1 and SP1 [48]. A more specific perspective was given by a recent work, which found that lnc *NR2F1-AS1* was directly correlated to poor prognosis, as its inhibition significantly inhibited the potential of breast cancer cells to metastasize [49]. This finding not only marked the lnc as a prognostic factor but probably as a therapeutic factor as well. In another interesting scientific work, a cytoplasmic-associated lncRNA (lacRNA) termed LINC00478-associated cytoplasmic RNA was derived from the nucleus-located lncRNA LINC00478, and it was found to pose a potential biomarker for breast cancer invasion and metastasis. This molecule's down-regulation was directly related to breast cancer's capability to metastasize both in vitro and in vivo [50]. The interesting finding in this study was the fact that this lnc is a regulator of *cMyc*, whose inhibition leads to a good prognosis.

35.2.3.3 circRNAs

Circular RNAs (circRNAs) have gained much attention in recent years, due to their presence in the eukaryotic transcriptome. Yet, their presence has been known for about the last 50 years, starting from the discovery of viral genomes, for example, the murine respirovirus [51]. circRNAs were experimentally verified through electron microscopy and found in the cytoplasm of HeLa cells (Fig. 35.5).

CircRNAs function as miRNA sponges, that is bind to miRNAs, not allowing them to further bind to their target genes. In addition, circRNAs can function as RNA stabilizers, targeting both mRNAs and lncRNAs, and they bind to RNA Binding Proteins (RBPs). An interesting example comes from the linking of circFOXO3, which binds to both p53 and E3 ubiquitin ligase MDM2, promoting the degradation of the p53 protein and the degradation of Foxo3, a pro-apoptotic protein [52].

Current literature, concerning the role of circRNAs in tumor biology and subsequently cutaneous metastases, is still scarce. Literature addressed this topic in two main subjects: the role of circRNAs in breast cancer and the tumor's potential to metastasize and the role of circRNAs in cutaneous neoplasms, for example, melanoma or squamous cell carcinoma.

In the case of breast cancer, one recent scientific work identified circPOKE as a biomarker for tumor invasion and metastasis. It was found that circPOKE was under-expressed in primary and metastatic breast cancer tissues, while the opposite effect (over-expression) "inhibited the metastatic potential but not the proliferative ability" of breast cancer cells both in vitro and in vivo [53]. This research work showed that circPOKE was able to competitively bind to USP10, inhibiting the downstream binding to the Snail protein, an important factor for epithelial-mesenchymal transition.

In the case of cutaneous malignancies, several circRNAs have been identified as potential biomarkers; for example, for squamous cell carcinoma, circPVT1 [54], circ_0067772 [55], circFADS2 [56], circ_0001821 [57], circ_006831 [58], circ_0005085 [59], and circIFFO1 [60]. Fewer reports have highlighted the role of circRNAs for melanoma; in particular, a recent review has summarized the potential circRNAs that are playing a role in melanoma progression, invasion, metastasis, and prognosis, which include circ_0083444, circ_0005320, circ_0067531, circ_0084043, circ_0000082, circ_0016418, circ_0085533, circ_0025039, circ_0001946, circ_0002770, circ_0079593, circ_0027247, circ_0017247, and circ_0020710 [61]. Finally, one more report found circZNF609 to play an inhibitory role in the progression and metastasis of cutaneous melanoma [62]. The circRNAs are summarized in Table 35.2.

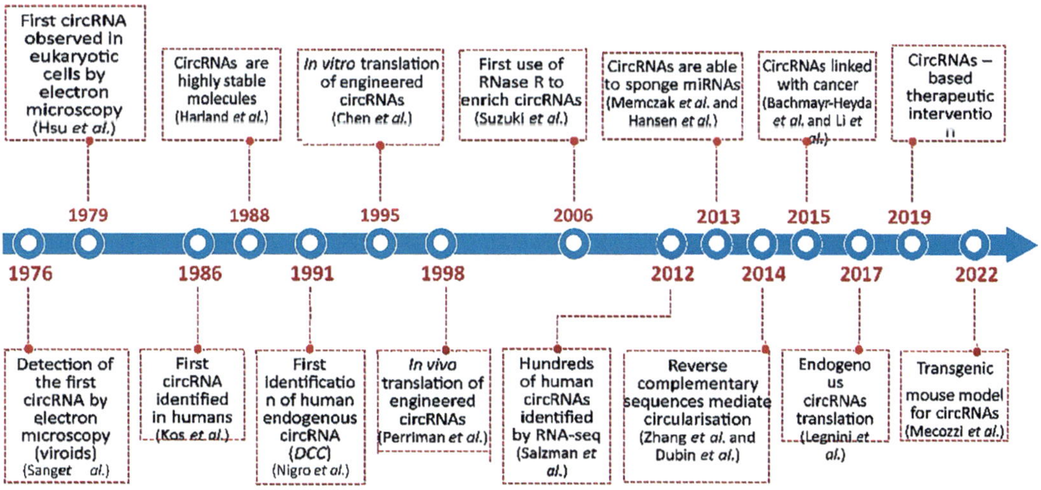

Fig. 35.5 The timeline and history of circular RNAs (circRNAs) . (Reproduced from Pisignano et al. (2023) [51], under the Creative Commons CC BY 4.0 License https://creativecommons.org/licenses/by/4.0/)

Table 35.2 Summary of circRNAs that are known to play a role in breast cancer, squamous cell carcinoma, and melanoma

CircRNA	Neoplasm	Regulation	Function in tumor progression	Function in metastasis	Ref.
circPOKE	BC	Down	Oncogene	Promotes	[53]
circPVT1	CSCC	Up	Oncogene	N/A	[54]
circ_0067772	CSCC	Up	Oncogene	Promotes	[55]
circFADS2	CSCC	Up	TS	Inhibits	[56]
circ_0001821	CSCC	Up	Oncogene	Promotes	[57]
circ_0068631	CSCC	Up	Oncogene	Promotes	[58]
circ_0005085	CSCC	Up	Oncogene	Promotes	[59]
circIFFO1	CSCC	Up	TS	Inhibits	[60]
circZNF609	MM	Up	TS	Inhibits	[62]
circ_0083444	MM	Up	Oncogene	Promotes	[61]
circ_0005320	MM	Up	Oncogene	Promotes	[63]
circ_0067531	MM	Up	Oncogene	Promotes	[63]
circ_0084043	MM	Up	Oncogene	Promotes	[64, 65]
circ_0000082	MM	Up	Oncogene	Promotes	[61]
circ_0016418	MM	Up	Oncogene	Promotes	[66]
circ_0085533	MM	Up	Oncogene	Promotes	[61]
circ_0025039	MM	Up	Oncogene	Promotes	[67]
circ_0001946	MM	Up	Oncogene	Promotes	[61]
circ_0002770	MM	Up	Oncogene	Promotes	[68]
circ_0079593	MM	Up	Oncogene	Promotes	[69, 70]
circ_0027247	MM	Up	Oncogene	Promotes	[64]
circ_0017247	MM	Up	Oncogene	Promotes	[71]
circ_0020710	MM	Up	Oncogene	Promotes	[72]

Legend: *BC* Breast Cancer, *CSCC* Cutaneous Squamous Cell Carcinoma, *Ref* Reference

35.3 Computational Methods as a Tool

The amazing progress of computational methods and the rapid development of the so-called "Artificial Intelligence" (AI) were made possible through a very simple fact: advances in computational power, memory, and storage capacities of modern computers. Today, the general public has been aware of AI capabilities with respect to Natural Language Processing (NLP), for example, "ChatGPT," and also has been very impressed by it.

However, AI has been around for a long time, before ChatGPT, and it has been used for different applications, including medical. It was apparent that computational approaches could provide an invaluable tool for the diagnosis, prognosis, and therapy of human disease, which includes skin disease of the neoplasmatic nature. There are several scientific works concerning the use of AI (with all its subdivisions) for the detection of cutaneous disease, not only neoplasmatic but also other skin conditions such as dermatitis [73], psoriasis [74], or even the diagnosis and stratification of osteosarcoma [75].

The first attempts for the use of AI in biomedicine were as early as the 1950s, where an automated assessment of symptoms was performed [76]. However, computational power was very limited, which posed obstacles to any such attempt. After the 1990s, the increase in computational power enabled the entry of AI into biomedicine. Automated evaluation of electrocardiograms (ECGs), the measurement of white blood cells in blood samples, and the analysis of retinal and skin conditions' photographs became aspects of potential analysis [77].

Thus, the main questions to be answered are whether computational methods and, in particular, AI, can provide an accurate tool for cutaneous neoplasmatic disease and especially cutaneous metastatic disease, but also could AI automate the diagnosis (and probably prognosis) of cutaneous medical imaging tests, contributing to a faster, more accurate, and more reliable decision-making process?

In this section, we will address the applications of AI, focusing mainly on machine learning, on cutaneous metastatic disease, and describe the up-to-date progress on the topic.

35.3.1 Medical Imaging: Old and New

The apparent advantage of cutaneous disease, neoplasmatic or not, has to do with the fact that cutaneous disease is apparent, i.e., readily approachable and relatively easy to observe, investigate, and record. In other words, it has to do with the visual information entailed in such a lesion. Medical imaging data have the ability to capture intricate details of the human body, which are essential for diagnosing, treating, and understanding many medical conditions. Such images can be produced from a variety of sources, such as radiological examinations, pathological specimens, endoscopies, photography, and others. Therefore, medical imaging data typically constitute the largest volume of medical data. Examples of medical imaging include X-ray, Computed Tomography (CT) scan, Magnetic Resonance Imaging (MRI), ultrasound, and photography. Yet, the remaining challenge is to combine the imaging information with other data (for example, clinical, genomic, transcriptomic, etc.) and use those in a holistic way to perform diagnosis or predict prognosis.

By capturing detailed images of organs, tissues, and biological processes, radiology is at the heart of modern healthcare. The field of radiodiagnostics began in 1895, with the accidental discovery of *Wilhelm Conrad Röntgen* [78]. This discovery consisted of a milestone for the beginning of radio-diagnostics. However, despite the initial enthusiasm, limitations were quickly realized, as the radiographs obtained were limited to two dimensions. A year after the discovery of X-rays, *E. Thompson* was already attempting to produce a three-dimensional radiograph, using stereoscopic techniques. However, at that time, the necessary computational power required was not available. Decades later, computational power and technological advancements made the "computed" or "axial" tomography (CT) possible.

A more modern imaging approach concerned the use of light for the purpose of obtaining biological and clinical images. One such method, dermatoscopy, represents a significant methodological breakthrough in the field of dermatology. This advanced technique allows the in vivo visualization of pigmented skin lesions, reaching a depth of up to the dermis, i.e., the network of collagen fibers located beneath the epidermis. The main idea behind this type of imaging is the use of light, both ultraviolet, visible, and infrared, which can detect cutaneous morphological features as well as features that come from the presence of melanin and hemoglobin under the various skin layers. Recent advances have utilized polarized light for dermatoscopy [79, 80]. Typically, dermatoscopes offer a 10× magnification, but more modern digital dermatoscopes are capable of producing images of up to 70×, while maintaining image clarity and sharpness. Unlike images obtained under the microscope, for histopathology, dermatoscope images are not focused on a single cutaneous plane, but consist of the superposition of multiple cutaneous planes.

35.3.2 Machine Learning

35.3.2.1 The "Classical Way of Things"

Machine learning is a field of AI that can potentially mimic human cognitive abilities, such as data analysis, problem solving, and ultimately decision making, including medical decision making. These functions are performed according to a predefined set of rules that have been previously defined. However, machine learning does not require any human intervention to enter "rules." Instead, an algorithm has the ability to "learn," or extract, on its own, the necessary rules by analyzing a set of data.

In order for the algorithm to actually work, it has to solve the so-called "learning problem." In general, learning is considered the process through which new knowledge, skills, or behaviors are acquired. Therefore, any computer system that can change its *modus operandi* and adapt based on new data entry can be considered to have the ability to "learn." In its simplest form, such a system memorizes every problem it encounters and recalls its solution whenever it is needed. However, in most cases, this function is not sufficient; the real goal is not to solve problems that have already occurred in the past, but to solve new, unknown problems that may appear in the future. Therefore, a machine learning system should be able to "generalize" the received information and inductively be led to a solution for an unknown problem.

Depending on the "learning" or "training" method, machine learning can be divided into three categories: (a) Supervised learning, where the system accepts data of a set of similar problems, as well as their final solutions, and attempts to predict the general rule underlying the set of problems. (b) Unsupervised learning, where the system "learns" on its own to analyze data and draw "conclusions," which, however, are not always clear, or even useful. The basic idea behind unsupervised learning is to group homogeneous data in order to discover hidden relationships and reduce their complexity. (c) Reinforcement learning, which is a special case of machine learning. This algorithm involves the interaction of an "intelligent" agent with its environment and monitors the outcome of the interaction. The environment feeds the agent with a positive or negative signal, and the agent adapts accordingly. Medical applications mainly concern the use of supervised and unsupervised learning. Their simplicity, interpretability, and proven effectiveness make them a very good alternative to more modern methods, which can actually lead to better results, especially when training data are limited.

Just to mention a few algorithms, utilized in machine learning approaches, these include: Support Vector Machines (SVM), Random Forests (RF), and k-Nearest Neighbors (k-NN). Support Vector Machines, often referred to as SVMs, are one of the most prominent methods of classical machine learning. Their basic operation is based on the concept of linear separability. More specifically, an SVM attempts to compute a hyperplane in the feature space that optimally separates the multidimensional samples of a data set into *n* categories [81]. A hyperplane is a flat, multidimensional surface that separates data points. In a two-dimensional space, a hyperplane is a straight line; in three dimensions, a two-dimensional surface, and so on. The goal of SVMs is to find the hyperplane that maximizes the margin between different classes, so that the model is more robust and generalizable to new data. However, SVMs are not only suitable for linear data. Although a data set may not be linearly separable in its original feature space, it could be linearly separable in a higher-dimensional feature space. Therefore, with the use of appropriate functions, SVMs can handle nonlinear data by mapping it to a higher-dimensional feature space. Although this is a very technical description, which makes almost no sense to the "non-expert," this is a formal description of SVMs.

Random forests are a powerful, combinatorial learning method. They are based on decision trees, which function by analyzing the decision-making process into a sequence of binary choices, i.e., a flowchart [82]. The main advantage of decision trees is their simple and easily interpretable approach. However, a decision tree by itself is prone to overfitting the data. Therefore, Random Forests combine multiple decision trees and leverage their collective intelligence to improve accuracy. This makes Random Forests to stand out concerning their robustness, scalability, and applicability to both classification and regression tasks.

The k-Nearest Neighbors (k-NN) algorithm is a simple but effective learning method. It works on the principle of proximity, classifying data points according to the majority class among their k-nearest neighbors in the feature space [83]. It is based on the idea that similar data points (samples) belonging to the same class exhibit similar properties, and therefore occupy adjacent positions in the feature space. k-NN is particularly useful for tasks involving clustering, classification, and regression. This is a very useful algorithm, especially in cases of multi-dimensional data.

35.3.2.2 Neural Networks

Having talked about machine learning, it would be negligent not to include a short description of Neural Networks (NNs). We are not going to get to the depths of it (since it is a very complicated technical matter), but we will mention some basic terms and characteristics. We could separate three NN methods: the "classical" NNs, the Deep Neural Networks (DNNs), and the Convolutional Neural Networks (CNNs).

In "classical" neural networks, a set of nodes interacts with each other, imitating biological neural networks. These nodes accept an input, and each one produces an output after solving a mathematical equation. This happens multiple times and under numerous layers, but the important part is that the "rules" must be given. The key concept is also the abundance of data. NNs can only function if there really is a lot of data!

On the other hand, Deep Neural Networks (DNNs) have the ability to automatically learn the necessary features from the input data, without relying on human factors. Their characteristic is their "deep" architecture, which includes multiple layers of interconnected neurons, i.e., non-linear computational structures. However, a prerequisite for training DNNs is the existence of a *sufficiently large* data set. The deeper and generally larger a network is, the greater the amount of data it requires for training. For example, today's DNNs used for image classification are trained on datasets such as ImageNet, which contains millions of images [84, 85]. Particularly in biomedical subjects, where available data are limited, training DNNs is a challenge.

Finally, Convolutional Neural Networks (CNNs) are considered one of the most cutting-edge approaches to neural networks to date. First reported in 2012 by Krizhevsky et al. [85]. This network used multiple convolutional layers, an architecture much deeper than previous neural networks used for image classification. This algorithm was considered a turning point in the field of computer vision and deep learning, since it demonstrated the effectiveness of deep neural networks in image analysis and classification, thus sparking a wave of research and developments in that field.

35.3.3 Disease Diagnosis and Prognosis

35.3.3.1 Application of Machine Learning to Malignancy Diagnosis and Prognosis

Having mentioned the whereabouts of machine learning, it is consequent to understand that research would have turned towards the automation of diagnosis in medical situations, for example, evaluating non-invasive imaging data. Such examples are dermatoscopy, computed tomography, magnetic resonance imaging, ultrasound, etc.

In dermatoscopy, the diagnosis of melanoma is of particular interest, where its early detection significantly increases patients' prognosis. However, melanoma can often mimic benign skin lesions, making it difficult to distinguish between harmless skin abnormalities and potentially malignant melanoma [86]. Therefore, machine learning approaches could potentially play a crucial role in early and accurate diagnosis. Towards that end, several systems have been proposed combining neural networks for melanoma diagnosis and segmentation [87, 88], some of them reaching a 76% accuracy. In another work by Yu et al., a double NN was proposed, which included a two-stage architecture [89]. This architecture included two deep NNs in series, which sequentially performed lesion segmentation and then diagnosis, achieving 95% accuracy. Another recent report proposed a fully automated method for melanoma diagnosis, which utilized region-based NNs (RCNN), combined with fuzzy k-means clustering (FKM) [90]. This method involved image pre-processing to enhance visual information, using RCNN for feature extraction, and using FKM for segmentation, achieving average accuracy 95.4%, 93.1%, and 95.6% in three different datasets.

In the same context, prognosis refers to the ability of a system to predict or assess the likely course and outcome of a disease in an individual patient. It includes the assessment of future development, possible complications, and the likelihood of recovery, deterioration, or death for the patient. Prognostic information is vital for both patients and healthcare professionals, as it guides therapeutic decisions for better disease management. A recent study used radiomic features in combination with clinical parameters to predict local recurrence and distant metastasis in patients with early non-small cell lung cancer after stereotactic body radiotherapy [91]. In particular, the study used patients' CT scans, in which the tumors were delineated by radiologists. Using the precise tumor boundaries, the authors extracted 944 radiomic features exclusively from these areas and combined them with clinical parameters. The clinical parameters included age, sex, body mass index, smoking history, and histological examination results. Using random survival forest, the authors were able to predict local recurrence and distant metastasis. In another recent report, CT scans were analyzed from patients with non-small cell lung cancer with the scope of predicting patient survival [92].

Another work used deep learning models to predict tumor morphological changes in metastatic colorectal cancer, based on CT scans, which could potentially allow for early adjustments during treatment [93]. Specifically, the study used a Spiking Neural Network (SNN) to extract features at multiple time points during treatment, and then a Recurrent Neural Network (RNN) to combine them and estimate the final outcome. As with diagnosis, prognosis can be investigated using a variety of imaging modalities.

35.3.3.2 Application of Machine Learning to Cutaneous Metastases

In the previous section, I addressed the use of machine learning approaches to the diagnosis or prognosis based on imaging data. Yet, there is another field of application for the use of machine learning. This concerns the investigation of transcriptomic and genomic profiles for the understanding of cutaneous metastases. This is an interesting approach, since the use of imaging data alone could not provide a complete perspective of the tumor machinery. In that sense, a recent report investigated the use of transcriptomic data to predict melanoma cutaneous metastatic potential, where it was found that distinctive gene signatures (for example, the over-expression of *ITGA4*, *ATF2*, and *CUL2* genes) are linked to the ability of melanoma to metastasize [94]. Another similar work found that *C7*, *MMP3*, *KRT14*, *LOC642587*, *CASP7*, *S100A7*, and miRNA hsa-mir-205 and hsa-mir-203b could be key genomic features contributing to the oncogenesis of melanoma. In addition, the same study found that *ESM1*, *NFATC3*, *C7orf4*, *CDK14*, *ZNF827*, and *ZSWIM7* could serve as potential biomarkers for cutaneous melanoma metastasis [95].

In a very interesting work, it has been reported that there is a direct correlation between cutaneous melanoma metastasis from an unknown primary tumor. In this study, gene expression profiling revealed that the transcriptomic profile was mostly linked to specific pathways such as autoimmunity, inflammation, immune cell infiltration, and immune activation. In addition, the same study showed that the metastatic tumor site was mostly infiltrated by CD8+ and CD4+ T cells, B cells, and NK cells, as well as significantly higher major histocompatibility complex (MHC)-I and MHC-II [96]. In addition, several works have dealt with the role of miRNAs in cutaneous melanoma and its metastatic potential. These studies indicate that miRNA signatures could prove very crucial for disease prognosis [97].

Most of the scientific literature deals with the issue of metastasis from the point of view where the cutaneous tumor is the primary source and has the potential to metastasize either internally or cutaneously, and not the other way around [98–100]. This is not peculiar, since internal metastases from primary cutaneous tumors are more frequent than cutaneous metastases from other primary tumors. Yet, as aforementioned, cutaneous metastases pose the advantage of easy and direct access; they can be detected by the patients themselves, and examination can be potentially non-invasive. This is the part where machine learning can assist in the integration of a huge amount of information for understanding cutaneous metastatic mechanisms.

35.4 Future Perspectives

Overall, the whole idea of integrating different and numerous biomedical data for disease diagnosis, prognosis, and therapy is still in its infancy. We are just starting to understand the interconnections of genomic, transcriptomic, radiomic, and clinical data. Especially, in the case of metastatic disease, prediction is of paramount importance, since it marks the line between life and probable death.

In the present chapter, we have addressed some novel aspects and tools concerning cutaneous metastases. It is apparent that there is not much knowledge concerning the topic. G-quadruplexes, lncRNAs, circRNAs, and miRNAs are molecules that play critical roles in tumorigenesis, tumor ontogenesis, and progression as well as metastasis. Apparently, more research is needed to understand those molecules' roles, but this is not only it. Future research should focus on the understanding of the complete network and towards the interpretation of what single molecules do. Although the personalized medicine trend is prevalent in recent times, it is deprived of something important; the understanding of the basic mechanisms behind tumor mechanics (or other disease mechanics).

Another challenge that still needs to be addressed is the use of non-invasive methods, such as dermatoscopy, and the interpretation of their results for disease prognosis. This field is still in its infancy, and this is a field where photometry, spectrometry, genomics, and transcriptomics could come together.

We have seen that in the case of cutaneous metastases, tumor has already progressed to such a point that makes prognosis dismal. Therefore, knowledge could also focus on the prediction of that condition and attempt to address it before it happens. This could be achieved, probably, not by analyzing one set or type of data at a time, but multiple. This is where machine learning comes in. It is a valuable tool that can help us integrate that kind of information into applicable knowledge.

Progress is slow, but hopeful!

References

1. Welfare AIoHa. Cancer in Australia: actual incidence data from 1982 to 2013 and mortality data from 1982 to 2014 with projections to 2017. Asia Pac J Clin Oncol. 2018;14(1):5–15. https://doi.org/10.1111/ajco.12761.
2. Chatzistergos T, Krivova NA, Yeo KL. Long-term changes in solar activity and irradiance. J Atmos Sol Terr Phys. 2023;252:106150. https://doi.org/10.1016/j.jastp.2023.106150.
3. Habermehl G, Ko J. Cutaneous metastases: a review and diagnostic approach to tumors of unknown origin. Arch Pathol Lab Med. 2019;143(8):943–57. https://doi.org/10.5858/arpa.2018-0051-RA.
4. Schwartz RA. Cutaneous metastatic disease. J Am Acad Dermatol. 1995;33(2 Pt 1):161–82; quiz 83–6. https://doi.org/10.1016/0190-9622(95)90231-7.
5. Kaplan RP. Specific cutaneous manifestations of internal malignancy. Adv Dermatol. 1986;1:3–42.
6. Martin CF, Hamilton WF. Two cases of sarcomatosis with purpura haemorrhagica. J Exp Med. 1896;1(4):595–612. https://doi.org/10.1084/jem.1.4.595.
7. Saeed S, Keehn CA, Morgan MB. Cutaneous metastasis: a clinical, pathological, and immunohistochemical appraisal. J Cutan Pathol. 2004;31(6):419–30. https://doi.org/10.1111/j.0303-6987.2004.00207.x.
8. Nashan D, Meiss F, Braun-Falco M, Reichenberger S. Cutaneous metastases from internal malignancies. Dermatol Ther. 2010;23(6):567–80. https://doi.org/10.1111/j.1529-8019.2010.01364.x.
9. Fitzgerald JE, Byrd BK, Patil RA, Strawbridge RR, Davis SC, Bellini C, et al. Heterogeneity of circulating tumor cell dissemination and lung metastases in a subcutaneous Lewis lung carcinoma model. Biomed Opt Express. 2020;11(7):3633–47. https://doi.org/10.1364/boe.395289.
10. Gurumurthi R, Thirumalai R, Easow JM, Mohan S. Tumor attributes predicting cutaneous metastatic destiny: a report of two interesting cases. Indian J Dermatol. 2014;59(4):422. https://doi.org/10.4103/0019-5154.135535.
11. Liu Q, Zhang H, Jiang X, Qian C, Liu Z, Luo D. Factors involved in cancer metastasis: a better understanding to "seed and soil" hypothesis. Mol Cancer. 2017;16(1):176. https://doi.org/10.1186/s12943-017-0742-4.

12. Otsuka I. Cutaneous metastasis after surgery, injury, lymphadenopathy, and peritonitis: possible mechanisms. Int J Mol Sci. 2019;20(13):3286.
13. Pantel K, Brakenhoff RH. Dissecting the metastatic cascade. Nat Rev. 2004;4(6):448–56. https://doi.org/10.1038/nrc1370.
14. Sundaram GM, Quah S, Sampath P. Cancer: the dark side of wound healing. FEBS J. 2018;285(24):4516–34. https://doi.org/10.1111/febs.14586.
15. Kalluri R. The biology and function of fibroblasts in cancer. Nat Rev. 2016;16(9):582–98. https://doi.org/10.1038/nrc.2016.73.
16. Kosiol N, Juranek S, Brossart P, Heine A, Paeschke K. G-quadruplexes: a promising target for cancer therapy. Mol Cancer. 2021;20(1):40. https://doi.org/10.1186/s12943-021-01328-4.
17. Burge S, Parkinson GN, Hazel P, Todd AK, Neidle S. Quadruplex DNA: sequence, topology and structure. Nucleic Acids Res. 2006;34(19):5402–15. https://doi.org/10.1093/nar/gkl655.
18. Capra JA, Paeschke K, Singh M, Zakian VA. G-quadruplex DNA sequences are evolutionarily conserved and associated with distinct genomic features in Saccharomyces cerevisiae. PLoS Comput Biol. 2010;6(7):e1000861. https://doi.org/10.1371/journal.pcbi.1000861.
19. Dai J, Punchihewa C, Ambrus A, Chen D, Jones RA, Yang D. Structure of the intramolecular human telomeric G-quadruplex in potassium solution: a novel adenine triple formation. Nucleic Acids Res. 2007;35(7):2440–50. https://doi.org/10.1093/nar/gkm009.
20. Chen FM. Sr2+ facilitates intermolecular G-quadruplex formation of telomeric sequences. Biochemistry. 1992;31(15):3769–76. https://doi.org/10.1021/bi00130a006.
21. Wang Y, de los Santos C, Gao XO, Greene K, Live D, Patel DJ. Multinuclear nuclear magnetic resonance studies of Na cation-stabilized complex formed by d(G-G-T-T-T-T-C-G-G) in solution. Implications for G-tetrad structures. J Mol Biol. 1991;222(3):819–32. https://doi.org/10.1016/0022-2836(91)90513-6.
22. Wang Y, Patel DJ. Guanine residues in d(T2AG3) and d(T2G4) form parallel-stranded potassium cation stabilized G-quadruplexes with anti glycosidic torsion angles in solution. Biochemistry. 1992;31(35):8112–9. https://doi.org/10.1021/bi00150a002.
23. Majumdar A, Gosser Y, Patel DJ. 1H-1H correlations across N-H...N hydrogen bonds in nucleic acids. J Biomol NMR. 2001;21(4):289–306. https://doi.org/10.1023/a:1013340227140.
24. Shafer RH, Smirnov I. Biological aspects of DNA/RNA quadruplexes. Biopolymers. 2000;56(3):209–27. https://doi.org/10.1002/1097-0282(2000/2001)56:3<209::aid-bip10018>3.0.-co;2-y.
25. Chambers VS, Marsico G, Boutell JM, Di Antonio M, Smith GP, Balasubramanian S. High-throughput sequencing of DNA G-quadruplex structures in the human genome. Nat Biotechnol. 2015;33(8):877–81. https://doi.org/10.1038/nbt.3295.
26. Marsico G, Chambers VS, Sahakyan AB, McCauley P, Boutell JM, Antonio MD, et al. Whole genome experimental maps of DNA G-quadruplexes in multiple species. Nucleic Acids Res. 2019;47(8):3862–74. https://doi.org/10.1093/nar/gkz179.
27. Kaplan OI, Berber B, Hekim N, Doluca O. G-quadruplex prediction in E. coli genome reveals a conserved putative G-quadruplex-Hairpin-Duplex switch. Nucleic Acids Res. 2016;44(19):9083–95. https://doi.org/10.1093/nar/gkw769.
28. Lavezzo E, Berselli M, Frasson I, Perrone R, Palù G, Brazzale AR, et al. G-quadruplex forming sequences in the genome of all known human viruses: a comprehensive guide. PLoS Comput Biol. 2018;14(12):e1006675. https://doi.org/10.1371/journal.pcbi.1006675.
29. Lane AN, Chaires JB, Gray RD, Trent JO. Stability and kinetics of G-quadruplex structures. Nucleic Acids Res. 2008;36(17):5482–515. https://doi.org/10.1093/nar/gkn517.
30. Ruggiero E, Richter SN. G-quadruplexes and G-quadruplex ligands: targets and tools in antiviral therapy. Nucleic Acids Res. 2018;46(7):3270–83. https://doi.org/10.1093/nar/gky187.
31. Kim NW, Piatyszek MA, Prowse KR, Harley CB, West MD, Ho PL, et al. Specific association of human telomerase activity with immortal cells and cancer. Science (New York, NY). 1994;266(5193):2011–5. https://doi.org/10.1126/science.7605428.
32. Tauchi T, Shin-Ya K, Sashida G, Sumi M, Nakajima A, Shimamoto T, et al. Activity of a novel G-quadruplex-interactive telomerase inhibitor, telomestatin (SOT-095), against human leukemia cells: involvement of ATM-dependent DNA damage response pathways. Oncogene. 2003;22(34):5338–47. https://doi.org/10.1038/sj.onc.1206833.
33. Sun JW, Zou J, Zheng Y, Yuan H, Xie YZ, Wang XN, et al. Design, synthesis, and evaluation of novel quindoline derivatives with fork-shaped side chains as RNA G-quadruplex stabilizers for repressing oncogene NRAS translation. Eur J Med Chem. 2024;271:116406. https://doi.org/10.1016/j.ejmech.2024.116406.
34. Guillon J, Denevault-Sabourin C, Chevret E, Brachet-Botineau M, Milano V, Guédin-Beaurepaire A, et al. Design, synthesis, and antiproliferative effect of 2,9-bis[4-(pyridinylalkylaminomethyl) phenyl]-1,10-phenanthroline derivatives on human leukemic cells by targeting G-quadruplex. Arch Pharm. 2021;354(8):e2000450. https://doi.org/10.1002/ardp.202000450.
35. Das RN, Chevret E, Desplat V, Rubio S, Mergny JL, Guillon J. Design, synthesis and biological evaluation of new substituted diquinolinyl-pyridine ligands as anticancer agents by targeting G-Quadruplex. Molecules (Basel, Switzerland). 2017;23(1):81. https://doi.org/10.3390/molecules23010081.

36. Monnerat C, Chompret A, Kannengiesser C, Avril MF, Janin N, Spatz A, et al. BRCA1, BRCA2, TP53, and CDKN2A germline mutations in patients with breast cancer and cutaneous melanoma. Fam Cancer. 2007;6(4):453–61. https://doi.org/10.1007/s10689-007-9143-y.
37. Grimaldi AM, Cassidy PB, Leachmann S, Ascierto PA. Novel approaches in melanoma prevention and therapy. Cancer Treat Res. 2014;159:443–55. https://doi.org/10.1007/978-3-642-38007-5_25.
38. Raimo M, Orso F, Grassi E, Cimino D, Penna E, De Pittà C, et al. miR-146a exerts differential effects on melanoma growth and metastatization. Mol Cancer Res. 2016;14(6):548–62. https://doi.org/10.1158/1541-7786.mcr-15-0425-t.
39. Vivacqua A, Muoio MG, Miglietta AM, Maggiolini M. Differential MicroRNA landscape triggered by estrogens in cancer associated fibroblasts (CAFs) of primary and metastatic breast tumors. Cancer. 2019;11(3):412.
40. Kaushik SB, Kaushik N. Non-coding RNAs in skin cancers: an update. Noncoding RNA Res. 2016;1(1):83–6. https://doi.org/10.1016/j.ncrna.2016.11.003.
41. Khan AQ, Ahmad F, Raza SS, Zarif L, Siveen KS, Sher G, et al. Role of non-coding RNAs in the progression and resistance of cutaneous malignancies and autoimmune diseases. Semin Cancer Biol. 2022;83:208–26. https://doi.org/10.1016/j.semcancer.2020.07.003.
42. Liu F, Li S. Non-coding RNAs in skin cancers: biological roles and molecular mechanisms. Front Pharmacol. 2022;13:934396. https://doi.org/10.3389/fphar.2022.934396.
43. Bone M, Schreyer D, Treanor-Taylor M, Proby CM, Harwood CA, Leigh IM, et al. The landscape of long non-coding RNA during cSCC progression. Br J Dermatol. 2025; https://doi.org/10.1093/bjd/ljaf108.
44. Qiu J, Guo Y, Wang S, Ren Q, Dong Z, Gao M, et al. Newly identified lncRNA-45 promotes breast cancer metastasis through activating the mTOR signaling pathway. Biochem Biophys Res Commun. 2023;640:40–9. https://doi.org/10.1016/j.bbrc.2022.11.099.
45. Nissinen L, Haalisto J, Riihilä P, Piipponen M, Kähäri VM. Clustering of RNA co-expression network identifies novel long non-coding RNA biomarkers in squamous cell carcinoma. Sci Rep. 2024;14(1):16864. https://doi.org/10.1038/s41598-024-67808-x.
46. Shi HZ, Tian CC, Wu MY, Ma L, Sun JF, Chen H. m6A- and m5C- modified lncRNAs orchestrate the prognosis in cutaneous melanoma and m6A- modified LINC00893 regulates cutaneous melanoma cell metastasis. Skin Res Technol. 2024;30(7):e13842. https://doi.org/10.1111/srt.13842.
47. Xu X, Ju Y, Zhao X, Yang P, Zhu F, Fang B. SMG7-AS1 as a prognostic biomarker and predictor of immunotherapy responses for skin cutaneous melanoma. Genomics. 2023;115(3):110614. https://doi.org/10.1016/j.ygeno.2023.110614.
48. Chakraborty S, Banerjee S. Multidimensional computational study to understand non-coding RNA interactions in breast cancer metastasis. Sci Rep. 2023;13(1):15771. https://doi.org/10.1038/s41598-023-42904-6.
49. Zhai D, Zhou Y, Kuang X, Shao F, Zhen T, Lin Y, et al. Lnc NR2F1-AS1 promotes breast cancer metastasis by targeting the MiR-25-3p/ZEB2 Axis. Int J Med Sci. 2023;20(9):1152–62. https://doi.org/10.7150/ijms.86969.
50. Guo R, Su Y, Zhang Q, Xiu B, Huang S, Chi W, et al. LINC00478-derived novel cytoplasmic lncRNA LacRNA stabilizes PHB2 and suppresses breast cancer metastasis via repressing MYC targets. J Transl Med. 2023;21(1):120. https://doi.org/10.1186/s12967-023-03967-1.
51. Pisignano G, Michael DC, Visal TH, Pirlog R, Ladomery M, Calin GA. Going circular: history, present, and future of circRNAs in cancer. Oncogene. 2023;42(38):2783–800. https://doi.org/10.1038/s41388-023-02780-w.
52. Du WW, Fang L, Yang W, Wu N, Awan FM, Yang Z, et al. Induction of tumor apoptosis through a circular RNA enhancing Foxo3 activity. Cell Death Differ. 2017;24(2):357–70. https://doi.org/10.1038/cdd.2016.133.
53. Luo Y, Zhu Q, Xiang S, Wang Q, Li J, Chen X, et al. Downregulated circPOKE promotes breast cancer metastasis through activation of the USP10-Snail axis. Oncogene. 2023;42(44):3236–51. https://doi.org/10.1038/s41388-023-02823-2.
54. Chen S, Ding J, Wang Y, Lu T, Wang L, Gao X, et al. RNA-Seq profiling of circular RNAs and the oncogenic role of circPVT1 in cutaneous squamous cell carcinoma. Onco Targets Ther. 2020;13:6777–88. https://doi.org/10.2147/ott.s252233.
55. Li X, Kong Y, Li H, Xu M, Jiang M, Sun W, et al. CircRNA circ_0067772 aggravates the malignant progression of cutaneous squamous cell carcinoma by regulating miR-1238-3p/FOXG1 axis. Genes Genomics. 2021;43(5):491–501. https://doi.org/10.1007/s13258-021-01074-3.
56. Zhang Z, Sun H, Hou J, Li L, Wu L. Circular RNA circFADS2 inhibits the progression of cutaneous squamous cell carcinoma by regulating miR-766-3p/HOXA9 axis. Histol Histopathol. 2022;37(4):335–48. https://doi.org/10.14670/hh-18-409.
57. Zhang Z, Deng X. circ_0001821 contributes to the development of cutaneous squamous cell carcinoma by regulating MicroRNA-148a-3p/EGFR axis and activating phosphatidylinositol 3-kinase/Akt pathway. Mol Cell Biol. 2022;42(3):e0008921. https://doi.org/10.1128/mcb.00089-21.
58. Ji J, Xiong C, Peng J, Zhang N, Zhang Y, Yang H, et al. Circ_0068631 sponges miR-139-5p to promote the growth and metastasis of cutaneous squamous cell carcinoma by upregulating HOXB7. Skin Res Technol. 2023;29(2):e13248. https://doi.org/10.1111/srt.13248.

59. Wang L, Liu Y, Gao Q, Hu R. Hsa_circ_0005085 may suppress cutaneous squamous cell carcinoma growth and metastasis through targeting the miR-186-5p/LAMC1 axis. Skin Res Technol. 2023;29(6):e13321. https://doi.org/10.1111/srt.13321.
60. Yu H, Liu P, Chen T. CircIFFO1 suppresses tumor growth and metastasis of cutaneous squamous cell carcinoma by targeting the miR-424-5p/NFIB axis. Arch Dermatol Res. 2023;315(9):2585–96. https://doi.org/10.1007/s00403-023-02659-6.
61. Cong L, Yang H, Sun H, Hao M, Liu C, Zheng Y, et al. Role of circular RNAs in the pathogenesis of malignant melanoma. Crit Rev Eukaryot Gene Expr. 2022;32(3):21–30. https://doi.org/10.1615/CritRevEukaryotGeneExpr.2021040319.
62. Shang Q, Du H, Wu X, Guo Q, Zhang F, Gong Z, et al. FMRP ligand circZNF609 destabilizes RAC1 mRNA to reduce metastasis in acral melanoma and cutaneous melanoma. J Exp Clin Cancer Res. 2022;41(1):170. https://doi.org/10.1186/s13046-022-02357-7.
63. Ju H, Zhang L, Mao L, Liu S, Xia W, Hu J, et al. Altered expression pattern of circular RNAs in metastatic oral mucosal melanoma. Am J Cancer Res. 2018;8(9):1788–800.
64. Chen Z, Chen J, Wa Q, He M, Wang X, Zhou J, et al. Knockdown of circ_0084043 suppresses the development of human melanoma cells through miR-429/tribbles homolog 2 axis and Wnt/β-catenin pathway. Life Sci. 2020;243:117323. https://doi.org/10.1016/j.lfs.2020.117323.
65. Wu S, Tang Y, Liu W. Circ_0084043 promotes cell proliferation and glycolysis but blocks cell apoptosis in melanoma via circ_0084043-miR-31-KLF3 axis. Open Life Sci. 2020;15(1):774–86. https://doi.org/10.1515/biol-2020-0071.
66. Lu R, Zhang X, Li X, Wan X. Circ_0016418 promotes melanoma development and glutamine catabolism by regulating the miR-605-5p/GLS axis. Int J Clin Exp Pathol. 2020;13(7):1791–801.
67. Bian D, Wu Y, Song G. Novel circular RNA, hsa_circ_0025039 promotes cell growth, invasion and glucose metabolism in malignant melanoma via the miR-198/CDK4 axis. Biomed Pharmacother. 2018;108:165–76. https://doi.org/10.1016/j.biopha.2018.08.152.
68. Qian P, Linbo L, Xiaomei Z, Hui P. Circ_0002770, acting as a competitive endogenous RNA, promotes proliferation and invasion by targeting miR-331-3p in melanoma. Cell Death Dis. 2020;11(4):264. https://doi.org/10.1038/s41419-020-2444-x.
69. Hao YL, Wang XQ. Circ-0079593 promotes proliferation and migration of melanoma cells by sponging microRNA-433 and elevating EGFR expression. Eur Rev Med Pharmacol Sci. 2021;25(2):779–86. https://doi.org/10.26355/eurrev_202101_24639.
70. Zhao F, Jia Z, Feng Y, Li Z, Feng J. Circular RNA circ_0079593 enhances malignant melanoma progression by the regulation of the miR-573/ABHD2 axis. J Dermatol Sci. 2021;102(1):7–15. https://doi.org/10.1016/j.jdermsci.2021.01.008.
71. Chen Z, Kang K, Chen S, Wang S, Zhang J, Zhang XY, et al. Circular RNA circ_0017247 promotes melanoma migration and invasion via targeting miR-145. Eur Rev Med Pharmacol Sci. 2020;24(17):8630. https://doi.org/10.26355/eurrev_202009_22778.
72. Wei CY, Zhu MX, Lu NH, Liu JQ, Yang YW, Zhang Y, et al. Circular RNA circ_0020710 drives tumor progression and immune evasion by regulating the miR-370-3p/CXCL12 axis in melanoma. Mol Cancer. 2020;19(1):84. https://doi.org/10.1186/s12943-020-01191-9.
73. Vezakis IA, Lambrou GI, Kyritsi A, Tagka A, Chatziioannou A, Matsopoulos GK. Detecting skin reactions in epicutaneous patch testing with deep learning: an evaluation of pre-processing and modality performance. Bioengineering (Basel, Switzerland). 2023;10(8):924. https://doi.org/10.3390/bioengineering10080924.
74. Li H, Chen G, Zhang L, Xu C, Wen J. A review of psoriasis image analysis based on machine learning. Front Med. 2024;11:1414582. https://doi.org/10.3389/fmed.2024.1414582.
75. Vezakis IA, Lambrou GI, Matsopoulos GK. Deep learning approaches to osteosarcoma diagnosis and classification: a comparative methodological approach. Cancers (Basel). 2023;15(8):2290. https://doi.org/10.3390/cancers15082290.
76. Brodman K, van Woerkom AJ, Erdmann AJ Jr, Goldstein LS. Interpretation of symptoms with a data-processing machine. 1959. MD Comput. 1996;13(2):173–9.
77. Haug CJ, Drazen JM. Artificial intelligence and machine learning in clinical medicine, 2023. N Engl J Med. 2023;388(13):1201–8. https://doi.org/10.1056/NEJMra2302038.
78. Nolan DJ. 100 years of x rays. BMJ (Clinical Research ed). 1995;310(6980):614–5. https://doi.org/10.1136/bmj.310.6980.614.
79. Bhat YJ, Ul Islam MS, Errichetti E. Ultraviolet-induced fluorescence dermoscopy, a novel diagnostic technique in dermatological practice: a systematic review. Indian Dermatol Online J. 2025;16(1):25–39. https://doi.org/10.4103/idoj.idoj_299_24.
80. Plozner N, Enechukwu NA, Bhat YJ, Behera B, Pietkiewicz P, Errichetti E. Diagnostic accuracy of polarized and ultraviolet fluorescence-induced dermoscopy in scarring and nonscarring alopecias: a retrospective observational multicentric study. Dermatol Ther. 2025;15(3):697–705. https://doi.org/10.1007/s13555-025-01355-9.
81. Noble WS. What is a support vector machine? Nat Biotechnol. 2006;24(12):1565–7. https://doi.org/10.1038/nbt1206-1565.
82. Breiman L. Random forests. Mach Learn. 2001;45(1):5–32. https://doi.org/10.1023/A:1010933404324.
83. Kramer O. K-Nearest neighbors. In: Dimensionality reduction with unsupervised nearest neighbors. Berlin, Heidelberg: Springer Berlin Heidelberg; 2013. p. 13–23.

84. Deng J, Dong W, Socher R, Li LJ, Kai L, Li F-F. ImageNet: a large-scale hierarchical image database. In: 2009 IEEE conference on computer vision and pattern recognition; 2009. p. 248–55.
85. Krizhevsky A, Sutskever I, Hinton GE. ImageNet classification with deep convolutional neural networks. Commun ACM. 2017;60(6):84–90. https://doi.org/10.1145/3065386.
86. Bishop JN, Bataille V, Gavin A, Lens M, Marsden J, Mathews T, et al. The prevention, diagnosis, referral and management of melanoma of the skin: concise guidelines. Clin Med (Lond). 2007;7(3):283–90. https://doi.org/10.7861/clinmedicine.7-3-283.
87. Codella NCF, Nguyen QB, Pankanti S, Gutman DA, Helba B, Halpern AC, et al. Deep learning ensembles for melanoma recognition in dermoscopy images. IBM J Res Dev. 2017;61(4/5):5:1–5:15. https://doi.org/10.1147/JRD.2017.2708299.
88. Osowski S, Les T. Deep learning ensemble for melanoma recognition. In: 2020 International Joint Conference on Neural Networks (IJCNN); 2020. p. 1–7.
89. Yu L, Chen H, Dou Q, Qin J, Heng PA. Automated melanoma recognition in dermoscopy images via very deep residual networks. IEEE Trans Med Imaging. 2017;36(4):994–1004. https://doi.org/10.1109/tmi.2016.2642839.
90. Nawaz M, Mehmood Z, Nazir T, Naqvi RA, Rehman A, Iqbal M, et al. Skin cancer detection from dermoscopic images using deep learning and fuzzy k-means clustering. Microsc Res Tech. 2022;85(1):339–51. https://doi.org/10.1002/jemt.23908.
91. Kakino R, Nakamura M, Mitsuyoshi T, Shintani T, Kokubo M, Negoro Y, et al. Application and limitation of radiomics approach to prognostic prediction for lung stereotactic body radiotherapy using breath-hold CT images with random survival forest: a multi-institutional study. Med Phys. 2020;47(9):4634–43. https://doi.org/10.1002/mp.14380.
92. Xu Y, Hosny A, Zeleznik R, Parmar C, Coroller T, Franco I, et al. Deep learning predicts lung cancer treatment response from serial medical imaging. Clin Cancer Res. 2019;25(11):3266–75. https://doi.org/10.1158/1078-0432.ccr-18-2495.
93. Lu L, Dercle L, Zhao B, Schwartz LH. Deep learning for the prediction of early on-treatment response in metastatic colorectal cancer from serial medical imaging. Nat Commun. 2021;12(1):6654. https://doi.org/10.1038/s41467-021-26990-6.
94. Wei D. A multigene support vector machine predictor for metastasis of cutaneous melanoma. Mol Med Rep. 2018;17(2):2907–14. https://doi.org/10.3892/mmr.2017.8219.
95. Bhalla S, Kaur H, Dhall A, Raghava GPS. Prediction and analysis of skin cancer progression using genomics profiles of patients. Sci Rep. 2019;9(1):15790. https://doi.org/10.1038/s41598-019-52134-4.
96. Tarhini AA, Lee SJ, Tan AC, El Naqa IM, Stephen Hodi F, Butterfield LH, et al. Improved prognosis and evidence of enhanced immunogenicity in tumor and circulation of high-risk melanoma patients with unknown primary. J Immunother Cancer. 2022;10(1):e004310. https://doi.org/10.1136/jitc-2021-004310.
97. Korfiati A, Grafanaki K, Kyriakopoulos GC, Skeparnias I, Georgiou S, Sakellaropoulos G, et al. Revisiting miRNA association with melanoma recurrence and metastasis from a machine learning point of view. Int J Mol Sci. 2022;23(3):1299. https://doi.org/10.3390/ijms23031299.
98. Aprati TJ, Day CP, Lee D, Pan A, Jee J, Tarantino G, et al. Clinico-genomic features predict distinct metastatic phenotypes in cutaneous melanoma. bioRxiv [preprint]. 2025; https://doi.org/10.1101/2025.01.24.633441.
99. Lan LF, Kai YL, Xu XL, Zhang JK, Xu GB, Dai YB, et al. Construction and validation of machine learning models for predicting lymph node metastasis in cutaneous malignant melanoma: a large population-based study. Transl Cancer Res. 2025;14(2):706–16. https://doi.org/10.21037/tcr-24-1672.
100. Shahwan KT, Walker TD, Tan A, Ruiz E, Ran N, Granger EE, et al. Identifying the impact of minor risk factors in Brigham and Women's Hospital stage T1 cutaneous squamous cell carcinomas on risk of poor outcomes: a retrospective cohort study. J Am Acad Dermatol. 2025;92(6):1319–26. https://doi.org/10.1016/j.jaad.2025.02.052.

Part XIX

Case Studies of Cutaneous Metastasis

36 Second Primary Cancers Related to the Skin

Despina Exadaktylou

Abstract

A second primary cancer (SPC) is defined as the appearance of a new, distinct malignancy in a patient already diagnosed with a first primary cancer (FPC).

We present two case reports: The first involves a 79-year-old female patient with a hypomelanotic malignant melanoma of the skin who developed breast cancer as an SPC 6 months later. The second case entails a 63-year-old male patient initially diagnosed with papillary urothelial carcinoma of the bladder who subsequently developed three SPCs 2 years later: one cutaneous malignant melanoma and two basal cell carcinomas.

Although the relationship between FPCs and SPCs has been documented in numerous reports in the literature, it remains a subject of debate. Large-scale population studies are needed to further investigate and confirm the existence of a potential causal connection.

Keywords

Second Primary Cancer (SPC) · First Primary Cancer (FPC) · Malignant Melanoma (MM) · Papillary Urothelial Carcinoma (PUC)

36.1 Introduction

The term "second primary cancer" (SPC)refers to the development of a new malignancy in a different organ or tissue in a patient with a prior history of a first primary cancer (FPC). SPCs arise from mutations in different cells, may occur months or years after the FPC—whether treated or untreated—and can present as either single or multiple tumors (Table 36.1) [1–3].

The emergence of a new malignancy is more common in individuals with a previously diagnosed malignancy compared to the general population. This possibility coexists with the ongoing risk of recurrence or metastasis of the first primary carcinoma [3].

In recent years, the development of new targeted treatment modalities as well as the advanced diagnostic procedures and population screenings have resulted in decreasing cancer mortality. The increasing life expectancy of patients with malignancies makes them prone to developing a second primary cancer [3, 4].

Nowadays, it is estimated that approximately one in five cancer diagnoses occur in a patient with a history of a prior malignancy [5].

D. Exadaktylou (✉)
Dermatology Department, General Hospital of Nikaia, Piraeus, Greece

D. Koumaki et al. (eds.), *Cutaneous Metastases*, https://doi.org/10.1007/978-3-032-26764-1_36

Table 36.1 Differences between primary cancer (PC), metastatic cancer (MC), and second primary cancer (SPC)

	PC	MC	SPC
Originating cells	Cells in a specific organ	Cells from the primary tumor	Cells in a different organ
Immune response	Immune suppression	Increasing immune suppression	Immune suppression
Progression of the disease	Risk of recurrence and/or metastasis	Systemic disease—multiorgan invasion	Risk of recurrence and/or metastasis as PC
Treatment	Therapy response	Therapy resistance	Therapy response as PC

36.2 Case 1: Hypomelanotic Skin Melanoma and Breast Cancer as Sēcond Primary Cancer

A 79-year-old female patient presented to the Dermatology clinic with a 1-year history of a slowly growing, asymptomatic lesion on her right arm. Clinical examination revealed a light red, indurated plaque with irregular borders, peripheral foci of grey-brown pigmentation, and superficial scaling, measuring 1.3 × 1.5 cm (Fig. 36.1a).

The clinical differential diagnosis included Bowen's disease (BD), basal cell carcinoma (BCC), and amelanotic–hypomelanotic melanoma (AHM).

Upon dermoscopy, detailed findings included asymmetric shape, multiple colors, scaling, and central scar-like depigmentation. Vessels were observed as polymorphic with centrally located linear, irregular vessels and peripheral dotted vessels. Finally, pigmentation was focal, irregular and located at the periphery with an atypical pigment network and atypical globules (Fig. 36.1b). The combination of these findings excluded the diagnosis of BCC and pointed to the differential diagnosis of AHM and BD.

Although dotted vessels, scaling and pigmentation are common dermoscopic findings in both BD and AHM, there are minor differences that could help orientate the diagnosis. According to literature, vessels in BD are often "glomerular," a term that attributes to larger size, looped appearance, and regular arrangement in clusters. In addition, BD pigmentation usually presents as smaller globules that are scattered throughout the lesion [6].

In case of AHM, due to scarcity of pigment, dermoscopy is mainly based on the vasculature characteristics, with the main finding being atypical distribution in the periphery of both dotted and irregular linear vessels. The form of the vessels is thought to be indicative of tumor progression, with dotted vessels mainly present in early AM and linear vessels appearing increasingly as the tumor progresses [7].

In our patient, the presence of both peripheral dotted vessels and central linear irregular vessels was an important clue towards the diagnosis of AHM.

Further dermoscopic features of AHM include an asymmetric shape, multiple colors, scar-like depigmentation, ulceration, blue-white veil, multiple blue-gray dots and milky red-pink areas. In our patient, we observed asymmetric shape, multiple colors, central scar-like depigmentation, and peripheral foci of atypical pigment network and atypical globules [8–10].

Scaling of the lesion, as in our case, has been reported in both AHM and BD. In AHM, scaly appearance is attributed to increased differentiation and proliferation of keratinocytes triggered by neoplastic melanocytes [6, 7].

The lesion was excised with a 2.0-mm peripheral skin margin. Histological and immunohistochemical examination confirmed the diagnosis of AHM Breslow 0.55 mm, one mitosis/mm^2, diffuse lymphocytic infiltration, absence of histological ulcerations, Melan-A (+), and HMB45 (+) (Fig. 36.1c).

The malignant melanoma (MM) was staged as T1a/N0/M0. The patient underwent surgical re-excision with a 1.0 cm peripheral skin margin and was thereafter regularly followed up.

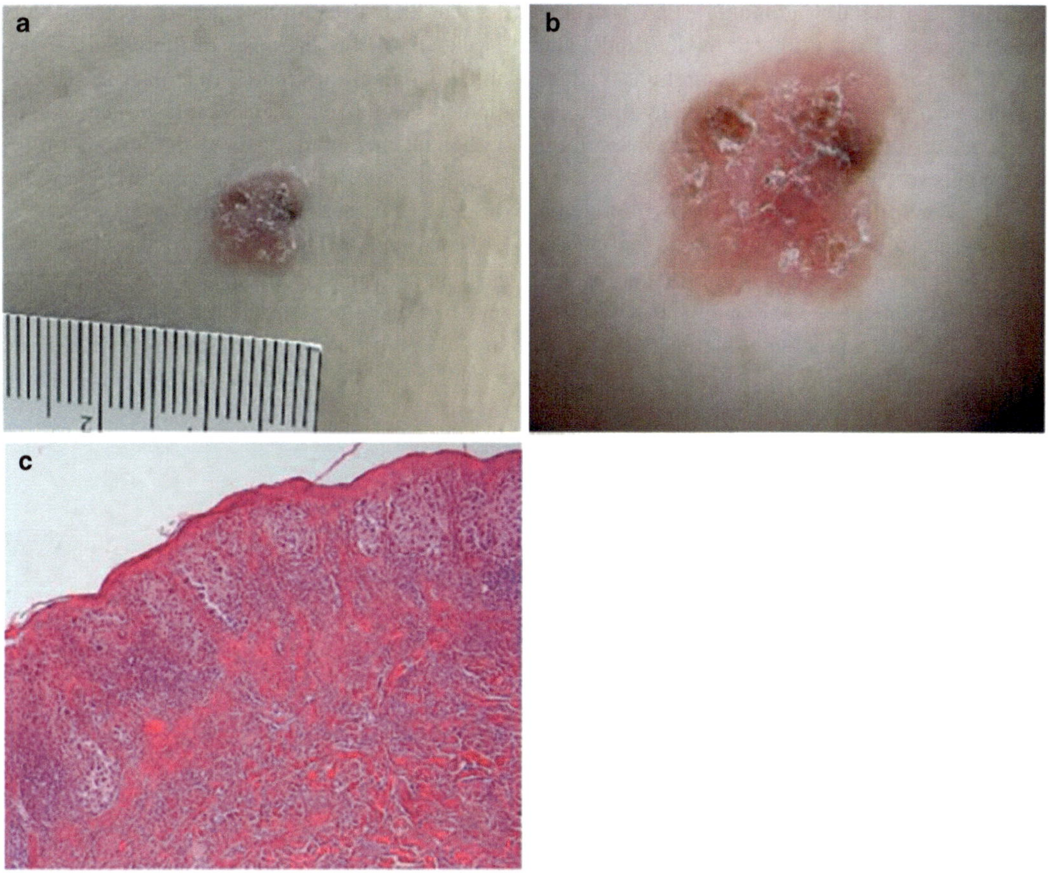

Fig. 36.1 (**a**) Clinical photo of the lesion on the right arm. Light red, 0.8 × 1.0 cm, indurated plaque with irregular borders, peripheral pigmentation, and superficial scaling. (**b**) Dermoscopic findings of the lesion on the right arm: asymmetric shape, scaling, polymorphic vessels, central depigmentation, and peripheral focal pigmentation. (**c**) Histological examination of the lesion on the right arm: atypical melanocytes infiltrating the papillary dermis as nests and solitary units with a pagetoid pattern. Malignant melanoma, Breslow 0.55 mm, one mitosis/mm^2 with diffuse lymphocytic infiltration and absence of histological ulcerations. Hematoxylin and eosin (H&E) stain, magnification ×10

Six months after the initial diagnosis of HM, a suspicious tumor was detected in the right breast during routine mammography. The lesion was surgically removed. Histological and immunohistochemical examination revealed malignant ductal carcinoma of non-specific type, 9.0 mm diameter, stage 2, with negative local lymph nodes.

36.3 Case 2: Bladder Carcinoma and Melanoma Second Primary Cancer

A 63-year-old male patient presented to the outpatient Dermatology clinic for a 1-year history of three skin lesions. Three years prior to the dermatology visit, the patient was diagnosed with

Papillary Urothelial Carcinoma (PUC) of the bladder, grade 2 according to WHO/ISUP. The neoplasm was treated with transurethral bladder tumor resection (TURBT) followed by immunotherapy with BCG vaccine 240 mg transurethral injections every 6 months.

The skin lesions included an asymptomatic pigmented plaque measuring 2.0 × 1.2 cm on the back (Fig. 36.2a), a pearly white plaque on the right temporal region measuring 0.9 × 0.9 cm (Fig. 36.3a), and a reddish eroded plaque on the right arm measuring 2.7 × 2.0 cm (Fig. 36.4a).

The patient reported that these lesions occurred within the last 12 months prior to his dermatological examination and approximately 2 years after the diagnosis of the bladder carcinoma. Clinical differential diagnosis of the pigmented lesion included dysplastic nevus and malignant melanoma, and of the lesions on the right arm and the temporal region BCC, bowen's disease (BD), and trichoepithelioma.

Dermoscopy of the pigmented plaque revealed asymmetry, irregular shape and structure, central scar-like depigmentation, blue–white veil, radial streaming, pseudopods, negative network, and irregular vascularity. These findings were indicative of MM (Fig. 36.2b).

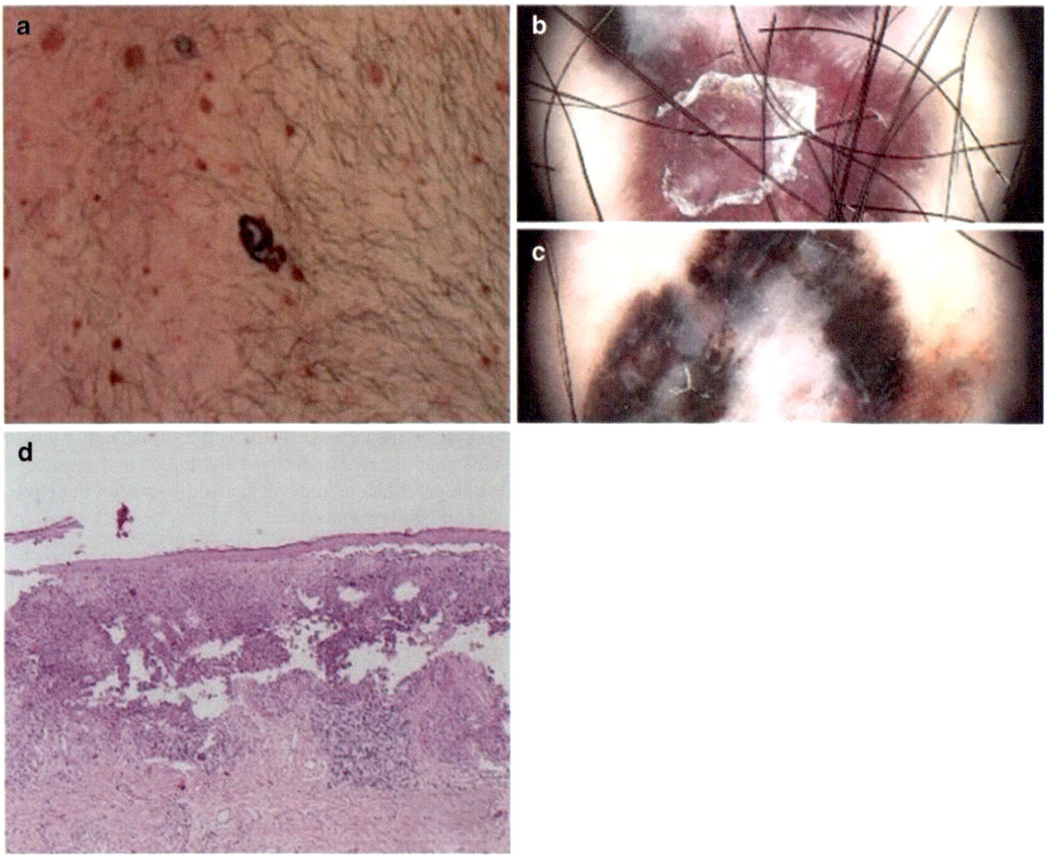

Fig. 36.2 (**a**) Pigmented, 2.0 × 1.2 cm, indurated plaque with marked asymmetry, irregular borders, and variation in color on the upper right back—clinical view. (**b** and **c**) Dermoscopic findings of the pigmented lesion: asymmetric shape, irregular structure and vascularity, atypical network, central scar-like depigmentation, blue-white veil, peripheral gray-brown irregular pigmentation with radial streaming and pseudopods. (**d**) Histological examination of the pigmented lesion: papillary dermis is infiltrated by atypical melanocytes with a pagetoid pattern as nests and solitary units. Superficial Spreading Malignant Melanoma (ssMM) , Breslow 1.3 mm—Clark III, 2 mitoses/mm^2, with regression <75%. Hematoxylin and eosin (H&E) stain, magnification ×40

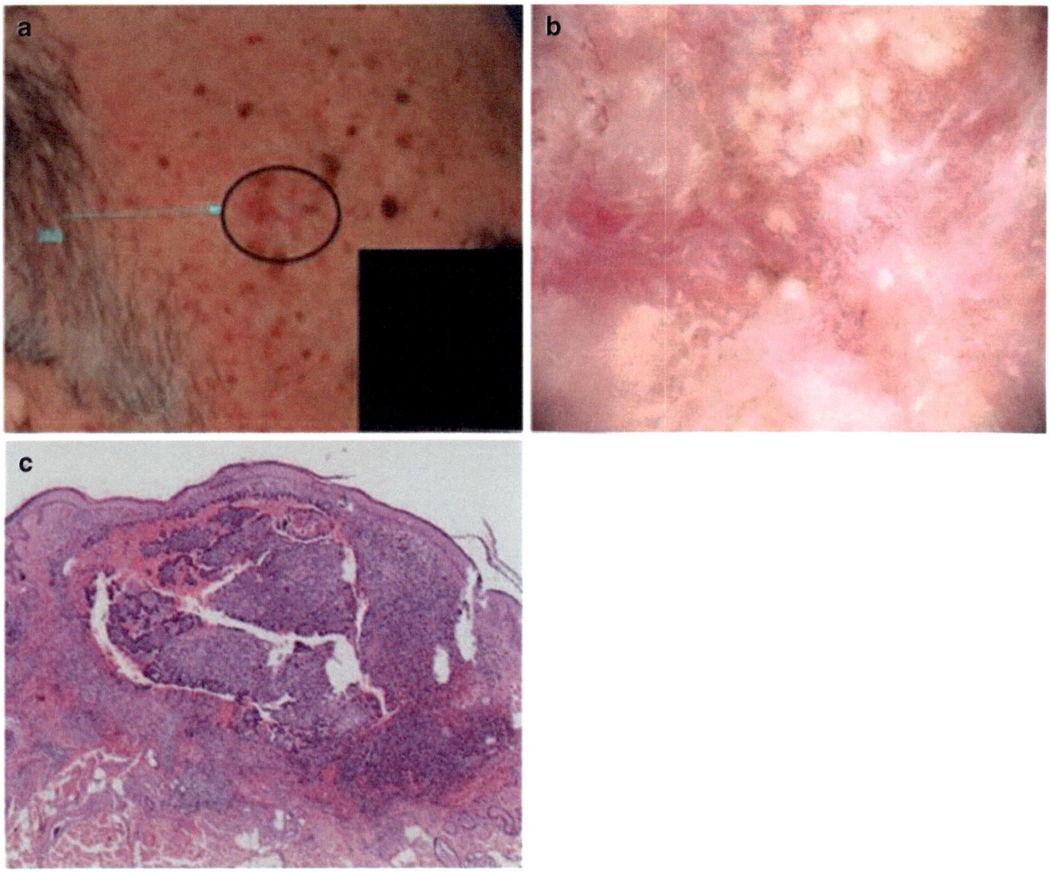

Fig. 36.3 (**a**) Pearly white, 0.9 × 0.9 cm, indurated skin plaque with irregular borders on the right temporal region—clinical view. (**b**) Dermoscopic findings of the lesion on the temporal area: branching vessels and white shimmering lines in an irregular erythematous background. (**c**) Histological examination of the lesion on the right temporal area: basaloid lobules with peripheral nuclear palisade in a fibromyxoid stroma infiltrating the papillary and partially the reticular dermis. Hematoxylin and eosin (H&E) stain, magnification ×40

The two lesions on the right arm and right temporal region revealed dermatoscopic characteristics of BCCs. The lesion on the temporal area showed well-focused branching vessels, white shimmering lines and irregular erythematous background (Fig. 36.3b). Accordingly, the lesion on the R arm demonstrated large-size central erosion (fiber sign), peripheral well-focused branching vessels and polymorphic vessels in an erythematous background (Fig. 36.4b).

The clinical and dermatoscopical differential diagnosis of the melanocytic plaque included MM, and thus the lesion was excised with a peripheral skin margin of 2.0 mm down to fascia.

The lesion on the temporal region was located in the high-risk "H area" of the face and was surgically removed with a peripheral skin margin of 5.0 mm down to fascia.

Finally, the lesion on the right arm had a maximum diameter of more than 2.0 cm, which is also considered a high-risk factor and it was excised with a peripheral skin margin of 10.0 mm down to fascia.

Histological examination of the melanotic lesion confirmed the diagnosis of Superficial Spreading Malignant Melanoma (ssMM), Breslow 1.3 mm—Clark III, 2 mitoses/mm^2, with regression <75%, MelanA+, HMB45 mild and focal diffuse positivity, p16 clonal loss of expression, PRAME score 1, Ki67: 8–10% (Fig. 36.2c).

Histological examination of the lesions on the right temporal area (Fig. 36.3c) and the right arm

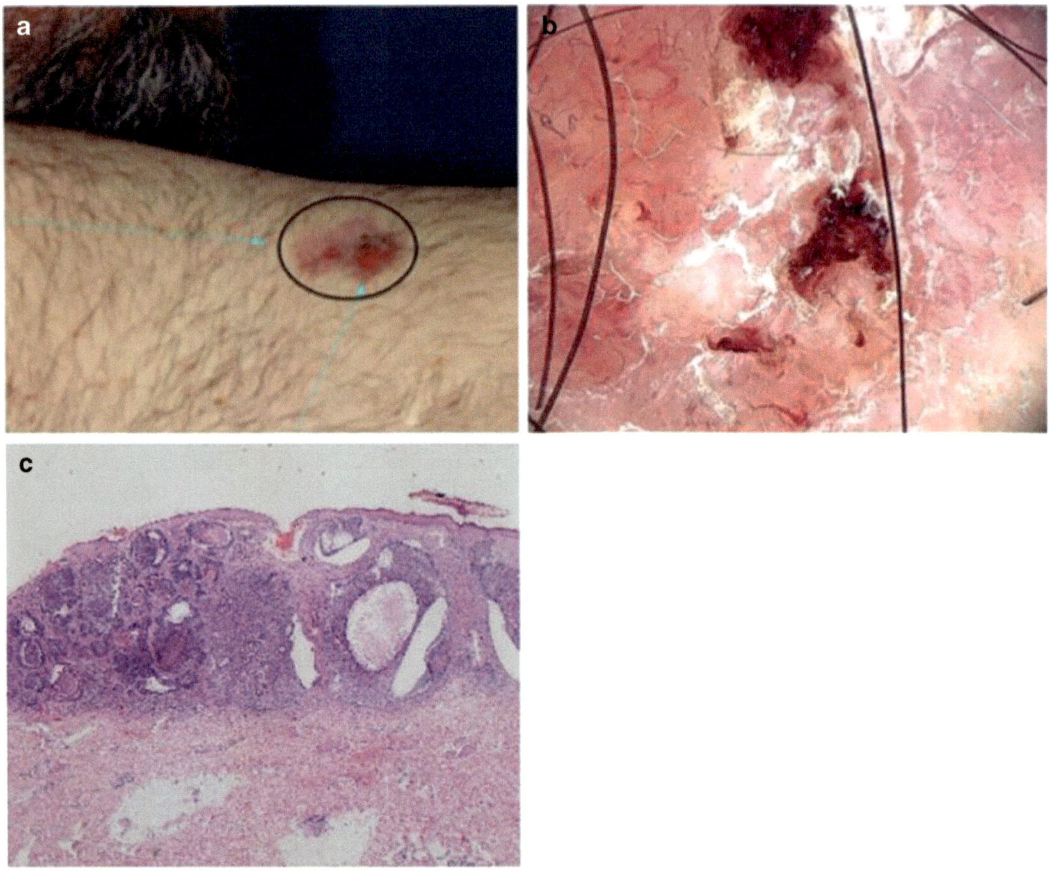

Fig. 36.4 (**a**) Light red, 2.7 × 2.0 cm, indurated skin plaque with irregular borders and marked erosion on the right arm- clinical view. (**b**) Dermoscopic findings of the lesion on the R arm: large-size central erosion (fiber sign), peripheral branching, and polymorphic vessels in an erythematous background. (**c**) Histological examination of the lesion on the right arm: basaloid lobules with peripheral nuclear palisade in a fibromyxoid stroma infiltrating the papillary and partially the reticular dermis. Hematoxylin and eosin (H&E) stain, magnification ×20

(Fig. 36.4c) confirmed the diagnosis of two nodular BCCs that infiltrate the papillary and reticular dermis.

All lesions were excised with clear histological margins.

Following the histological confirmation of the diagnosis of MM, the patient underwent central nervous system MRI, chest and upper-lower abdomen CT, regional lymph node U/S and no metastatic disease was found. He was then referred for sentinel lymph node biopsy and wide re-excision of the MM. Both the 2.0 cm re-excision and the sentinel lymph node did not show malignant infiltration. Thus, the MM was staged as T2a/N0/M0 and the patient is currently under long-term follow-up.

36.4 Discussion

Second primary cancers (SPCs) are more frequent in patients with a diagnosed first primary cancer (FPC) than in the general population, in parallel with the recurrence and metastasis risk of the FPC [2].

Most studies describe associations rather than casual relationships between FPCs and SPCs and are often based on cancer registry data that may not reflect the general population. Factors influencing SPC detection include increased surveillance in cancer patients, treatment-related risks (e.g., radiation, chemotherapy), follow-up variability, environmental exposures and genetic predisposition. Patients with FPCs have more frequent screenings compared to the general population and indolent cancers (e.g., thyroid and prostate cancer) could have been over-reported. Different medical facilities demonstrate different treatment options such as radiation therapy and chemotherapy that could influence the risk of developing SPCs. Moreover, follow-up visits are variable and could have an impact on the time of detection of SPCs. In addition, comorbidities and environmental factors also affect the associations between FPCs and SPCs [1].

In dermatology, SPCs involving malignant melanoma and breast cancer are frequently cited and described as amphidromous, i.e., bidirectional. Standardized incidence ratios range from 1.03 to 4.10 for primary breast carcinoma (BC) developing after cutaneous malignant melanoma (cMM) and 1.16 to 5.13 for cMM developing after BC. The risk is highest within the first year after FPC diagnosis and in younger patients [11, 12].

Theories supporting this association include shared susceptibility genes such as BRCA2 and CDK2NA, biological factors such as estrogen exposure and surveillance bias [11].

However, not all studies support this association. In a recent review, research was conducted about both SPC cutaneous malignant melanoma (cMM) after breast cancer (BC) and SPC BC after cMM. Although some studies report findings strongly suggestive of the link between the two neoplasms, others suggest insignificant or no increase in hazard ratio [11].

In our case, the elderly patient was not subjected to estrogen, and the possible explanations for developing breast cancer as SPC subsequent to MM are surveillance bias and genetic factors.

The second patient developed three SPCs: one ssMM and two BCCs, two years following the diagnosis and treatment of papillary urothelial neoplasm (PUN).

In a study by the Surveillance, Epidemiology, and End Results registry, SPCs following bladder Ca are reported at a 42% higher risk compared to the general population. The most common SPCs in these patients are prostate, lung, and bladder cancers, with the latter having the highest relative risk, while the occurrence of melanoma was not common [13].

Moreover, in patients with primary malignancies of more than 5 years, the incidence of melanoma was recorded with a significant reduction compared to the general population [14, 15].

In our patient, no common risk factor was found for all three malignancies. The relationship between cancer of the bladder and cutaneous malignancies has not been investigated, and possible risk factors for their connection have not been identified.

Genetic predisposition to developing cancers is often associated with multigene alteration. Genetic mutations known to increase cancer risk include BAP1, CDKN2A, nucleotide repair pathway NER pathway defects, and TP53, which is mutated in approximately 50% of all cancers, including BCC, MM, and bladder cancer [16–20].

The relative risk of developing SPC was increased in patients who underwent chemotherapy or radiation therapy for prior primary malignancy [2, 3, 21].

Our patient was not administered chemotherapy or radiation therapy for the treatment of bladder Ca. Instead, he underwent transurethral bladder tumor resection (TURBT) with subsequent transurethral injections of BCG vaccine to date. None of the treatments he received can be considered to induce carcinogenicity.

Our patient had never undergone a dermatological examination and came 3 years after the bladder Ca, because he was aesthetically disturbed by numerous Seborrheic Keratoses (SebKs). He had not realized the seriousness of the lesions that we identified as suspicious of malignancy. Therefore, our patient was not aware of the need for secondary prevention of skin cancers [22].

36.5 Conclusion

The association of FPCs and SPCs remains inconclusive and is not universally accepted. Nevertheless, it is a compelling aspect of cancer biology and warrants attention from healthcare providers. Large-scale population studies are necessary to clarify these associations and guide follow-up strategies for cancer survivors.

References

1. Ruan X, Huang D, Zhan Y, et al. Risk of second primary cancers after a diagnosis of first primary cancer: a pan-cancer analysis and Mendelian randomization study. elife. 2023;12:e86379. https://doi.org/10.7554/eLife.86379.
2. Vogt A, Schmid S, Heinimann K, et al. Multiple primary tumours: challenges and approaches, a review. ESMO Open. 2017;2(2):e000172. https://doi.org/10.1136/esmoopen-2017-000172.
3. Donin N, Filson C, Drakaki A, et al. Risk of second primary malignancies among cancer survivors in the United States, 1992 through 2008. Cancer. 2016;122(19):3075–86. https://doi.org/10.1002/cncr.30164.
4. Siegel RL, Miller KD, Jemal A. Cancer statistics, 2015. CA Cancer J Clin. 2015;65:5–29.
5. NIH National Cancer Institute Division on Cancer Epidemiology & Genetics. Available online: https://dceg.cancer.gov/research/what-we-study/second--cancers
6. Zalaudek I, Argenziano G, Leinweber B, et al. Dermoscopy of Bowen's disease. Br J Dermatol. 2004;150(6):1112–6. https://doi.org/10.1111/j.1365-2133.2004.05924.x.
7. Kaizer-Salk KA, Herten RJ, Ragsdale BD, Sengelmann RD. Amelanotic melanoma: a unique case study and review of the literature. BMJ Case Rep. 2018;2018:bcr2017222751. https://doi.org/10.1136/bcr-2017-222751.
8. Cabrera R, Recule F. Unusual clinical presentations of malignant melanoma: a review of clinical and histologic features with special emphasis on dermatoscopic findings. Am J Clin Dermatol. 2018;19(Suppl 1):15–23. https://doi.org/10.1007/s40257-018-0373-6.
9. Chiaravalloti A, Banki A. An elusive amelanotic melanoma and review of dermoscopic findings. J Drugs Dermatol. 2017;16(11):1164–5.
10. Ogawa S, Namiki T, Uchida C, et al. Hypomelanotic melanoma simulating pigmented Bowen's disease and its challenging dermoscopic features. J Dermatol. 2019;46(5):e173–5. https://doi.org/10.1111/1346-8138.14687.
11. Jeyakumar A, Chua TC, Lam AK-Y, Gopalan V. The melanoma and breast cancer association: an overview of their 'second primary cancers' and the epidemiological, genetic and biological correlations. Crit Rev Oncol Hematol. 2020;152:102989.
12. Kashyap D, Pal D, Sharma R, et al. Global increase in breast cancer incidence: risk factors and preventive measures. Biomed Res Int. 2022;2022:9605439. https://doi.org/10.1155/2022/9605439. eCollection 2022
13. Khanal A, Budhathoki N, Singh VP, et al. Second primary malignancy in bladder carcinoma - a population-based study. Anticancer Res. 2017;37(4):2033–6. https://doi.org/10.21873/anticanres.11548.
14. Strashilov S, Yordanov A. Aetiology and pathogenesis of cutaneous melanoma: current concepts and advances. Int J Mol Sci. 2021;22(12):6395. https://doi.org/10.3390/ijms22126395.
15. Rohan TZ, Mandel JL, Yang HY, et al. Identifying subsets of cancer patients with an increased risk of developing cutaneous melanoma: a surveillance, epidemiology, and end results–based analysis. JID Innov. 2024;5(1):100323. https://doi.org/10.1016/jxjidi2024100323. eCollection 2025 Jan
16. Ragusa R, Torrisi A, Di Prima AA, et al. Cancer prevention for survivors: incidence of second primary cancers and sex differences-a population-based study from an Italian cancer registry. Int J Environ Res Public Health. 2022;19(19):12201. https://doi.org/10.3390/ijerph191912201.
17. de Snoo FA, Bishop DT, Bergman W, et al. Increased risk of cancer other than melanoma in CDKN2A founder mutation (p16-Leiden)-positive melanoma families. Clin Cancer Res. 2008;14(21):7151–7. https://doi.org/10.1158/1078-0432.CCR-08-0403.
18. Foretová L, Navrátilová M, Svoboda M, et al. BAP1 syndrome - predisposition to malignant mesothelioma, skin and uveal melanoma, renal and other cancers. Klin Onkol. 2019;32(Suppl 2):118–22. https://doi.org/10.14735/amko2019S118.
19. Giglia-Mari G, Sarasin A. TP53 mutations in human skin cancers. Hum Mutat. 2003;21(3):217–28. https://doi.org/10.1002/humu.10179.
20. Sarkis AS, Dalbagni G, Cordon-Cardo C, et al. Nuclear overexpression of p53 protein in transitional cell bladder carcinoma: a marker for disease progression. J Natl Cancer Inst. 1993;85(1):53–9. https://doi.org/10.1093/jnci/85.1.53.
21. Starace M, Rapparini L, Cedirian S. Skin malignancies due to anti-cancer therapies. Cancers (Basel). 2024;16(11):1960. https://doi.org/10.3390/cancers16111960.
22. Corkum M, Hayden JA, Kephart G, et al. Screening for new primary cancers in cancer survivors compared to non-cancer controls: a systematic review and meta-analysis. J Cancer Surviv. 2013;7(3):455–63. https://doi.org/10.1007/s11764-013-0278-6. Epub 2013 May 5

37 Case Presentations of Cutaneous Metastases from Different Primary Tumors Part I (Breast, Unknown Origin, Bladder, and Urothelial Cancer)

Dimitra Koumaki, Ioannis Kokkinakis, Eleni Lappa, and Eleni Lagoudaki

Abstract

Cutaneous metastases are a rare but serious presentation of advanced visceral neoplasms, typically indicating widespread disease and poor prognosis. The current chapter documents a series of cases demonstrating the diverse clinical and histopathological manifestations of cutaneous metastases from breast, bladder, and urothelial carcinomas. Breast carcinoma, the most common origin of skin metastases in women, typically presents as firm, nontender erythematous to violaceous papules and nodules that are found predominantly over the front of the chest, abdomen, and scalp. Skin metastases from bladder cancer, while less frequent, are erythematous to violaceous nodules or plaques, found most commonly on the lower abdomen and genital mucosa, consistent with lymphatic or hematogenous spread. Unusual urothelial carcinoma metastatic deposits appear as nodules in the abdomen and head and neck in the initial phase. Clinical suspicion, dermoscopic and histopathologic correlation, and immunohistochemical profiling with markers such as GATA3, estrogen receptors (ER), progesterone receptors (PR), CK7, CK20, p63, and E-Cadherin are emphasized in the chapter to prevent misdiagnosis. Early biopsy diagnosis makes it possible to have timely multidisciplinary treatment. The cases demonstrate the polymorphic presentation, diagnostic challenge, and prognostic value of cutaneous metastases from different urogenital and breast carcinomas.

Keywords

Cutaneous metastasis · Breast cancer · Bladder cancer · Urothelial carcinoma · Skin nodules · Histopathology · Immunohistochemistry · Dermoscopy · Metastatic cancer

37.1 Cutaneous Metastasis from Breast Cancer Cases

37.1.1 Skin Metastasis from Breast Cancer: Case 1

A 50-year-old female patient with a history of invasive breast cancer presented with multiple palpable, firm, erythematous to violaceous papules and nodules on the front chest, abdomen,

D. Koumaki (✉)
Dermatology Department, University Hospital of Heraklion, Heraklion, Greece

I. Kokkinakis · E. Lappa · E. Lagoudaki
Pathology Department, University Hospital of Heraklion, Heraklion, Greece

D. Koumaki et al. (eds.), *Cutaneous Metastases*, https://doi.org/10.1007/978-3-032-26764-1_37

and thorax. The lesions were painless, appeared quickly, and were spread predominantly over the trunk (Fig. 37.1). A biopsy of skin, right submammary region, revealed a spindle-shaped tissue sample (1 × 0.7 cm, 0.9 cm thick) with extensive involvement of the dermis and subcutis by a carcinomatous infiltrate (Fig. 37.2a, b). The neoplastic cells were arranged in files, cords, clusters, aggregates of ≥20 cells, and as single cells. Immunohistochemical evaluation revealed a negative/focal weak membranous E-Cadherin expression; ER positivity (Allred score 4) was negative for PR, and it was equivocal for HER2 expression (score 2); and it had a low Ki-67 index, an immunophenotype compatible with lobular breast carcinoma.

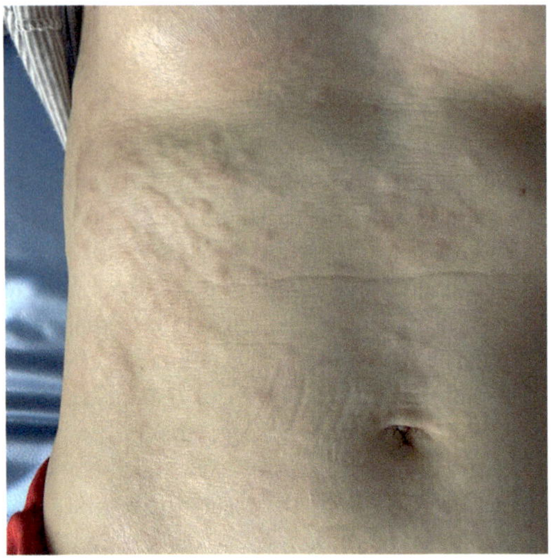

Fig. 37.1 Multiple erythematous to skin-colored firm papules and nodules dispersed across the anterior chest wall and abdominal wall, consistent with cutaneous metastases from invasive breast carcinoma in a 50-year-old female patient with metastatic breast cancer

Cutaneous metastases from breast carcinoma present clinically as firm, painless, erythematous to violaceous papules or nodules, mostly on the anterior chest and abdomen, along lymphatic drainage and proximity to the original tumor site [1–5]. They may also present as mimickers of benign dermatologic lesions and hence lead to diagnostic delay. Histopathology is that of an adenocarcinoma with various degrees of differentiation, and it is important to utilize immunohistochemical profiling to determine the breast's primary origin.

Epidemiologically, cutaneous metastases present in 0.6–10.4% of patients with cancer of any form, the most frequent source among women being breast cancer, accounting for up to 70% of all cases [6]. Cutaneous metastasis is seen in approximately 2–5% of patients with breast cancer. Metastatic skin lesions are seen in poor prognosis and advanced disease, and median survival upon diagnosis has been reported to be 8 months [7–9]. Prompt recognition and biopsy of any suspected skin lesions are critical to accurate diagnosis and treatment.

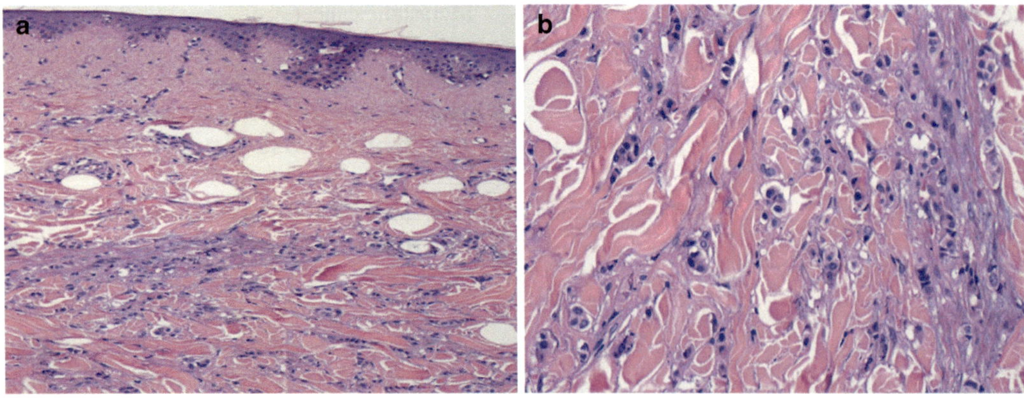

Fig. 37.2 Biopsy of a skin-colored papule in a 50-year-old female patient with a history of metastatic breast cancer. (**a**) The dermis is infiltrated by a poorly differentiated adenocarcinoma. (**b**) The neoplastic cells infiltrate the dermis as isolated cells, forming trabecular structures, small aggregates, and focal gland-like structures

37.1.2 Cutaneous Metastasis from Breast Cancer: Case 2

A 69-year-old female patient with a history of breast carcinoma, presenting with stage IV disease and known metastatic lung, liver, kidney, and bone lesions. On follow-up, she had developed two typical cutaneous lesions.

The original lesion was a violaceous, centrally ulcerated nodule on the right chest wall (Fig. 37.3a). The lesion was firm, nontender, and increasing gradually. The violaceous coloration and ulceration raised suspicion of secondary neoplastic involvement but also mimicked vascular or adnexal tumors.

The second lesion was on the scalp as a dome-shaped, pink to skin-colored nodule that appeared over 3 weeks (Fig. 37.4a). The nodule was firm and not tender. Differential diagnoses based on location and clinical morphology were adnexal neoplasms, cysts, or primary skin tumors. The aspect that both lesions have occurred at different anatomical locations is a testament to the heterogeneity in clinical presentations of cutaneous metastases.

37.1.2.1 Dermoscopic Features

On dermoscopy of the chest wall nodule, a polymorphous vascular pattern, including irregular linear and arborizing vessels on a diffuse erythematous base (Fig. 37.3b), was observed. A central ulcerated area with hemorrhagic crust was noted, which is consistent with necrosis and ulceration. Such features, while not pathognomonic, are strongly suggestive of cutaneous metastasis in the context of known malignancy.

The scalp lesion, however, had multiple dermoscopic features. It had a homogenous pinkish background and diffuse fine linear vessels and superimposed white shiny streaks (Fig. 37.4b). In contrast to the chest lesion, ulceration and hemorrhage were not observed. The above-stated facts highlight the dermoscopic variability of cutaneous metastasis from vascular-rich, ulcerated nodules to smooth, structureless, pink nodules depending upon the location of the tumor and dermal depth of invasion.

37.1.2.2 Histopathological Correlation

Biopsies of the chest wall as well as scalp nodules were diagnostic of metastatic breast carci-

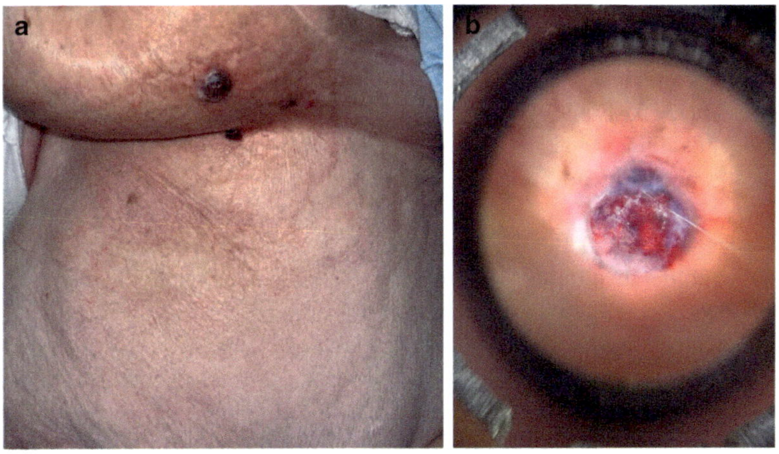

Fig. 37.3 Clinical and dermoscopic images of skin metastasis of breast carcinoma in a 68-year-old female patient. (Left) (**a**) Clinical image of the right chest wall of a 69-year-old woman with advanced breast carcinoma, showing a violaceous nodule with central ulceration on the skin surface. (Right) (**b**) Dermoscopy of this violaceous nodule on the right breast reveals a polymorphous vascular pattern with arborizing and linear irregular vessels, a diffuse erythematous background, and central ulceration with hemorrhagic crust, consistent with metastatic skin involvement

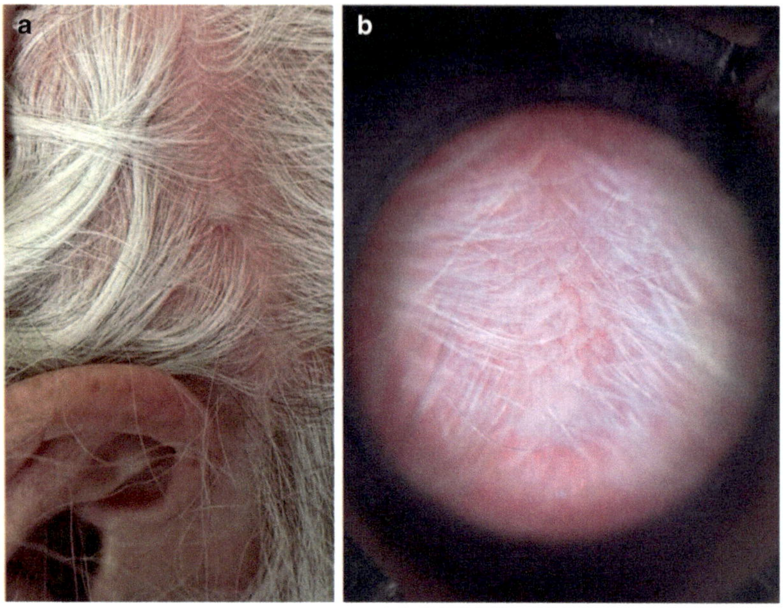

Fig. 37.4 Clinical and dermoscopic images of skin metastasis of breast carcinoma on the scalp of a 68-year-old female patient with breast cancer. (Left) (**a**) Clinical image of a dome-shaped, skin-colored to pink nodule on the left parietal scalp. (Right) (**b**) Dermoscopy reveals a pinkish, structureless background with thin linear vessels and overlying white shiny streaks, consistent with dermal metastatic infiltration

noma. Histology showed poorly differentiated adenocarcinoma with increased nuclear atypia, numerous mitotic figures, and necrosis. Coalescing solid carcinomatous blasts, with foci of necrosis and hemorrhaging infiltrates (Fig. 37.5a) showing no connection with the overlying epidermis or with skin adnexa (Fig. 37.5b). Immunohistochemically, the neoplastic cells expressed GATA3 (Fig. 37.5c) while showing no expression for ER, PR, or HER2 (not shown), characteristic of triple-negative breast carcinoma. On the basis of GATA3 expression and the patient's clinical history, the diagnosis of metastatic breast adenocarcinoma was assigned.

The Ki-67 index was extremely high (~95%), which was a very proliferative tumor. The histopathological findings concurred with the dermoscopic findings of ulceration, hemorrhage, and vascular proliferation.

37.1.2.3 Clinical Course

Cutaneous metastasis formation in this patient predicted widespread dissemination and a poor prognosis. Palliative therapy aside, her disease progressed rapidly, and she succumbed shortly thereafter. The short interval between the development of cutaneous metastases and death is consistent with the natural history of advanced metastatic breast carcinoma.

37.1.3 Cutaneous Metastasis of Breast Cancer: Case 3

Case 3 is a 69-year-old woman presenting with advanced invasive ductal breast carcinoma and multifocal systemic metastatic disease, including cutaneous manifestations on the scalp, regional nodes, and pulmonary locations.

37.1.3.1 Clinical and Systemic Presentation

The patient had initially had the diagnosis of moderately to poorly differentiated ductal breast carcinoma and was initially treated with surgery and neoadjuvant chemotherapy. Her illness had advanced to stage IV despite treatment, characterized by metastasis to lungs, regional lymph nodes, bones, and cutaneous lesions. Interestingly, she also had a dome-shaped, firm, skin-colored to pink nodule on the left parietal scalp, which appeared approximately 3 weeks prior to dermatologic evaluation.

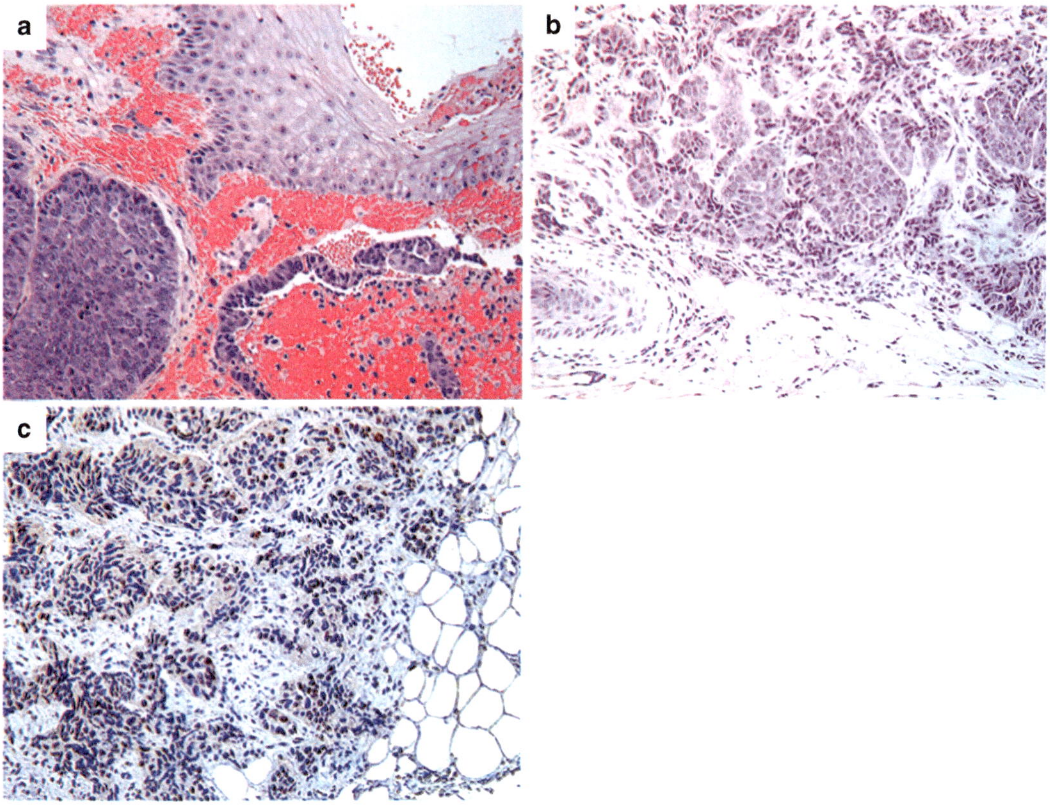

Fig. 37.5 Microscopic examination of the excised cutaneous lesion of the scalp of this 68-year-old female patient with breast cancer showed infiltration of the dermis and of the subcutaneous tissue from coalescing solid carcinomatous blasts, with foci of necrosis and hemorrhaging infiltrates (**a**, **b**) showing no connection with the overlying epidermis or with skin adnexa. Immunohistochemically, the neoplastic cells expressed GATA3 (**c**) while showing no expression for ER, PR, or Her-2 (not shown). On the basis of GATA3 expression and the patient's clinical history, the diagnosis of metastatic breast adenocarcinoma was assigned. (**a**, **b**): H/E ×100 magnification, (**c**): GATA3 ×100 magnification

The acutely developing scalp nodule raised a clinical suspicion of cutaneous metastasis in the context of the patient's known disseminated carcinoma. She had also had enlarged supraclavicular and axillary lymph nodes and pulmonary nodules on imaging that were consistent with metastatic disease, underlining the systemic burden of disease. These are the features of advanced metastatic breast cancer of poor prognosis.

37.1.3.2 Histopathological Findings

Scalp lesion biopsy revealed dermal invasion by a moderately to poorly differentiated adenocarcinoma. Hematoxylin and eosin staining revealed neoplastic cells arranged in tubular, solid, or cribriform architectural patterns with invasion of the dermis but without epidermal or adnexal involvement (Fig. 37.6). The tumor cells were of medium size, had dark, oval-to-atypical nuclei with prominent nucleoli, and were full of lumina containing multiple mitotic figures, reflecting aggressive proliferative activity.

Immunohistochemical study demonstrated strong positivity for E-Cadherin (Fig. 37.7a) and cytokeratin 19 (CK19) (Fig. 37.7b), an epithelial marker of ductal lineage. The tumor cells were negative for CK20 and TTF-1 markers, hence excluding other possible primary sites such as colorectal or pulmonary carcinoma. Hormone receptor status was negative for ER and PR and

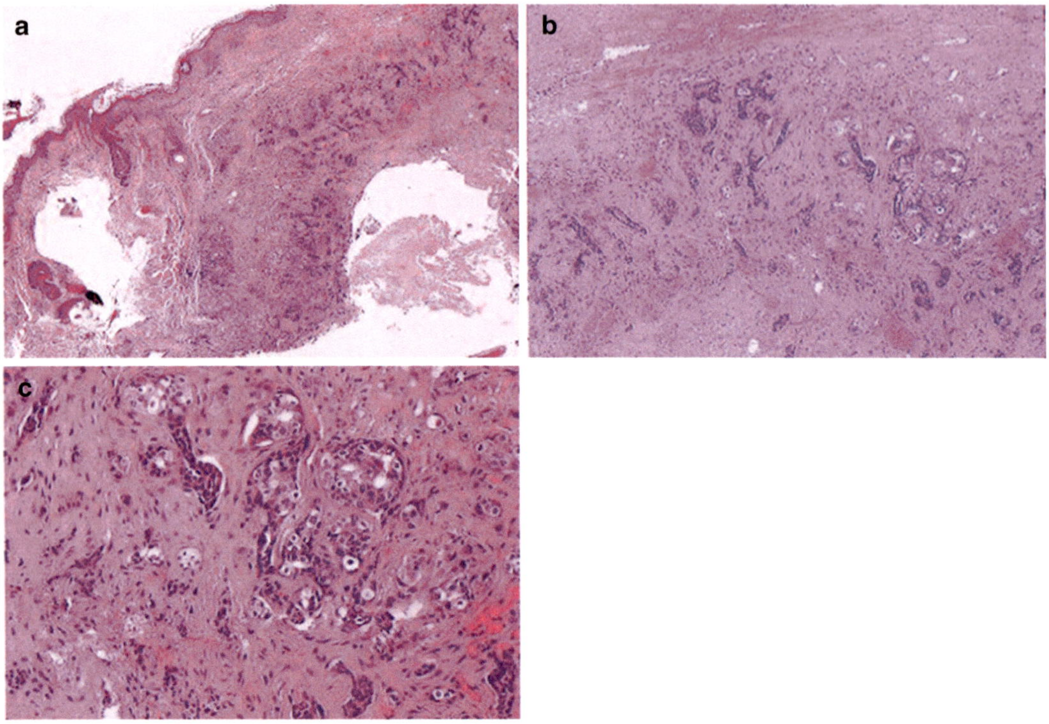

Fig. 37.6 Histopathological and immunohistochemical features of the cutaneous metastasis lesion on the scalp of a 69-year-old female patient with breast cancer. Hematoxylin and eosin (H&E) staining demonstrates dermal infiltration by a moderately to poorly differentiated carcinoma composed of medium-sized neoplastic cells forming tubular, solid, and cribriform structures. The cells exhibit dark oval or atypical nuclei, prominent nucleoli, and numerous mitoses. Areas of dermal invasion show no connection to the epidermis or cutaneous adnexa. H&E staining: (**a**) ×40, (**b**) ×100, and (**c**) ×200

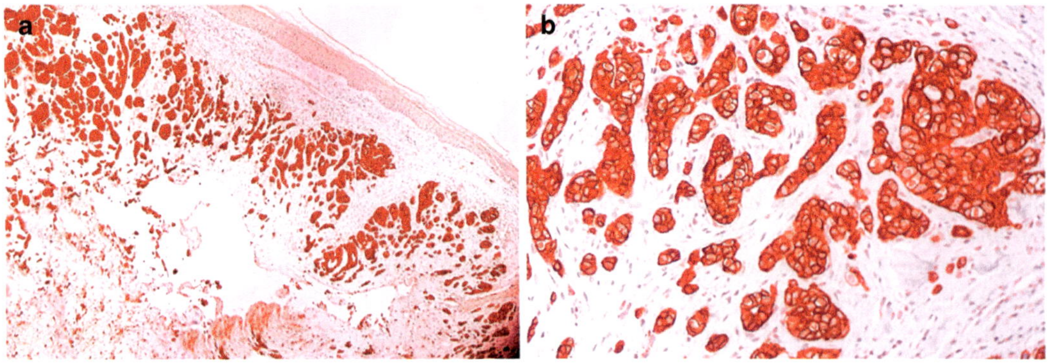

Fig. 37.7 Immunohistochemistry of the cutaneous metastasis lesion on the scalp of a 69-year-old female patient with breast cancer showing strong cytoplasmic positivity for cytokeratin 19 (CK19) at ×40 (**a**) and ×200 (**b**), consistent with metastatic breast adenocarcinoma

showed a low HER-2 score, creating a profile of triple-negative breast carcinoma. A focally positive Alcian blue staining demonstrated limited mucin production by the tumor cells.

In addition to the above, histopathological examination of a synchronous lung nodule and of a pathological regional lymph node also revealed metastatic deposits of low-grade carcinoma of primary breast origin. Secondary locations also had similar histology and immunoprofiles (E-Cadherin and CK19 positive, TTF-1 and calretinin negative), proving systemic metastatic spread from the original breast carcinoma.

37.1.3.3 Pathophysiological Considerations

Cutaneous metastases of breast cancer most commonly follow lymphatic or hematogenous routes. The scalp, although a rare location, can be involved owing to its vascular character and proximity to regional lymphatic drainage pathways. Regional nodal and lung involvement illustrate the multifocal pattern of extensive disease.

The histologic grade of differentiation and immunohistochemical phenotype provide information on tumor aggressiveness and dictate treatment management. The triple-negative pattern in this situation is associated with poor prognosis, virulent clinical behavior, and limited possibilities for targeted therapy.

37.1.3.4 Clinical and Dermoscopic Correlation

Clinically, metastatic scalp lesions may appear as nodules or plaques, resembling the dome-shaped tumor of the patient. The absence of epidermal attachment on histology correlates with metastatic deposits derived from the dermal matrix, distinguishing such lesions from primary cutaneous neoplasms. Dermoscopy typically reveals structureless pink backgrounds with fine linear vessels and shiny white streaks, indicating infiltration by the tumor and stromal change.

37.1.3.5 Prognosis and Management

The development of skin metastases with concomitant pulmonary and lymph node metastases is indicative of systemic disease progression and is prognostically associated with decreasing survival. Therapy remains largely palliative, including systemic chemotherapy or receptor status-directed immunotherapy. Local treatments like surgical extirpation or irradiation may be attempted for symptom control, but do not significantly alter the prognosis as a whole.

37.1.4 Cutaneous Metastasis of Breast Cancer: Case 4

A 62-year-old female with a long-standing history of carcinoma of the breast presented with multiple violaceous to skin-colored papules and nodules over the neck, chest, and anterior thorax—clinically suggestive of cutaneous metastases. From her past medical history, she had invasive ductal carcinoma of the breast, which had been diagnosed in 2012. During the course of her disease, she had received multiple lines of systemic therapy. In 2023, she was treated with sacituzumab govitecan for metastatic triple-negative breast cancer. She was referred to our department in November 2023 with a new onset of skin lesions over the neck. Clinically, the most notable feature was a firm, erythematous metastatic nodule over the left cervical region (Fig. 37.8a). The lesion measured approximately 1.5–2 cm in diameter, was elevated, and had an infiltrative base characteristic of cutaneous metastatic deposits. Apart from this huge dominant lesion, several small satellite nodules were scattered on the neck, upper thoracic, and presternal regions. These nodules ranged from a few millimeters to 1 cm in diameter and were firm on palpation (Fig. 37.8b). Furthermore, the patient also presented with hyperkeratotic plaques in the inframammary folds and on the abdomen. These lesions were erythematous, irregular, thickened, and manifested overlying hyperkeratosis—characteristic of extensive secondary cutaneous metastasis. The coexistence of both nodular metastases and hyperkeratotic plaques emphasized the polymorphic clinical presentation of cutaneous dissemination in advanced breast cancer.

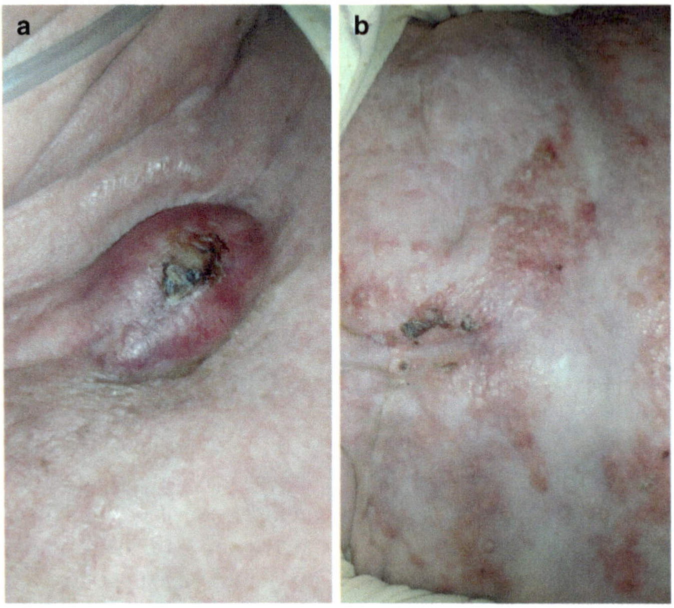

Fig. 37.8 (**a**) Clinical image of a metastatic nodule in the left cervical region of a 62-year-old female with triple-negative breast cancer and known cutaneous metastases. The nodule appears erythematous to violaceous, firm, and ulcerated with central necrosis. Multiple smaller nodular and papular lesions are noted along the neck and thorax, as well as hyperkeratotic plaques in the inframammary and abdominal regions (**b**)

A biopsy of one of the nodular lesions of the anterior thoracic wall was done. Macroscopically, the tissue was a piece of skin with a spindle shape measuring 2.1 × 0.8 cm in dimensions and with a dermal-subcutaneous layer thickness of 0.4 cm. Microscopic examination revealed dermal infiltration from a poorly differentiated carcinoma. The neoplasm consisted of pleomorphic large cells with irregular, vesicular, and partly angulated nuclei; visible nucleoli; and multiple mitotic figures (Fig. 37.9a, b). The tumor cells were arranged in trabecular and linear patterns, small groups, and scattered single cells. There was also a moderate chronic inflammatory infiltrate. Immunohistochemistry demonstrated strong positivity for CK19 and E-Cadherin in the neoplastic cells. GCDFP-15 was positive in isolated cells. ER, PR, and HER2 were negative (score 1+). The proliferative index (Ki-67) was around 40–50% (Fig. 37.9). Immunophenotypic pattern and morphology overall were in accordance with the cutaneous metastasis of the patient's known invasive ductal breast carcinoma (Fig. 37.9c, d, and e).

Clinically, the presentation illustrates the polymorphic appearance of cutaneous metastases of advanced breast cancer. The cervical site is fairly rare in contrast to the more common chest wall, inframammary, and abdominal sites. The presence of discrete nodules and keratotic plaques within the same patient illustrates the heterogeneity of skin metastatic disease. Detection of such lesions is important because they can be the first sign of progression or resistance to therapy, and they typically are associated with a poor prognosis.

This case illustrates the need to have a high index of suspicion for cutaneous metastases in advanced breast cancer patients, especially those with triple-negative breast cancer, whose cutaneous spread can be diffuse and aggressive.

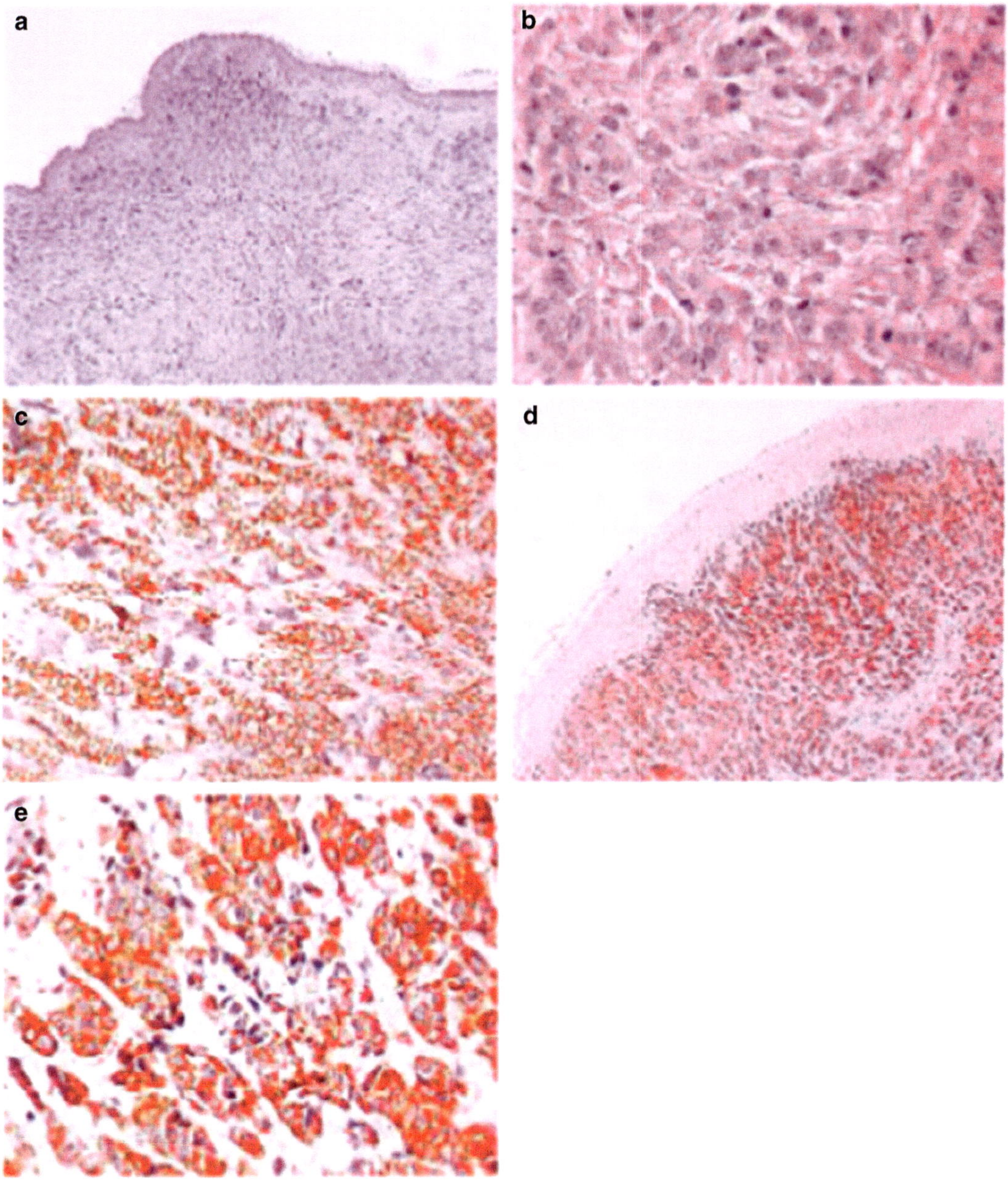

Fig. 37.9 Histopathological and immunohistochemical findings of skin metastasis from breast carcinoma. (**a**) H&E ×20: Invasion of the skin dermis by a poorly differentiated carcinoma. (**b**) H&E ×400: Small groups of large neoplastic cells with abnormal, pleomorphic nuclei, prominent nucleoli, and numerous mitotic figures. (**c**) E-Cadherin ×400: Strong membranous expression of E-cadherin by tumor cells. (**d**) CK19 ×40: Diffuse cytoplasmic staining for CK19 in tumor nests. (**e**) CK19 ×400: High-power view confirming strong CK19 positivity in individual neoplastic cells

37.1.5 Cutaneous Metastasis of Unknown Origin with the Original Primary Cancer Being Bladder Cancer: Case 5

The patient is a 69-year-old male with a history of long-standing bladder cancer diagnosed in 2005 and who subsequently developed massive cutaneous metastases across the lower abdominal wall in 2022. The patient came to the gastroenterology ward due to ascitic fluid accumulation, a feature of advanced malignancy. His oncologic past included surgical management of bladder cancer with urinary diversion (left ureterostomy) and adjuvant therapy, though precise protocols before the onset of skin lesions were not documented in the reports seen.

In January 2022, the patient had multiple erythematous to violaceous plaques and nodules on the lower abdomen. Lesions were progressively enlarging, with some demonstrating superficial ulceration and crusting. The lesions were painful and occasionally produced a burning sensation (Fig. 37.10). There were no other areas of cutaneous involvement at presentation.

A biopsy of the erythematous nodule in the lower abdomen was performed to arrive at a definitive diagnosis. The dermis is diffusely infiltrated by angulated tubular carcinomatous blasts (Fig. 37.11a) exhibiting no connection with the overlying epidermis or with skin adnexa. Immunohistochemical staining was positive for CDX2 (Fig. 37.11b) and CK7 (Fig. 37.11c) and only focally positive for CK20 (Fig. 37.11d), while it resulted in a negative for p63 (Fig. 37.11e). Histochemical staining with Alcian blue highlighted the presence of intracytoplasmic mucin droplets in several neoplastic cells as well as the presence of extracellular mucin within the lumens of the neoplastic glandular formations (Fig. 37.11f). The immunophenotype was compatible with adenocarcinoma but was not diagnostic of its primary origin.

Cutaneous metastases of unknown origin herald advanced systemic dissemination and poor prognosis. The lesions may have polymorphous morphology—plaques, nodules, and ulcerations—which reflects aggressive tumor biology and extensive dermal infiltration.

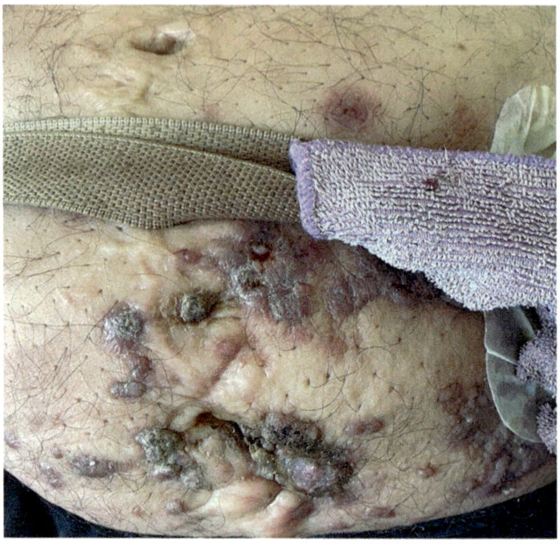

Fig. 37.10 Clinical image illustrating multiple metastatic nodules and plaques on the lower abdominal skin of a 69-year-old male patient with a history of bladder cancer diagnosed in 2005. The lesions appear erythematous to violaceous, with several well-demarcated firm nodules, some exhibiting crusting and ulceration. The skin shows induration with areas of sclerosis and hyperpigmentation, consistent with extensive cutaneous infiltration. The patient was hospitalized for ascitic fluid collection and had a skin biopsy confirming metastatic adenocarcinoma of moderate differentiation

A history of urinary diversion and prior urologic surgery is not rare in survivors of bladder cancer, with resultant close long-term follow-up mandated because of a risk for local recurrence and metastasis. Ascites development paralleled the natural history of systemic disease.

The case emphasizes the requirement of multidisciplinary management by oncologists, dermatologists, gastroenterologists, and pathologists for managing advanced cutaneous metastasis of unknown origin. Other systemic therapies like chemotherapy or immunotherapy may be added based on the overall condition of the patient and tumor behavior.

In conclusion, this case is a reminder of the clinical, histological, and immunophenotypic manifestation of cutaneous metastases of unknown origin, highlighting the significance of high clinical suspicion, early biopsy, and exten-

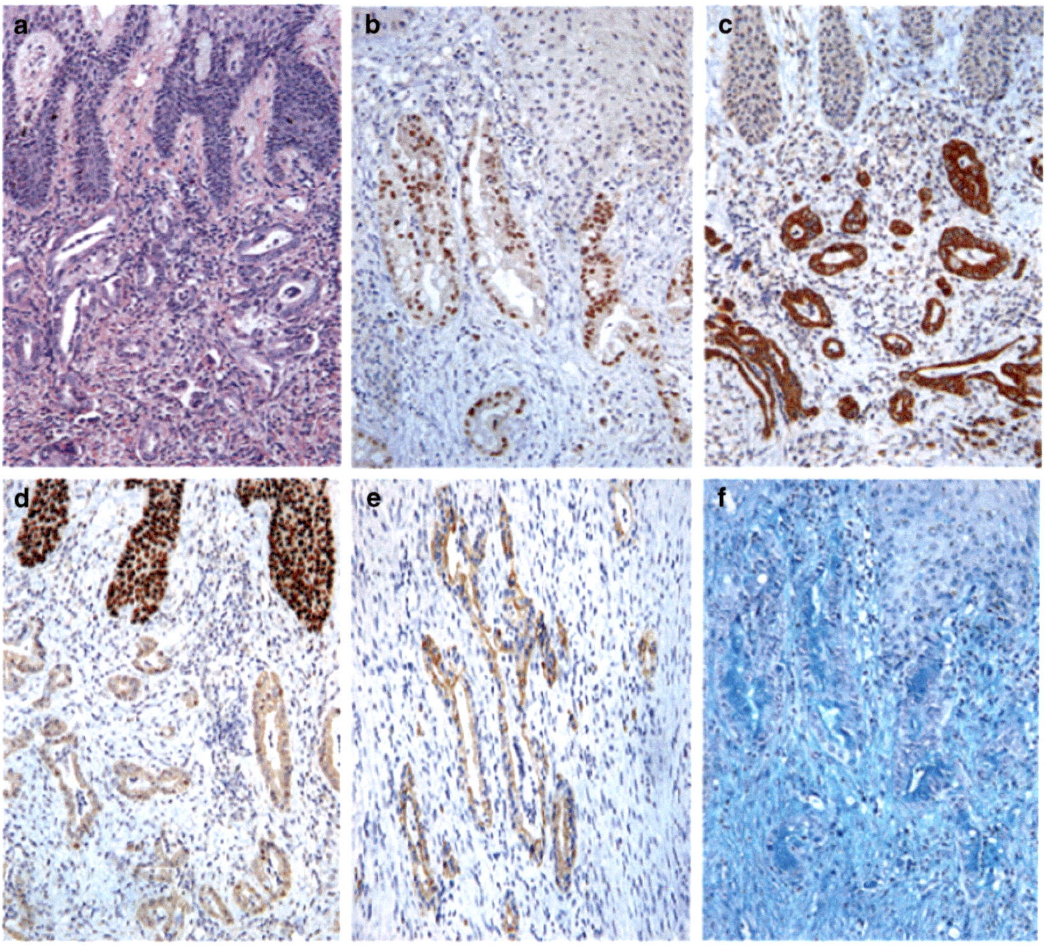

Fig. 37.11 Skin biopsy from a violaceous nodule on the lower abdominal skin of a 69-year-old male patient with a history of bladder cancer. Histological examination revealed diffuse infiltration of the dermis by angulated tubular carcinomatous cells (**a**), with no connection to the overlying epidermis or adnexal structures. Immunohistochemistry showed strong positivity for CDX2 (**b**) and CK7 (**c**), focal positivity for CK20 (**d**), and negativity for p63 (**e**). Histochemical staining highlighted intracytoplasmic mucin droplets in several neoplastic cells, as well as extracellular mucin within the lumina of glandular tumor formations. The immunophenotypic profile was consistent with adenocarcinoma but was not diagnostic of its primary origin. (**a**) H&E, ×100; (**b**) CDX2, ×100; (**c**) CK7, ×100; (**d**) CK20, ×100; (**e**) p63, ×100.

sive diagnostic evaluation in individuals presenting with new skin lesions and a history of cancer.

37.1.6 Cutaneous Metastasis of Bladder Cancer: Case 6

A 74-year-old male patient with past bladder cancer and a left nephrostomy presented in the oncology clinic with multiple subcutaneous nodules that have developed on the left lower abdomen close to the nephrostomy site. The nodular lesions appeared around a month ago, prior to the evaluation, initially noted on November 20, 2022. The patient underwent a skin biopsy of one of the subcutaneous nodules on December 9, 2022, in order to establish a histopathological diagnosis.

The history of the patient with bladder malignancy was invasive urothelial carcinoma with previous treatment and now surveillance in the oncology clinic. A nephrostomy is a chronic urinary diversion secondary to tumor progression-related ureteral obstruction.

Histological examination of bladder tissue showed massive aggregates of invasion of the mucosal lamina propria and different locations of involvement of muscularis propria by solid, low-differentiation urothelial carcinoma. Locations of intact urothelial covering had in situ carcinoma changes. Pathological stage was pT2. The mucosal lamina propria also showed focal edema, perivascular dense lymphocytic aggregates, and vascular dilatation with hyperemia.

The excised subcutaneous tumor measured 1.6 × 0.7 centimeters with a thickness of 1.1 centimeters, made up of the dermis and subcutis. Macroscopically, an ill-defined white patch was noticed. Microscopically, some compact and sheet-like groups of carcinoma cells were noted scattered in the deep dermis and subcutis. The neoplastic cells were bulky with marked atypia of nuclei and a high number of mitoses (Fig. 37.12a). Immunophenotyping was CK20, p63, and Cam5.2 positive, consistent with urothelial carcinoma of established primary bladder origin (Fig. 37.12b, c, and d). Perineural invasion, lymphovascular emboli, and fibrosis were identified.

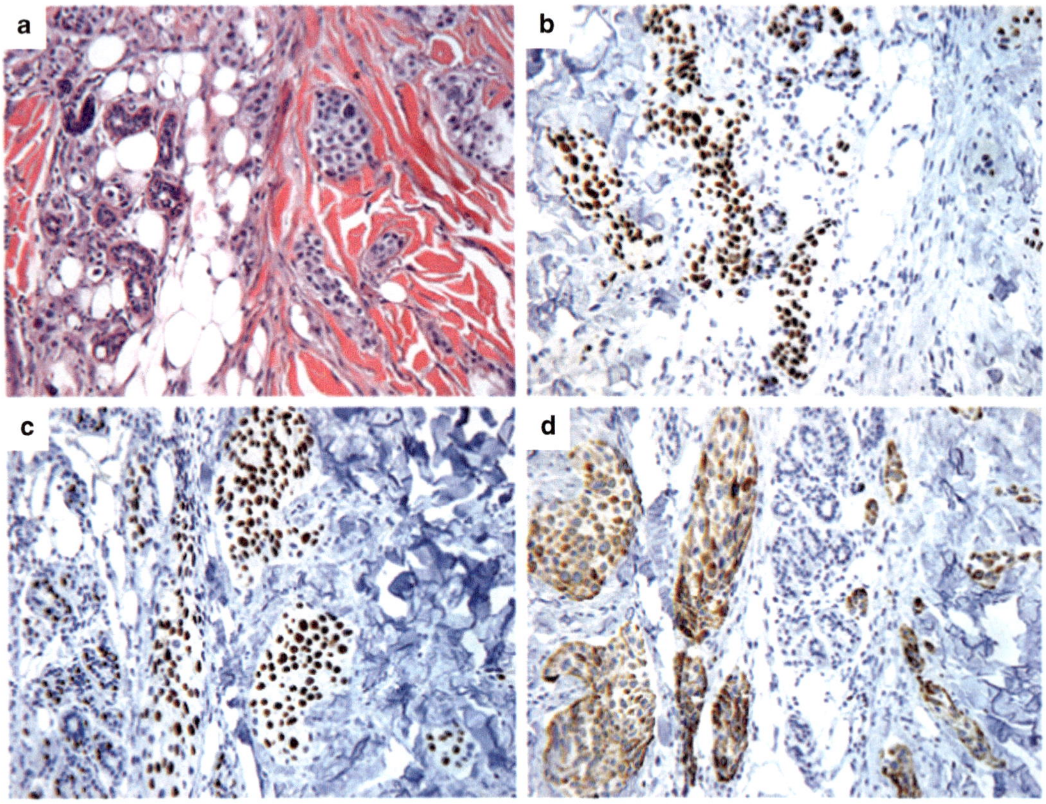

Fig. 37.12 Microscopic examination of the excised cutaneous nodule showed infiltration of the deep dermis and the subcutaneous fat by variably sized solid neoplastic blasts showing no connection with the epidermis or with the skin adnexa. Picture (**a**) shows the metastatic blasts in the deep dermis around the coiled secretory segment of a sweat gland. Immunohistochemically, the neoplastic cells expressed GATA3 (**b**), p63 (**c**), and CK20 (**d**). The immunohistochemical and morphologic characteristics were compatible with cutaneous metastasis from urothelial carcinoma. (**a**): H/E ×100 magnification; (**b**): GATA3 ×100 magnification; (**c**): p63 ×100 magnification; (**d**): CK20 ×100 magnification

The overlying epidermis and superficial dermis were free of tumors. Tumor cells extended to the surgical margins, indicating incomplete excision. Clinical and imaging correlation was recommended. Microscopic photos showed aggregates of metastatic carcinoma cells surrounding sweat gland secretory coils within the deep dermis with no epidermal or skin adnexal attachment. Immunohistochemical profiles were GATA3, p63, and CK20 positive. These findings confirmed cutaneous metastasis from urothelial carcinoma. Clinically, the occurrence of multiple subcutaneous nodules over surgical sites such as nephrostomies suggests implications of mechanisms, including lymphatic spread or iatrogenic seeding of tumors. Cutaneous metastasis from bladder carcinoma is rare, representing less than 3% of metastases, and typically indicates widespread systemic dissemination with a bad prognosis. Diagnosis hinges upon a high index of suspicion and histological evidence to differentiate from other cutaneous lesions.

37.1.7 Cutaneous Metastasis of Bladder Cancer: Case 7

A 58-year-old woman patient with a history of known bladder urothelial carcinoma presented with new lesions over the genitalia. She had initially been diagnosed with cancer of the bladder 2 years back, following hematuria and pelvic discomfort. Diagnoses by cystoscopy and transurethral resection were of high-grade urothelial carcinoma, and she underwent radical treatment, including systemic chemotherapy.

Though early in onset, she developed metastatic disease, both at regional nodes and later at distant visceral sites. On a follow-up visit, she had complained of the development of tender nodules and erythematous plaques over the vulvar and perineal area. On inspection, there were multiple firm nodules over the skin and mucosa of the genitalia. The nodules were erythematous to violaceous, palpable, tender, and varied in diameter from 0.5 cm to 2 cm. Some of them were discrete, but others blended to give irregular, indurated plaques. The mucosa over the nodules was edematous and inflamed, causing significant pain, particularly when walking and voiding.

Given her oncologic history, the clinical suspicion for cutaneous and mucosal metastases was high. One of the vulvar nodules was biopsied with a punch biopsy for histopathological examination.

Histology revealed dermis infiltration by malignant epithelioid cells in a nested and diffuse manner (Fig. 37.13a, b, and c). The tumor cells had ovoid to round nuclei with vesicular chromatin, large nucleoli, and moderate eosinophilic cytoplasm. There were numerous mitotic figures and necrosis as well. The overlying epidermis was normal, and the tumor growth was restricted to the dermis and submucosa.

Immunohistochemical staining was performed in an attempt to further characterize the neoplasm. The neoplastic cells were GATA3 and CK20-positive with intense nuclear and cytoplasmic positivity, respectively. They also showed p63 positivity. Such an immunophenotypic pattern, along with the morphologic features and history, resulted in the diagnosis of cutaneous and mucosal metastasis of urothelial carcinoma of the bladder.

Clinically, cutaneous metastasis of urothelial carcinoma is rare and happens in less than 1% of cases [10–12]. Genitalia are not a common site of involvement but may be present by lymphatic spread, hematogenous dissemination, or direct extension from pelvic cancer. Genital cutaneous and mucosal metastases in this patient were an indication of far-advanced systemic disease [13–18].

Management was mostly symptomatic, highlighting relief of symptoms, pain control, and protection against secondary infection. Therapeutic options were conceptualized in terms of her overall disease course and past therapies. Cutaneous metastasis from bladder cancer in general has a poor prognosis, reflecting aggressive tumor biology and limited remaining therapeutic options.

This case illustrates the clinical heterogeneity of cutaneous metastases, their ability to involve unusual sites such as genital mucosa, and the utility of confirmation by biopsy. Dermatologists

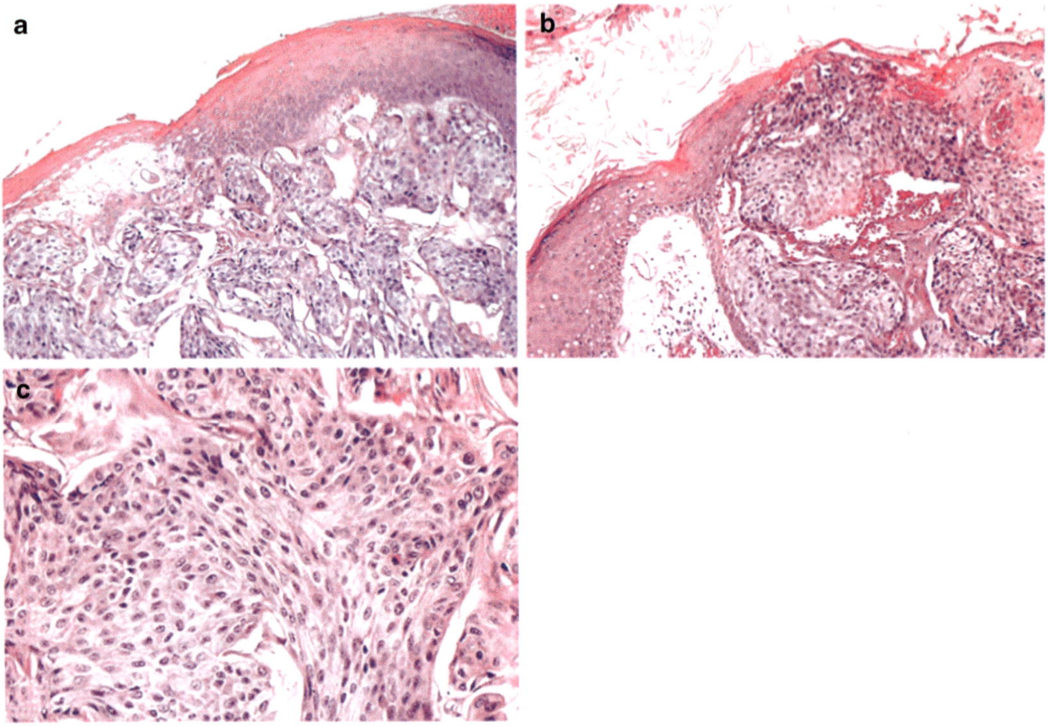

Fig. 37.13 Histopathological findings of a cutaneous metastasis on the genital area and genital mucosa from urothelial carcinoma in a 58-year-old female patient. (**a**, **b**) The dermis is infiltrated by malignant epithelioid cells arranged in nested and diffuse patterns. (**c**) High magnification: tumor cells with round to ovoid nuclei, vesicular chromatin, prominent nucleoli, and moderate amounts of eosinophilic cytoplasm. These morphologic features, together with the immunophenotypic profile, are consistent with metastatic urothelial carcinoma

and oncologists should recognize such presentations since they might be the presenting sign of progression in patients with established urothelial carcinoma.

Cutaneous metastases of bladder carcinoma are a rare but clinically significant condition, with a reported incidence varying from 0.2% to 2.9% among patients with bladder malignancies. They constitute 0.1% to 2% of all cutaneous metastases from visceral cancers. Bladder cancer is one of the most common urogenital malignancies worldwide—fourth and tenth in men and women, respectively—but cutaneous metastasis is a rare manifestation of an advanced disease with poor prognosis.

The majority of reported cases are of urothelial (transitional cell) carcinoma (approximately 72.8%), the remaining being adenocarcinoma, poorly differentiated carcinoma, sarcomatoid carcinoma, and other rare histologies. Cutaneous metastases may occur many years after the initial diagnosis of the cancer, although sometimes the skin lesions may occur before or simultaneously with the bladder cancer diagnosis.

Patient demographics are predominantly male (about 85%) with an age range from 33 to 88 years. Clinical presentation is generally associated with firm, painless erythematous to violaceous nodules (65–75%), plaques, or ulcerated lesions and may be accompanied by crusting and necrosis at times. The most frequent anatomic sites are the abdomen (lower abdominal wall especially), chest, upper extremities (axillae and shoulders), back, neck, and inguinal area, with lesions frequently present in association with the relative area of recent or old surgical sites, including stomas or incision scars. They vary from a solitary nodule to polymorphic cutaneous lesions, causing pain locally and functional impairment.

Histopathologic examination is typically defined by dermal invasion by malignant urothelial cells with nuclear atypia, high mitotic activity, and variable degrees of differentiation. The immunohistochemical profile is frequently positive for CK7, CK20, GATA3, and p63 and aids in determining urothelial origin (Fig. 37.13). Cutaneous metastasis results from one or more mechanisms: direct intradermal extension of the tumor, hematogenous seeding, lymphatic spread, or iatrogenic implantation following surgical or diagnostic manipulations.

Laboratory examinations, when performed, may reveal anemia, elevated creatinine, or abnormal urinalysis with hematuria, indicative of systemic extension of disease. The presence of cutaneous metastases normally follows metastases to other structures like lungs, liver, bones, and adrenals.

Treatment options are diverse and may involve systemic chemotherapy, immunotherapy, radiotherapy, excision of metastatic skin lesions, or palliative treatment, with little overall survival reported. Median survival after the detection of cutaneous metastasis is often less than 1 year. Due to disparate clinical manifestations, skin metastases may mimic infections, drug reactions, or benign cutaneous conditions, emphasizing the importance of biopsy in correct diagnosis.

In conclusion, skin metastases in patients with bladder cancer represent advanced-stage disease. Early detection, accurate histopathologic diagnosis, and multidisciplinary management by oncologists, dermatologists, and pathologists are required to optimize patient treatment and guide therapy [19–21].

37.1.8 Cutaneous Metastasis from Urothelial Carcinoma of the Renal Pelvis (Upper Tract Urothelial Carcinoma/ UTUC): Case 8

A 68-year-old man with a known history of urothelial carcinoma of the renal pelvis (upper tract urothelial carcinoma/UTUC) presented with a new skin lesion on the abdominal wall. The patient had been diagnosed with a urothelial carcinoma, measuring 6.5 × 5 cm, following symptoms of hematuria and flank pain. Imaging studies at the time of diagnosis confirmed a urothelial mass without obvious cutaneous involvement, and he underwent surgical and oncological evaluation for further management.

Approximately 1 year after his initial diagnosis, the patient noticed the gradual appearance of a solitary erythematous to skin-colored nodule on the left lower abdominal area. The lesion was firm, dome-shaped, and erythematous to skin colored, measuring about 4 cm in diameter. Over subsequent weeks, the nodule increased in size and became tender. No ulceration or bleeding was noted, but the lesion raised clinical concern for metastatic spread, particularly given the patient's oncologic background.

On dermatological examination, the abdominal lesion appeared to be a well-circumscribed, firm, reddish to violaceous nodule located on the left lower quadrant. The surface was smooth, without secondary changes, but the rapid growth and induration suggested an underlying malignant process. Given the suspicion of cutaneous metastasis, an excisional biopsy was performed.

Histological examination of the skin specimen revealed infiltration of the dermis by solid sheets and nests of carcinoma, showing areas of necrosis, the latter suggesting aggressive growth (Fig. 37.14a, b). The tumor cells were poorly differentiated, with large, irregular nuclei, prominent nucleoli, and abundant eosinophilic cytoplasm. Importantly, there was no connection between the tumor and the overlying epidermis, excluding a primary cutaneous carcinoma.

Immunohistochemical studies were carried out to characterize the neoplasm further. Tumor cells' immunophenotype was characterized by the combined positive expression for GATA3, CK7, and CK20, validating their urothelial origin. The phenotypic features, together with the immunoprofile and the patient's clinical history, supported the diagnosis of cutaneous metastasis from urothelial carcinoma.

From a clinical standpoint, cutaneous metastases from urothelial cancers are relatively uncommon, representing only a small fraction of

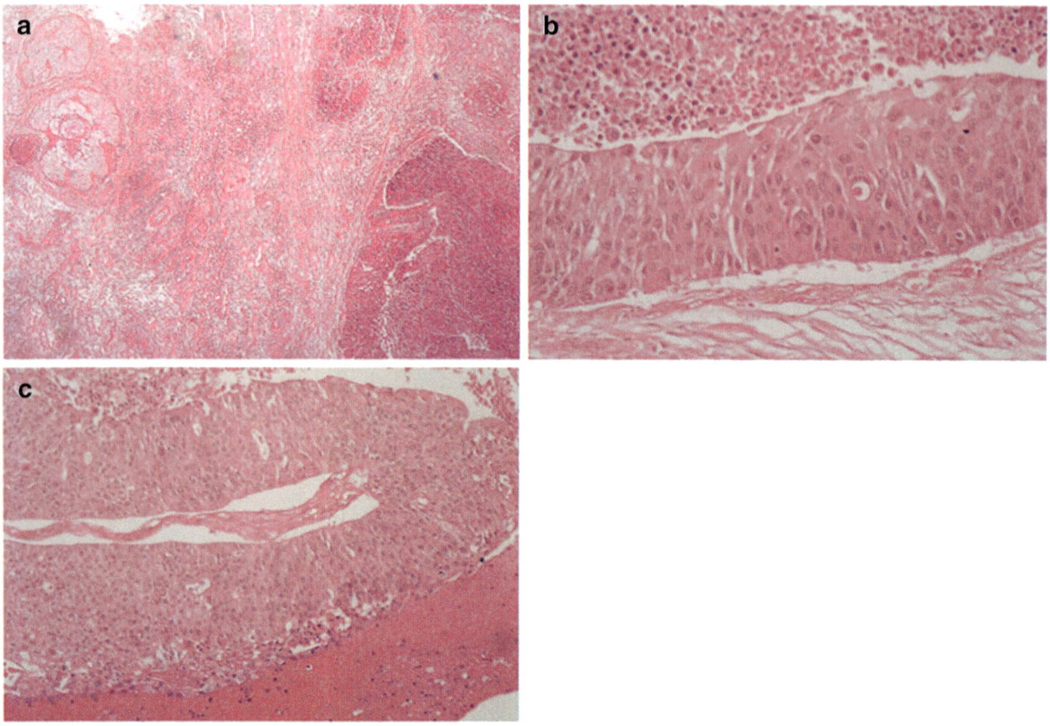

Fig. 37.14 Cutaneous metastasis from urothelial carcinoma in a 68-year-old male. (**a**, **b**) At the upper left, a pilosebaceous unit is visible, while the adjacent dermis on the right side is infiltrated by malignant tumor cells. (**c**) High magnification: poorly differentiated carcinoma infiltrating the dermis with areas of necrosis. The morphologic and immunohistochemical findings were consistent with cutaneous metastasis from urothelial carcinoma

metastatic urinary bladder carcinoma cases. When present, they typically manifest as solitary or multiple nodules, most frequently involving the scalp, trunk, or abdominal wall. The abdominal localization in this patient is consistent with reported patterns of hematogenous dissemination.

The appearance of cutaneous metastasis in urothelial carcinoma generally signals advanced systemic disease and is associated with a poor prognosis. For this patient, the finding prompted reassessment of systemic disease burden, including imaging studies to evaluate for visceral metastases [21–23].

Management was primarily palliative, focusing on local excision of symptomatic cutaneous lesions and systemic oncologic therapies. Unfortunately, cutaneous metastasis often reflects aggressive tumor biology, with limited curative treatment options available.

This case emphasizes the importance of careful cutaneous examination in patients with a known history of urothelial carcinoma. Even small or seemingly innocuous nodules may represent metastatic disease, and biopsy remains essential for diagnosis. Recognition of such lesions can guide staging, prognosis, and treatment planning in patients with renal malignancies.

Cutaneous metastasis from bladder cancer is less common than the skin metastasis from breast cancer (Fig. 37.15a-c), most often presents as nodules or infiltrated plaques on the abdominal wall or lower extremities, and similarly indicates advanced disease with poor prognosis.

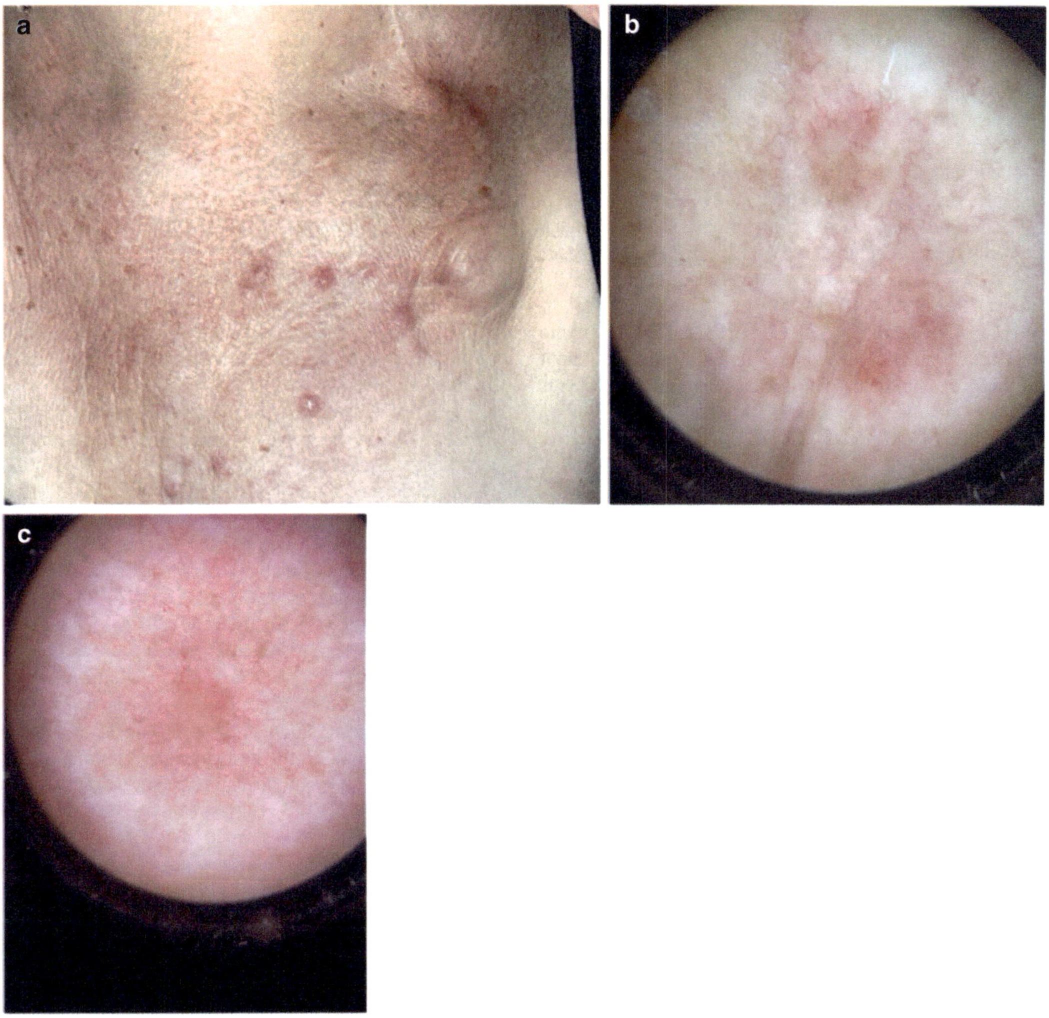

Fig. 37.15 (a) Cutaneous metastasis from breast cancer presenting as violaceous to erythematous nodules on the frontal thoracic area in a woman with breast cancer and (**b** + **c**) Dermoscopic features reveal irregular linear and branching (arborizing) vessels on an erythematous background

Acknowledgments "The authors would like to thank Professor Elias Drakos, MD, PhD, Department of Pathology, Medical School, University of Crete, Heraklion, Greece, for providing the histological images and slides for some of the cases."

"The authors would also like to thank Dr. Georgios Evangelou, Consultant Dermatologist-Venereologist, MD, PhD, Department of Dermatology, University Hospital of Heraklion, Heraklion, Greece, for providing clinical and dermoscopic images for some of the cases."

References

1. Gu W, Yuan J, Dong M, Sheng J, Jiang K. Case report: advanced breast invasive ductal carcinoma with erysipeloid cutaneous metastasis misdiagnosed as erysipelas. Front Oncol. 2025;15:1535421. https://doi.org/10.3389/fonc.2025.1535421. eCollection 2025. PMID: 40727474.
2. Mandli S, Surani A, Doshi YJ, Shah B. Cutaneous presentations of metastatic carcinoma breast: a case

series. Indian Dermatol Online J. 2025;16(4):595–600. https://doi.org/10.4103/idoj.idoj_712_24. eCollection 2025 Jul-Aug. PMID: 40688163.

3. Russano F, Corrado G, Bonadies A, Migliano E, di Giacomo R, Esposito E, Zamagni C, Ala A, Campana L, Fabrizio T, Ghilli M, Palli D, Renne M, Cabula R, Pelle F, Silvestri B, Dieci MV, Guarneri V, Rastrelli M. Prospective multicentre study of patients with cutaneous metastases from breast cancer treated with electrochemotherapy. Clin Exp Metastasis. 2025;42(4):32. https://doi.org/10.1007/s10585-025-10350-5. PMID: 40439892.
4. Chen R, Shalhout SZ, Gerber AA, Ly A, Hoang MP. Carcinoma en cuirasse is an independent poor survival predictor in breast carcinoma patients with cutaneous metastasis. J Am Acad Dermatol. 2025;93(3):784–6. https://doi.org/10.1016/j.jaad.2025.05.004. Epub 2025 May 7. PMID: 40345541.
5. Flindris S, Margioula-Siarkou C, Margioula-Siarkou G, Gouta C, Styliara E, Navrozoglou I, Petousis S, Dinas K. Cutaneous metastasis of triple negative breast cancer: a case report and review of literature. Cureus. 2025;17(3):e79926. https://doi.org/10.7759/cureus.79926. eCollection 2025 Mar. PMID: 40171370.
6. Custer MK, Nessel T, Aron JL, Israeli AF, Nash KT, Graves E. Cutaneous scalp metastasis from mammary ductal carcinoma. Cureus. 2025;17(1):e77187. https://doi.org/10.7759/cureus.77187. eCollection 2025 Jan. PMID: 39925600.
7. Albalawi IAS, Nukaly HY, Said MI, Moharram L, Elgazzar K. Cutaneous metastasis of breast carcinoma in the distal phalanx of the left little finger: a case report. Plast Reconstr Surg Glob Open. 2024;12(11):e6274. https://doi.org/10.1097/GOX0000000000006274. eCollection 2024 Nov. PMID: 39534372.
8. Jamjoum G, Arab FS, Tayeb R, Samkari A, Johari AA, Ashkar L, Akbar J. Cutaneous metastasis in breast cancer: a case report. Am J Case Rep. 2024;25:e943999. https://doi.org/10.12659/AJCR.943999. PMID: 38992932.
9. Xu Y, Ding L, Li C, Hua B, Wang S, Zhang J, Liu C, Guo R, Zhang Y. Molecular alterations and prognosis of breast cancer with cutaneous metastasis. Diagn Pathol. 2024;19(1):93. https://doi.org/10.1186/s13000-024-01509-x. PMID: 38970069.
10. Raghavan D. Cutaneous manifestations of genitourinary malignancy. Semin Oncol. 2016;43(3):347–52. https://doi.org/10.1053/j.seminoncol.2016.02.027. Epub 2016 Feb 23. PMID: 27178687.
11. Truong H, Parsons TM, Trabulsi EJ. Cutaneous metastasis of micropapillary urothelial carcinoma. Urology. 2015;85(2):e7–8. https://doi.org/10.1016/j.urology.2014.10.015. Epub 2015 Jan 2. PMID: 25559725.
12. Zangrilli A, Saraceno R, Sarmati L, Orlandi A, Bianchi L, Chimenti S. Erysipeloid cutaneous metastasis from bladder carcinoma. Eur J Dermatol. 2007;17(6):534–6. https://doi.org/10.1684/ejd.2007.0271. Epub 2007 Oct 19. PMID: 17951136.
13. Swick BL, Gordon JR. Superficially invasive transitional cell carcinoma of the bladder associated with distant cutaneous metastases. J Cutan Pathol. 2010;37(12):1245–50. https://doi.org/10.1111/j.1600-0560.2009.01471.x. PMID: 19919656
14. Akman Y, Cam K, Kavak A, Alper M. Extensive cutaneous metastasis of transitional cell carcinoma of the bladder. Int J Urol. 2003;10(2):103–4. https://doi.org/10.1046/j.1442-2042.2003.00571.x. PMID: 12588608.
15. Zaouak A, Ebdelli W, Slimène MB, Smida W, Debbiche A, Jannet SB, Hammami H, Fenniche S. Cutaneous metastases: clinicopathologic study of 30 patients. Skinmed. 2024;22(1):30–4. eCollection 2024. PMID: 38494612.
16. Lees AN. Cutaneous metastasis of transitional cell carcinoma of the urinary bladder eight years after the primary: a case report. J Med Case Rep. 2015;9:102. https://doi.org/10.1186/s13256-015-0585-9. PMID: 25943325.
17. Bazzi N, Jaber S, Saad WA, Al Hassan S, Dbouk S, Alhousseini A. Cutaneous metastasis of bladder cancer: a systematic review. Cureus. 2024;16(11):e74439. https://doi.org/10.7759/cureus.74439. eCollection 2024 Nov. PMID: 39726500.
18. Izzo P, Izzo L, Lai S, D'Onghia G, Giancontieri P, Gabriele R, Polistena A, Sibio S, Costanzo ML, De Intinis C, Izzo S. Nodular cutaneous metastasis of the leg in advanced urothelial bladder carcinoma: a case report and systematic literature review. Front Oncol. 2023;13:1216725. https://doi.org/10.3389/fonc.2023.1216725. eCollection 2023. PMID: 37675233.
19. Mueller TJ, Wu H, Greenberg RE, Hudes G, Topham N, Lessin SR, Uzzo RG. Cutaneous metastases from genitourinary malignancies. Urology. 2004;63(6):1021–6. https://doi.org/10.1016/j.urology.2004.01.014. PMID: 15183939.
20. Somani BK, Prita D, Grant S, Nabi G, N'dow J. Herpetiform cutaneous metastases from transitional cell carcinoma of the urinary bladder: immunohistochemical analysis. J Clin Pathol. 2006;59(12):1331–3. https://doi.org/10.1136/jcp.2005.031500. PMID: 17142578.
21. Kuritza V, Pei S. Zosteriform cutaneous metastases from urothelial carcinoma: report of a rare case and literature review. J Cutan Pathol. 2023;50(10):890–6. https://doi.org/10.1111/cup.14471. Epub 2023 May 29. PMID: 37246593.
22. Osen ER, Warren AY. Rare abdominal cutaneous presentation of clear cell renal cell carcinoma: a case report. Urology. 2019;127:e8–9. https://doi.org/10.1016/j.urology.2019.01.028. Epub 2019 Feb 8. PMID: 30738883.
23. Wang W, Kang Y, Qu X, Li Y, Zhou H. A rare case report of renal clear cell carcinoma with multiple skin metastases and a review of the literature. Front Oncol. 2024;14:1461791. https://doi.org/10.3389/fonc.2024.1461791. eCollection 2024. PMID: 39697235.

38 Case Presentations of Cutaneous Metastases from Different Primary Tumors, Part II (Lung Cancer, Unknown Primary Cancer, and Colon Adenocarcinoma Cases)

Dimitra Koumaki, Ioannis Kokkinakis, Eleni Lappa, and Eleni Lagoudaki

Abstract

Skin metastases represent a rare but clinically significant manifestation of internal malignancies, typically indicating advanced disease and poor prognosis. This report illustrates a few cases of skin metastases from two kinds of primary tumors: lung cancer and colon adenocarcinoma. In lung cancers, patients presented with diverse cutaneous lesions, including solitary nodules, ulcerating plaques, telangiectatic patches, and lymphangitic carcinomatosis. Histopathologic examination of the lesions revealed invasion of the dermis by atypical epithelial cells with glandular or poorly differentiated morphology. Immunohistochemistry was extremely helpful in validating pulmonary primary origin, with the standard markers thyroid transcription factor 1 (TTF-1) and CK7 showing positive expression and CK20 and CDX2 negative. High proliferative rates (Ki-67 up to 100%) and aberrant expression patterns consistent with aggressive tumor behavior were seen in some cases. Dermoscopic analysis showed classic irregular vascular patterns and necrosis areas, facilitating early clinical suspicion. Cutaneous lymphangitic carcinomatous spread was highlighted as a rare but aggressive pattern of skin involvement.

Similarly, a case of skin metastasis from a colon adenocarcinoma was described, presenting with violaceous thoracic nodules and glandular histological infiltration of the dermis by malignant glandular and cribriform blasts compatible with colorectal origin. Immunoprofiling was in the differential diagnosis from a prior anal squamous cell carcinoma, emphasizing the diagnostic challenge in patients with synchronous cancers.

D. Koumaki (✉)
Dermatology Department, University Hospital of Heraklion, Heraklion, Greece

I. Kokkinakis · E. Lappa · E. Lagoudaki
Pathology Department, University Hospital of Heraklion, Heraklion, Greece

D. Koumaki et al. (eds.), *Cutaneous Metastases*, https://doi.org/10.1007/978-3-032-26764-1_38

Epidemiologically, skin metastases from lung cancer occur in 0.6–12% of patients, and metastatic skin lesions from colorectal adenocarcinoma account for approximately 3% of cases with advanced disease. Clinically, these metastases often present disguised as benign dermatoses, underlining the importance of biopsy and immunohistochemistry for their definitive diagnosis. Prognosis for these patients with cutaneous metastases remains poor, with median survival measured in months from diagnosis. Understanding of clinical, dermoscopic, histologic, and immunophenotypic features is essential to recognizing skin metastasis as a sign of advanced disease, enabling early multidisciplinary care. The case series contributes to growing evidence on the diverse presentations and diagnostic pitfalls of cutaneous metastases from lung and colon cancers.

Keywords

Cutaneous metastasis · Lung cancer · Non-small cell carcinoma · Colon adenocarcinoma · Dermoscopy · Immunohistochemistry · TTF-1 · CK7 · Lymphangitic carcinomatosis · Poorly differentiated carcinoma · Prognosis · Metastatic disease

38.1 Cutaneous Metastasis from Lung Cancer: Case 1

A 72-year-old male with a known history of pulmonary adenocarcinoma presented with an erythematous nodule of the scalp. The swelling was present for 1 month and was growing quickly. During clinical examination at the time of biopsy, a firm nodular swelling that was rounded was present, and part of it was excised for histological examination.

Histopathological examination of the excised sample revealed diffuse infiltration of the dermis by atypical epithelial cells arranged in glandular structures showing no association with the overlying epidermis or with adnexal structures. The neoplastic cells were of medium size with oval to irregular nuclei and eosinophilic cytoplasm in adenoid and cribriform patterns (Fig. 38.1a). Immunohistochemistry revealed strong expression of thyroid transcription factor-1 (TTF-1) (Fig. 38.1b), and cytokeratin 7 (CK7) (Fig. 38.1c), while staining for cytokeratin 20 (CK20) (Fig. 38.1d), and caudal type homeobox 2 (CDX2) was negative. These findings were consistent with the diagnosis of cutaneous metastasis of lung adenocarcinoma. The patient's clinical course was severe, and he expired a few months after cutaneous involvement was diagnosed, as expected with the poor prognosis of cutaneous metastasis with lung cancer.

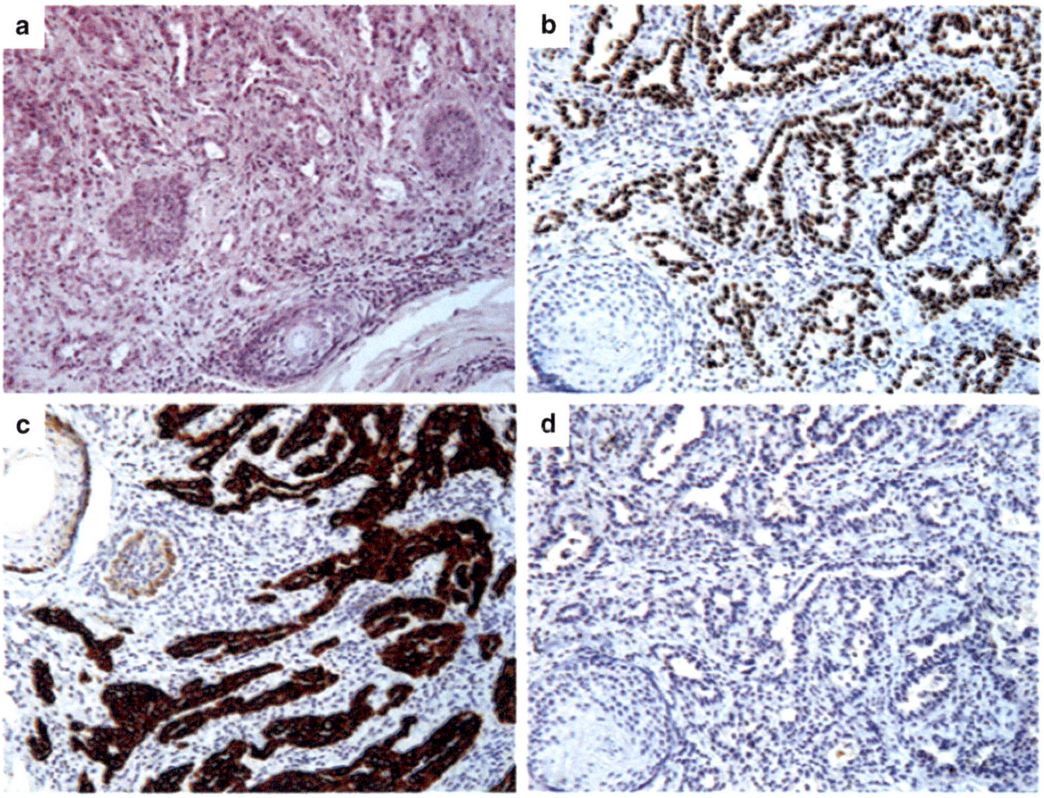

Fig. 38.1 Histological and immunohistochemical features of the excised nodule on the scalp in a 72-year-old patient with lung adenocarcinoma. The dermis of the excised lesion of the scalp displayed diffuse infiltration from glandular blasts of adenocarcinoma with no connection with the overlying epidermis or the adnexa (**a**). Immunohistochemical staining of the neoplastic cells was positive for the expression of TTF-1 (**b**) and CK7 (**c**), while it was negative for CDX2 (**d**) and CK20 (not shown). The immunophenotype was consistent with metastatic lung adenocarcinoma. (**a**): H/E X100 magnification, (**b**): TTF-1 X 100 magnification, (**c**): CK7 X 100 magnification, (**d**): CDX2 X 100 magnification

38.2 Cutaneous Metastasis from Unknown Primary Cancer: Case 2

A 47-year-old female patient with a history of lung carcinoma presented with the development of a tender, enlarging nodule on the front of the neck. Clinically, the lesion was an erythematous-violaceous infiltrated plaque with ulceration and necrotic areas spreading onto the upper chest (Fig. 38.2a). Dermoscopy revealed irregular linear and arborizing vessels on a reddish background, ulceration, hemorrhagic crusts, and necrotic whitish-yellow patches, suggestive of secondary skin involvement by a malignant neoplasm (Fig. 38.2b). Histopathological examination of the skin biopsy revealed dermal infiltration from a poorly differentiated carcinoma with overlapping morphological features of large cell carcinoma (Fig. 38.3a). The tumor consisted of large atypical epithelioid cells with marked nucleoli, moderate cytoplasm, high mitosis frequency (up to 10 per high-power field), and extensive necrosis (Fig. 38.3b). Immunohistochemical examina-

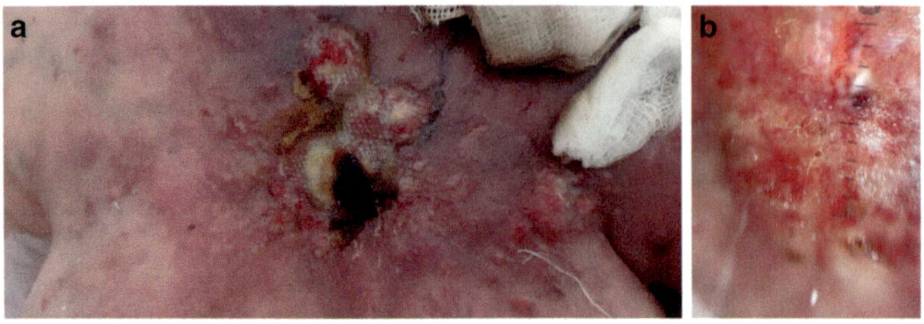

Fig. 38.2 (**a**) Clinical photograph showing an erythematous-violaceous infiltrated plaque with ulceration, central necrosis, and multiple nodular components on the anterior neck and upper chest in a patient with metastatic lung carcinoma. (**b**) Dermoscopic view demonstrating polymorphic vascular structures, including irregular linear and arborizing vessels, over a reddish background with ulceration, hemorrhagic crusts, and whitish-yellow structureless areas consistent with necrosis

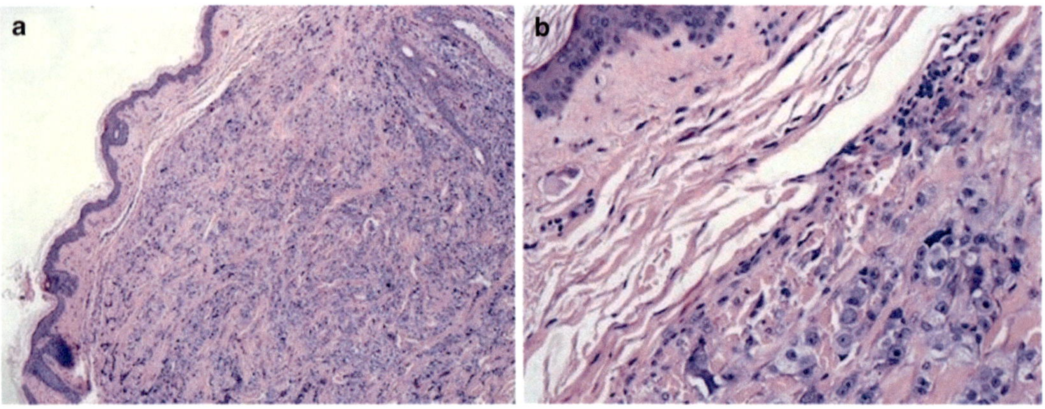

Fig. 38.3 The histology of a biopsy of the nodule on the anterior neck of a 47-year-old female patient with metastatic lung cancer showed that the dermis is diffusely infiltrated by a poorly differentiated carcinoma (*asterisk*), with destruction of dermal architecture. Immunohistochemical analysis confirmed a large cell lung carcinoma

tion revealed positive expression for E-cadherin, CAM5.2, CK7, CK19 (partially), 34βE12 (partially), INI1, and showed strong p53 nuclear positivity; however, TTF-1, p40, synaptophysin, and other lineage markers were negative. PD-L1 expression was present in approximately 25–30% of the tumor cells (TPS and CPS 25–30). Proliferation rate, Ki-67, was high (~70–75%). The diagnosis was large cell carcinoma of unknown primary origin, but SMARCA4-deficient thoracic tumor and NUT carcinoma were also in the differential diagnosis. The patient had been treated with pembrolizumab, paclitaxel, carboplatin, and peg filgrastim as part of her systemic oncologic therapy. Cutaneous metastasis at presentation was an indicator of advanced disease with an unfavorable prognosis and emphasized the importance of diagnosing skin involvement as a manifestation of advanced cancer.

38.2.1 Epidemiology and Incidence of Cutaneous Metastasis in Lung Cancer

Cutaneous metastases from lung carcinoma are observed in approximately 0.6% to 12% of patients with lung carcinoma [1]. They may either present as the first sign of an underlying associated malignancy or as an indicator of advanced disease. Lung cancer is one of the most frequent causes of cutaneous metastases in men and has a poor prognosis [2]. Median survival at the time of diagnosis of skin metastasis is usually limited to a few months, and it is noted with emphasis on the aggressive nature of this presentation.

38.2.2 Clinical Presentation of Cutaneous Metastasis in Lung Cancer

Cutaneous metastasis is most commonly reported by firm, non-tender, flesh-colored to erythematous nodules or tumors. They are either single or multiple lesions and are ulcerated. Metastases to the skin occur most frequently on the chest, back, abdomen, and extremities but are also known to occur in the neck and head area [3]. Due to the variability of clinical presentations, lesions can appear as imitations of benign skin lesions, and hence, the diagnosis can be made only after biopsy (Figs. 38.4 and 38.5).

38.2.3 Dermoscopic Features of Skin Metastasis in Lung Carcinoma

The dermoscopic hallmark of lung cancer metastases to the skin is an unsystematic vascular pattern, typically observed as serpiginous or linear irregular vessels within most nonpigmented lesions. Structureless white, pink, or red spots are common and likely represent neoplastic invasion and necrosis [4]. Pigmented lesions are rare in lung cancer metastases but may be seen in metastases from other primaries, such as melanoma or breast carcinoma. Dermoscopy may be a valuable noninvasive method to raise the suspicion of skin metastasis in a patient with a history of malignancy [5–10].

38.2.4 Histology and Immunohistochemistry of Cutaneous Metastasis of Lung Cancer

Histologic examination of the skin biopsy reveals the dermis diffusely infiltrated by poorly differentiated carcinoma composed of large epithelioid cells with eosinophilic nucleoli, numerous mitoses, and extensive necrosis. Immunohistochemical examination is typically positive for markers such as E-cadherin, CAM5.2, CK7, and partial positivity for CK19 and PD-L1. Tumor markers known to be present in other tumor lineages (e.g., CK20, TTF1, p63, melanocytic markers) are negative, making other neoplasms less likely. Characterized by increased proliferation index (Ki67 ~ 70–75%) and strong p53 expression, which is common, consistent with aggressive tumor behavior [11–14].

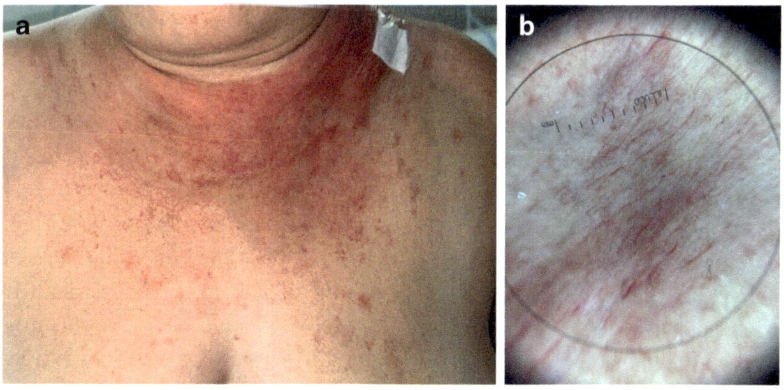

Fig. 38.4 (**a**) *Clinical presentation*. Erythematous patches with prominent telangiectasias and diffuse, irregular macules distributed over the upper chest and lower neck region of a 52-year-old female patient with stage IV lung cancer. The lesion's vascular features and erythema suggest cutaneous metastatic involvement (lymphangitic carcinomatosis of the skin secondary to lung carcinoma). (**b**) *Dermoscopic findings*. Close-up dermoscopic image revealing irregular linear and serpentine telangiectasias against a pinkish background without pigmentation, consistent with vascular proliferation in cutaneous metastasis from lung carcinoma

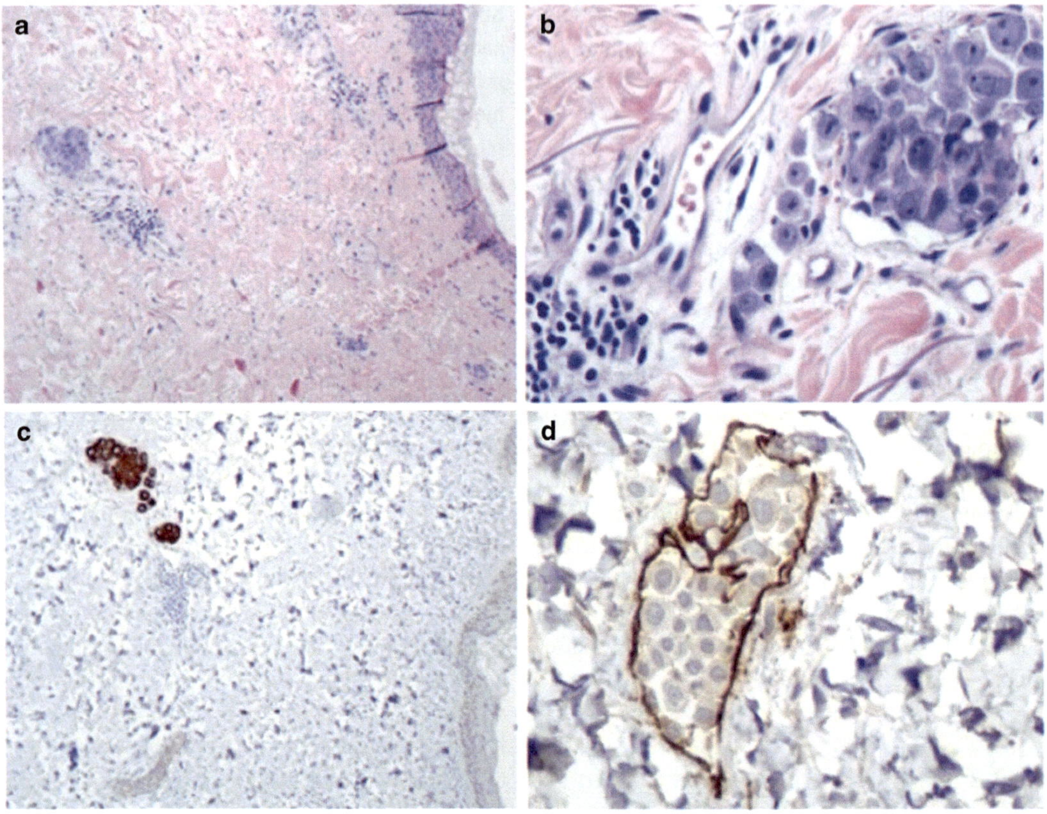

Fig. 38.5 Skin biopsy from a 52-year-old female patient with stage IV lung cancer showing cutaneous lymphangitic metastasis. *Histology and immunohistochemistry*. (**a**) Hematoxylin and eosin stain showing small clusters of large malignant epithelial cells within dermal lymphatic vessels (arrows), indicating lymphatic invasion by metastatic carcinoma (original magnifications: X40 left a, X400 b). (**c**) Immunohistochemical staining with cytokeratin 7 confirms cytoplasmic positivity of metastatic tumor cells, while podoplanin highlights the lymphatic endothelial lining (**d**). The tumor cells are also TTF1 positive, confirming pulmonary origin. PD-L1 expression is negative (TPS 0%, CPS 0%), as demonstrated by immunostaining with clone 9A11

38.3 Cutaneous Lymphangitis Carcinomatosa as a Cutaneous Manifestation in a Patient with Lung Adenocarcinoma: Case 3

A 52-year-old female with a known history of chronic obstructive pulmonary disease presented with progressive erythematous, telangiectatic patches localized on the anterior chest and lower neck. These cutaneous lesions were initially asymptomatic but progressively raised clinical concern due to their persistent, vascular appearance. Dermoscopic examination demonstrated irregular linear and serpentine telangiectasias over a pink background, suggestive of neoplastic vascular proliferation.

Skin biopsy was performed, revealing small clusters of large malignant epithelial cells confined within the lymphatic vessels of the dermis. Immunohistochemical analysis showed strong cytoplasmic positivity for CK7 and nuclear positivity for TTF1, consistent with the pulmonary origin of the tumor. Podoplanin highlighted the lymphatic endothelium, confirming lymphangitic spread. PD-L1 expression was negative.

The diagnosis of cutaneous lymphangitic metastasis secondary to stage IV lung carcinoma was established. Despite initiation of systemic chemotherapy with pemetrexed and carboplatin, the patient's disease progression was rapid, and she succumbed to the illness within months. This case illustrates the importance of recognizing cutaneous lymphangitic metastases as a manifestation of advanced lung cancer, facilitating prompt diagnosis and multidisciplinary management.

38.4 Cutaneous Metastasis from Poorly Differentiated Non-small Cell Carcinoma, Most Likely from Lung Cancer: Case 4

A 78-year-old male developed a new firm nodule on the left side of his back. Skin biopsy revealed a poorly differentiated non-small cell carcinoma infiltrating the dermis diffusely in sheets. The neoplastic cells were pleomorphic with eosinophilic to clear cytoplasm and one or more prominent nucleoli, along with numerous mitotic and apoptotic figures (Fig. 38.6a–c). Immunohistochemistry was positive for MFN-116, TTF-1, and CK7, while staining for CD68, p63, CK20, and 760/B was negative.

High molecular weight cytokeratin highlighted the stratified squamous epithelium, while the neoplastic cells remained negative (Fig. 38.6d).

The case demonstrates the aggressive nature of poorly differentiated lung cancer and its propensity to present as cutaneous metastasis in the form of an isolated skin nodule. Recognition of such lesions is necessary for early diagnosis and treatment.

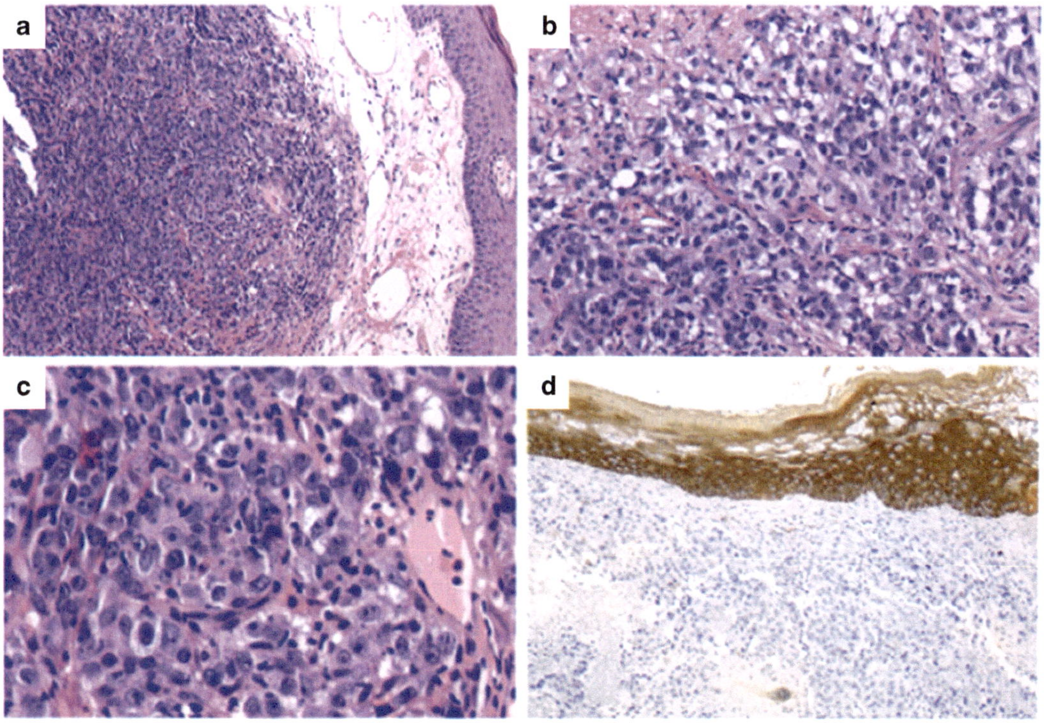

Fig. 38.6 Histological features of a skin biopsy of a nodule on the back of a 78-year-old man showed poorly differentiated non-small cell carcinoma metastatic to the skin. The dermis is being infiltrated by a diffuse sheet of neoplastic cells (**a**). The neoplastic cells are pleomorphic and contain medium amounts of eosinophilic to clear cytoplasm, one or multiple prominent nucleoli, and numerous mitotic and apoptotic figures (**b**). The neoplastic cells are pleomorphic, contain medium amounts of eosinophilic to clear cytoplasm, and have one or multiple prominent nucleoli (**c**). High molecular weight cytokeratin highlights the stratified squamous epithelium. The neoplastic cells are negative (**d**)

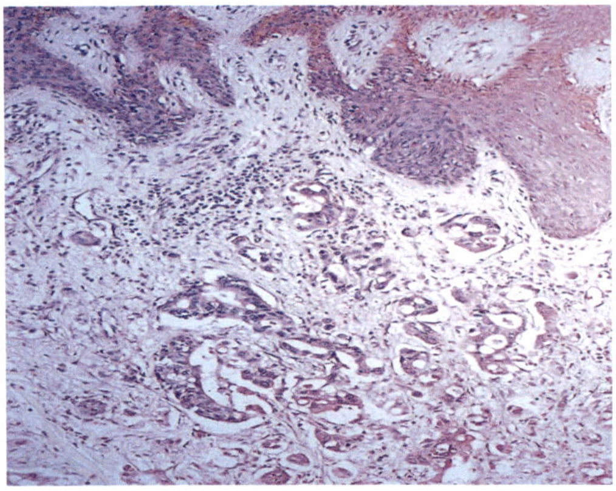

Fig. 38.7 Histology of skin biopsy from frontal thoracic nodule in a 50-year-old female with a history of colon adenocarcinoma. The dermis is infiltrated by malignant cells that form glandular structures

38.5 Cutaneous Metastasis from Colon Adenocarcinoma: Case 5

A 50-year-old female with a remote history of low-grade anal squamous cell carcinoma, treated surgically a decade ago, followed by adjuvant chemotherapy, presented with a new violaceous nodule on the frontal thoracic area. She had a history of lymph node metastases treated 3 years prior and was undergoing chemotherapy for anal cancer recurrence.

Thoracic skin biopsy revealed dermal invasion by malignant cells in glandular structures consistent with adenocarcinoma histology (Fig. 38.7). The biopsy specimen revealed a brown, nodular lesion with areas of necrosis involving the subcutaneous tissue completely. An immunohistochemical panel of MNF-116, Cam5.2, p63, HMW, Desmin, INI1, SMA, S100, HMB45, Melan-A, and S-100 was performed to exclude other neoplastic processes; metastatic colorectal adenocarcinoma was favored. The lesion was completely excised.

Immunohistochemical stains confirmed the diagnosis of skin metastasis from colon adenocarcinoma, a second primary tumor distinct from her prior anal squamous cell carcinoma. The case represents the diagnostic challenge of skin metastases in patients with multiple prior malignancies [15–20].

Skin metastasis of colorectal adenocarcinoma is rare and typically signifies widespread disease with poor prognosis. The clinical presentation can be unusual, often with nodular violaceous lesions, such as in the present patient. Histology typically reveals dermal infiltration by malignant gland-forming cells mimicking the primary colon cancer. Vigilance and histopathologic diagnosis are necessary for proper diagnosis and management [21].

Skin metastasis from colorectal adenocarcinoma is uncommon, occurring in approximately 3% of patients with advanced colorectal cancer, and is typically in the setting of widespread metastatic disease and unfavorable prognosis.

In men, colorectal cancer is one of the more frequent sources of skin metastases, following lung and melanoma cancer.

The median survival after the diagnosis of cutaneous metastasis is typically measured in months, reflecting the late stage at presentation.

Clinically, these metastases most frequently manifest as firm, non-tender, flesh-colored to erythematous nodules or tumors, which may be single or multiple. They can also appear as papules, plaques, or ulcers and can mimic benign conditions such as cysts, lipomas, or cellulitis. The most common anatomical sites are the abdominal wall, perineum, and surgical scars, but distant sites can be affected. Lesions can be the first manifestation of an occult colorectal cancer or represent recurrence after treatment [22–28].

Dermoscopy of cutaneous metastases of colorectal adenocarcinoma typically shows prominent vascular patterns, such as serpentine or linear irregular vessels, and structureless pink, red, or white areas. These are not of colorectal nature but are highly suggestive of metastatic disease in the appropriate clinical setting. Pigmented structures are rare in colorectal metastases, and vascular structures should always arouse suspicion for biopsy in patients with a history of internal malignancy.

Acknowledgments "The authors would like to thank Professor Elias Drakos, MD, PhD, Department of Pathology, Medical School, University of Crete, Heraklion, Greece, for providing the histological images and slides for some of the cases."

"The authors would also like to thank Dr. Georgios Evangelou, Consultant Dermatologist-Venereologist, MD, PhD, Department of Dermatology, University Hospital of Heraklion, Heraklion, Greece, for providing clinical and dermoscopic images for some of the cases."

References

1. Dhambri S, Zendah I, Ayadi-Kaddour A, Adouni O, El Mezni F. Cutaneous metastasis of lung carcinoma: a retrospective study of 12 cases. J Eur Acad Dermatol Venereol. 2011;25(6):722–6. https://doi.org/10.1111/j.1468-3083.2010.03818.x. Epub 2010 Aug 23. PMID: 20735519.
2. Snow K, Moody R, Kremer M, Chaudhry S. Metastatic lung cancer mimicking varicella-zoster virus. Dermatol Online J. 2025;31(1). https://doi.org/10.5070/D331164970. PMID: 40526944.
3. Owen CE. Cutaneous manifestations of lung cancer. Semin Oncol. 2016;43(3):366–9. https://doi.org/10.1053/j.seminoncol.2016.02.025. Epub 2016 Feb 23. PMID: 27178690.
4. Simionescu O, Petrică M, Avram AM, Costache M, Scurtu LG, Tudorache SI, Iorga PG, Grigore M. Dermoscopy of skin metastases in advanced cancer-systemic (visceral, hematologic) and cutaneous. Front Med (Lausanne). 2024;11:1445811. https://doi.org/10.3389/fmed.2024.1445811. eCollection 2024. PMID: 39139791.
5. Kerrouch H, Danset M, Hjira N, Kanitakis J. Metastatic adenocarcinoma of the lung presenting as a presternal cutaneous mass: case report and brief literature review. Anticancer Res. 2023;43(5):2367–70. https://doi.org/10.21873/anticanres.16402. PMID: 37097655.
6. Paul D, Bhardwaj S, Soni A, Chauhan A, Dhankhar R, Kaur P. Carcinoma lung with cutaneous metastasis: experience from an Indian institute. Rep Pract Oncol Radiother. 2025;29(6):690–9. https://doi.org/10.5603/rpor.103526. eCollection 2024. PMID: 40104658.
7. Mollet TW, Garcia CA, Koester G. Skin metastases from lung cancer. Dermatol Online J. 2009;15(5):1. PMID: 19624979.
8. Marcoval J, Penín RM, Llatjós R, Martínez-Ballarín I. Cutaneous metastasis from lung cancer: retrospective analysis of 30 patients. Australas J Dermatol. 2012;53(4):288–90. https://doi.org/10.1111/j.1440-0960.2011.00828.x. Epub 2011 Nov 15. PMID: 23157780.
9. Chun SM, Kim YC, Lee JB, Kim SJ, Lee SC, Won YH, Yun SJ. Nasal tip cutaneous metastases secondary to lung carcinoma: three case reports and a review of the literature. Acta Derm Venereol. 2013;93(5):569–72. https://doi.org/10.2340/00015555-1529. PMID: 23303432.
10. Ardavanis A, Orphanos G, Ioannidis G, Rigatos G. Skin metastases from primary lung cancer. Report of three cases and a brief review. In Vivo. 2006;20(5):671–3. PMID: 17091776.
11. Song Z, Lin B, Shao L, Zhang Y. Cutaneous metastasis as a initial presentation in advanced non-small cell lung cancer and its poor survival prognosis. J Cancer Res Clin Oncol. 2012;138(10):1613–7. https://doi.org/10.1007/s00432-012-1239-6. Epub 2012 May 13. PMID: 22581263.
12. Bhattarai B, Schmidt MF, Ghosh M, Sinha Ray A, Manhas S, Oke V, Agu CC, Basunia MR, Enriquez D, Quist J, Bianchi C, Hans R, Kandel S. Lung cancer with skin and breast metastasis: a case report and literature review. Case Rep Pulmonol. 2015;2015:136970. https://doi.org/10.1155/2015/136970. Epub 2015 Mar 16. PMID: 25861506.
13. Prat L, Chouaid C, Kettaneh A, Fardet L. Cutaneous lymphangitis carcinomatosa in a patient with lung adenocarcinoma: case report and literature review. Lung Cancer. 2013;79(1):91–3. https://doi.org/10.1016/j.lungcan.2012.09.009. Epub 2012 Nov 17. PMID: 23164553.
14. Homler HJ, Goetz CS, Weisenburger DD. Lymphangitic cutaneous metastases from lung cancer mimicking cellulitis. Carcinoma erysipeloides. West J Med. 1986;144(5):610–2. PMID: 3716421.
15. Krathen RA, Orengo IF, Rosen T. Cutaneous metastasis: a meta-analysis of data. South Med J. 2003;96(2):164–7. https://doi.org/10.1097/01.SMJ.0000053676.73249.E5. PMID: 12630642.
16. Wong CY, Helm MA, Helm TN, Zeitouni N. Patterns of skin metastases: a review of 25 years' experience at a single cancer center. Int J Dermatol. 2014;53(1):56–60. https://doi.org/10.1111/j.1365-4632.2012.05635.x. Epub 2013 Feb 22. PMID: 23432658.
17. Chernoff KA, Marghoob AA, Lacouture ME, Deng L, Busam KJ, Myskowski PL. Dermoscopic findings in cutaneous metastases. JAMA Dermatol. 2014;150(4):429–33. https://doi.org/10.1001/jamadermatol.2013.8502. PMID: 24430974.
18. Parente P, Covelli C, Parrella P, Latiano TP, Fiordelisi F, Pellico MT, Maiello E, Graziano P. Intestinal adenosquamous carcinoma with a synchronous skin metastasis: a immunohistochemical and molecular analysis. Int J Color Dis. 2020;35(2):337–41. https://doi.org/10.1007/s00384-019-03464-2. Epub 2019 Dec 10. PMID: 31823050.
19. Shah N, Ali MA, Patel AV. Cutaneous metastases of colon adenocarcinoma. Dig Liver Dis. 2025;57(2):636–7. https://doi.org/10.1016/j.dld.2024.10.017. Epub 2024 Nov 8. PMID: 39521671.
20. Yamai D, Shimada Y, Ozeki H, Matsumoto A, Abe K, Tajima Y, Nakano M, Ichikawa H, Sakata J, Wakai T. Axillary cutaneous metastasis of colon cancer with microsatellite instability-high and BRAF V600E mutation treated with curative-intent surgery: a case

report. Surg Case Rep. 2023;9(1):196. https://doi.org/10.1186/s40792-023-01780-y. PMID: 37962682.
21. Omiya M, Murata T, Sawaki A, Teshima S, Kawachi J. Cutaneous metastasis of transverse colon cancer with an aberrant pattern of CK7/CK20/CDX2 and high microsatellite instability. Intern Med. 2023;62(24):3625–30. https://doi.org/10.2169/internalmedicine.1629-23. Epub 2023 May 10. PMID: 37164671.
22. Jimenez A, Winsett F, Kelly B, Goodwin B. Epidermotropic cutaneous metastasis of colonic adenocarcinoma presenting as a Sister Mary Joseph Nodule. Am J Dermatopathol. 2022;44(11):828–30. https://doi.org/10.1097/DAD.0000000000002253. Epub 2022 Jul 28.
23. Correia P, Correia JF, Scigliano H, Nora M. Unusual Cutaneous Metastases From Colon Adenocarcinoma. Cureus. 2021;13(3):e14065. https://doi.org/10.7759/cureus.14065. PMID: 33898148.
24. Junak M, Jecius H, Erdrich J. Cutaneous metastasis in the setting of both colon and breast primary malignancies. Case Rep Gastrointest Med. 2020;2020:8852459. https://doi.org/10.1155/2020/8852459. eCollection 2020. PMID: 33062353.
25. Yang Y, Chen R, Zhang R. Cutaneous metastasis of a colon adenocarcinoma presenting as an unusual manifestation: a report of one case. Int J Clin Exp Pathol. 2020;13(7):1897–901. eCollection 2020. PMID: 32782720.
26. Randall G, Abrahams J. Cutaneous colon cancer metastases in a surgical scar. N Engl J Med. 2020;382(24):e90. https://doi.org/10.1056/NEJMicm1910443. PMID: 32521137.
27. Liao L, Cheng Q, Zhu G, Pei F, Ye S. Cutaneous metastasis of ascending colon cancer harboring a BRAF V600E mutation: a rare case report. Medicine (Baltimore). 2020;99(21):e20026. https://doi.org/10.1097/MD.0000000000020026. PMID: 32481270.
28. Faenza M, Del Torto G, Di Costanzo P, Pieretti G, Lamberti R, Franco R, Ferraro GA, Nicoletti GF. Large single cutaneous metastasis of colon adenocarcinoma mimicking a squamous cell carcinoma of the skin: a case report. Int J Surg Case Rep. 2019;56:96–100. https://doi.org/10.1016/j.ijscr.2019.02.043. Epub 2019 Mar 7. PMID: 30870738.

Index

D. Koumaki et al. (eds.), *Cutaneous Metastases*, https://doi.org/10.1007/978-3-032-26764-1

N

T